NETTER'S
NEUROSCIENCE COLORING BOOK

2

SECOND EDITION

NETTER'S NEUROSCIENCE COLORING BOOK

David L. Felten, MD, PhD
Associate Dean of Clinical Sciences
Professor of Neuroscience
University of Medicine and Health Sciences
New York, New York

Mary Summo Maida, PhD
Adjunct Professor of Neurobiology and Anatomy
University of Rochester School of Medicine
Rochester, New York

ARTISTS
Art based on the works of the Frank H. Netter, MD collection
www.netterimages.com

Modified for coloring by
Dragonfly Media Group

ELSEVIER

Elsevier
1600 John F. Kennedy Blvd.
Ste 1800
Philadelphia, PA 19103-2899

NETTER'S NEUROSCIENCE COLORING BOOK, SECOND EDITION ISBN: 978-0-443-11731-2

Publisher: Elyse O'Grady
Senior *Content Development Specialist:* Kate Mannix
Publishing Services Manager: Shereen Jameel
Senior *Project Manager:* Beula Christopher
Design Direction: Patrick Ferguson

Printed in India

Last digit is the print number: 9 8 7 6 5 4 3 2 1

Dedication

In loving memory of my mother, Jane E. Felten (1915–1989)

Paralyzed with polio at the age of 8 and faced with daunting medical challenges all of her life, she took great joy in her family and friends, her faith, and her intellectual pursuits, including helping edit an elementary school series of English books, never complaining of her lot in life.

Her happiness and success in life, her incredible willpower, and her indomitable spirit sparked my lifetime interest in how the nervous system works, what happens in nervous system diseases, and how personal determination and a positive, grateful attitude can powerfully influence the quality of life.

She gave me an early appreciation of activities with colored pencils and the value of using flash cards, which continues to this day through these Netter projects.

AND

In loving memory of my father, Harold D. Felten (1916–2016)

A man of unshakable integrity, kindness, caring, and spiritual depth, he truly lived what he preached. He provided a lifetime of love and care for his wife without ever complaining.

Even though he had family obligations that prevented him from obtaining a college education, he was a wise man, and he strongly encouraged my academic pursuits. His sage advice and outstanding personal example were inspirational and guided me through difficult challenges.

He passed away 10 days shy of his 100th birthday, a rich life well lived.

David L. Felten

To my parents, Dr. Anthony Summo and Mary Summo

My greatest gift is to call you Dad and Mom. I'm even more privileged to have always known the forever happy place of being loved, valued, and disciplined when needed, and of having you as my biggest cheerleaders.

Thank you for modeling and teaching me that, whether my current interests center on science, medicine, music, arts, community service, or all other topics that captured my time and interest, it's most fun when one thinks out of the box or colors outside the lines. This presupposes that one has first been taught where the box is and where the lines are at the outset, and, when moving beyond those boundaries, when it's beneficial and when it's not, because no one makes choices that don't impact others.

I thank you and love you for having lived and modeled parenthood at its finest.

Mary Summo Maida

About the Artists

Frank H. Netter, MD

Frank H. Netter was born in 1906 in New York City. He studied art at the Art Students League and the National Academy of Design before entering medical school at New York University, where he received his MD degree in 1931. During his student years, Dr. Netter's notebook sketches attracted the attention of the medical faculty and other physicians, allowing him to augment his income by illustrating articles and textbooks. He continued illustrating as a sideline after establishing a surgical practice in 1933, but he ultimately opted to give up his practice in favor of a full-time commitment to art. After service in the United States Army during World War II, Dr. Netter began his long collaboration with the CIBA Pharmaceutical Company (now Novartis Pharmaceuticals). This 45-year partnership resulted in the production of the extraordinary collection of medical art so familiar to physicians and other medical professionals worldwide.

In 2005, Elsevier, Inc. purchased the Netter collection and all publications from Icon Learning Systems. There are now over 50 publications featuring the art of Dr. Netter available through Elsevier, Inc. (in the United States: www.us.elsevierhealth.com/Netter; outside the United States: www.elsevierhealth.com).

Dr. Netter's works are among the finest examples of the use of illustration in the teaching of medical concepts. The 13-book *Netter Collection of Medical Illustrations*, which includes the greater part of the more than 20,000 paintings created by Dr. Netter, became and remains one of the most famous medical works ever published. The *Netter Atlas of Human Anatomy*, first published in 1989, presents the anatomical paintings from the Netter collection. Now translated into 16 languages, it is the anatomy atlas of choice among medical- and health-professions students the world over.

The Netter illustrations are appreciated not only for their aesthetic qualities but, more importantly, for their intellectual content. As Dr. Netter wrote in 1949, "Clarification of a subject is the aim and goal of illustration. No matter how beautifully painted, how delicately and subtly rendered a subject may be, it is of little value as a *medical illustration* if it does not serve to make clear some medical point." Dr. Netter's planning, conception, point of view, and approach are what inform his paintings and what make them so intellectually valuable.

Frank H. Netter, MD, physician and artist, died in 1991.

Learn more about the physician-artist whose work has inspired the Netter Reference collection:
https://www.netterimages.com/artist-frank-h-netter.html

Carlos Machado, MD

Carlos Machado was chosen by Novartis to be Dr. Netter's successor. He continues to be the main artist who contributes to the Netter collection of medical illustrations.

Self-taught in medical illustration, cardiologist Carlos Machado has contributed meticulous updates to some of Dr. Netter's original plates and has created many paintings of his own in the style of Netter as an extension of the Netter collection. Dr. Machado's photorealistic expertise and his keen insight into the physician–patient relationship inform his vivid and unforgettable visual style. His dedication to researching each topic and subject he paints places him among the premier medical illustrators at work today.

Learn more about his background and see more of his art at:
https://www.netterimages.com/artist-carlos-a-g-machado.html

James A. Perkins, CMI, FAMI

James A. Perkins, MFA, CMI, FAMI, is Distinguished Professor and Graduate Director, Medical Illustrations, and Head of the Department of Medical Sciences, Health, & Management in the College of Health Sciences & Technology, Rochester Institute of Technology (RIT). He also teaches courses in anatomy, digital illustration, and scientific visualization. He is a Board-Certified Medical Illustrator and Fellow of the Association of Medical Illustrators.

An expert in visualizing biological processes, Prof. Perkins has illustrated more than 40 medical textbooks, particularly in the areas of pathology, physiology, neuroscience, and molecular biology. For over 20 years, he has been the sole illustrator of the *Robbins* series of pathology texts published by Elsevier, including the flagship of the series, *Robbins and Cotran Pathologic Basis of Disease.* He has been a contributor to the Netter collection since 2001, creating most of the new art for *Netter's Atlas of Human Physiology, Netter's Illustrated Pharmacology*, and *Netter's Atlas of Neuroscience*, and contributing to many other titles.

Prof. Perkins received a bachelor's degree in biology and geology from Cornell University and studied vertebrate paleontology and anatomy at the University of Texas and University of Rochester. He received a Master of Fine Arts degree in medical illustration from RIT and spent several years working in medical publishing and the medical legal exhibit field before returning to RIT to join the faculty.

Learn more about his background and see more of his art at:
https://www.netterimages.com/artist-james-a-perkins.html

About the Authors

DAVID L. FELTEN, MD, PhD, is currently Associate Dean of Clinical Sciences and professor of neuroscience at the University of Medicine and Health Sciences, New York, New York, and Distinguished Scholar in Residence, Division of Applied Health and Wellness, Keuka College, Keuka Park, New York. He was formerly Vice President for Research and Medical Director of the Research Institute at William Beaumont Health System in Royal Oak, Michigan, and the founding associate dean for research at Oakland University William Beaumont School of Medicine. He previously served as Dean of the School of Graduate Medical Education at Seton Hall University in South Orange, New Jersey; the founding Executive Director of the Susan Samueli Center for Integrative Medicine; professor of anatomy and neurobiology at the University of California, Irvine School of Medicine; the founding director of the Center for Neuroimmunology at Loma Linda School of Medicine; the Kilian J. and Caroline F. Schmitt professor and Chair of the Department of Neurobiology; and Director of the Markey Charitable Trust Institute for Neurobiology and Neurodegenerative Diseases and Aging at the University of Rochester School of Medicine in Rochester, New York. He received a Bachelor of Science from Massachusetts Institute of Technology and an MD and PhD from the University of Pennsylvania School of Medicine. Dr. Felten carried out pioneering studies of autonomic innervation of immunocytes in lymphoid organs, and neural-immune signaling that underlies the mechanistic foundations for psychoneuroimmunology and many aspects of integrative medicine.

Dr. Felten is the recipient of numerous honors and awards, including the prestigious John D. and Catherine T. MacArthur Foundation Prize Fellowship, two simultaneous NIH MERIT Awards from the National Institutes of Mental Health and the National Institute on Aging, an Alfred P. Sloan Foundation Fellowship, an Andrew W. Mellon Foundation Fellowship, a Robert Wood Johnson Dean's Senior Teaching Scholar Award, the Norman Cousins Award in Mind-Body Medicine, the Building Bridges of Integration Award from the Traditional Chinese Medicine World Foundation, and numerous teaching awards.

Dr. Felten cowrote the definitive scholarly text in the field of neural-immune interactions, *Psychoneuroimmunology* (Academic Press, 3rd edition, 2001), and was a founding coeditor of the major journal in the field, *Brain, Behavior, and Immunity*, with Drs. Robert Ader and Nicholas Cohen of the University of Rochester School of Medicine. Dr. Felten is the author of over 210 peer-reviewed journal articles and reviews, many on links between the nervous system and immune system. His work has been featured on Bill Moyer's PBS series, in his book, *Healing and the Mind*, on *20/20*, and on many other media venues. He served for over a decade on the National Board of Medical Examiners, including chair of the Neurosciences Committee for the US Medical Licensure Examination.

Dr. Felten is the author (with M. Kerry O'Banion, MD, PhD, and Mary S. Maida, PhD) of *Netter's Atlas of Neuroscience,* 4th edition, 2022, Elsevier, and is author of *Netter's Neuroscience Flash Cards,* 4th edition, 2022, Elsevier.

About the Authors - Continued

MARY SUMMO MAIDA, PhD. Dr. Maida's background includes bachelor's degrees in microbiology, finance, and operations management. She holds a master's degree in neurobiology and anatomy and a PhD in molecular neuroscience, each earned at the University of Rochester School of Medicine and Dentistry, Rochester, New York. Before her return to medical school, Dr. Maida served as CFO for a privately held consulting firm involved in developing shopping malls and other commercial properties throughout the United States.

After thoroughly enjoying her most crucial role as a stay-at-home mom, a sports coach to her sons' teams, and a school and community volunteer, Dr. Maida returned to the University of Rochester School of Medicine to complete her medical research degree after her youngest son entered his second year of college. Her initial studies focused on research in Parkinson's disease and neuroimmunology. After completing her core rotations, Dr. Maida focused her energy and research on molecular neuroscience in the laboratory of Dr. M. Kerry O'Banion, best known for his pioneering research and discovery of cyclooxygenase-2 (COX-2), a significant component of inflammatory diseases. Dr. Maida's research concentrated particularly on conditions where neuroinflammation appears to be a significant disease component. These include Alzheimer's disease, amyotrophic lateral sclerosis (ALS), radiation exposure, and chronic psychiatric disease. As part of her academic career, Dr. Maida remains a senior advisor and teaching professor to many graduate and medical students.

While completing her postdoctoral fellowship, Dr. Maida became particularly interested in the emerging field of technology transfer. Because of her background in science, medicine, and business, Dr. Maida founded The Medingen Group, LLC. This business incubator assists medical professionals who are inventors of health care products through all phases from concept to commercial readiness, with the goal of either licensing or entering full-scale production. In her role as CEO of Medingen, she developed a uniquely innovative intranasal drug delivery device invented by Drs. DeWitt and Patsy Reed.

In 2006, Dr. Maida established a second company, Clerisy Corp, to complete the research and development, international patenting, FDA approvals, and market testing to bring this intranasal drug delivery device to market. Products with over-the-counter applications were introduced to the marketplace in 2013. In 2017, Dr. Maida sold the company to a private corporation.

Her current academic appointments include an adjunct professorship at the University of Rochester School of Medicine and Dentistry (Rochester, New York), a visiting professorship at the University of Medical Health Sciences (St. Kitts and New York, New York), and an adjunct professorship at Simon School of Business, University of Rochester (Rochester, New York).

Dr. Maida has received several honors and awards across many disciplines, including the Outstanding Alumni of Distinction Award from Excelsior College, the New York State Hall of Distinction Award, the Partners in Lifelong Learning Award, Greater Rochester Excellence in Achievement Technology Award, Winning Mentor for Mark Ain Business Competition, 43North Semifinalist distinction, and winning finalist in several Open Invitation Awards.

Dr. Maida lives in the Finger Lakes region of upstate New York with her husband, Dr. David Felten (MD, PhD), and their adult sons live nearby in neighboring communities. In her leisure time, Dr. Maida enjoys participating in "anything and everything sports or comedy," reading, singing in a cappella groups and church choirs, playing the piano, learning the bass guitar, boating, and (her favorite hobby) fishing. She rarely passes on an opportunity to participate in all fun social events and continues to serve on not-for-profit boards in Monroe and Ontario Counties.

Preface

Foundations for *Netter's Neuroscience Coloring Book*

Netter's Neuroscience Coloring Book is based on some of the illustrations in *Netter's Atlas of Neuroscience,* 4th edition, which combines the richness and beauty of Dr. Frank Netter's illustrations with key information about the many regions and systems of the brain, spinal cord, and periphery. Jim Perkins and John Craig have contributed additional outstanding illustrations to complement the original Netter illustrations.

Netter's Atlas of Neuroscience, 4th edition, provides a comprehensive view of the entire nervous system, including the peripheral nerves and their target tissues, the central nervous system, the ventricular system, the meninges, the cerebral vascular system, developmental neuroscience, and neuroendocrine regulation. We have provided substantial but not exhaustive details and labels so that the reader can understand the basics of human neuroscience, including information presented in medical neurosciences courses, the nervous system components of anatomy courses, and neural components of physiology courses in medical school.

Netter's Neuroscience Coloring Book is organized similar to the 4th edition of *Netter's Atlas of Neuroscience:* (1) Overview; (2) Regional Neurosciences; (3) Systemic Neurosciences; and (4) Global Brain Function. The Overview is a presentation of the basic components and organization of the nervous system, a "view from 30,000 feet"; this view is an essential foundation for understanding the details of regional and systemic neurosciences. The Overview includes chapters/sections on neurons and their properties, an introduction to the forebrain, brainstem and cerebellum, spinal cord, meninges, ventricular system, cerebral vasculature, and neurodevelopment.

The Regional Neurosciences section provides the structural components of the peripheral nervous system, the spinal cord, the brainstem and cerebellum, and the forebrain (diencephalon and telencephalon). We begin in the periphery and move from caudal to rostral. The peripheral nervous system section includes details about the somatic and autonomic innervation of peripheral nerves; we do not leave the learner at the boundary of CNS and PNS and hope that they can find out about peripheral and autonomic nerves from a gross anatomy course or text. This detailed regional understanding is necessary to diagnose and understand the consequences of a host of lesions whose localization depends on regional knowledge; this includes strokes, local effects of tumors, injuries, specific demyelinating lesions, inflammatory reactions, and many other localized problems. In this section, many of the clinical correlations assist the reader in integrating a knowledge of the vascular supply with the consequences of infarcts (e.g., brainstem syndromes), which requires a detailed understanding of brainstem anatomy and relationships.

The Systemic Neurosciences section evaluates the sensory systems, motor systems (including cerebellum and basal ganglia, acknowledging that they also are involved in many other spheres of activity besides motor), autonomic-hypothalamic-limbic systems (including neuroendocrine), and higher cortical functions. Within this section, we have organized each sensory system, when appropriate, with a sequential presentation of the secondary sensory reflex channels, cerebellar channels, and lemniscal channels. For the motor systems, we begin with lower motor neurons and then show the various systems of upper motor neurons followed by cerebellum and basal ganglia, whose major motor influences are ultimately exerted through regulation of upper motor neuronal systems. For the autonomic-hypothalamic-limbic system, we begin with the autonomic preganglionic and postganglionic organization and then present brainstem and hypothalamic regulation of autonomic outflow, and finally limbic and cortical regulation of the hypothalamus and autonomic outflow. This section includes new plates on prefrontal cortex and other limbic forebrain structures. The systemic neurosciences constitute the basis for carrying out and interpreting the neurological examination. We believe that it is necessary for a student of neuroscience to understand both regional organization and systemic organization. Without this dual understanding, clinical evaluation of a patient with a neurological problem would be incomplete.

The Global Brain Function section was added to the 4th edition to provide students with an understanding of dementias, especially Alzheimer's disease; several important neuropsychiatric disorders, including posttraumatic stress; brain substrates of addictive behaviors; traumatic brain injury (TBI) and chronic traumatic encephalopathy (CTE); the aphasias and nondominant hemispheric disorders; memory circuits; consciousness and coma; and aging and the nervous system. Several new illustrations in the 2nd edition of *Netter's Neuroscience Coloring Book* are derived from this new section of the Atlas.

We appreciate that the 3rd edition of *Netter's Atlas of Neuroscience* has been recognized with three international awards, a British Medical Association Book Award (Highly Commended, Neurology), an Association of Medical Illustrators Award (Award of Merit), and a Wiki Award (Top 10 Neurosciences Textbooks, #2). We believe that our audience for *Netter's Neuroscience Coloring Book*, 2nd edition, will find the organization helpful for their study of the nervous system and that those seeking more detailed colored full illustrations will benefit from the availability of *Netter's Atlas of Neuroscience*, 4th edition, organized in a similar fashion.

How to Use This Coloring Book

We have benefited from the example and advice from our friend and colleague, Dr. John Hansen, from the University of Rochester School of Medicine, author of *Netter's Anatomy Coloring Book* (2nd ed, 2015, Elsevier). This coloring book is a highly acclaimed tool for hands-on, active learning of anatomy. It provides the enjoyment of the lasting pursuit of colored pencil exercises with the knowledge and clinical applications of the illustrations. *Netter's Neuroscience Coloring Book,* 2nd edition, follows a similar format. We have selected 145 illustrations, or sets of illustrations, organized according to the four sections mentioned above: (1) Overview, (2) Regional Neuroscience, (3) Systemic Neuroscience, and (4) Global Brain Function.

Preface - Continued

For each illustration, there are three components: (1) introductory information about the illustration, including some organizational points, summaries of key information, charts or tables, and observations on the anatomical and physiological importance of the illustration(s); (2) coloring instructions for approximately 12 structures in each illustration; and (3) a clinical note, which discusses the clinical importance of one or more structures in the illustration, an important related disease, or observations of therapeutic insights based on knowledge gained from the illustration. The clinical note is not intended as a simplistic "sound bite," nor is it intended as a scholarly neurological discourse. It is intended to provide useful and intriguing information to show the value of underlying anatomy and physiology to the understanding of human neurological diseases and dysfunction. A summary of the organization of these plates is (1) What is it, and what does it do?; (2) What do we consider the most important structures? Color them; and (3) What is the clinical significance or organizational significance of the plate?

Each user should feel free to use his/her own imagination and interests in the coloring exercises. We offer approximately 12 structures, based on the recommendation of study groups; there is always a balance between too few and too many structures. The object is not to obfuscate or produce the neuroanatomical equivalent of a mind-bending metabolic pathways chart. If you see additional structures that interest or intrigue you, color them. If you encounter very small structures (e.g., dendritic spines), feel free to point to them with a colored arrow rather than to try to color them. For anatomical pathways and tracts, they can be traced over with a conspicuous color. In some cases, you may recognize that our instructions for coloring individual regions (e.g., medulla, pons, and midbrain) with separate colors provide somewhat artificial anatomical separation of functional units that span the entire brainstem (e.g., reticular formation, raphe nuclei).

The authors provided their own perspectives, with necessary compromise. Dr. Felten enjoys outlines, summaries, and the many details that they entail. Dr. Maida likes to take complex arrays of structures and processes and make them succinct and understandable. And we both needed to work with the thoughtful guidelines provided by the editors to produce a usable and enjoyable coloring book. For some users, this coloring book will be their first introduction to the nervous system. We hope that you will see the extraordinary beauty and organization of this amazingly complex system, the source of all human behavior and endeavors. Delving into the neurosciences can be a lifetime challenge and a most rewarding pursuit. The most sobering realization is that even after a lifetime of intensive research, teaching, clinical activities, and reading about the nervous system, at the end of the day, even the most knowledgeable "expert" knows, at best, 1 mL in an ocean of potential understanding.

For users who are medical students or health care professionals who have already been introduced to aspects of the neurosciences, we hope that you can solidify your organizational understanding of the nervous system and come to appreciate how readily the anatomical and physiological aspects translate into lasting appreciation of their clinical importance. We hope that you will use your own creativity to select whatever interests you, above and beyond "color that structure" instructions, and let an active learning process guide you to the joy of discovery in the nervous system.

Acknowledgments

For decades, Dr. Frank Netter's beautiful and informative artwork has provided the visual basis for understanding anatomy, physiology, and relationships of great importance in medicine. Generations of physicians and health care professionals have "learned from the master" and have carried Dr. Netter's legacy forward through their own knowledge and contributions to patient care. There is no way to compare Dr. Netter's artwork to anything else because it stands in a class of its own. For many decades, the Netter collection volume on the nervous system has been a flagship for the medical profession and for students of neuroscience. It was a great honor to provide the framework, organization, and new information for the updated first, second, third, and fourth editions of *Netter's Atlas of Neuroscience*, components of which are adapted for this coloring book. The opportunity to make a lasting contribution to the next generation of physicians and health care professionals is perhaps the greatest honor anyone could receive.

I thank our outstanding artist and medical illustrator, James Perkins, MS, MFA, for his clear, creative, and beautiful contributions to *Netter's Atlas of Neuroscience*, all editions; his color images are used as the starting point in this coloring book. We also thank Rob Duckwell, the artist who created the black-and-white illustrations for this coloring book.

Special thanks go to the outstanding editors at Elsevier: Elyse O'Grady, Publisher; Kate Mannix, Senior Content Development Specialist; and Beula Christopher, Senior Project Manager. They helped to guide the process of this challenging task from start to finished publication, kept me from doing anything too drastic or unsuited for the coloring book, and gave us the latitude to introduce new components.

David L. Felten

Contents

Contents - Continued

Contents - Continued

Chapter 1 Neurons and Their Properties

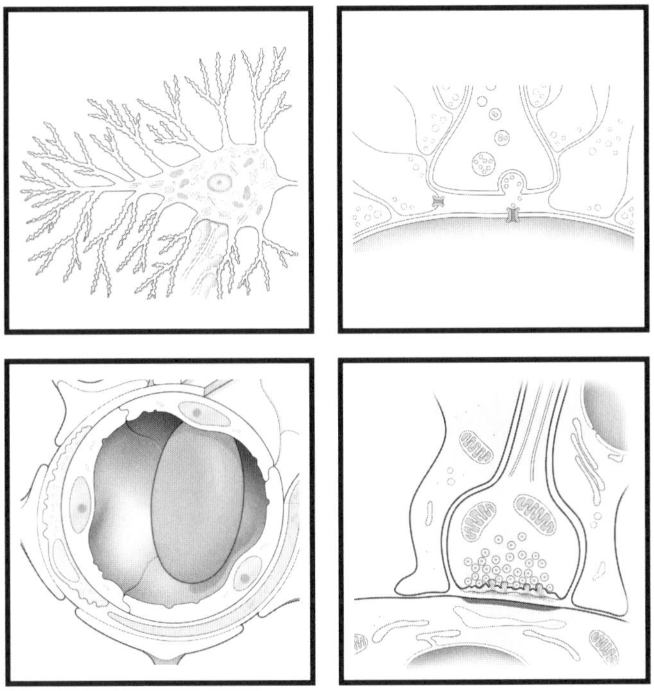

1 Neuronal Structure

A **neuron** is the individual anatomical, physiological, genetic, and trophic unit of the nervous system. Each neuron is an individual cell, separated from adjacent neurons (the neuron doctrine). The components of a neuron are the **cell body**, the **dendrites**, and one (or occasionally no) **axon**. The cell body contains the **nucleus** (and its **nucleolus**) with the neuronal genome, extensive **mitochondria** needed for aerobic metabolism, abundant **rough endoplasmic reticulum** necessary for the synthesis of proteins for neuronal structural integrity and function, **Golgi apparatus** needed for packaging molecules for transport down the axon, and other essential organelles. Anatomical processes, dendrites and an axon, extend from the cell body. The dendrites are extensively branched processes that emerge from the cell body and are sites where incoming axons terminate and provide neurotransmitter influences on the neuron (sometimes ending on the **dendritic spines**). The axon tapers from the cell body at the **axon hillock** and initiates the all-or-none electrical message, the self-reinforcing action potential (AP), at the **initial segment**. The AP propagates by reinitiating at each node of Ranvier, where bare axon membrane with sodium channels is found. Axons may branch profusely (called axonal projections), making contact with millions of target neuronal cell bodies **(axosomatic synapses)** and dendrites (**axodendritic synapses**; e.g., locus coeruleus noradrenergic neurons), or may provide targeted, direct contact with only a few neurons (e.g., primary sensory neurons with Ia afferent monosynaptic muscle stretch reflex connections or lower motor neurons [LMNs] with muscle fibers at the neuromuscular junction [NMJ]). While this pattern for neuronal components is the general pattern, there are exceptions: primary sensory neurons in the dorsal root ganglion and some cranial nerve ganglia have cell bodies with no dendrites (the sensory receptor acts as a dendrite), some neurons possess no axon (amacrine cells), and some neuronal systems have extensive networks of dendrodendritic synaptic interactions (e.g., the dendrite bundles of the serotonergic raphe nuclei in the brainstem and the phrenic motor nucleus in the spinal cord).

COLOR each of the following structures, using a separate color for each structure.

☐ 1. **Dendrites**
☐ 2. **Dendritic spines**
☐ 3. **Rough endoplasmic reticulum**
☐ 4. **Mitochondria**
☐ 5. **Nucleus**
☐ 6. **Nucleolus**
☐ 7. **Axon hillock**
☐ 8. **Axon**
☐ 9. **Initial segment of the axon**
☐ 10. **Cell body (soma)**
☐ 11. **Axosomatic synapse**
☐ 12. **Axodendritic synapse**

Clinical Note

Neurons are metabolically very active obligatory aerobic cells and have high demand for glucose and oxygen, consuming far more resources than predicted by percent body weight. Neurons have very little energy reserve and depend on continuous delivery of oxygen and glucose for proper function. If an ischemic episode occurs, neuronal dysfunction can occur rapidly, and within 5 minutes following an ischemic stroke or a heart attack, some neurons become irreversibly damaged. Sites such as the CA1 sector of the hippocampus are highly sensitive to ischemic damage and subsequent neuronal death (apoptosis), leaving serious functional deficits such as loss of short-term memory and inability to consolidate short-term memory into long-term traces.

Neurons also are highly active genomically, expressing genes for needed protein synthesis for required functions. The local milieu also influences the individual neuronal genome. Following insult or injury, the genome shifts to protein synthesis for reparative processes.

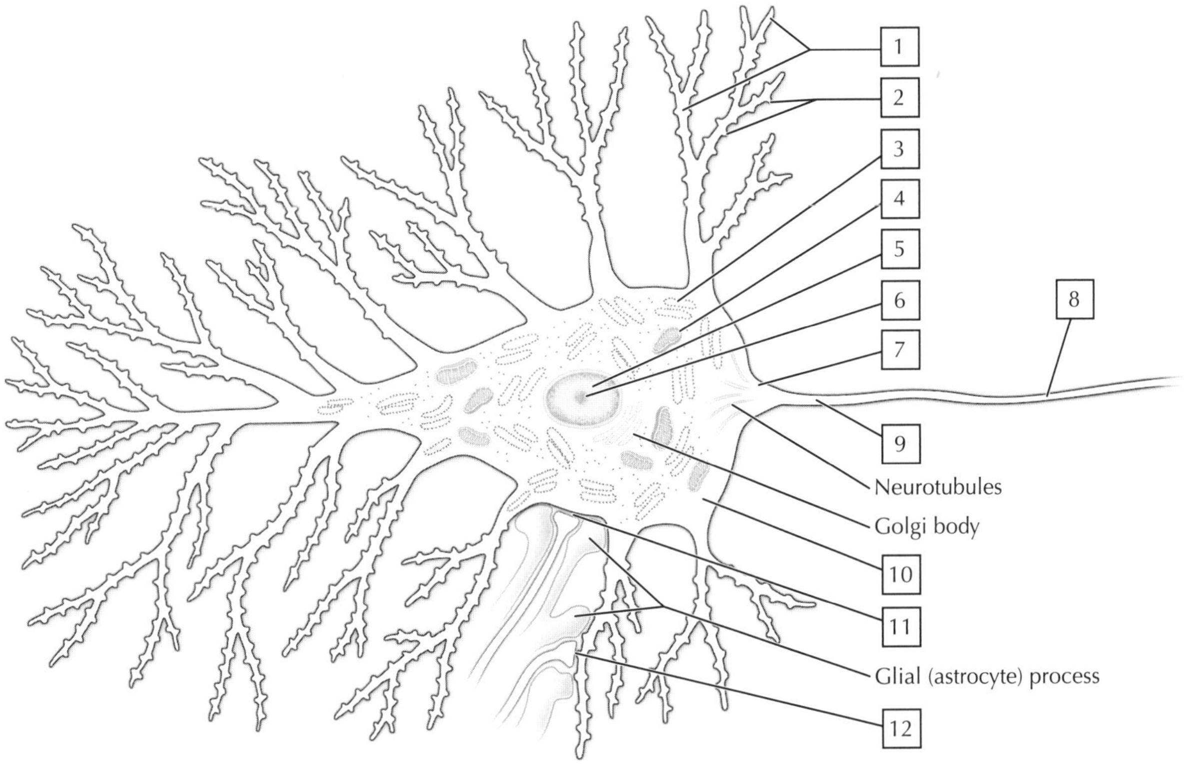

A. Large multipolar neuron

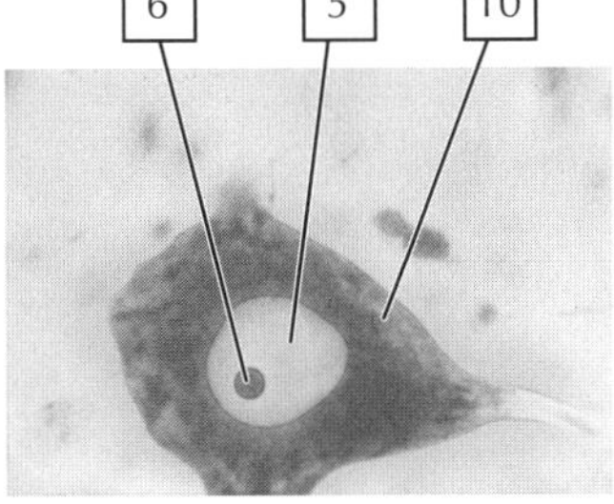

B. Spinal cord lower motor neuron

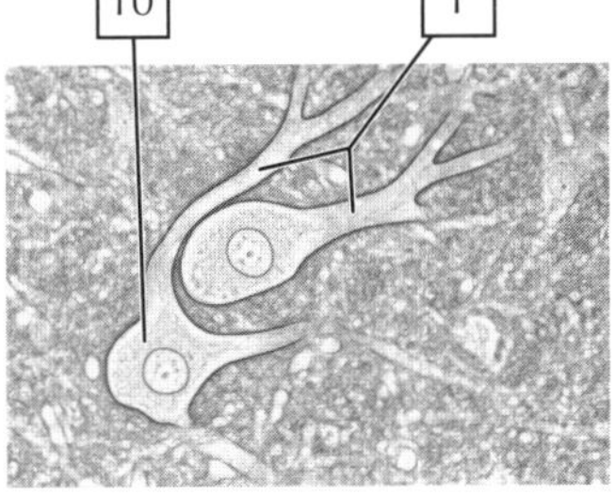

C. Cerebellar Purkinje neurons

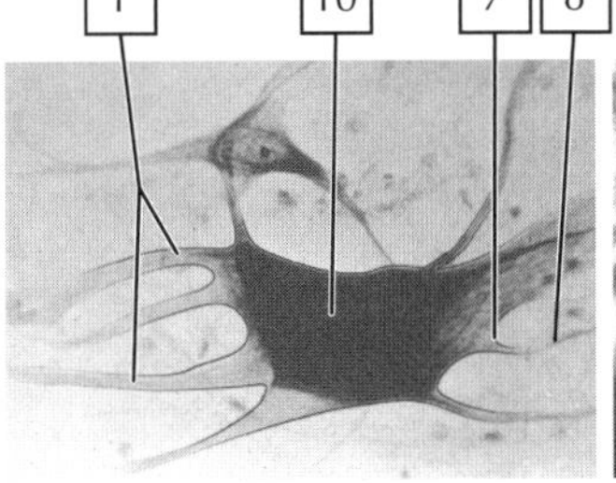

D. Spinal cord neuron

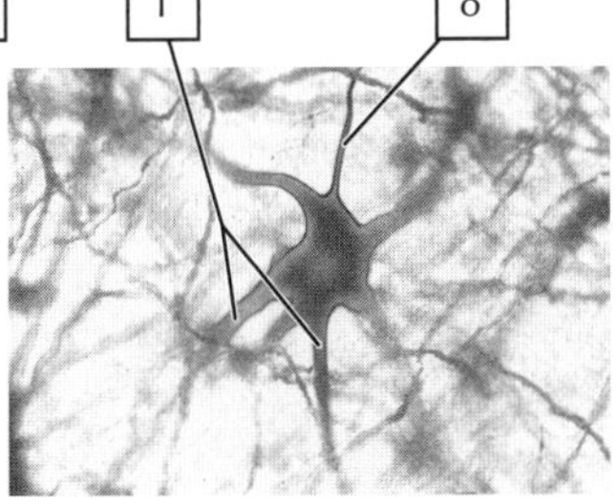

E. Reticular formation neuron

1 Types of Synapses

A **synapse** is a structural site of communication between a component of one neuron (cell body, dendrite, axon) with one or more components of either a single neuron or a more complex array of neuronal structures. The most commonly encountered synaptic arrangements are the **axosomatic** (axon with cell body of target neuron) and **axodendritic** (axon with dendrite[s] or dendritic spines of target neuron) synapses. These synaptic influences usually add a small increment to the cell body or dendritic membrane potential, either **depolarization** or **hyperpolarization**, but rarely single-handedly cause the initiation or blockage of an action potential (AP). Synapses that terminate on the axon hillock are close enough to the site of initiation of the AP (initial segment) that a single depolarizing influence may lead to the firing of an AP by the axon. Some axonal synapses target other axon terminals (**axoaxonic** synapses); these contacts can prevent the target axon terminal from releasing its neurotransmitter, thereby causing presynaptic inhibition. Some synapses are "**reciprocal synapses**" because each neuronal element communicates with its counterpart. A **serial synapse** involves multiple sites in a single axon where clusters of synaptic vesicles are found at many adjacent sites, providing transmitter release along a long stretch of target membrane; these serial synapses provide sufficient stimulation to the target membrane to guarantee a desired synaptic effect. Some axons form small bead-like accumulations of synaptic vesicles (called **varicosities**, or boutons en passage), which provide large numbers of sites of release of neurotransmitter, such as those found with the noradrenergic, dopaminergic, and serotonergic axons. These sites of contact are useful for general secretion (paracrine secretion) into a given vicinity, rather than a precisely targeted anatomical contact. Some structures have highly complex synaptic interactions among three or more neuronal elements, termed "glomeruli," found in the retina, cerebellum, olfactory bulb, and elsewhere. See the upper two figures on Plate 1.15 for further examples of synapses.

COLOR the following structures, using a separate color for each structure.

- ☐ **1. Axosomatic or axodendritic synapse**
- ☐ **2. Axodendritic synapse on a dendritic spine**
- ☐ **3. Axoaxonic synapse on a terminal which is forming an axodendritic synapse**
- ☐ **4. Combined axodendritic and axoaxonic synapse**
- ☐ **5. Axonal varicosities**
- ☐ **6. Dendrodendritic synapse**
- ☐ **7. Reciprocal synapse**
- ☐ **8. Serial synapse**

Clinical Note

The structural configuration of synapses on a given neuron provides information about how that neuron is controlled. At the NMJ, cholinergic synapses from the motor axon terminate in troughs adjacent to infolded regions of the muscle membrane, making extensive connections with a single target. Usually, sufficient acetylcholine (ACh) is released from these terminals during a single motor AP to bring the muscle membrane to threshold, thereby causing the contraction of the muscle fibers in that motor unit. In the central nervous system (CNS), some upper motor neuron synapses, such as corticospinal synapses on an LMN membrane near the axon hillock, bring the LMN to threshold and fire an AP, permitting successful initiation of voluntary movements. In many cases, collective synapses converging on a target neuron, such as a neuron in the reticular formation, will converge on dendrites and the cell body, with no single axon or group of axons having sufficient depolarizing capacity to fire an AP in that neuron's axon. Bringing such an axon to threshold requires either spatial summation (excitation by many axons) or temporal summation (excitation by multiple inputs recurring over time). Some complex synaptic interactions, such as arrays of **dendrodendritic synapses** in dendrite bundles, occur among LMNs supplying motor axons to the diaphragm and help to pulse the activity of arrays of neurons to provide coordinated activation of their targets. Some modulatory neurotransmitters, such as norepinephrine, change the threshold or excitability of other systems of inputs, such as excitatory glutamate inputs and inhibitory γ-aminobutyric acid (GABA) inputs, even on a single neuron (e.g., Purkinje cells in the cerebellum).

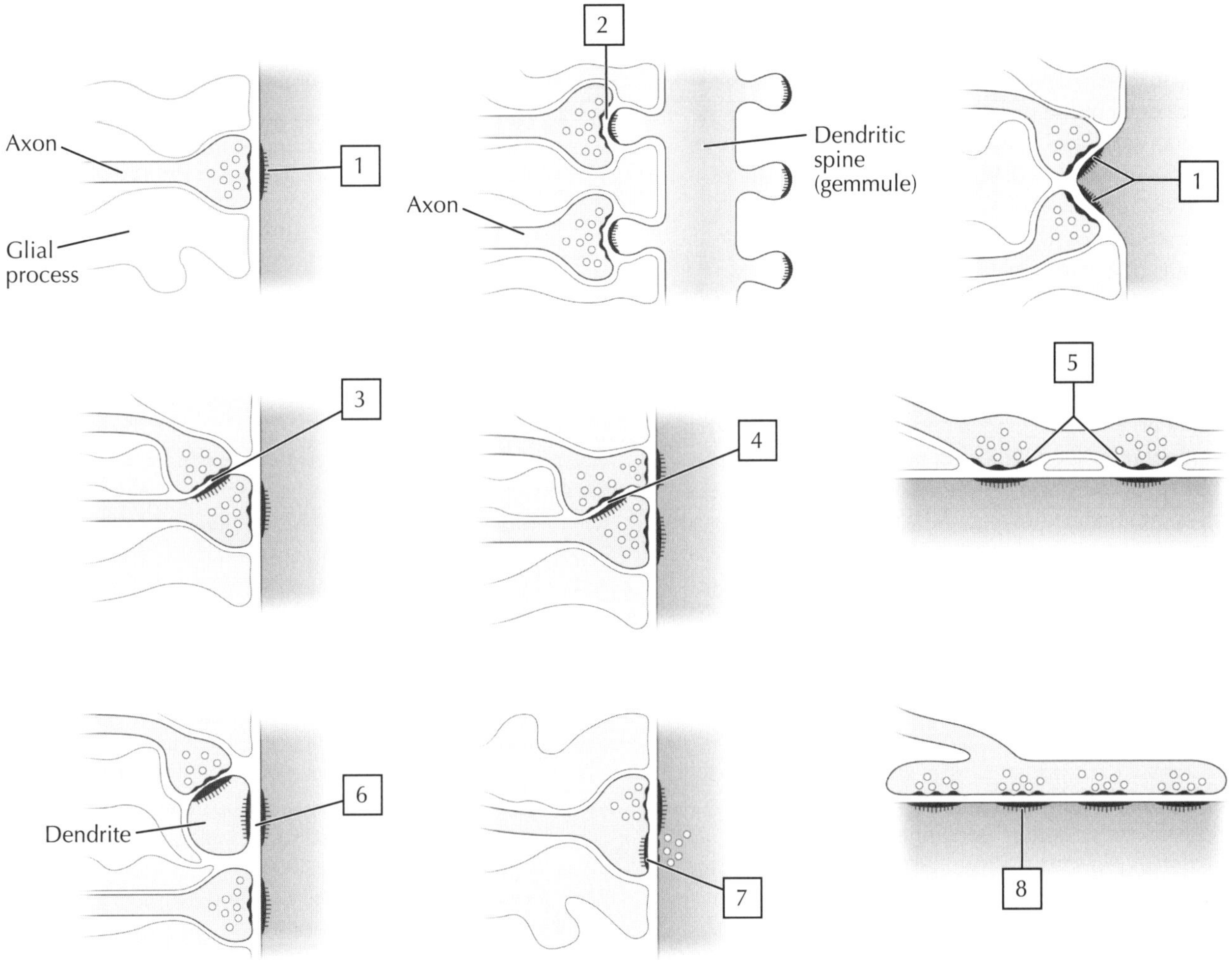
Axon
Glial process
1
2
Dendritic spine (gemmule)
Axon
1
3
4
5
Dendrite
6
7
8

Neuronal Cell Types

Neuronal size, structure, dendritic arborizations, and axonal projection patterns reveal the functional role for these neurons. In the CNS (depicted by the dashed lines; the lower region depicts the spinal cord and the upper region the brain), the **lower motor neurons** (LMNs) have large cell bodies with extensive dendritic arborizations, reflecting the extensive **upper motor neuronal** input converging upon them from the brain, from interneurons, and from sensory inputs. The LMNs have axons that exit through the ventral roots, targeted specifically to a group of muscle fibers, constituting a motor unit. The **preganglionic autonomic neurons**, found in the brainstem and sacral spinal cord for the parasympathetic system and the thoracolumbar spinal cord for the sympathetic system, also have large cell bodies with extensive dendritic branching. Their axons target autonomic ganglion cells in the periphery. Some CNS neurons, such as the **pyramidal cells of the cerebral cortex,** have systems of apical dendrites and basolateral dendrites receiving extensive inputs from many CNS structures. Their axons distribute to other cortical neurons (commissural and association fibers) or subcortical structures (projection fibers), including LMNs. Reticular formation neurons and Purkinje cells of the cerebellum have unique dendritic trees that are characteristic of these neurons. Many **interneurons** are smaller **multipolar neurons,** which interact with specific larger neurons, such as LMNs.

In the peripheral nervous system (PNS), primary sensory neurons of the **dorsal root ganglia** and **cranial nerve ganglia** are either **unipolar** (a single axon and no dendrites) or **bipolar** (an axon both proximally and distally, and no dendrites). These axons convey information (trains of APs) from peripheral sensory receptors to secondary sensory neurons in the CNS that inform the CNS target neurons of transduced sensory modalities. The **autonomic ganglion cells** are multipolar neurons acting as both recipients of preganglionic input and integrative activities for subsequent regulation of target structures (cardiac muscle, smooth muscle, secretory glands, metabolic cells, immunocytes).

CNS neurons are supported by glia, including **astrocytes**, **microglia**, and **oligodendrocytes** (myelin-producing glia), and PNS neurons are supported by **Schwann cells**.

This illustration provides the hierarchical neuronal substrate for understanding the inputs (sensory) and outputs (motor, autonomic) of the brain, the fundamental basis for neuronal organization.

COLOR the following structures, using a single color for each structure.

- ☐ **1. Bipolar primary sensory neuron (in a cranial nerve ganglion)**
- ☐ **2. Unipolar primary sensory neuron (in a cranial nerve ganglion)**
- ☐ **3. Schwann cell**
- ☐ **4. Unipolar primary sensory neuron (in a dorsal root ganglion)**
- ☐ **5. CNS interneuron (in the spinal cord)**
- ☐ **6. Astrocyte**
- ☐ **7. Autonomic ganglion neuron (postganglionic)**
- ☐ **8. Lower motor neuron (somatic motor cell of the anterior horn of the spinal cord)**
- ☐ **9. Oligodendrocyte**
- ☐ **10. Multipolar somatic motor cell (of motor cranial nerve nuclei)**
- ☐ **11. Pyramidal neuron (in the cerebral cortex)**

Clinical Note

Neurons are organized into sensory, motor, and autonomic hierarchies, with each cell type in each hierarchy reflecting its role through its unique neuronal configuration and connections. In the sensory hierarchy, primary sensory neurons (unipolar and bipolar) transduce specific sensory stimuli in the periphery into axon potentials that are conveyed without prior modification to secondary sensory neurons in the CNS. In the motor system the LMNs are large, multipolar neurons receiving huge convergence of inputs, including inputs from upper motor neurons in the cortex and brainstem, interneurons in the spinal cord, and sensory inputs conveyed directly (monosynaptic muscle stretch reflex) or indirectly (other somatic reflexes). In the autonomic hierarchy, both preganglionic neurons in the CNS and ganglion cells in the PNS are large multipolar neurons with extensive converging influence (for preganglionics, from spinal cord interneurons, from brainstem autonomic centers, from hypothalamic connections, and from limbic forebrain connections).

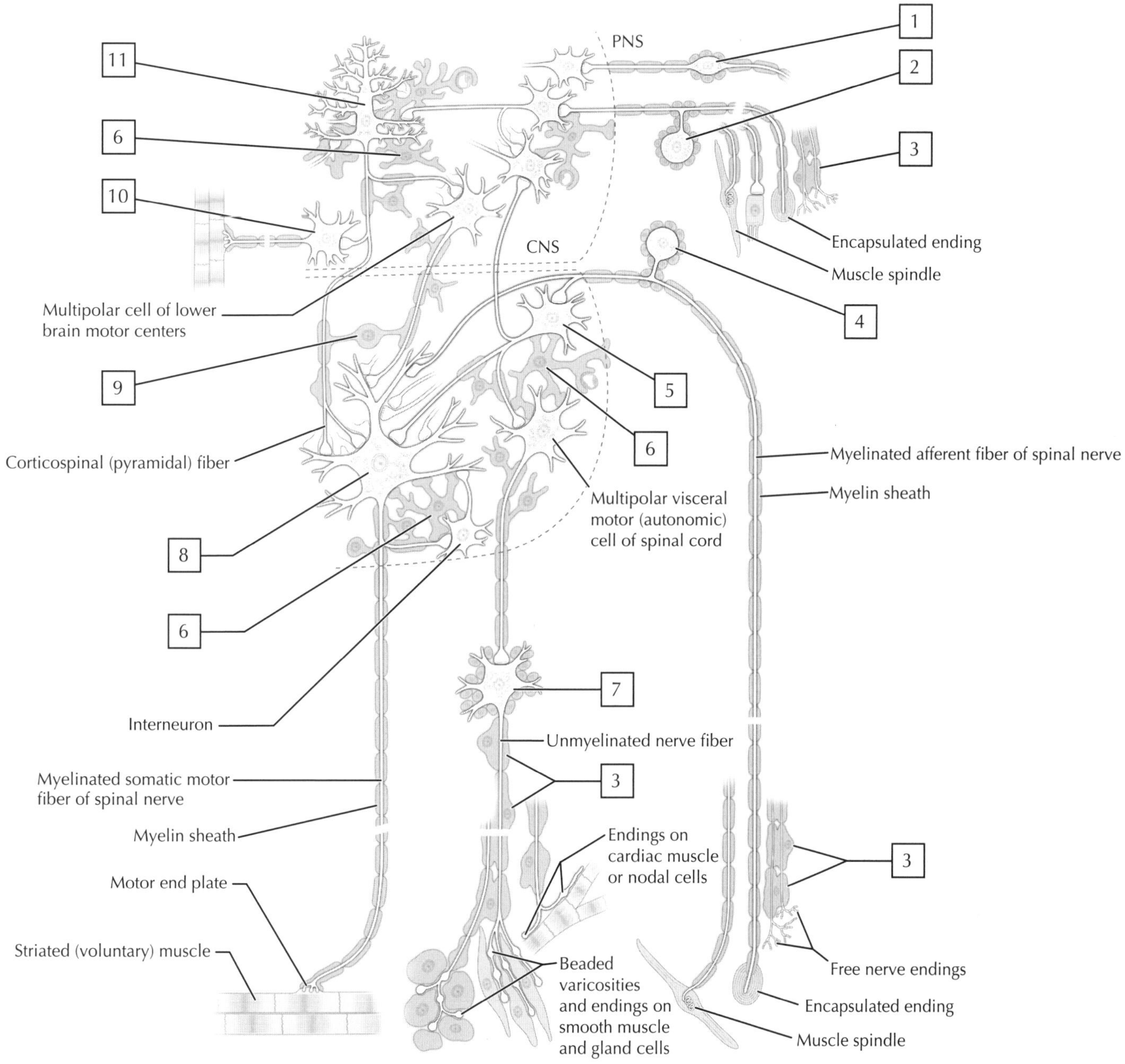

4 *CNS,* Central nervous system; *PNS,* peripheral nervous system.

1 Glial Cell Types

Three major glial cell types provide extensive support for **neurons** in the CNS. **Astrocytes** and **oligodendrocytes** are derived from neural tube cells, while most **microglial cells** are derived from specialized mesenchymal cells infiltrating from the yolk sac. Some anatomists call gray matter astrocytes "protoplasmic astrocytes" and white matter astrocytes "fibrous astrocytes." Astrocytes provide structural support for neurons; they wall off zones of synaptic interaction (e.g., axo-somatic synapses) and protect the neuronal cell membranes in the CNS. **Astrocyte end foot processes** also contact pial cells of the **pia mater** and form a **pial–glial membrane** to protect the entire outer surface of the brain. They also form **end foot processes** to provide support for the capillary endothelial cells and their tight junctions that constitute the major anatomical component of the blood-brain barrier. Astrocytes sequester K^+, provide metabolic and trophic support, and support for growth and signaling functions of neurons.

Microglia act as scavenger cells of the CNS and can invade the CNS from the periphery. They play prominent roles in phagocytosis of debris, initiation and participation in inflammatory responses of the brain, secretion of some growth factors and cytokines in the brain, and participation in some immune functions in the brain, such as antigen recognition and presentation. Some **perivascular cells** can participate in similar functions.

The main function of oligodendrocytes is the myelination of **central axons.** Each oligodendrocyte can myelinate a single segment of many axons. **Ependymal cells** line the ventricles of the brain, separating the cerebrospinal fluid from the extracellular space. Some specialized ependymal cells, called **tanycytes**, can sequester substances from the cerebrospinal fluid and transport them through extensive processes that end in specific CNS sites, where they may be released to influence CNS neurons.

COLOR each of the following structures, using a separate color for each structure.

- ☐ **1. Neuron**
- ☐ **2. Ependymal cell**
- ☐ **3. Tanycyte**
- ☐ **4. Microglia**
- ☐ **5. Axon**
- ☐ **6. Oligodendrocyte**
- ☐ **7. Axosomatic synapse**
- ☐ **8. Perivascular cell (pericyte)**
- ☐ **9. Astrocyte end foot process**
- ☐ **10. Astrocyte**
- ☐ **11. Pia mater**

Clinical Note

Glial cells are approximately 10 times more abundant than neurons in the CNS. Astrocytes have their own zone for neuronal support, and oligodendrocytes have their own segments of multiple axons provided with protective myelin. Microglia are present in the CNS (resident microglia) but also can invade the CNS when needed. They can become converted to reactive microglia and initiate inflammatory responses, carry out immune functions, phagocytose debris, and release reactive ions and molecules.

Glial cells are the main source of brain tumors. Astrocytomas, oligodendrogliomas, ependymomas, glioblastomas, and other glial-derived tumors can be highly invasive and destructive tumors, damaging neurons, acting as space-occupying masses, and resulting in death. Many glial tumors are quite resistant to chemotherapy and radiation therapy. Meningiomas are benign tumors that are frequently found adherent to dural structures, such as the falx cerebri. They can cause damage by local invasion and space-occupying effects but are not malignant and invasive. Meningiomas often can be removed successfully by surgical means.

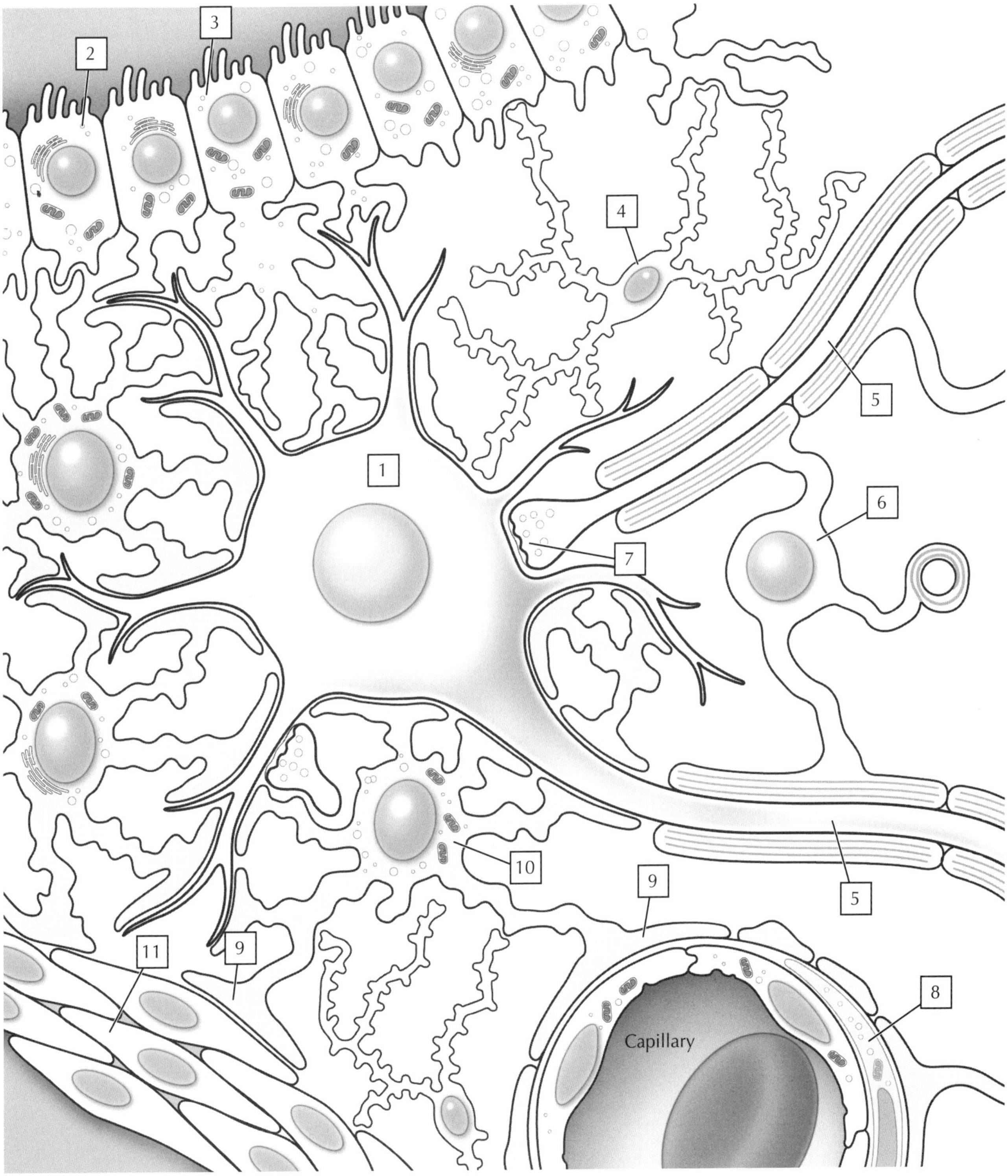
2
3
4
5
1
6
7
5
10
9
9
11
8
Capillary

1 Astrocyte Biology

Astrocytes are abundant glial cells, organized in **nonoverlapping 3D polyhedral domains**. Large numbers of **bushy processes** fill in the spaces within these domains. Astrocytic processes form **gap junctions** between adjacent astrocytes, which form a syncytium. They are highly effective at **insulating synapses**, walling off incoming axon terminals, and the synaptic sites on which they terminate. Astrocytes also form **end foot processes**, which ensheath arterioles and capillaries (and assist in the formation of the blood-brain barrier), end adjacent to **vascular smooth muscle cells** or endothelial cells, regulate the formation of endothelial tight junctions, and regulate water transport via aquaporin 4. The end feet also can release bioactive molecules such as glutamate, adenosine triphosphate (ATP), and adenosine, sometimes called **gliotransmitters**. Astrocyte processes surround and insulate synapses, provide **ionic support** (**K^+ sequestration** and pH buffering), **uptake glutamate and GABA** from the synaptic cleft, and inactivate glutamate to glutamine. Other metabolic support provided by astrocytes includes providing lactate to neurons, secreting neural growth factors, and laying down glial scar tissue following an injury.

COLOR each of the following structures, using a separate color for each structure.

- ☐ 1. **Nonoverlapping three-dimensional polyhedral domains**
- ☐ 2. **Bushy processes (filling in spaces in the domains)**
- ☐ 3. **Astrocytic insulation of synapses**
- ☐ 4. **Site of K^+ sequestration and ionic balance**
- ☐ 5. **Site of glutamate and GABA reuptake by astrocytes**
- ☐ 6. **Vascular smooth muscle cells**
- ☐ 7. **Astrocyte end foot processes**
- ☐ 8. **Endothelial cells**
- ☐ 9. **Gap junction (between adjacent astrocytic processes)**

Clinical Note

Astrocytes provide a host of supportive activities to help neurons with metabolic functions, to insulate synapses and keep unwanted interference away from specific synaptic interactions, to help **endothelial cells** form their tight junctions in support of the blood-brain barrier, to provide the supportive pial–glial membrane along the entire exterior of the brain surface, and to assist in the inactivation (through uptake) of potentially highly damaging neurotransmitters, glutamate and GABA. One reactive function of astrocytes is to respond to damage and insult by laying down glial scar tissue. This helps to provide the CNS equivalent of scar formation. One potential unwanted function of such central astrocytic scar formation is the possible irritative foci from the scar tissue, which can initiate seizure activity. Surgical treatment of the scar tissue is often not successful; antiseizure treatments are needed.

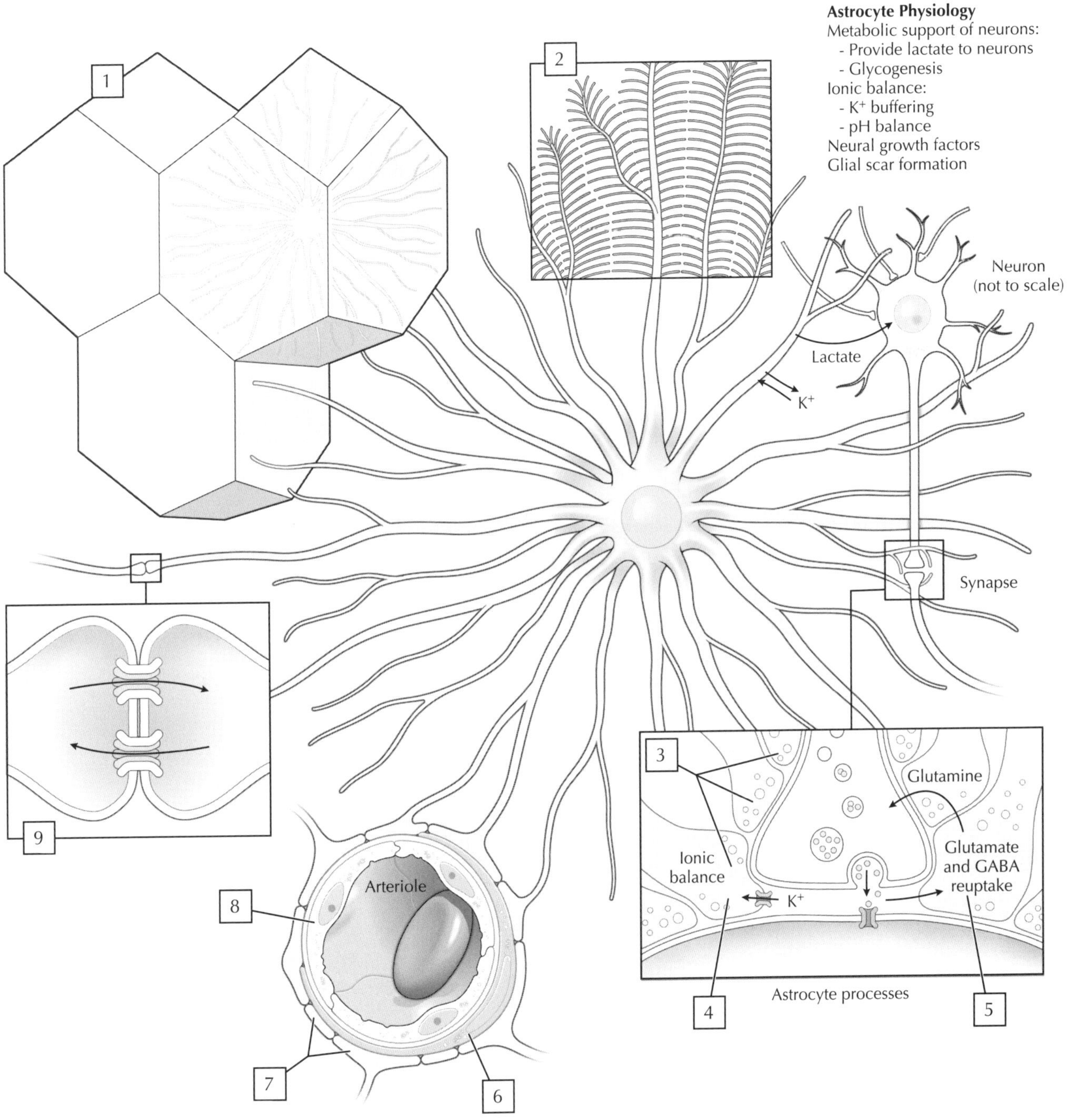
Astrocyte Physiology
Metabolic support of neurons:
- Provide lactate to neurons
- Glycogenesis
Ionic balance:
- K+ buffering
- pH balance
Neural growth factors
Glial scar formation
1
2
Neuron
(not to scale)
Lactate
K+
Synapse
9
3
Glutamine
Ionic balance
Glutamate and GABA reuptake
K+
Astrocyte processes
4
5
8
Arteriole
7
6

Microglial Biology

Resident microglia are present in the CNS, where their **processes constantly sample the local microenvironment** by moving back and forth. Approximately once per hour, the **processes make contact with synapses and sense synaptic activity**. The microglia are capable of stripping synapses that are not needed; they can **remodel synaptic sites** of interaction, and play an important role in synaptic plasticity. **Microglia respond to cell injury and apoptosis** of neurons through secreting damage-associated molecular patterns (DAMPs), also called alarmins, which activate toll-like receptors (TLRs) to bring about the genomic expression of cytokines such as interleukin 1-beta (IL-1β), which activates the microglial cell. Microglia initiate a similar **activational response to pathogens** (viruses, bacteria, cytokine-like stimuli) through secretion of pathogen-associated molecular patterns (PAMPs) and subsequent activation of TLRs.

When microglia are activated, they take on an ameboid shape, retract their processes to become shorter and thicker, and **release signal molecules**, including reactive oxygen species and nitrogen species, proinflammatory cytokines, matrix metalloproteinases, and neurotrophic factors. Activated microglia also **phagocytize pathogens and cellular debris**. The **release of interleukins and cytokines from activated microglia** can activate T cells for **antigen presentation and initiation of an immune response**. Invading microglia may add to this process.

COLOR each of the following structures, using a separate color for each structure.

- ☐ 1. **Microglial processes sampling the microenvironment**
- ☐ 2. **Microglial processes making contact with synapses**
- ☐ 3. **Microglia remodeling synapses and aiding in synaptic plasticity**
- ☐ 4. **Microglial response to injury and apoptosis**
- ☐ 5. **Microglial response to pathogens**
- ☐ 6. **Microglial release of signal molecules and reactive ion species**
- ☐ 7. **Microglial phagocytosis of pathogens and debris**
- ☐ 8. **Microglia release of cytokines**
- ☐ 9. **Microglia antigen presentation**

Clinical Note

Microglia have an important role in surveying synaptic activity, remodeling synapses, culling out unneeded interactions, and playing a continuing role in synaptic plasticity. By surveying the local microenvironment, microglia can provide a quick response.

Microglia are both resident populations and traversing populations from the periphery. They have the capability of becoming activated in the presence of cell injury, neuronal apoptosis, and the presence of pathogens. Activated microglia release a host of mediators, including reactive oxygen species and reactive nitrogen species, as well as proinflammatory cytokines and matrix metalloproteinases. These mediators can produce damaging inflammatory responses, leading to neuronal injury and apoptosis. This process is involved in the ongoing damage and destruction of neurons in Alzheimer disease. The inflammatory damage occurs from both microglial reactivity and astrocytic reactivity. Some recent experimental data suggest that radiation may reduce this inflammatory response and may enhance the clearance of aberrant beta-amyloid (Aβ) protein.

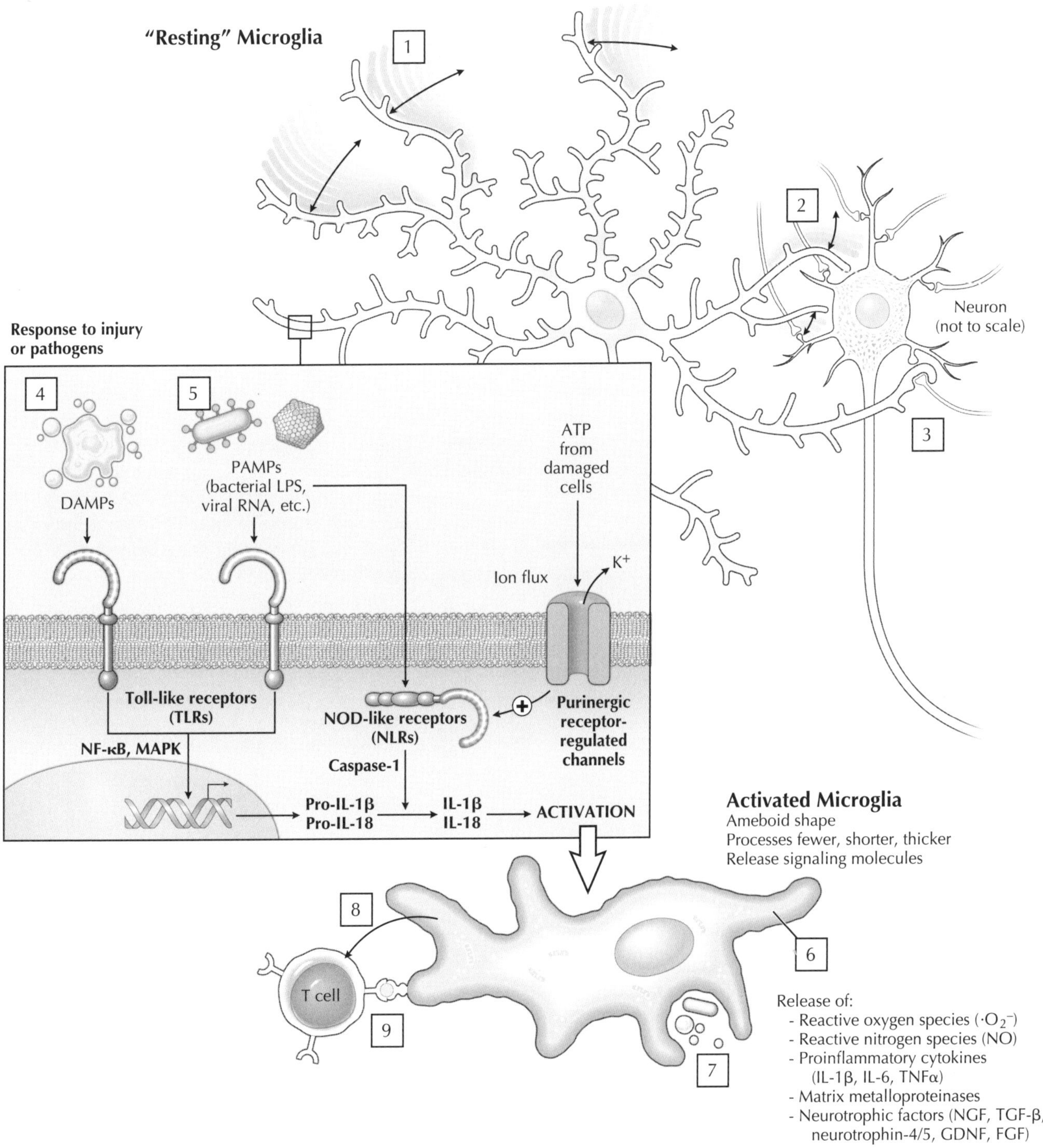
"Resting" Microglia
1
2
Neuron
(not to scale)
3
Response to injury
or pathogens
4
5
DAMPs
PAMPs
(bacterial LPS,
viral RNA, etc.)
ATP
from
damaged
cells
Ion flux
K^+
Toll-like receptors
(TLRs)
NOD-like receptors
(NLRs)
Purinergic
receptor-
regulated
channels
NF-κB, MAPK
Caspase-1
Pro-IL-1β
Pro-IL-18
IL-1β
IL-18
ACTIVATION
Activated Microglia
Ameboid shape
Processes fewer, shorter, thicker
Release signaling molecules
8
6
T cell
9
7
Release of:
- Reactive oxygen species ($\cdot O_2^-$)
- Reactive nitrogen species (NO)
- Proinflammatory cytokines
(IL-1β, IL-6, TNFα)
- Matrix metalloproteinases
- Neurotrophic factors (NGF, TGF-β,
neurotrophin-4/5, GDNF, FGF)

1 Oligodendrocyte Biology

Oligodendrocytes are neural tube–derived supportive cells whose key role is to provide myelination for axons in the CNS. These cells have processes extending from the cell body, which then **enwrap a single segment of axon for a single neuron** for each process; a single oligodendrocyte may myelinate a single axonal segment for each of 30 or more axons. A single axon may have dozens of oligodendrocytes myelinating adjacent segments of axon. There is a **trophic interaction** whereby a central axon **signals oligodendrocytes to myelinate the axon**; these signals may include ATP, potassium ion, glutamate, GABA, and cell adhesion molecules. Axon diameter may be an important factor, as large corticospinal tract axons are myelinated, but noradrenergic axons of locus coeruleus neurons, which give rise to substantial numbers of varicosities from small diameter axons, do not signal oligodendrocytes for myelination. The myelin sheath consists of lamella of **fused layers of oligodendrocyte cell membrane** wrapped concentrically around the segment of axon. Very small volumes of cytoplasm are trapped between fused membrane layers. **Monocarboxylate transporter 1 (MCT1)** delivers lactate, pyruvate, and ketone bodies from the oligodendrocyte through the myelin sheath. The adjacent **nodes of Ranvier** remain bare and possess the axonal membrane with its accumulated **sodium channels**, the site at which the AP is reinitiated as it moves down the axonal membrane (saltatory conduction).

COLOR each of the following structures, using a separate color for each structure.

- ☐ 1. **Site of trophic signal that provokes an oligodendrocyte to myelinate a segment of axon**
- ☐ 2. **Oligodendrocyte enwrapping a single segment of a single axon**
- ☐ 3. **Adjacent segments of CNS axon myelinated by different oligodendrocytes**
- ☐ 4. **Oligodendrocyte myelinating a single segment of multiple axons**
- ☐ 5. **Node of Ranvier**
- ☐ 6. **Site of sodium channels**
- ☐ 7. **Monocarboxylate transporter 1 in oligodendrocyte membrane**
- ☐ 8. **Fused layers of oligodendrocyte membrane**

Clinical Note

Oligodendrocyte myelination of CNS axons is essential for the rapid AP communication between hundreds of millions of neurons in the CNS. Any disruption in myelination will result in neuronal dysfunction and neurological deficits. The classic example of oligodendrocyte dysfunction in the CNS is multiple sclerosis (MS). In this disease, an autoimmune reaction results in an immune-mediated attack on the oligodendrocyte, producing segmental demyelination, slowed axonal conduction, and neurological dysfunction, including motor activity, sensation, vision, emotional reactivity, eye movements, and many others. MS often shows a course of remissions and exacerbations, or occasionally a progressive downhill course. In some situations of MS, the oligodendrocytes can replicate, remyelinate the central axons, and at least partially restore function, although conduction velocity rarely recovers to the full pre-MS rate. It is clear that, under the right circumstances, oligodendrocytes can replicate, thus providing more cells to participate in the remyelination process. Stressful life circumstances have been noted sometimes to exacerbate MS episodes in this condition, which is characterized by exacerbations and remissions. It appears that the most likely time for exacerbations is shortly following a high-stress situation; steady lifestyle events, without periods of very high stress, appear to provide the best opportunity for fewer exacerbations. Following MS demyelination, many patients recover, while some individuals continue with deficits. Infrequently, some individuals experience a steady downhill course for MS dysfunction.

A. Oligodendrocyte Maturation

Functional activity in neurons triggers myelination by oligodendrocyte precursor cells (OPCs)

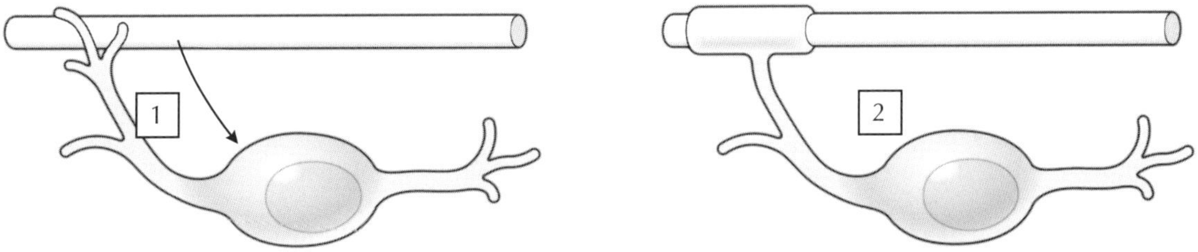

B. Oligodendrocyte Physiology

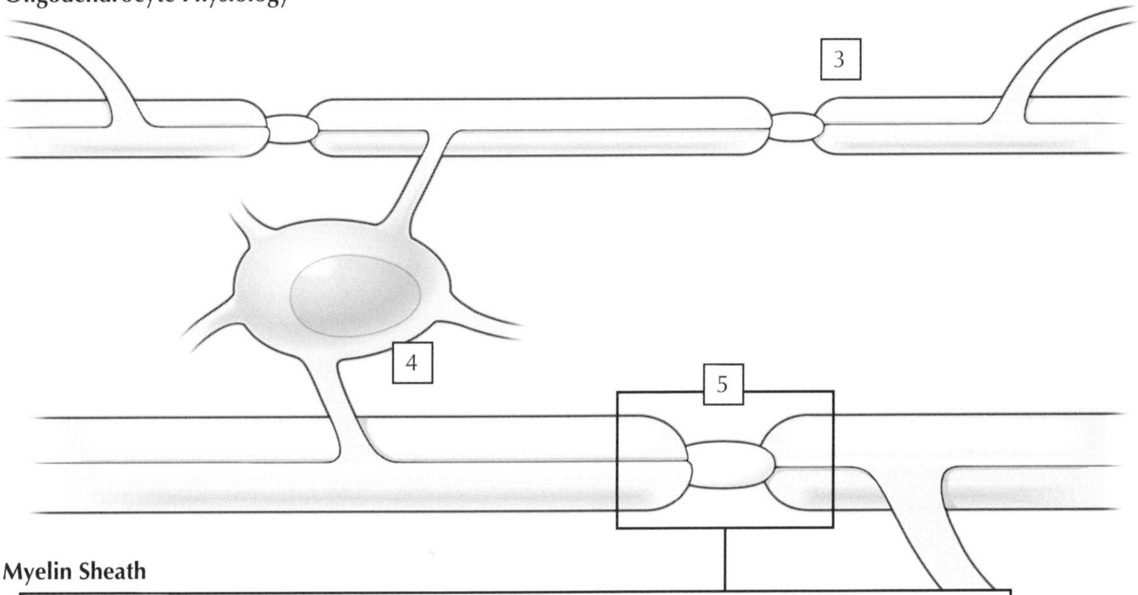

C. Myelin Sheath

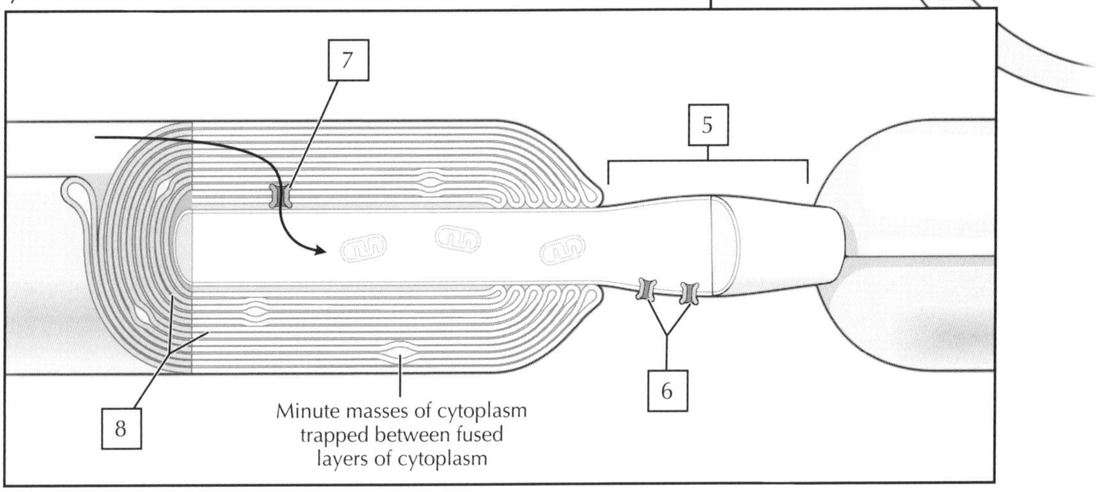

1 The Blood-Brain Barrier

The **blood-brain barrier** is the protective interface between the peripheral circulation and the CNS. The cellular components that allow this protective barrier include the **capillary endothelial cells** and their elaborate network of **tight junctions** and associated cells, such as the **astrocytes** and their **astrocytic end feet**, which abut the endothelial cells and their **basement membranes** and assist in the presence and maintenance of the **endothelial tight junctions**. The perivascular pericytes wrap around the capillaries and help to prevent leakage and extravasation. Perivascular macrophages act as resident microglia and help to regulate vessel barrier integrity and vascular permeability. The astrocytic end feet help to transport some important metabolites from the blood to neurons and also help to clear K^+ and some neurotransmitters (glutamate and GABA) from the adjacent extracellular space. These cellular elements exclude many large molecules and prevent potentially toxic substances in the peripheral circulation from damaging the neuronal and glial elements of the CNS. The endothelial cells demonstrate low levels of pinocytotic activity, further restricting easy access into the CNS for the peripheral molecules. The endothelial cells do possess some specialized transport systems, such as carrier molecules for transporting essential molecules for energy production and amino acid metabolism into the CNS. As an example, there is a competitive transport system for moving tyrosine, tryptophan, leucine, isoleucine, and valine into the brain. During a high-protein diet, tyrosine will competitively gain entrance into the brain, enhancing metabolism of catecholamines (dopamine, norepinephrine); during a low-protein diet, tryptophan will competitively gain entrance into the brain, enhancing metabolism of serotonin.

COLOR the following structures, using a separate color for each structure.

- ☐ 1. **Perivascular macrophage**
- ☐ 2. **Endothelial cell tight junction**
- ☐ 3. **Capillary endothelial cell**
- ☐ 4. **Perivascular pericyte**
- ☐ 5. **Astrocyte**
- ☐ 6. **Astrocytic end foot processes**
- ☐ 7. **Basement membrane**
- ☐ 8. **Tight junction proteins**

Clinical Note

The presence of a blood-brain barrier has many advantages and some disadvantages. The conspicuous advantage is the protective function of keeping potentially toxic molecules and unwanted large molecules out of the CNS and away from the neurons, which they could harm. Toxic damage to large neurons (not replaceable) could result in irreparable functional brain damage. The blood-brain barrier also has endothelial cells with specialized transport systems, such as that for the aforementioned amino acids. This allows regulation of some specific neurotransmitter expression, allowing a protein-rich diet to provide the essential catecholamines during development to contribute to neuronal connectivity and enrichment.

A major disadvantage of a blood-brain barrier is the likelihood that large therapeutic molecules are excluded from access to the brain. Many antibiotics, chemotherapeutic agents, and other medications are excluded from access to the brain, requiring intrathecal injection if they are to be of therapeutic use. A newer alternative is the coupling of larger therapeutic molecules to carrier molecules, which can gain access to the brain through the blood-brain barrier. One danger of some neurological disorders such as CNS tumors, infections, trauma, stroke, and other disruptions is the physical breakdown of the blood-brain barrier, allowing some molecules to cross into the brain and exert damaging effects on neurons. These effects on neurons can be fatal, leading to significant and irreversible neurological deficits. Nonfatal but damaging effects can create chronic inflammatory reactions that leave the brain susceptible to further damage.

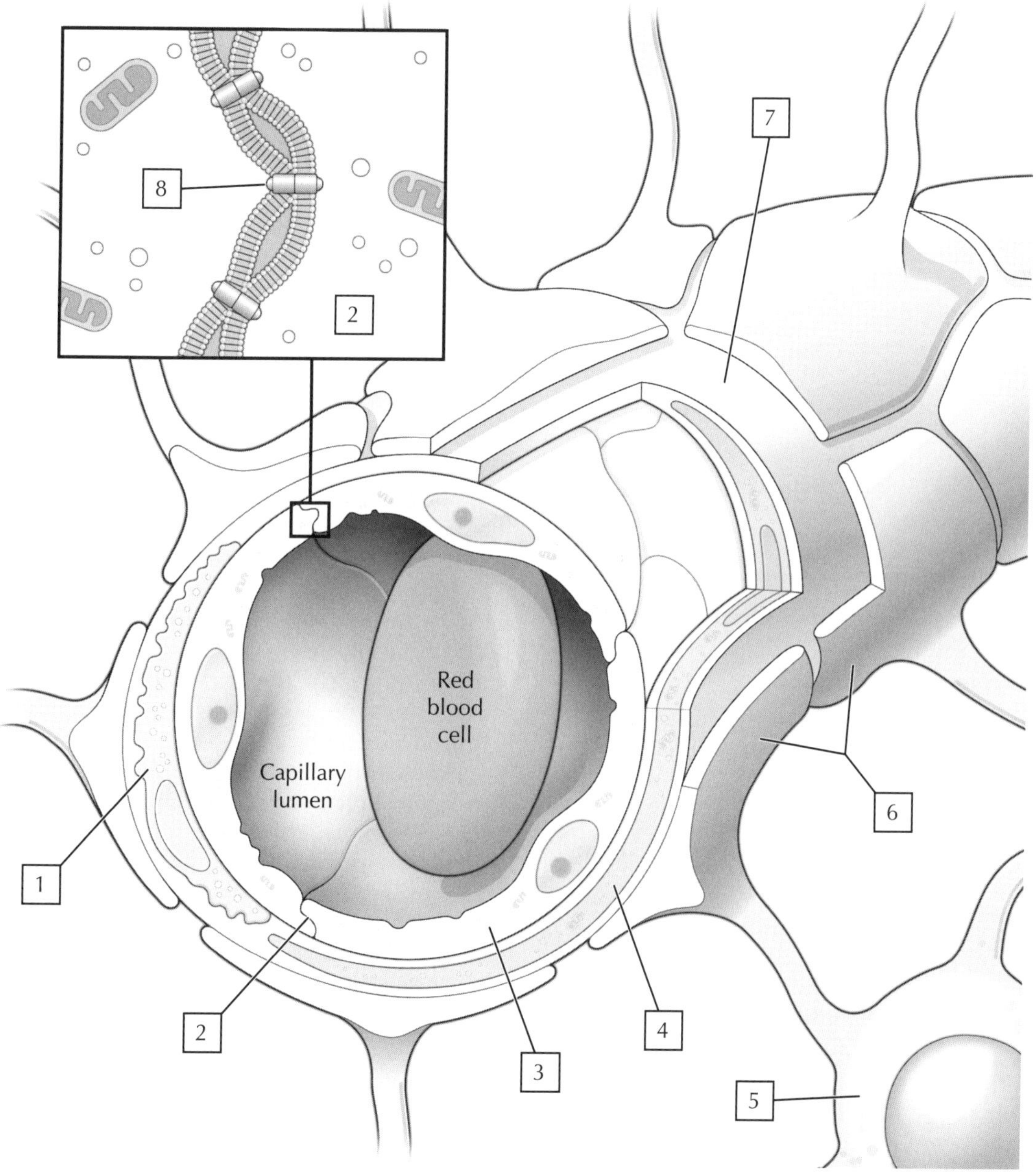
8
2
7
Red
blood
cell
Capillary
lumen
6
1
2
3
4
5

1 Axonal Transport in the Central Nervous System and Peripheral Nervous System

Proteins, intracellular organelles, and other substances are transported along the **axon**, both away from the cell body (anterograde) and toward the cell body (retrograde). The transport systems are either fast **(fast anterograde axonal transport, fast retrograde axonal transport)** or slow (**slow axonal transport**, anterograde only). Fast anterograde transport moves **vesicles, mitochondria,** organelles, membrane proteins, smooth endoplasmic reticulum, and components of neurotransmitter systems at a rate varying from 100 to 400 mm/day. These components move in a saltatory (stop-start) fashion, using **kinesin** as a transport mechanism. Fast retrograde transport moves damaged organelles, **endosomes**, some viruses and toxins, growth factors, and trophic factors toward the cell body at a rate of 200 to 270 mm/day, using **dynein** as a transport mechanism. Slow anterograde transport moves **microtubules**, **neurofilaments**, and some cytoskeletal proteins at 0.2–2.5 mm/day (slow Component a) and moves some enzymes and proteins at 5.0–6.0 mm/day (slow Component b). Some cellular organelles, such as **rough endoplasmic reticulum**, remain in the cell body and dendrites and are not transported.

COLOR the following structures, using a separate color for each structure.

- ☐ **1. Rough endoplasmic reticulum**
- ☐ **2. Mitochondrion**
- ☐ **3. Vesicle**
- ☐ **4. Kinesin**
- ☐ **5. Microtubule**
- ☐ **6. Axon**
- ☐ **7. Endosome**
- ☐ **8. Dynein**
- ☐ **9. Transport of neurofilaments**

Clinical Note

Axonal transport is essential for the normal shipment of organelles, proteins, and other molecules from the cell body (anterograde transport) along the axon (and also along dendrites); and for the shipment of organelles and proteins back to the cell body for disposal or modification. Retrograde axonal transport also is used for the ability of a neuron to sample the local environment in the region of its axonal terminals. In some cases, signal molecules (e.g., cytokines) can be taken up into the terminals and retrogradely transported back to the cell body, where alterations in nuclear transcription are induced; this alters genomic expression and allows the neuron to modify its protein synthesis. The same process occurs if the axon or nerve terminals are damaged. Signal molecules are transported back to the cell body, and altered protein synthesis allows repair and remodeling to occur to restore the structural and functional integrity of the axon and its terminals.

On some occasions, a virus or toxin can gain access to the nerve terminals (e.g., polio virus or herpes zoster virus), utilize the retrograde axonal transport system, and gain access to the machinery of the cell body. In some cases, the virus kills the neuron (polio), and in other cases, it lies dormant (herpes zoster), activating at a much later time, perhaps in response to immune dysfunction or immune signals during a period of high stress, producing painful blistering and reactivation of the virus at the sites of distribution of the nerve terminals or sensory receptor distribution.

The systems of anterograde and retrograde transport have been utilized for tracing axonal connections in experimental models. A retrogradely transported dye can be taken up by the nerve terminals in a region of distribution and transported back to the cell bodies, revealing the cells of origin for those terminals. Labeled substances can be injected into the region of neuronal cell bodies, taken up, and transported down the axon, thereby revealing the distribution of axonal terminals derived from those neurons. Use of multiple agents can reveal whether a single neuron can provide multiple branches to several distant structures or whether separate neurons each give rise to axons destined for a single region.

Faulty axonal transport may contribute to clinical deficits such as hyperphosphorylation of tau protein, leading to microtubule and cytoskeletal collapse in Alzheimer disease.

A. Fast Anterograde Axonal Transport

100–400 mm/day in a saltatory fashion (start–stop–start)

Cargo includes:
- Synaptic vesicles and synaptic vesicle precursors
- Mitochondria and other membrane organelles
- Integral membrane proteins
- Secretory polypeptides
- Neurotransmitters
- Elements of smooth endoplasmic reticulum

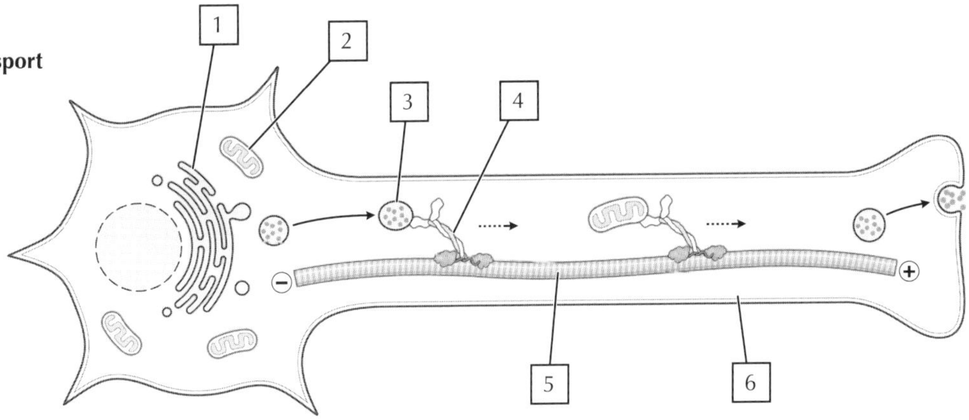

B. Fast Retrograde Axonal Transport

200–270 mm/day

Cargo includes:
- Endosomes
- Damaged mitochondria and other organelles
- Elements of smooth endoplasmic reticulum
- Regulatory signals (growth factors and neurotrophins)
- Viruses and toxins (e.g., tetanus, herpes simplex, rabies, polio)

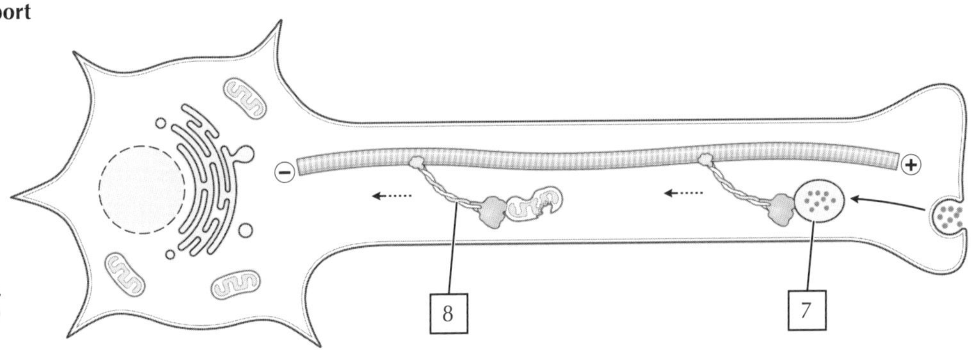

C. Slow Axonal Transport (Anterograde Only)

Different substances move at two different speeds:

Slow Component a (SCa)
0.2–2.5 mm/day (rate of neurite elongation)
- Microtubules
- Neurofilaments
- Cytoskeletal proteins (e.g., α and β tubulin)

Slow Component b (SCb)
5.0–6.0 mm/day
- Cytosolic proteins
- Clathrin
- Calmodulin
- Soluble enzymes and other proteins

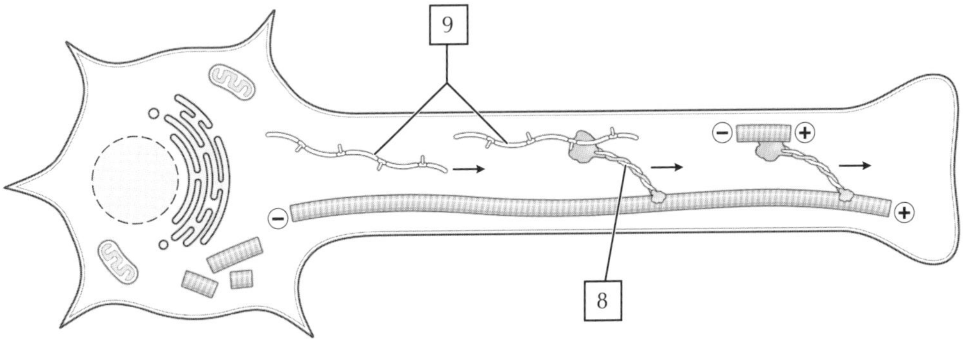

1 Myelination of Central Nervous System and Peripheral Nervous System Axons

Myelination of central axons is provided by **oligodendrocytes**, which enwrap a single segment of each of several axons (30 or more) with lamellae (concentric layers) of oligodendrocyte membrane. Size appears to be a trigger for myelination, with axons of 1 to 2 μm diameter, providing a signal for myelination. A single central axon is myelinated by many oligodendrocytes, one per segment. The intervening **nodes of Ranvier** are sites of bare axon containing the sodium channels, which permit the reinitiation of the AP as it propagates down the axon (saltatory conduction).

Peripheral axons (PNS) are myelinated by **Schwann cells** and also have a size threshold of 1 to 2 μm diameter triggering the myelination. A single Schwann cell enwraps a single segment of one axon with lamellae of cell membrane. Schwann cells myelinate axons of **lower motor neurons** (peripheral portion only), **primary sensory axons** other than C fibers (peripheral portion only), **preganglionic autonomic axons** (peripheral portion only), and a few **postganglionic autonomic axons**. In the PNS, all unmyelinated axons are surrounded by a Schwann cell sheath, arms of Schwann cell cytoplasm that protect them.

COLOR the following structures, using a separate color for each structure.

- ☐ 1. **Oligodendrocyte**
- ☐ 2. **Primary sensory cell body**
- ☐ 3. **Schwann cells (associated with the myelin sheaths of myelinated PNS axons)**
- ☐ 4. **Astrocytes**
- ☐ 5. **Axosomatic synapses on central neurons**
- ☐ 6. **Postganglionic neuron of an autonomic ganglion**
- ☐ 7. **Node of Ranvier**
- ☐ 8. **Axons terminating on striated muscle in a motor end plate**

Clinical Note

The myelin sheath around both central and peripheral axons permits rapid conduction of the AP at speeds of 100 m/s or more. Without the myelin sheath, the functional activities of these axons are lost, and severe neurological dysfunction occurs. Central demyelination can occur when the oligodendrocytes are attacked in an autoimmune process such as multiple sclerosis (MS). As oligodendrocytes are damaged and their myelinated segments lose their insulation, functional deficits in many sites may occur, such as blindness, diplopia from loss of coordination of eye muscles, weakness, sensory losses, loss of coordination, cognitive and emotional changes, and others. Oligodendrocytes can replicate and often remyelinate denuded segments of central axons, thereby providing some recovery of function. In some cases, functional recovery is either incomplete or does not occur.

Peripheral demyelination may occur during an autoimmune attack on the myelin (Guillain-Barré syndrome) following an infectious process such as a gastrointestinal infection (Campylobacter jejuni) or a viral infection (Zika virus), resulting in paresis and loss of epicritic sensation in the affected regions. Paresis frequently begins distally and moves proximally. Gradual recovery and remyelination may occur but may take many months. In some cases, residual deficits remain, or recovery does not occur. The ability of both oligodendrocytes and Schwann cells to replicate and initiate remyelination is critical to their ability to repair the damage left by these autoimmune attacks.

Myelination of Central Nervous System and Peripheral Nervous System Axons

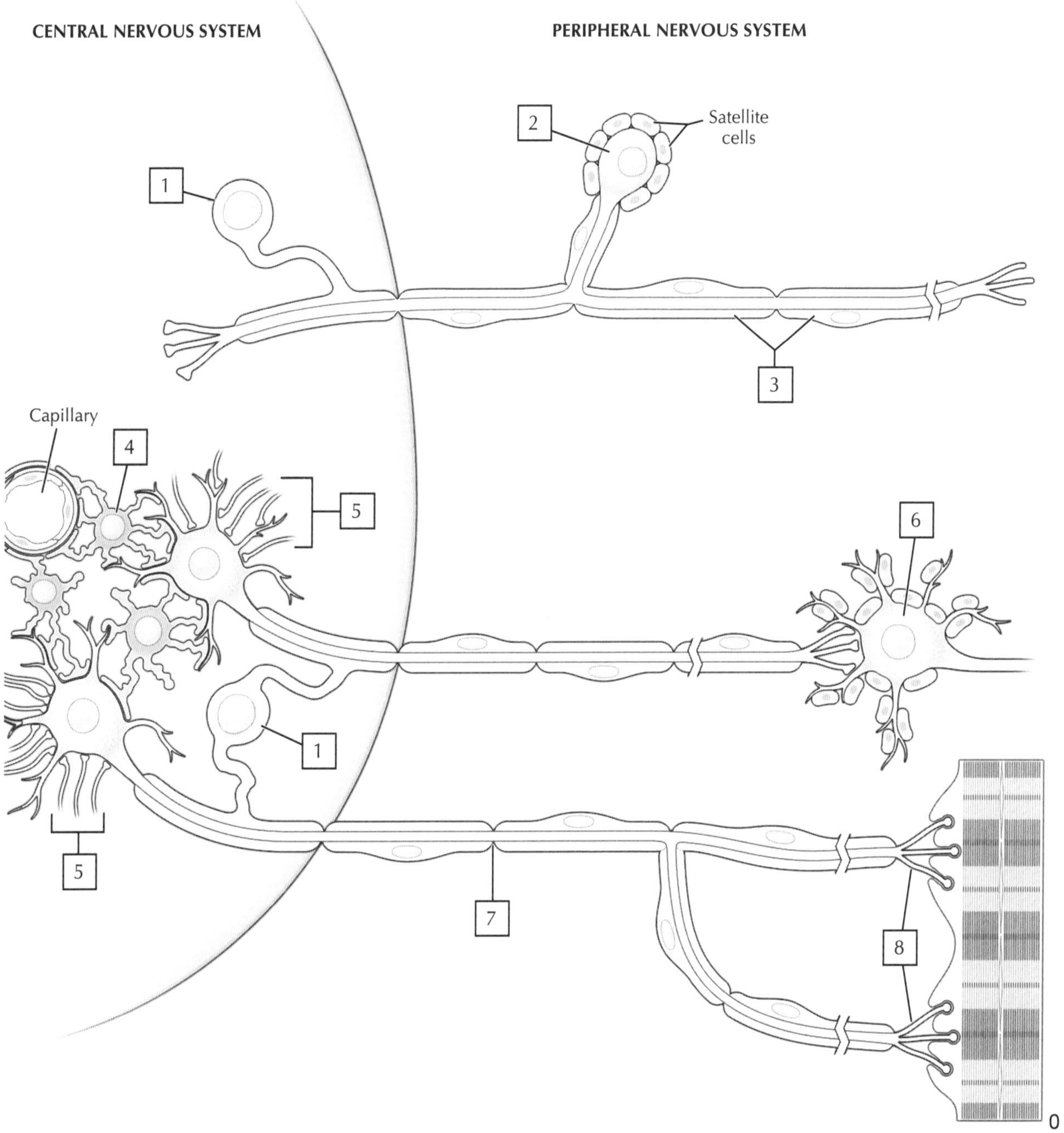

1 Neuronal Resting Potential

The **neuronal membrane (a lipid bilayer)** is a differentially permeable membrane, with the **major cations (Na^+, K^+)** and **anions (Cl^- and intracellular anions)** distributed unevenly on the outside and inside of the neuron. The two major forces that cause this uneven distribution are the **separation of charges** and the **diffusion of specific ion species**. The neuronal membrane changes its permeability to the major ions depending on the state of **depolarization**. At rest, the membrane resting potential is approximately –70 to –90 mV with respect to the **extracellular fluid**; at this stage, the membrane is near the **K^+ equilibrium potential** (point at which only K^+ is permeable through the membrane). At rest, the extracellular Na^+ concentration (145 mEq/L) and Cl^- concentration (105 mEq/L) are high compared with the intracellular concentrations of Na^+ (15 mEq/L) and Cl^- (8 mEq/L). The extracellular concentration of K^+ is low (3.5 mEq/L) compared with the intracellular concentration (130 mEq/L). These uneven ion distributions establish diffusion gradients. Na^+ is actively pumped out of the neuron, and K^+ is actively pumped into the neuron by the **Na^+–K^+–ATPase membrane pump**. At rest, the distribution of **intracellular and extracellular concentrations** of the major ions reflects the differential permeability of the membrane, its alteration as depolarization occurs (charge moving toward 0 mV), and the resultant separation of charges and diffusion of ion species.

Clinical Note

The differential permeability of the neuronal lipid bilayer membrane and its ATPase-dependent pumps keeps the ions separated by charge and diffusion; this process is very expensive from the point of view of energy consumption by the neurons. The CNS uses far more oxygen and glucose than expected (approximately 20%) from size and weight alone (2%). Without the effectiveness of the ion pumps and changes in Na^+ entry into the neuron during depolarization (causing the axonal AP when more Na^+ influx occurs than can be countered by K^+ efflux), neuronal electrical activity and communication with other neurons via axons would cease. The Na^+ channels are distributed along the membrane in unmyelinated axons but are found only at the nodes of Ranvier in myelinated axons. Blocking of the Na^+ channel at the nodes of Ranvier stops axonal conduction of APs; local anesthetics block nerve conductance by blocking consecutive nodes (e.g., mandibular nerve block for dental work).

There are many diseases related to ion channel malfunctions and mutations, including physiological disorders, neuronal disorders, kidney disorders, secretion disorders, vision disorders, and others. For a review, see Dworakowska B, Dołowy K. Ion channels-related diseases. *Acta Biochem Pol.* 2000;47(3):685-703.

COLOR the following structures, using a separate color for each structure.

- ☐ 1. **Axoplasm (intracellular space) (note with a small region of color)**
- ☐ 2. **Neuronal membrane**
- ☐ 3. **Extracellular space (note with a small region of color)**
- ☐ 4. **Na^+ diffusion gradient**
- ☐ 5. **K^+ diffusion gradient**
- ☐ 6. **Cl^- diffusion gradient**
- ☐ 7. **Intracellular anions**
- ☐ 8. **K^+ concentration gradient**
- ☐ 9. **K^+ diffusion from electrical potential difference**
- ☐ 10. **Na^+ channel resting**
- ☐ 11. **Na^+ channel activated (open) during depolarization**
- ☐ 12. **Na^+ channel inactivated during repolarization**

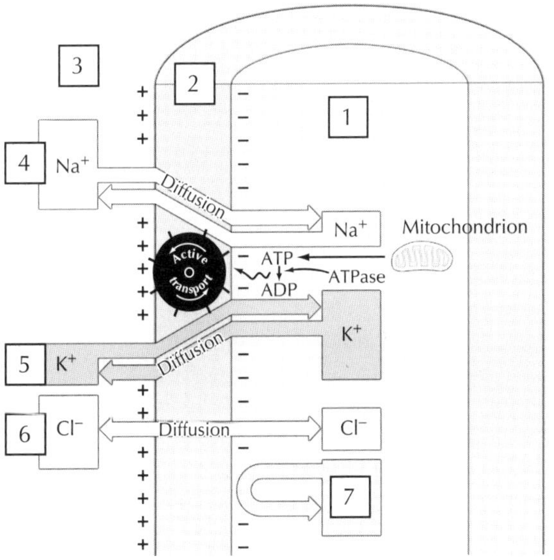

A. Distribution of ions in an axon by charge separation and diffusion

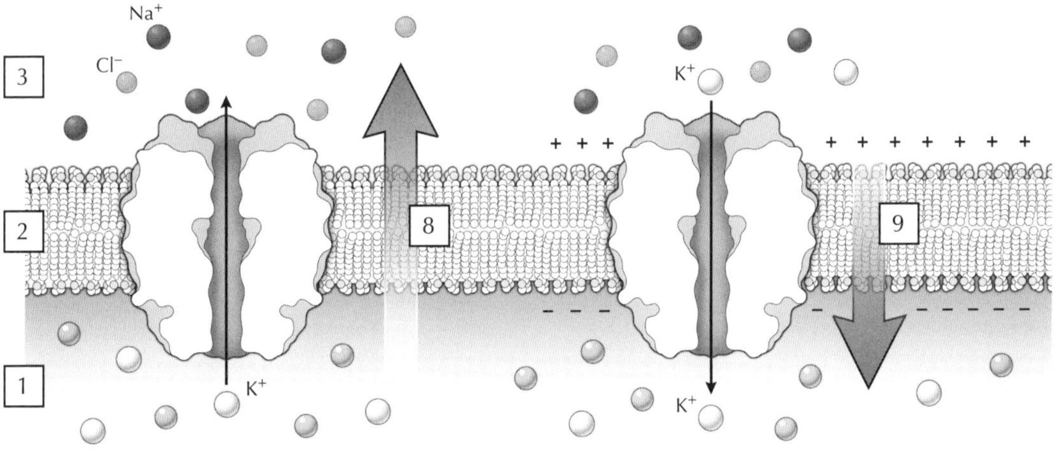

B. Movement of ions across the axonal cell membrane

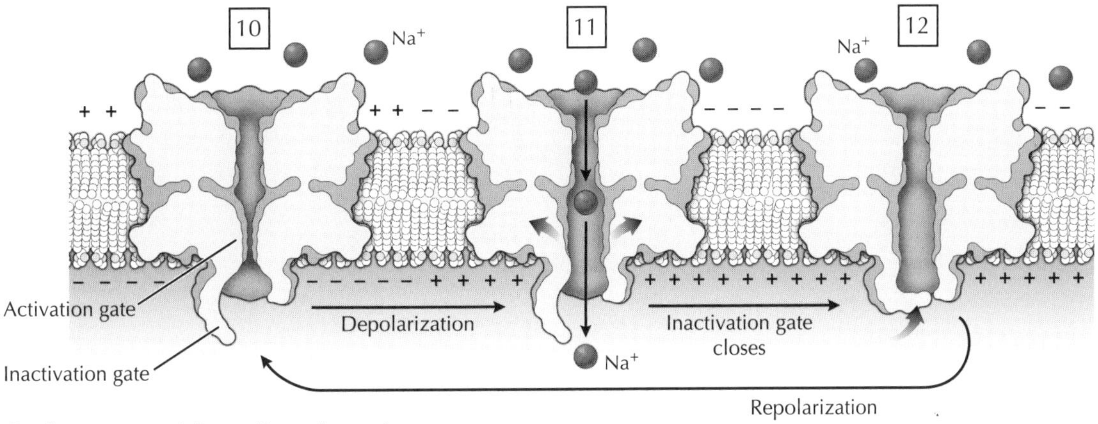

C. Three states of the sodium channel

1 Graded Potentials in Neurons

Neuronal membrane perturbations (**depolarization,** toward 0 mV; **hyperpolarization**, away from 0 mV) can be induced by the action of **neurotransmitters** (released from **synaptic vesicles** in the **presynaptic nerve ending**) on their **cognate receptors** on the surface of the postsynaptic membrane. The neurotransmitter–receptor interaction **can alter the membrane potential (via ligand-gated ion channels)** and also can **activate intracellular signal transduction pathways (via metabotropic receptors)** that influence genomic expression and other intracellular neuronal functions. In the patch of membrane at which the neurotransmitter–receptor interaction occurs, either a **depolarizing excitatory response** (influx of Na^+ from increased membrane permeability to positively charged ions) or a **hyperpolarizing inhibitory response** (influx of Cl^- ion) is seen. These changes in membrane potential are called **graded potentials** and are named **excitatory postsynaptic potentials (EPSPs)** and **inhibitory postsynaptic potentials (IPSPs)**. These local EPSPs and IPSPs exert local effects that dissipate over space and time. It is unusual for an EPSP to depolarize the axonal membrane sufficiently to bring it to **threshold for the initiation of an action potential at the initial segment of the axon**. EPSPs can accumulate over space **(spatial summation)** and time **(temporal summation)** to achieve such a depolarization to threshold. Strategically placed IPSPs can block depolarization and prevent the firing of an AP. This process of neurotransmission, with release of excitatory and inhibitory neurotransmitters, usually takes place from axon terminal release of neurotransmitter to act on the neuronal membrane of the postsynaptic cell body and dendrites; however, axonal release of neurotransmitter can act on other nerve terminals (e.g., presynaptic inhibition), and dendrites also can release neurotransmitter adjacent to other axon terminals and dendrites. Note that whether a neurotransmitter is excitatory or inhibitory depends on the effects it exerts through its postsynaptic receptor(s).

Clinical Note

Convergence of inputs is a general principle of neural communication. Many functionally important neurons (LMNs, preganglionic autonomic neurons, secondary sensory neurons, cerebellar Purkinje cells, cortical pyramidal cells, and hundreds of other cell types) receive input from thousands of axons deriving from many sources, sometimes from many diverse neuronal cell groups. The axons from these inputs terminate on a variety of anatomical sites of the target neurons, including the cell body, dendrites, dendritic spines, and even other incoming axon terminals. These incoming influences usually require spatial summation and temporal summation of EPSPs to significantly depolarize the neuronal membrane near the axon hillock, the site adjacent to the initial segment, the place of initiation of the AP in the axon. IPSPs can balance out or prevent such depolarization. Depending on the intensity of inputs to a given site on a target neuron, the excitability of the target neuronal membrane is changed. With a more intense AP train from a given set of inputs, there may be altered concentration of neurotransmitters released; many axon terminals contain more than one neurotransmitter, and release is usually nonlinear with respect to AP frequency. Some molecules present in the extracellular fluid may either alter the structural configuration of another neurotransmitter (e.g., dopamine, serotonin, and norepinephrine altering the three-dimensional conformation of some neuropeptides) or may change the interaction of another neurotransmitter with its cognate receptors (e.g., norepinephrine altering the response of Purkinje cells to both GABA and glutamate neurotransmission).

The balance of neuronal inputs and the graded potentials they elicit is essential for appropriate neuronal function. If these inputs are lost or become reorganized, as occurs with lower motor neurons following spinal cord damage, those neurons may show aberrant responses such as hypertonia and hyperreflexia.

COLOR the following structures, using a separate color for each structure.

- ☐ 1. **Synaptic vesicles in nerve endings**
- ☐ 2. **Presynaptic membrane**
- ☐ 3. **Neurotransmitter in the synaptic cleft**
- ☐ 4. **Postsynaptic membrane**
- ☐ 5. **Presynaptic nerve ending**
- ☐ 6. **Site of current flow from graded potentials**
- ☐ 7. **Excitatory fiber using glutamate**
- ☐ 8. **Inhibitory fiber using GABA**
- ☐ 9. **Ca^{++} channels for the influx of Ca^{++} into the presynaptic nerve ending**
- ☐ 10. **Na^+ channels**

Chemical Synaptic Transmission

A. Ion movements

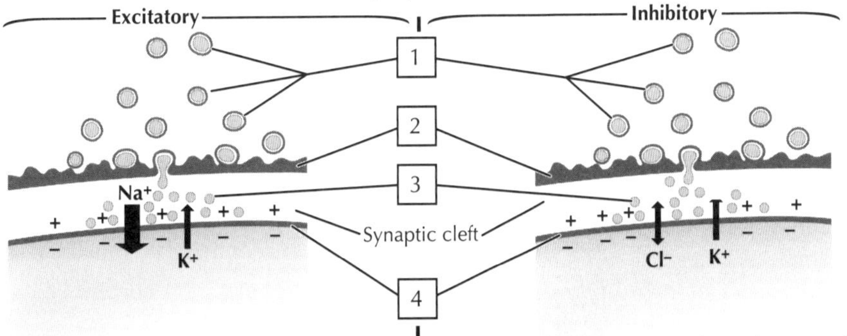

When impulse reaches excitatory synaptic bouton, it causes release of a transmitter substance into synaptic cleft. This increases permeability of postsynaptic membrane to Na^+ and K^+. More Na^+ moves into postsynaptic cell than K^+ moves out due to greater electrochemical gradient.

At inhibitory synapse, transmitter substance released by an impulse increases permeability of postsynaptic membrane to K^+ and Cl^- but not Na^+. K^+ moves out of postsynaptic cell.

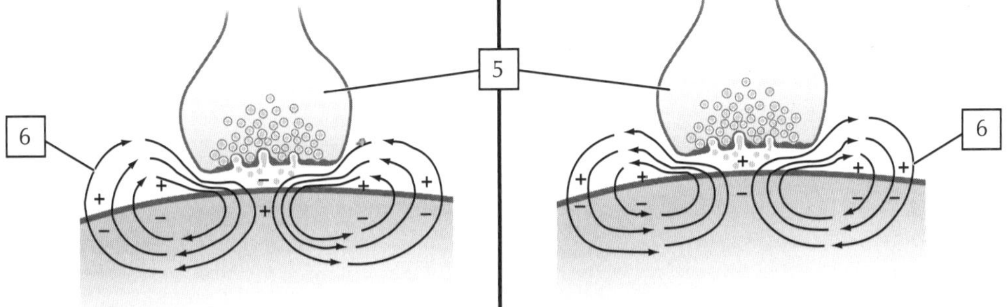

Resultant net ionic current flow is in a direction that tends to depolarize postsynaptic cell. If depolarization reaches firing threshold at the axon hillock, an impulse is generated in postsynaptic cell.

Resultant ionic current flow is in a direction that tends to hyperpolarize postsynaptic cell. This makes depolarization by excitatory synapses more difficult—more depolarization is required to reach threshold.

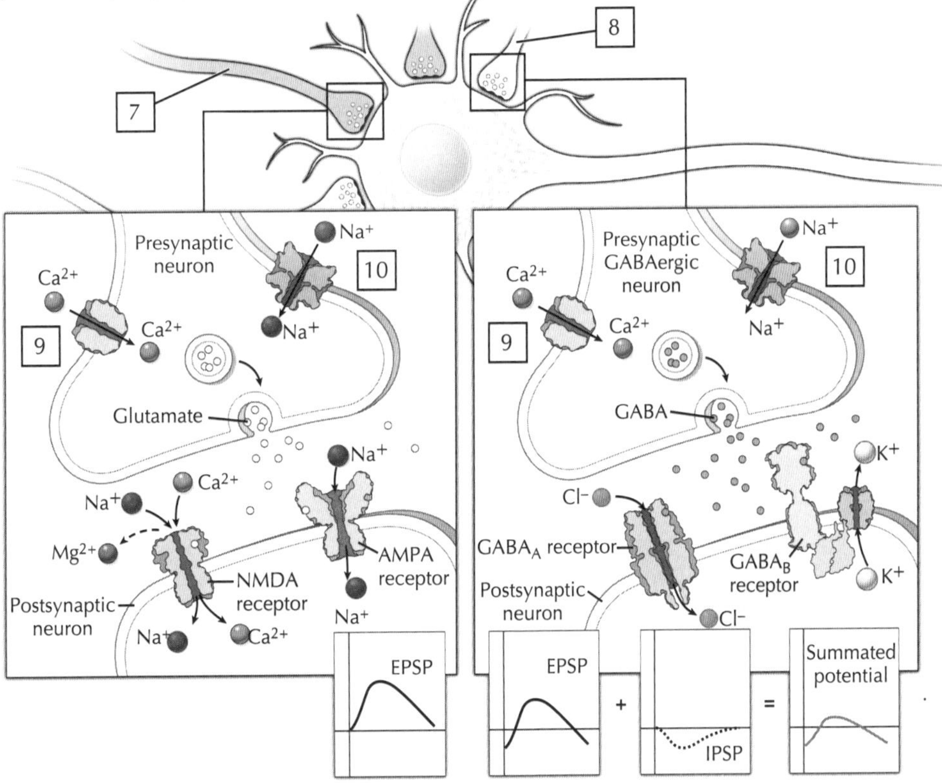

B. Excitatory and inhibitory fibers eliciting an EPSP and IPSP, respectively

Action Potentials

At rest, Na^+ concentration is far higher in the **extracellular fluid** than in the **axoplasm (intracellular fluid)**. It is actively pumped out of the axon by the **Na^+–K^+–ATPase membrane pumps**. The **resting potential** is approximately –70 to –90 mV. As axonal inputs impinge on various portions of the neuronal membrane, portions of the membrane depolarize (due to opening of channels for cations), bringing it closer to 0. As the membrane depolarizes, some **Na^+ channels** are opened, allowing Na^+ to enter the neuron **(Na^+ conductance)** as a **depolarizing current**. This influx of Na^+ can be countered by another cation, K^+, leaving the axon into the extracellular fluid **(K^+ conductance)**. The efflux of K^+ can counterbalance Na^+ influx up to a point. When the Na^+ influx reaches the point where K^+ efflux can no longer counterbalance, the membrane reaches threshold (between –40 and –55 mV) and Na^+ rapidly enters the neuron and brings the membrane potential to approximately + 20 mV, approaching the **equilibrium potential of Na^+ (+55 mV)**. This rapid influx of Na^+ and resultant depolarization is the **AP**. It is an all-or-none (only happens when threshold is reached), nondecremental electrical potential. As the Na^+ influx rapidly causes depolarization during the rising phase of the AP, this increases K^+ conductance, which then allows K^+ efflux to counter the depolarization and bring the membrane potential back toward its resting level **(repolarizing current)**. The all-important site for the initiation of the AP is the **initial segment** of the axon; influences near this site (**axon hillock**, adjacent membrane) have far greater influence over depolarization than inputs at more distant sites, such as distal dendrites.

COLOR the following structures, using a separate color for each structure.

- ☐ **1. Action potential**
- ☐ **2. Na^+ conductance**
- ☐ **3. K^+ conductance**
- ☐ **4. Extracellular fluid**
- ☐ **5. Axonal membrane**
- ☐ **6. Intracellular fluid (axoplasm)**
- ☐ **7. Repolarizing current**
- ☐ **8. Depolarizing current**

Clinical Note

The AP, involving the rapid nondecremental conductance of current down an axon, permits the rapid electrical transmission of information from a neuron to distant sites. The AP invades the nerve terminals and initiates an excitation–secretion coupling of neurotransmitter, thereby using electrochemical coupling to signal target neurons or effector tissue (in the periphery). The rapid conduction (up to 120 m/s) provides quick responses that are essential for proper functioning of neuronal systems and are essential for survival. Demyelination eliminates rapid conduction of APs and produces profound neuronal dysfunction in the affected systems. This demyelination process happens in autoimmune diseases (Guillain–Barré syndrome in the PNS, MS in the CNS), in peripheral neuropathies (e.g., diabetic neuropathy), and in other central demyelinating diseases.

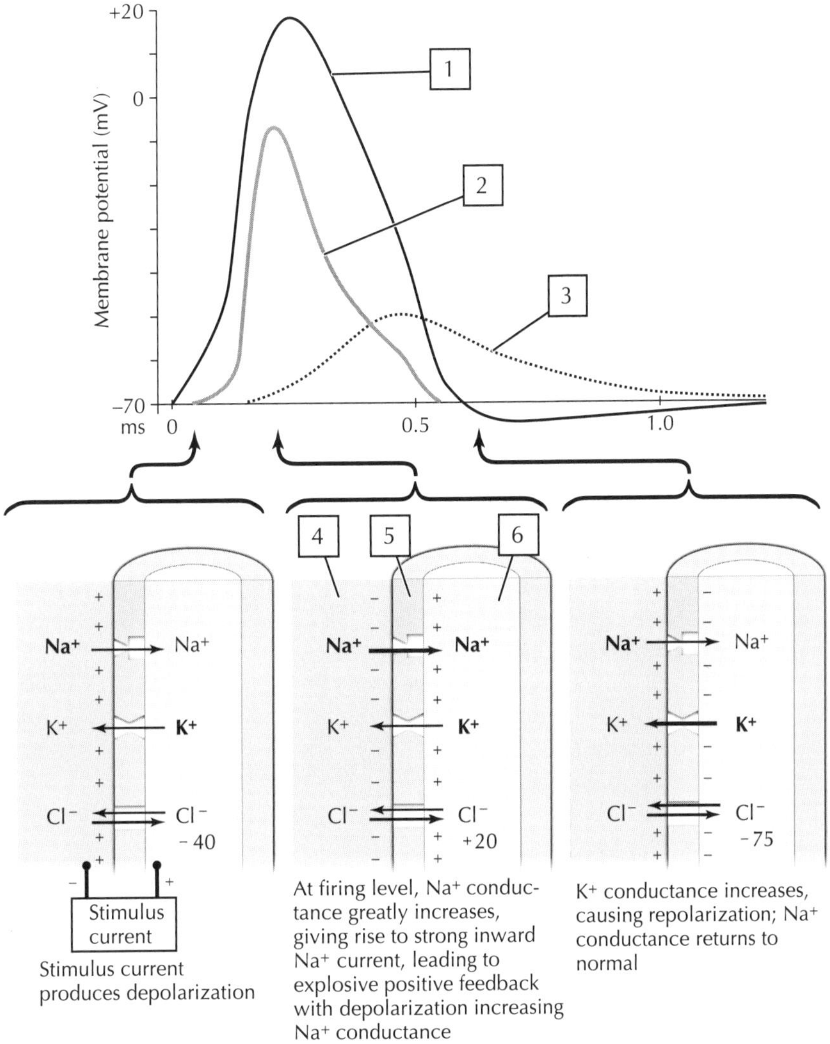

A. The action potential, ion conductances, and ion movements during an AP

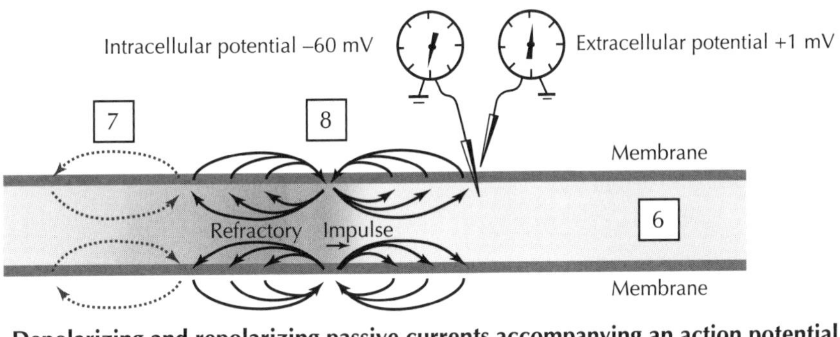

B. Depolarizing and repolarizing passive currents accompanying an action potential

Conduction Velocity

The rapid depolarization of the membrane during the rising phase of an AP causes **local current flow**, which can result in an adjacent patch of axonal membrane in an unmyelinated axon to reach **threshold** and **reinitiate the AP**. This causes the AP to move down the axonal membrane, called **propagation of the AP**. Conduction velocity increases with **increasing diameter** of an unmyelinated axon. In a myelinated axon, the **Na^+ channels** are confined to the **nodes of Ranvier**. The **local passive current flow** brings the next node to its threshold, thereby reinitiating the AP at the next node. This process gives the appearance of the AP skipping down the axon from node to node, called **saltatory conduction**. Conduction velocity increases with increasing axon diameter and extent of myelination.

Nerve size (diameter) is categorized by Roman numerals I–IV for sensory fibers (I is largest; IV is smallest), and by an A, B, C system for all fibers (motor, sensory, autonomic) (A is largest; C is smallest).

In a graph of **conduction velocity versus axon diameter**, the slowest conducting axons (1–2 m/s) are the small, **group IV unmyelinated axons** (**C fibers**: nociceptive axons and postganglionic autonomic unmyelinated axons), 1 to 2 μm in diameter. Axons over 2 μm in diameter (2–20 μm) trigger **myelination** in both the CNS and PNS. In the PNS, the fastest conducting axons are the **Ia muscle spindle afferents** (up to 120 m/s), followed by **lower motor neuron axons** and **group Ib Golgi tendon organ afferent axons** (60–100 m/s). **Group II afferents** (secondary muscle spindle afferents, **proprioceptive afferents** for touch and pressure) conduct at 30 to 70 m/s. **Group III fibers** (A-delta fibers) from some muscle and joint receptors, some touch and pressure receptors, visceral afferents, thermoreceptors, and others, conduct at 10 to 30 m/s. The **gamma motor neuron axons** overlap the group II and III categories and conduct at 20 to 40 m/s. **Autonomic preganglionic myelinated axons** conduct at 5 to 15 m/s.

COLOR the following structures, using a separate color for each structure.

- ☐ 1. **Node of Ranvier**
- ☐ 2. **Myelin sheath**
- ☐ 3. **Axonal bilipid membrane**
- ☐ 4. **Axoplasm (intracellular space) (denote with small patch of color)**
- ☐ 5. **Extracellular space (denote with small patch of color)**
- ☐ 6. **Ia afferent conduction velocities**
- ☐ 7. **Proprioceptive afferent conduction velocities**
- ☐ 8. **Lower motor neuron axon conduction velocities**
- ☐ 9. **Autonomic preganglionic axon conduction velocities**
- ☐ 10. **Nociceptive C-fiber conduction velocities**

Clinical Note

Peripheral conduction velocity measurements can be readily assessed in a clinical setting. Electromyography records electrical activity in muscles during voluntary contraction. These electromyographic recordings provide information about possible myopathies and axonal neuropathies, which may result in fibrillations and fasciculations. Fibrillation is the twitch of an individual muscle fiber, often occurring when that fiber loses contact with its incoming motor axon. Fasciculations are visible twitches of entire motor units, often benign, but sometimes indicative of a damaged LMN firing aberrant action potentials. Nerve conduction velocity studies provide information about the ability of myelinated axons to conduct electrically evoked APs in sensory and motor axons in the periphery, useful for assessing demyelinating diseases and neuropathies.

In the CNS, conduction velocity of many axonal pathways cannot be achieved. However, flow of information through a functional pathway, such as visual evoked potentials and auditory evoked potentials, can be assessed, and dysfunction in these systems may be detectable.

A. Myelinated fibers

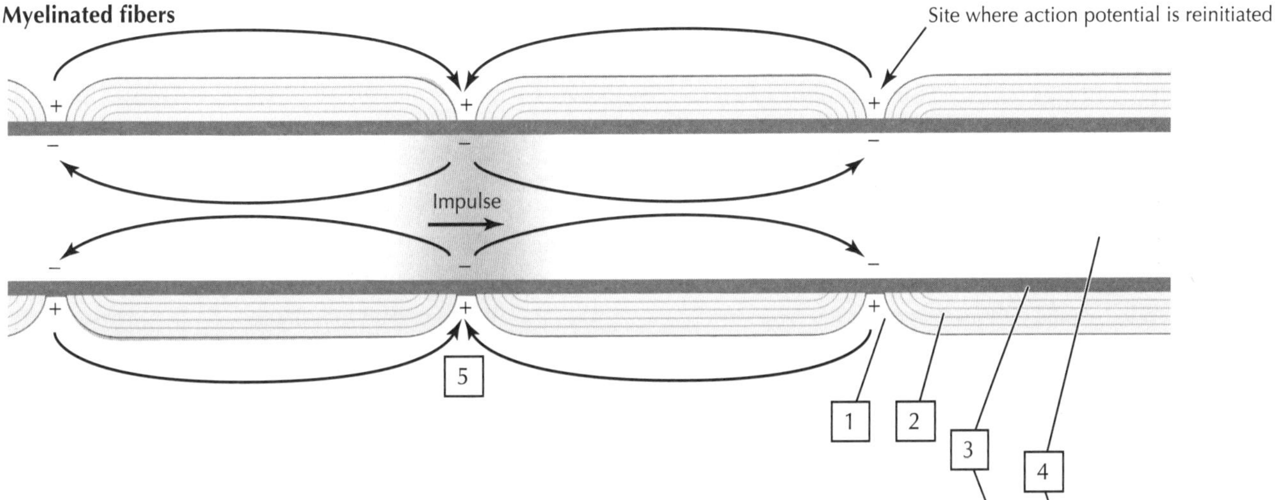

B. Unmyelinated fibers

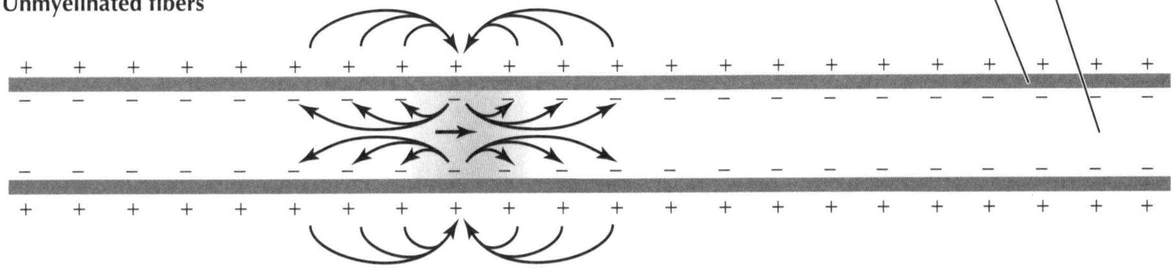

C. Classification of peripheral nerve fibers by size and conduction velocity

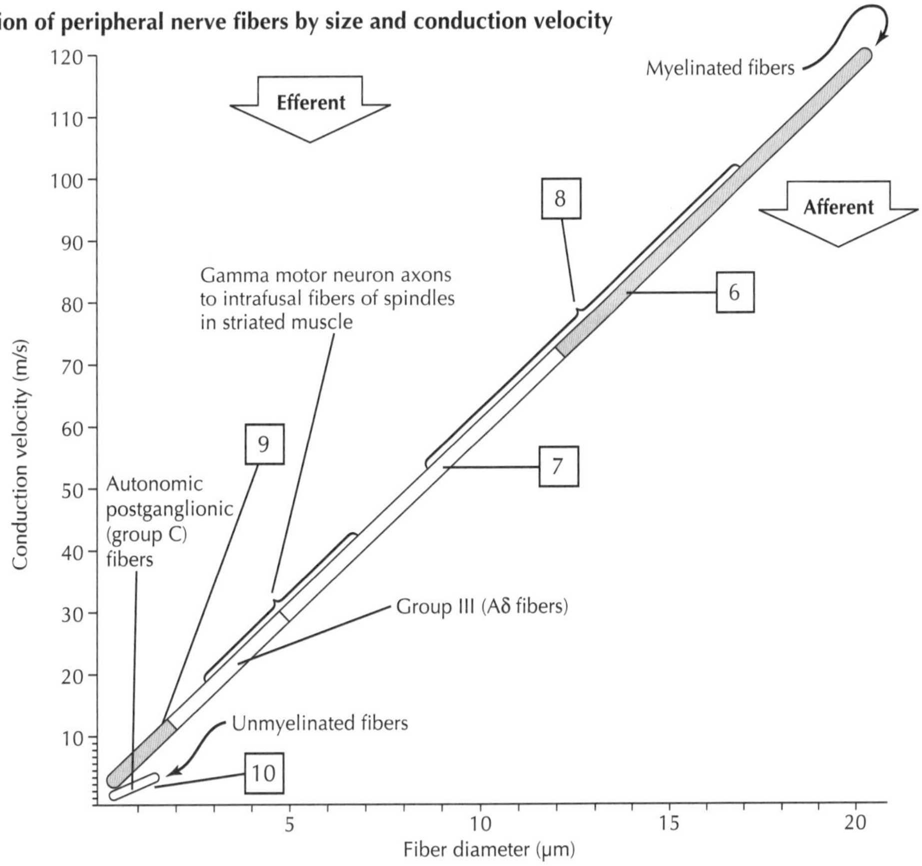

Neurotransmitter Release

Synapses are specialized sites where **nerve terminals** (and sometimes **dendrites** or the **cell body**) communicate with other neurons or target tissues. The nerve terminals are derived from both myelinated and unmyelinated **axons** and end on dendrites, the cell body, the **axon hillock**, or other nerve terminals. Synapses are protected and walled off by **astrocytic (glial) processes**. As an AP invades a nerve terminal, it causes the **influx of Ca^{2+},** which helps to mobilize the **synaptic vesicles** that contain one or more **neurotransmitters**. These vesicles fuse with the **presynaptic membrane** through the **SNARE complex** (docking proteins, membrane fusion, simultaneous vesicle release) and release their neurotransmitter "packet" (quantal content, quantal release) into the **synaptic cleft**. The neurotransmitter then acts on receptors of **ligand-gated ion channels** to affect **postsynaptic membrane** excitability or on **metabotropic postsynaptic receptors** to affect intracellular responses such as signal transduction cascades or genomic transcription factors. Synapses usually possess both presynaptic and postsynaptic neurotransmitter receptors; the **presynaptic autoreceptors** can influence subsequent neurotransmitter release or other activities in the presynaptic nerve terminal. Neurotransmitters are inactivated by presynaptic uptake through **high-affinity uptake carriers** (e.g., dopamine, norepinephrine, serotonin) by glial and presynaptic nonreceptor mechanisms (e.g., glutamate, GABA), by diffusion, or by enzymatic degradation (e.g., ACh, some peptides, catecholamines, serotonin). The high-affinity uptake carrier can reuptake both recently released neurotransmitter from the synaptic cleft and a nonsynaptic source of neurotransmitter (e.g., circulating norepinephrine and epinephrine), which can be subsequently released as a **"substitute" neurotransmitter**; this process allows circulating catecholamines to reinforce and augment sympathetic noradrenergic activation during a "fight-or-flight" response.

COLOR the following structures, using a separate color for each structure.

- ☐ 1. **Dendrite**
- ☐ 2. **Axon hillock**
- ☐ 3. **Glial (astrocyte) process**
- ☐ 4. **Synaptic vesicles**
- ☐ 5. **Synaptic cleft**
- ☐ 6. **Presynaptic membrane**
- ☐ 7. **Postsynaptic membrane**
- ☐ 8. **Ligand-gated Na^+ channel**
- ☐ 9. **SNARE complex**
- ☐ 10. **Metabotropic postsynaptic receptor**
- ☐ 11. **Presynaptic autoreceptor**
- ☐ 12. **High-affinity uptake carrier**

Clinical Point

The pattern of termination of axodendritic and axosomatic synapses on a target neuron will determine that neuron's responsiveness and activity to important sources of input. Thus an LMN responds to a combination of descending input from upper motor neurons, to incoming monosynaptic input from Ia muscle spindle primary afferents, to cascades of other local interneuronal inputs, and to recurrent connections from other adjacent LMNs. If one of these critical sources of input is damaged, such as some of the descending pathways (corticospinal, corticorubrospinal) with a stroke in the internal capsule or all of the upper motor neuronal descending connections in a spinal cord lesion, the LMNs will be devoid of this input, and the remaining nerve terminal sources will sprout to occupy the denuded sites on the dendrites and cell body. This will markedly change the responsiveness of the LMNs and will ultimately (after reorganization) make them hyperresponsive to muscle stretch reflexes (hyperreflexia), sensory stimuli (exaggerated withdrawal responses), and bowel and bladder responsiveness. This is the picture of spasticity seen following spinal cord injury.

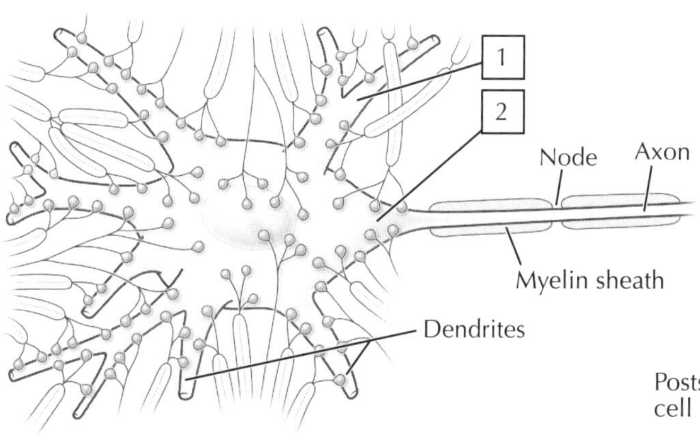

A. Numerous boutons (synaptic knobs) of presynaptic neurons terminating on a motor neuron and its dendrites

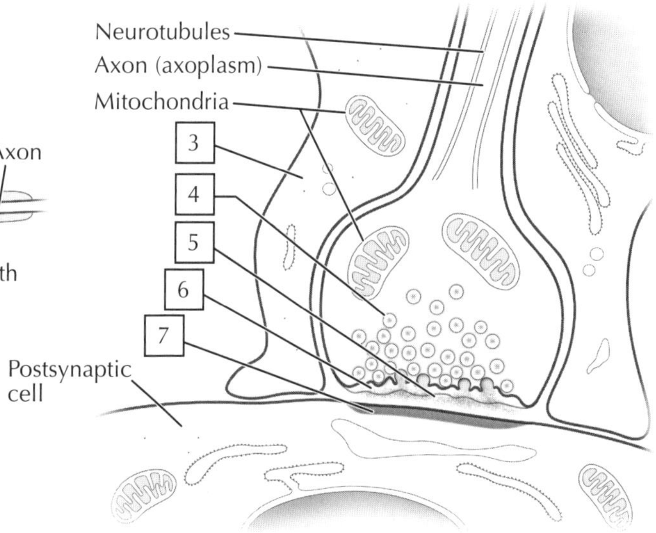

B. Morphology of a synapse in the CNS

C. Action potential

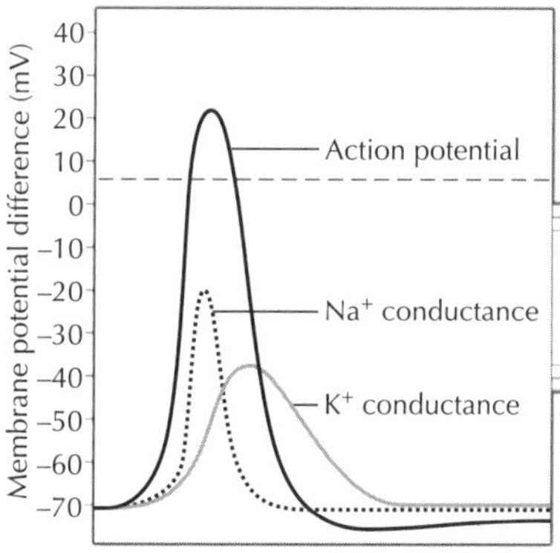

D. Ligand-gated channels

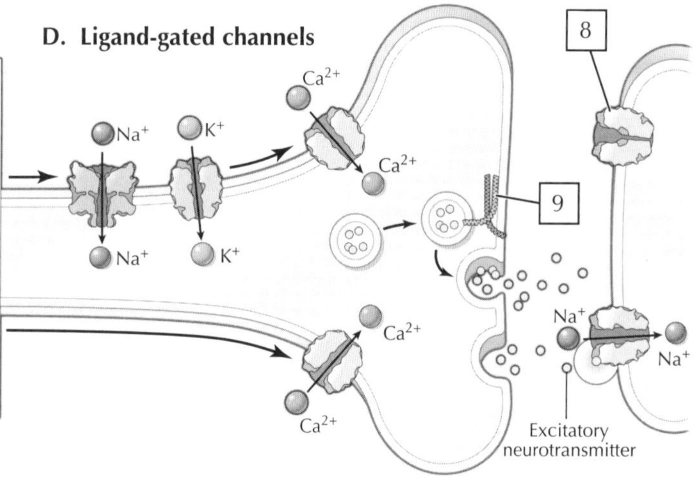

E. Metabotropic receptors

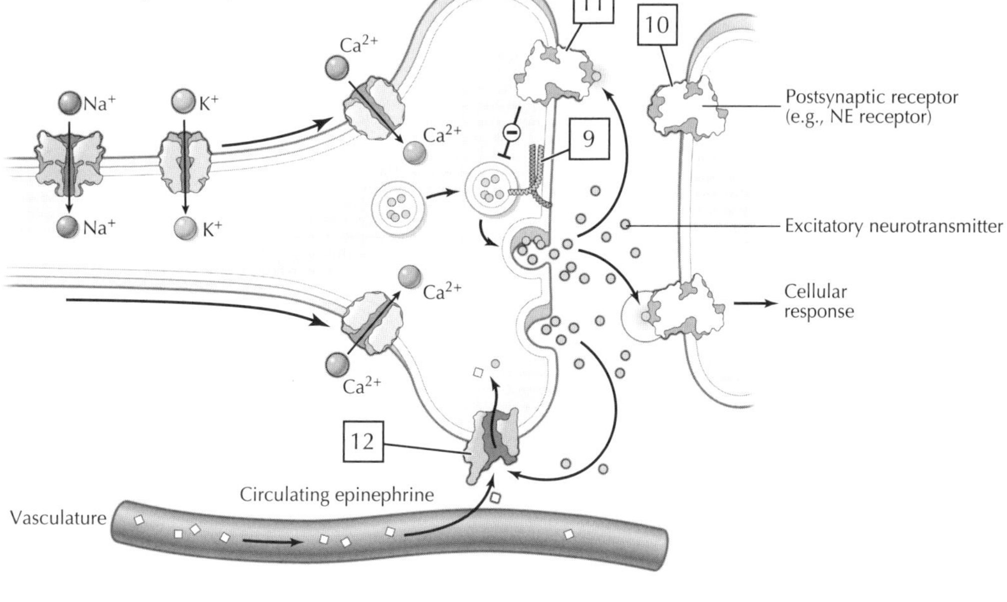

Multiple Neurotransmitter Synthesis, Release, and Signaling From Individual Neurons

Activation of neurotransmitter release is not necessarily linear with the frequency of APs invading the terminals; release is usually **nonlinear** and may also be accompanied by differential nonlinear release of **additional (multiple) neurotransmitters** in the nerve terminals (e.g., **norepinephrine** and **neuropeptide Y [NPY]**, **substance P**, and **calcitonin gene-related peptide [CGRP]**). Some neurons normally synthesize, store, and release several neurotransmitters, often in the same terminals (e.g., norepinephrine and NPY); however, some neurons, even in the same cell group, synthesize only norepinephrine or NPY, but not both. In some cases, the major branches synthesize and release one neurotransmitter (e.g., lower motor axons ending on skeletal muscle fibers at **neuromuscular junctions** releasing **acetylcholine)**, while another branch of that same axon (in the spinal cord) releases another neurotransmitter (**glutamate**). Signal molecules in the extracellular fluid near some nerve terminals (e.g., **cytokines** near noradrenergic nerve terminals innervating the parenchyma of secondary lymphoid organs) may be taken up by the nerve terminals, transported back to the cell body, act as, or induce, a **nuclear transcription factor**, and induce the synthesis of a new signal molecule (e.g., a cytokine such as **interleukin 1-β**), which can be subsequently transported anterogradely down the axon and released as a new "neurotransmitter" into the neural–immune zone of contact in the secondary lymphoid organ.

While the usual neurotransmitter model for both **ligand-gated** effects and **metabotropic** effects shows neurotransmitter release from nerve terminals and the presence of responsive receptors on the immediate postsynaptic site, this is sometimes not the case. The nearest responsive receptors may be long distances away, creating a significant **neurotransmitter–receptor mismatch** in localization. Thus predictions about the effects of neurotransmitter release and subsequent neuronal responses are both nonlinear and highly complex.

COLOR the following structures, using a separate color for each structure.

- ☐ **1. Nerve terminal using both norepinephrine and NPY**
- ☐ **2. Acetylcholine in terminals of a motor axon**
- ☐ **3. Glutamate in terminals of a motor axon**
- ☐ **4. Neuromuscular junction**
- ☐ **5. Nerve terminal showing diminished neurotransmitter release with increased action potential frequency**
- ☐ **6. Example of receptor demonstrating neurotransmitter–receptor mismatch**

Clinical Note

The frequency of AP firing of incoming axons may determine the amount and percentage of specific neurotransmitters released and available to interact with the target from an afferent. Thus it is not possible to provide a simple answer to the question "What does input A do when it contacts its target B?" The effect of input A depends on which co-released neurotransmitter(s) are released and in what quantities; what other neurotransmitters are released in the same vicinity at the same time from other afferents; what inhibitory signals are arriving to counter possible excitatory inputs; what autocrine, paracrine, or endocrine signals also are present; and what the electrical and metabolic state of the target neuron is. As a result, some neuronal systems act as "permissive" or neuromodulatory systems (dopamine, norepinephrine, serotonin); their presence alters the responsiveness of the postsynaptic sites to other systems. This may well account for the many side effects of antidepressive medications that alter the presence, release, or inactivation of these monoaminergic neurotransmitters, especially given the incredibly widespread distribution of the axonal varicosities to virtually every major subdivision of the CNS.

Multiple Neurotransmitter Synthesis, Release, and Signaling From Individual Neurons

A. Colocalization and Release

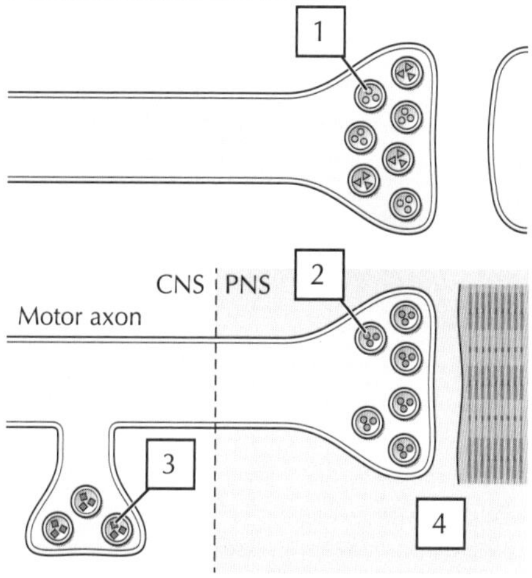

Neurotransmitter	Co-transmitters
DA	Glutamate, neurotensin, CCK or multiples + calbindin
NE (sympathetics)	Neuropeptide Y, somatostatin
NE (locus coeruleus)	Galanin
SP	CGRP (calcitonin gene-related peptide)
Serotonin (5-HT)	Glutamate, GABA
CRF	GABA
GHRH	DA, GABA
ACh	VIP
Met-enkephalin	Oxytocin (in magnocellular neurons of hypothalamus)

Fiber Type	Colocalized neurotransmitters
Motor axon	ACh at neuromuscular junction, glutamate in SC
Medial habenula	ACh, glutamate
Arcuate nucleus	DA, GABA, many others
Mossy fibers	GABA, glycine
Dorsal horn neurons	Met-enkephalin, GABA
Striatal neurons	Met-enkephalin, GABA

B. Nonlinearity of Release

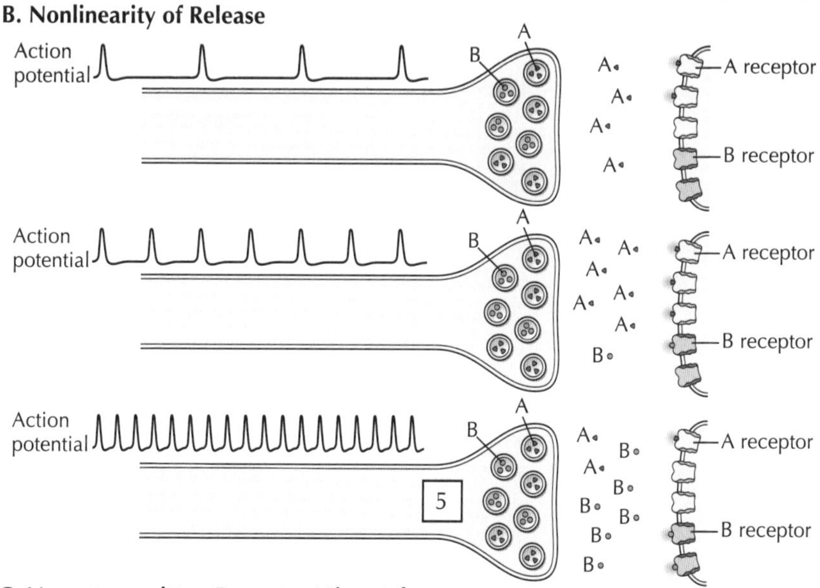

Diminishing release at high frequency due to:
1. Depletion of vesicles
2. Depletion of extracellular Ca^{2+}

C. Neurotransmitter–Receptor Mismatch

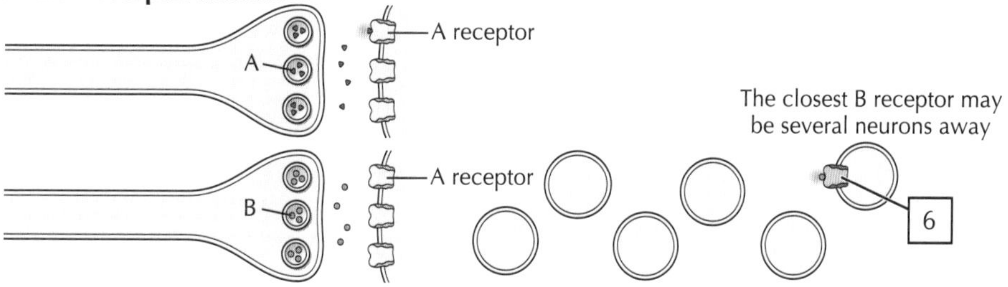

Chemical Neurotransmission

Neurotransmitters vary from very small molecules to very large molecules, from sites of synthesis and metabolic regulation, and from mechanisms of action and inactivation. Amino acid neurotransmitters (**glutamate** and **aspartate** as **excitatory**, **GABA** and **glycine** as inhibitory) are present in the cytoplasm in nerve endings and are taken up into synaptic **vesicles**. APs invading the nerve terminals evoke the release of the amino acid neurotransmitter (e.g., glutamate), which then acts on postsynaptic receptors (e.g., N-methyl-D-aspartate [NMDA], or α-amino-3-hydroxy-5-methyl-4-isoxazolepropionic acid [AMPA] receptors) to achieve a postsynaptic response.

Norepinephrine is synthesized in the nerve terminal by the action of **tyrosine hydroxylase**, the rate-limiting enzyme synthesized in the cell body, on the precursor **tyrosine** (obtained from the diet). The resultant L-dopa is converted to dopamine (by aromatic l-amino acid decarboxylase), the end-product in some terminals, or is further converted to norepinephrine by **dopamine-beta-hydroxylase**. The catecholamines are inactivated mainly by reuptake into the releasing terminal through the actions of a **high-affinity uptake carrier**.

Similarly, **serotonin** is synthesized in the nerve terminal by the action of **tryptophan hydroxylase (TrH),** the rate-limiting synthetic enzyme synthesized in the cell body, on the precursor tryptophan (obtained from the diet). The resultant 5-hydroxytryptophan is converted to 5-hydroxytryptamine (serotonin) by aromatic l-amino acid decarboxylase. Serotonin is inactivated mainly by reuptake into the releasing terminal through the actions of a high-affinity uptake carrier.

Peptide neurotransmitters are synthesized in the cell body through the actions of the rough endoplasmic reticulum sometimes posttranslatronally modified, packaged into vesicles, and transported anterogradely down the axon to the nerve terminals. Neuropeptides may diffuse after release from a peptidergic synapse and act on **neuropeptide receptors**. Peptide neurotransmitters are mainly inactivated by **peptidases**.

Cholinergic neurotransmission occurs through the actions of **choline acetyltransferase** on acetyl-CoA and choline in the nerve terminal. The resultant ACh is packaged in synaptic vesicles and is released upon APs invading the nerve terminals, acting on **cholinergic receptors** on target neurons or effector tissues. The ACh is rapidly inactivated (hydrolyzed) by **acetylcholinesterase (AChE)**, and both choline and acetyl CoA are recycled back into the nerve terminal for reuse.

COLOR the following structures, using a separate color for each structure.

- ☐ 1. **Amino acid synapse (terminal)**
- ☐ 2. **Glutamate**
- ☐ 3. **Catecholamine synapse (terminal)**
- ☐ 4. **Tyrosine hydroxylase**
- ☐ 5. **High-affinity uptake carrier for norepinephrine**
- ☐ 6. **Serotonin synapse (terminal)**
- ☐ 7. **Tryptophan hydroxylase**
- ☐ 8. **High-affinity uptake carrier for serotonin**
- ☐ 9. **Peptide synapse (terminal)**
- ☐ 10. **Peptidases**
- ☐ 11. **Acetylcholine synapse (terminal)**
- ☐ 12. **Choline**
- ☐ 13. **Choline acetyltransferase**
- ☐ 14. **Acetylcholinesterase**

Clinical Note

The release and subsequent postsynaptic actions of neurotransmitters are essential to successful physiological functioning of neuronal systems. Equally important is the **inactivation** of neurotransmitters after release into the synaptic cleft to prevent their possible prolonged and persistent toxic effect. ACh released at the NMJ is essential for muscle contraction following APs from LMNs. Enough ACh is usually released to bring the innervated muscle fibers to their threshold, guaranteeing a muscle contraction. AChE is essential for hydrolyzing ACh to choline and Coenzyme A. If AChE is blocked (e.g., by organophosphate or carbamate insecticides), ACh will persist at the NMJ and at autonomic cholinergic synapses. As a result, the patient will experience salivation, tearing, urination, diarrhea, and a wide range of autonomic activational effects. At the NMJ the patient will experience muscle twitching, fasciculations, weakness, respiratory depression, coma, and ultimately death (depending on the dosage of the AChE inhibitor agent). There are some agents, such as pralidoxime, that can reactivate AChE and permit some reversal of the effects of the AChE inhibition.

Glutamate also can persist at central synapses where it is released. In the hippocampus, high exposure to glucocorticoids can result in excess glutamate release, which may induce neuronal apoptosis, especially in sector CA3 of the hippocampus.

Selective serotonin reuptake inhibitors (SSRIs) prolong the activity of serotonin in the synaptic cleft. They are a mainstay for treatment of mood disorders.

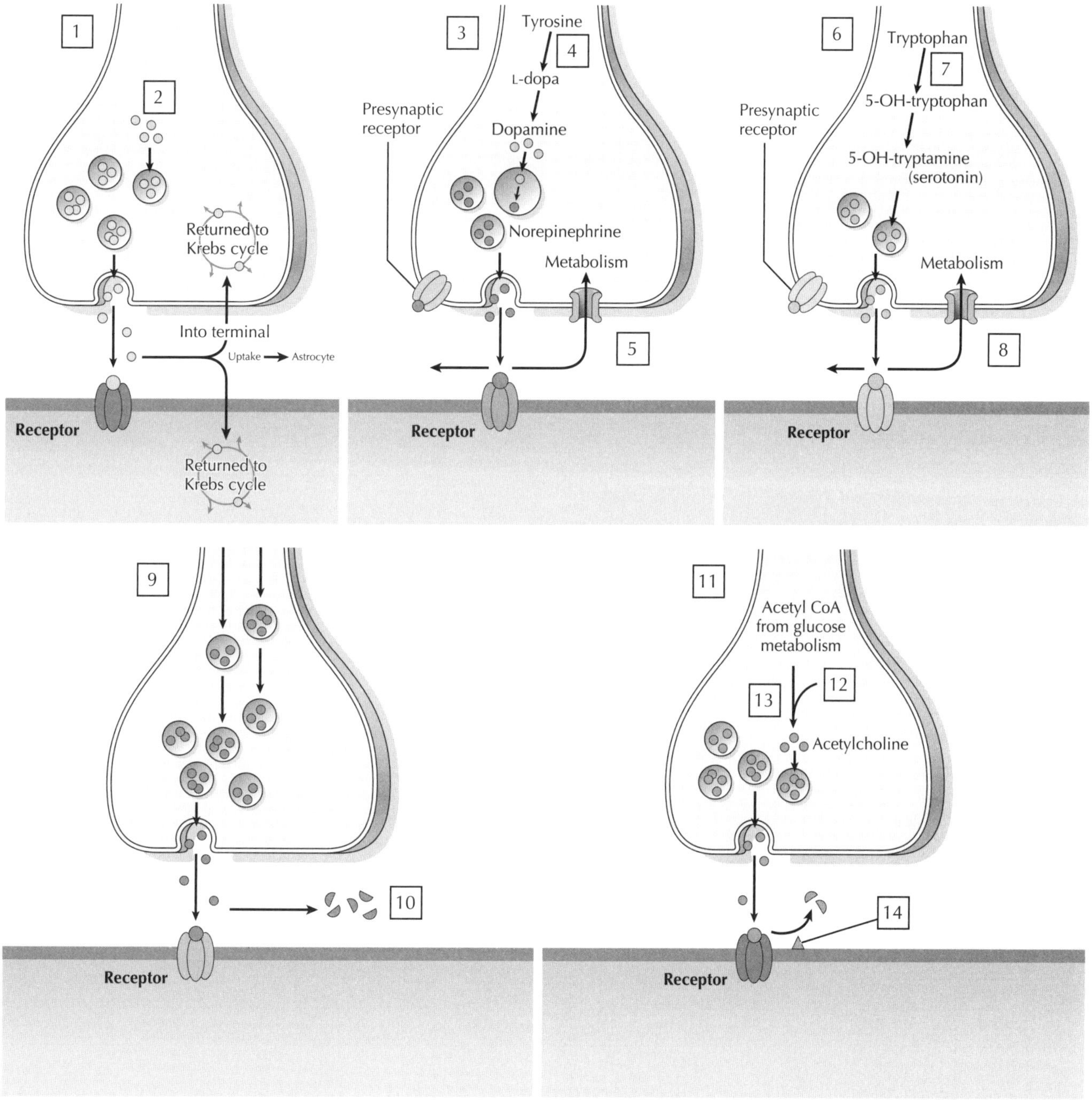
1
2
Returned to Krebs cycle
Into terminal
Uptake → Astrocyte
Receptor
Returned to Krebs cycle
3
Tyrosine
4
L-dopa
Presynaptic receptor
Dopamine
Norepinephrine
Metabolism
5
Receptor
6
Tryptophan
7
5-OH-tryptophan
Presynaptic receptor
5-OH-tryptamine (serotonin)
Metabolism
8
Receptor
9
10
Receptor
11
Acetyl CoA from glucose metabolism
12
13
Acetylcholine
14
Receptor

Chapter 2 Brain, Skull, and Meninges

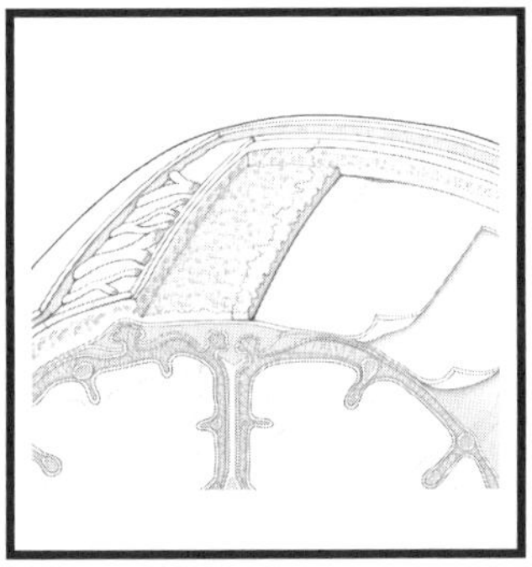
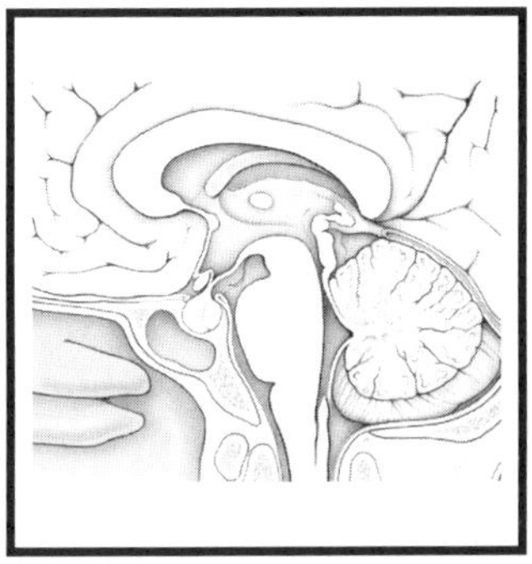
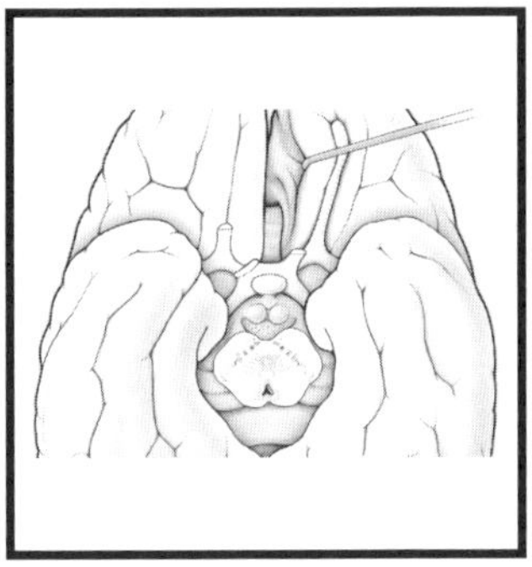
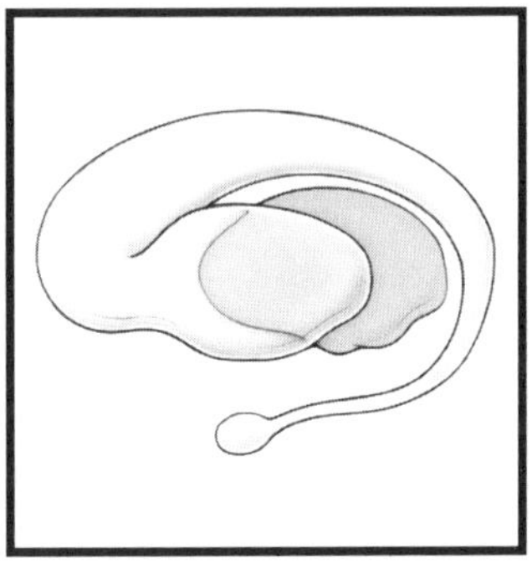

2 Meninges and Their Relationship to the Brain and Skull

The **meninges** protect and support the underlying neural tissue in the central nervous system (CNS). The **pia mater** adheres to every contour of the CNS, following the infoldings (sulci, folia). Astrocytic glial end feet intertwine with the pial cells of this membrane, forming the **pial–glial membrane**. The **arachnoid** is a delicate membrane external to the pia; it bridges across the sulci and folia. The space between the arachnoid and pial membranes is the **subarachnoid space**, in which the cerebrospinal fluid (CSF) is found. The CSF provides buoyancy and cushioning of the brain, protecting it from damage due to acceleratory and deceleratory movements. The **dura mater** is a tough, fibrous protective outer membrane, usually adherent to the arachnoid membrane inwardly and to the inner table of the **skull (calvaria)** outwardly. The dura splits into an **inner and outer layer** in some sites, forming dural sinuses, in which the returning venous blood flows on its way into the internal jugular system. The inner layers of the dura travel together into the midline between the cerebral hemispheres, forming the tough protective membrane, the **falx cerebri**. **Arachnoid granulations** protrude from the subarachnoid space into the venous sinuses, especially in the **superior sagittal sinus**, allowing the CSF to drain into the venous blood and return to the heart.

The cerebral veins travel in the subarachnoid space and drain venous blood from the brain into the dural sinuses. The **cerebral arteries** also travel in the subarachnoid space; a ruptured cerebral aneurysm can bleed into the subarachnoid space.

COLOR the three meninges using a different color for each.

☐ 1. **Dura mater**
- 1A. Falx cerebri
- 1B. Inner layer of the dura
- 1C. Outer layer of the dura
- 1D. Fused layers of the dura

☐ 2. **Arachnoid mater**

☐ 3. **Pia mater (pial–glial membrane)**

COLOR the protrusions that extend from the subarachnoid space into the dural sinuses, especially the superior sagittal sinus.

☐ 4. **Arachnoid granulations**

COLOR one of the major dural venous sinuses.

☐ 5. **Superior sagittal sinus**

COLOR the important:

☐ 6. **Subarachnoid space**

☐ 7. **Middle meningeal artery**

☐ 8. **Superior cerebral vein**

Clinical Note

The **cerebral arteries** are found traversing through the subarachnoid space. The rupture of a **cerebral aneurysm**, most often occurring at a site in or near the circle of Willis, results in **a subarachnoid hemorrhage**, causing an excruciating headache and sometimes, a loss of consciousness, or death. Bridging veins also traverse the subarachnoid space, including the large superior cerebral veins. If these bridging veins are torn, either by severe trauma in a young individual or by milder trauma in someone elderly (due to brain atrophy), the bridging veins can bleed into the subdural space, dissecting it free from the underlying arachnoid membrane because of the presence of blood. The resultant **subdural hematoma** can be acute (severe trauma) or more gradual (chronic). The subdural hematoma acts as a space-occupying lesion, can increase the intracranial pressure (ICP), can produce **cerebral edema**, and can produce brain herniation across the free edge of the tentorium cerebelli. The arachnoid granulations provide one-way valves for the drainage of CSF into the venous circulation. If these arachnoid granulations become blocked (e.g., acute purulent meningitis), the CSF pressure backs up, resulting in increased ICP. This increased ICP can result in pressure on the brain, brain herniation, and death. A **skull fracture** can tear associated vessels adherent to the skull, such as the **middle meningeal artery**. The arterial blood from a middle meningeal tear can dissect the outer dural membrane away from the inner table of the skull, producing an **epidural hematoma**, which acts as a space-occupying mass and a potential cause of brain herniation.

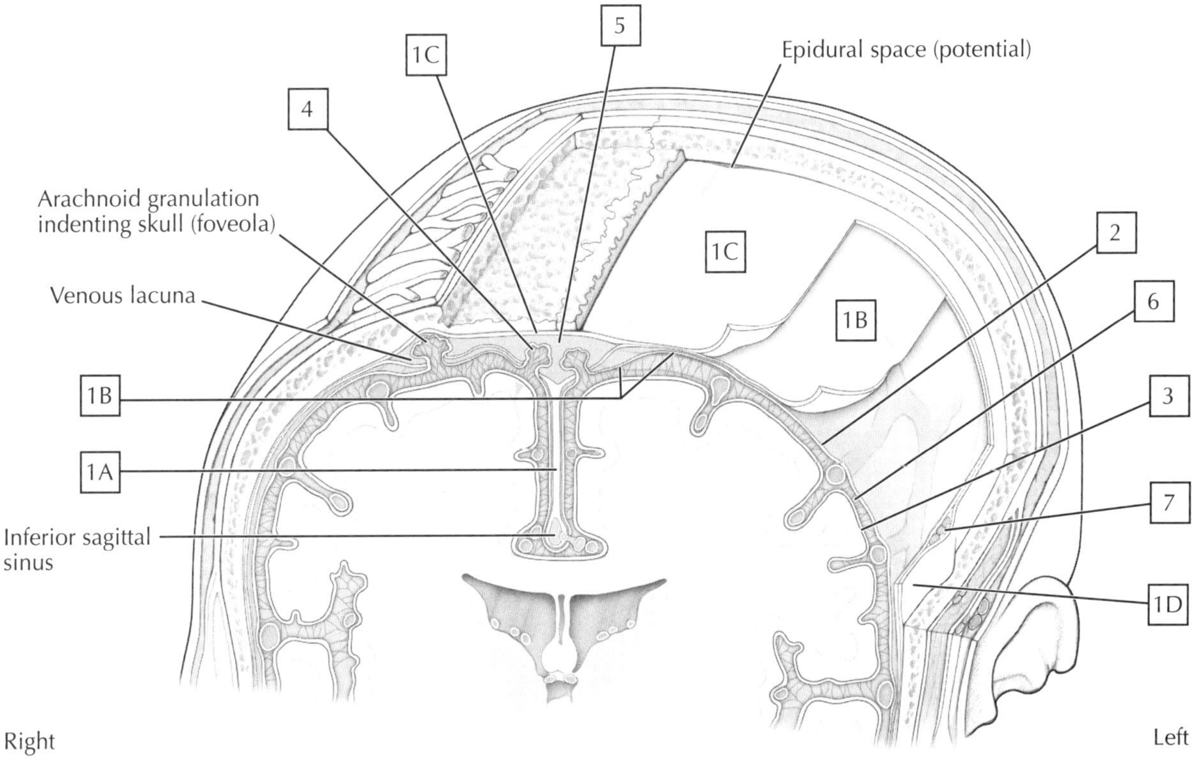

A. Scalp, skull, meningeal, and cerebral blood vessels

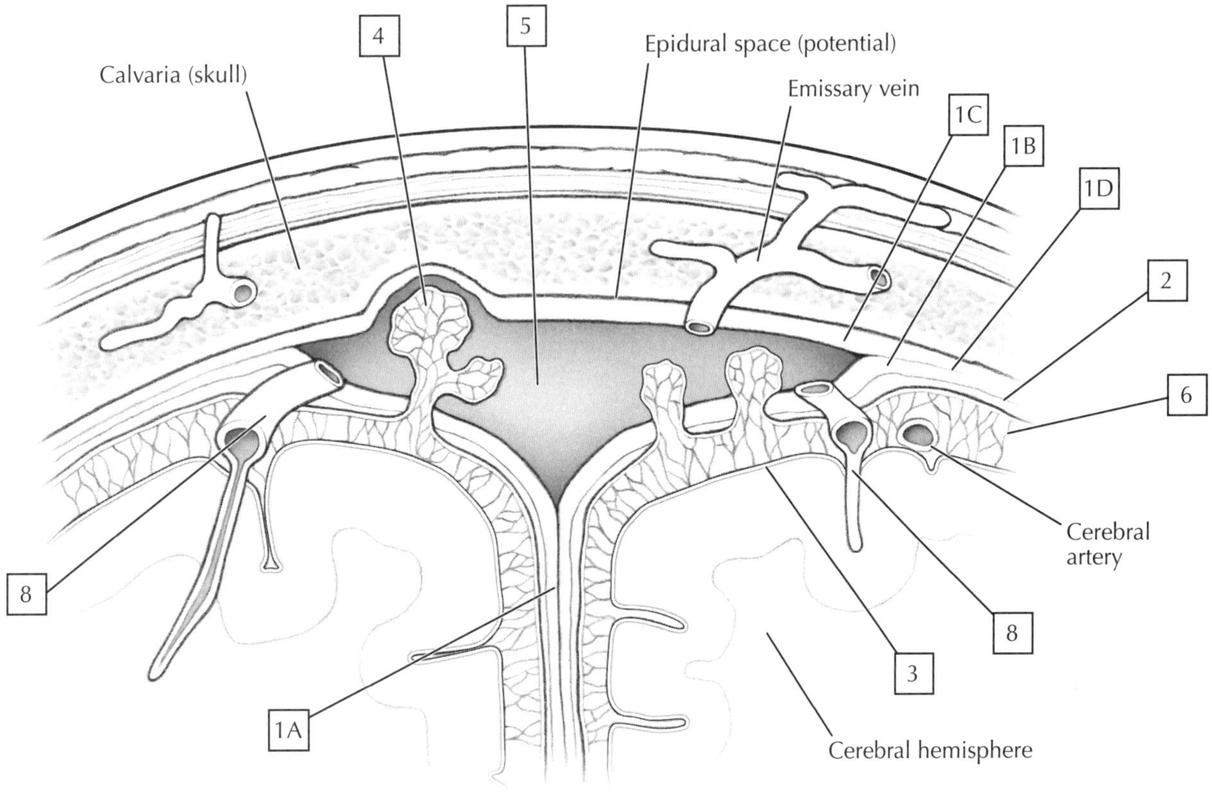

B. Meninges and superficial cerebral veins

2 Surface Anatomy of the Forebrain: Lateral View

The cerebral cortex is convoluted and folded into **sulci** (valleys) and **gyri** (hills). This arrangement permits the folding of large amounts of cerebral cortex into a small volume. Major sulci and gyri serve as important landmarks. The cortex of the brain is subdivided into four lobes: frontal, parietal, temporal, and occipital. The **lateral fissure** (sylvian fissure) separates the temporal lobe below from the frontal and parietal lobes above. The **central sulcus** separates the **frontal lobe** in front from the **parietal lobe** behind. The parietooccipital sulcus on the median surface separates the parietal lobe in front from the occipital lobe behind.

Several of the named gyri subserve specific functions. The **precentral gyrus** serves as the **primary motor cortex**. The **postcentral gyrus** serves as the **primary sensory cortex**. The **transverse gyrus of Heschl** on the upper portion of the superior temporal gyrus serves as the **primary auditory cortex**. The upper and lower **banks of the calcarine fissure** in the occipital lobe serve as the **primary visual cortex**.

On the left hemisphere, **Broca's area** on the inner portion of the **inferior frontal gyrus** serves as the center for expressive language function, and **Wernicke's area (supramarginal and angular gyri)** serves as the center for receptive language function. Some gyri, such as the **superior, middle, and inferior frontal and temporal gyri**, serve as anatomical landmarks rather than areas subserving specific functional modalities. The **superior parietal lobule** subserves spatial orientation and perception of body image. Some complex functions, such as long-term memory storage, involve many regions of cerebral cortex in multiple regions of the brain and cannot be specifically localized to one zone. Some deep regions of cortex, such as the **insular cortex**, subserve multiple visceral functions.

COLOR each region with a specific color.

- ☐ 1. **Lateral fissure**
- ☐ 2. **Inferior frontal gyrus**
- ☐ 3. **Precentral gyrus**
- ☐ 4. **Central sulcus**
- ☐ 5. **Postcentral gyrus**
- ☐ 6. **Supramarginal gyrus**
- ☐ 7. **Superior parietal lobule**
- ☐ 8. **Angular gyrus**
- ☐ 9. **Superior temporal gyrus**
- ☐ 10. **Insular cortex**
- ☐ 11. **Color each major lobe in Part B**

Clinical Note

Because of the localization of some specific brain functions to specific regions of the cerebral cortex, damage to that region of cortex, by trauma, mass lesions, or vascular insult, can result in the loss of the specific function. Damage to the precentral gyrus and the adjacent premotor cortex (e.g., middle cerebral artery infarct) on the lateral hemisphere can result in **contralateral spastic paresis** of the upper extremity and drooping of the contralateral lower face. Damage to the postcentral gyrus on the lateral hemisphere can result in loss of sensation in the contralateral upper body. Damage to the medial zone of the precentral gyrus and postcentral gyrus (the paracentral lobule) from an anterior cerebral artery infarct can result in contralateral spastic paresis and loss of sensation in the lower extremity. Damage to the upper and lower banks of the **calcarine fissure** (posterior cerebral artery infarct) can result in contralateral loss of vision **(contralateral hemianopia)**. Specific damage to some vision-related regions of the temporal lobe can result in **agnosia** (loss of knowing) for the recognition of faces, or the ability to identify animate versus inanimate objects.

Surface Anatomy of the Forebrain: Lateral View

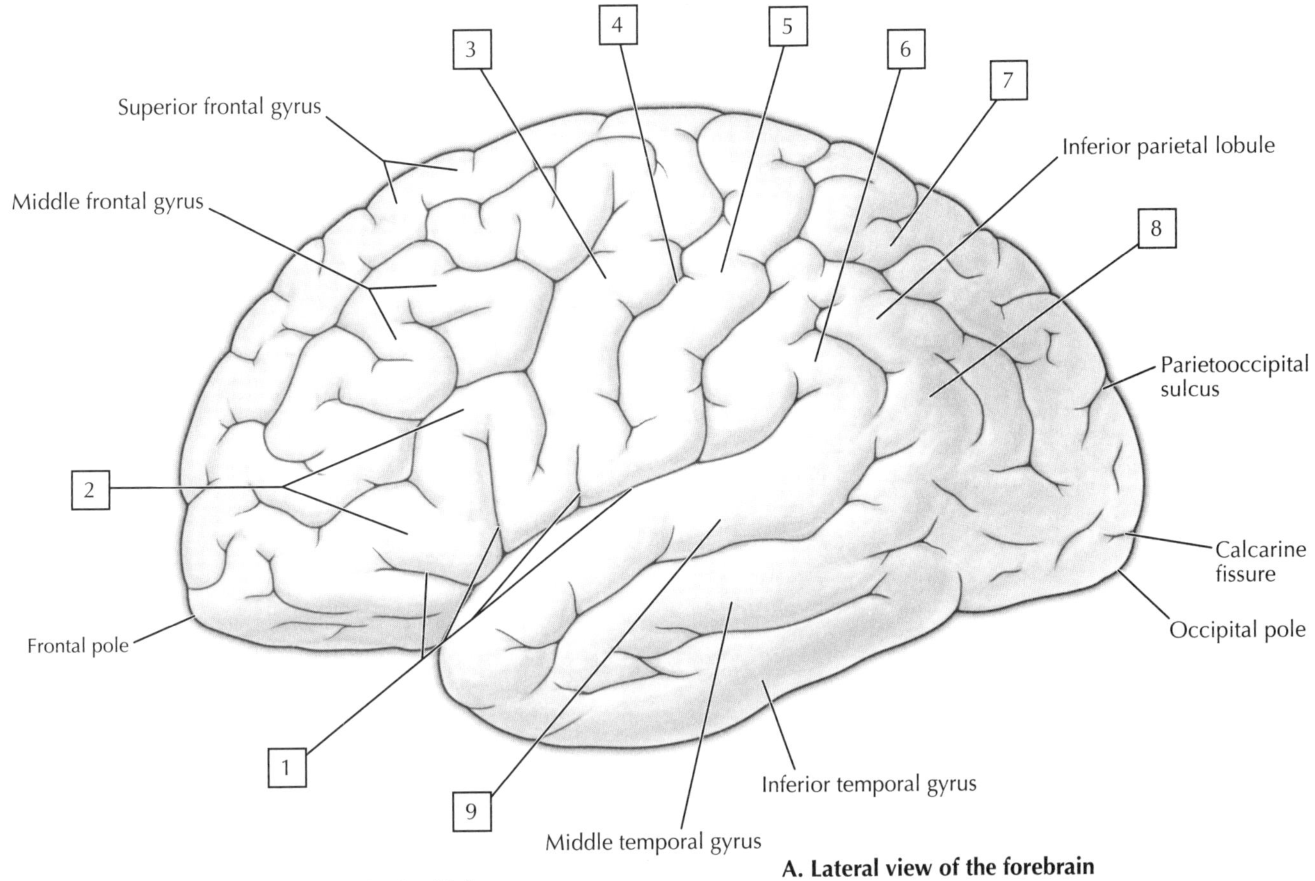

A. Lateral view of the forebrain

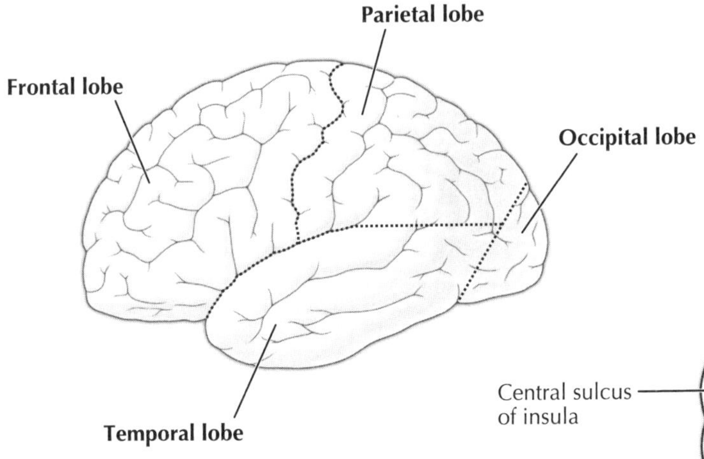

B. Major lobes of the cortex (lateral view)

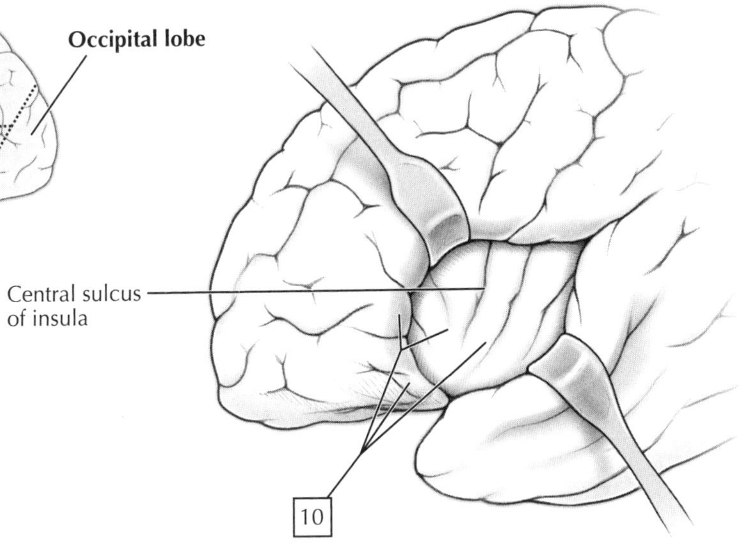

C. Insular cortex (lateral view)

2 Cerebral Cortex Anatomy and Functional Regions: Lateral View

The **cerebral cortex** (neocortex) consists of six horizontal layers of neurons, including pyramidal cells, granule cells, and other mixed populations of neurons. Some regions of the cerebral cortex are associated with specific functions, sometimes topographically organized through **"vertical columns"** of neurons that process specific information from specific regions of the body.

The well-organized regions of cerebral cortex are sometimes described as **"primary cortex"** (somatosensory cortex, trigeminal sensory cortex, visual cortex, auditory cortex, motor cortex) or **"secondary cortex"** (sensory modalities). For the primary somatosensory cortex and primary motor cortex, the lower extremity is represented medially, the body and upper extremity more laterally, and the head region far laterally, near the lateral fissure. Other regions of cortex are organized less specifically, especially integrative regions that receive multimodal inputs from a wide range of CNS regions.

CORTICAL REGION	FUNCTIONAL ROLE
Broca's area	Responsible for initiating expressive language
Lateral primary somatosensory cortex	Receives information related to touch from the upper contralateral extremity via the ventral posterolateral nucleus of the thalamus
Lateral primary motor cortex	Region from which movement of the contralateral hand and finger muscles occurs
Supplemental motor cortex	Becomes active when movement is anticipated but has not yet been initiated
Primary visual cortex	Receives visual information from the contralateral visual field
Frontal eye fields	Initiates contralateral conjugate movement of the eyes
Parietal cortex	Subserves analysis of movement and positional relationships of viewed objects
Superior parietal lobule	Provides integrated awareness of body regions and position
Primary auditory cortex	Receives bilateral auditory information
Middle temporal gyrus	Provides visual object recognition and form
Wernicke's area	Responsible for understanding of spoken language

COLOR the following functional regions, using a different color for each region.

- ☐ 1. **Broca's area**
- ☐ 2. **Frontal eye fields**
- ☐ 3. **Premotor and supplemental motor cortex**
- ☐ 4. **Lateral primary motor cortex**
- ☐ 5. **Lateral primary somatosensory cortex**
- ☐ 6. **Primary auditory cortex**
- ☐ 7. **Middle temporal gyrus**
- ☐ 8. **Wernicke's area**
- ☐ 9. **Superior parietal lobule**
- ☐ 10. **Primary visual cortex**

Clinical Note

Regions of cerebral cortex may be damaged by vascular lesions (hemorrhages, infarcts), by mass lesions that impinge on a specific cortical area, or by degenerative processes. **Ischemia** (lack of blood flow) or **anoxia** (lack of oxygen) may lead to more global dysfunction with serious cognitive consequences, including **coma**. Consciousness requires a functioning brainstem reticular activating system and at least one functioning hemisphere. The topographical organization of some primary cortical regions (e.g., somatosensory cortex and primary motor cortex) is important in the interpretation of neurological findings. A stroke in either the middle cerebral artery or the anterior cerebral artery on one side may lead to sensory and/or motor deficits in a specific region of the body on the contralateral side. Cortical damage in the dominant hemisphere (usually the left hemisphere in right-handed individuals and most left-handed individuals) may lead to **expressive aphasia** (Broca's area), **receptive aphasia** (Wernicke's area), or **global aphasia** (cortical zone supplied by the middle cerebral artery). The cerebral cortex on one side or both sides may be rendered dysfunctional by increased ICP.

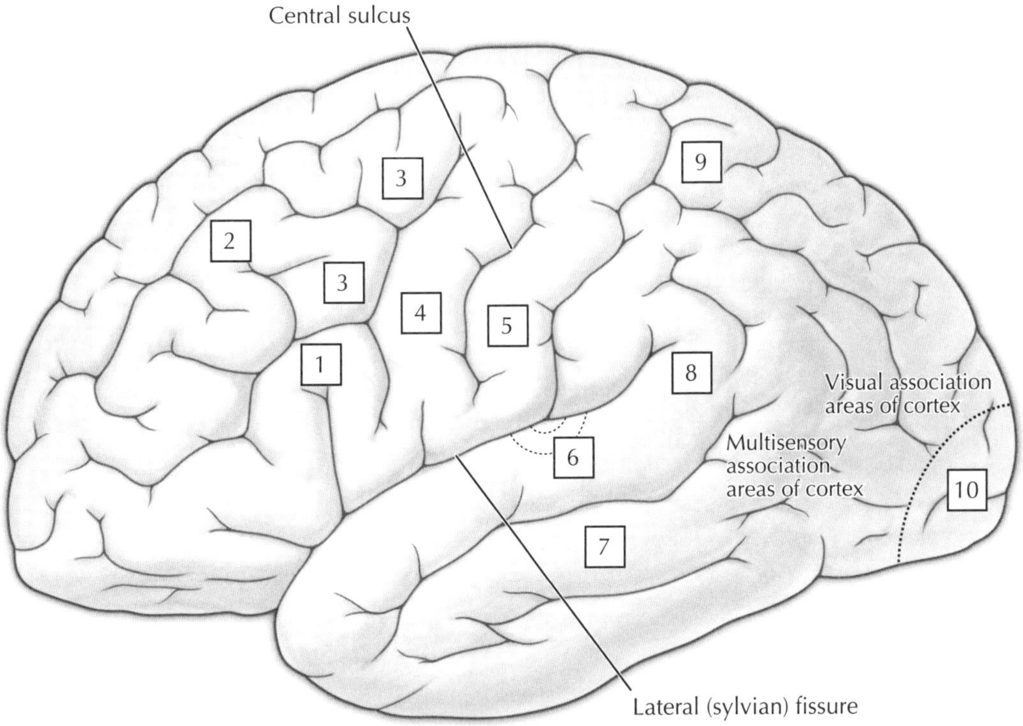

A. Lateral view of forebrain

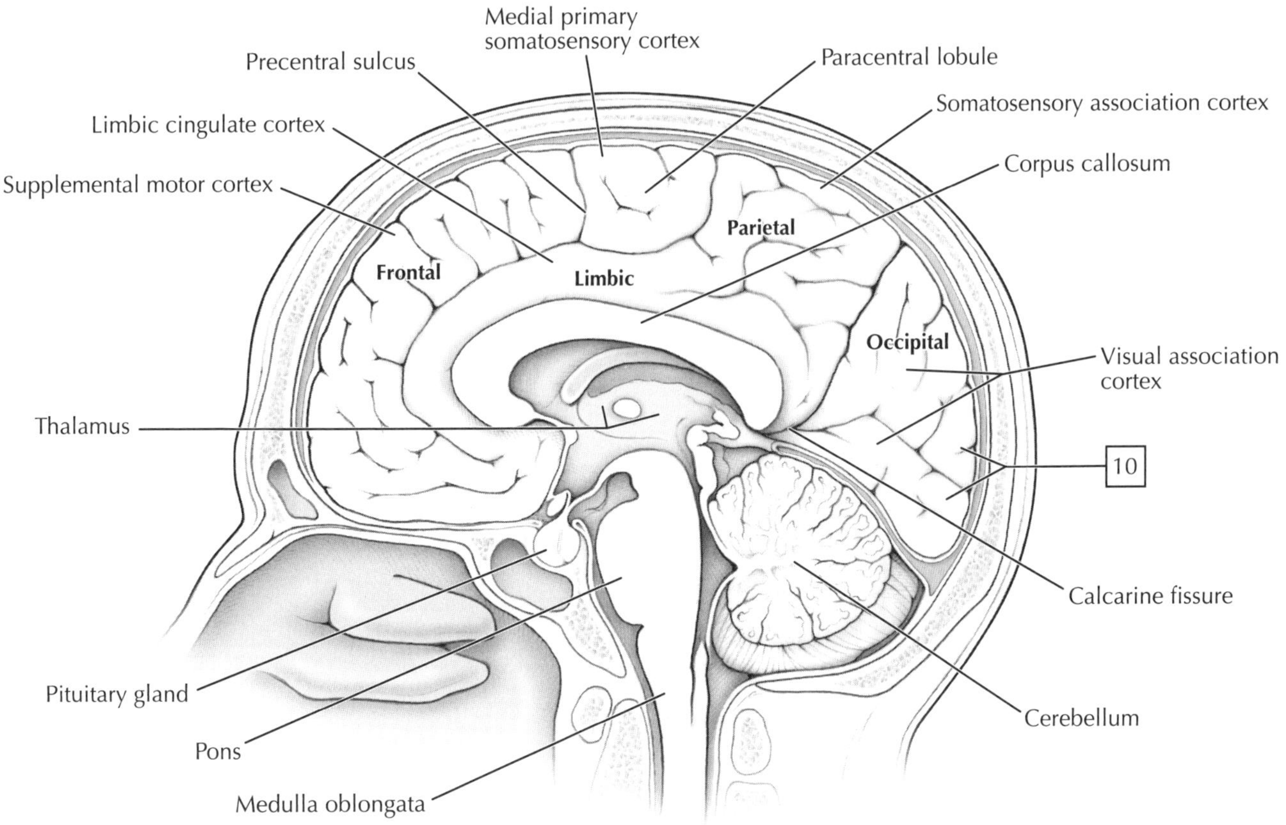

B. Medial (midsagittal) surface of the brain *in situ*

Cortical Architecture: Brodmann Areas

With the advent of neurohistological staining using dyes, early neuroanatomical pioneers such as Golgi and Cajal demonstrated a wide variety of neuronal shapes, sizes, branching patterns, and connectivity. The cerebral cortex, called **neocortex**, contains **six layers of neurons**, arranged horizontally, which vary in both thickness and layering; the **granule cell** layers (layers IV and II), composed of small neurons that receive extensive input, are abundant in somatosensory cortex, whereas **pyramidal cells** (layers V and III), which send axons to other regions of cortex on the same side **(association fibers)**, the opposite side **(callosal fibers)**, and subcortical areas **(projection fibers)**, are abundant in motor cortex. Because of the complexity of the neocortex, several neuroanatomists proposed descriptions of **different types of cortex**, varying from 40 to over 200 separate types of cortex. The system of nomenclature that endures is that proposed by Korbinian Brodmann in 1909, with which he provided numbers for different functional regions and types of cortex. These **Brodmann areas** are used widely in neurosciences to refer to functional zones of cortex.

BRODMANN AREAS	FUNCTIONAL ROLE OF CORTEX	ANATOMICAL SITE
Areas 3, 1, 2	Primary somatosensory cortex	Postcentral gyrus
Area 40 (vent)	Secondary somatosensory cortex	Ventral anterior lower parietal lobe
Areas 5, 7	Body perception, spatial orientation	Superior parietal lobule
Area 4	Primary motor cortex	Precentral gyrus
Area 6	Premotor, supplemental motor cortex	Middle frontal gyrus—upper part
Area 8	Frontal eye fields	Middle frontal gyrus—anterior upper
Areas 44, 45	Broca's area (left hemisphere)	Lateral inferior frontal gyrus
Area 40, 39	Wernicke's area (left hemisphere)	Anterior lower parietal lobe
Area 11	Orbitofrontal cortex	Base of lateral frontal lobe
Areas 41, 42	Primary auditory cortex	Transverse gyrus of Heschl (superior temporal gyrus)
Area 17	Primary visual cortex	Banks of the calcarine fissure (sulcus)
Areas 18, 19	Association visual cortex	Occipital cortex external to area 17
Areas 21, 22, 37	Polymodal sensory association cortex	Middle and superior temporal lobe

COLOR each region with a separate color and note the depiction of functional regions with Brodmann areas.

- ☐ 1. **Area 11**
- ☐ 2. **Area 8**
- ☐ 3. **Areas 44, 45**
- ☐ 4. **Area 6 (contributes to corticospinal tract, along with motor cortex)**
- ☐ 5. **Area 4**
- ☐ 6. **Areas 3, 1, 2**
- ☐ 7. **Areas 5, 7**
- ☐ 8. **Areas 40, 39**
- ☐ 9. **Area 40**
- ☐ 10. **Areas 41, 42**
- ☐ 11. **Areas 18, 19**
- ☐ 12. **Area 17**

Clinical Note

Damage to specific zones of cortex, denoted by Brodmann areas (numbers), results in specific clinical symptoms and findings. Damage to the primary somatosensory cortex results in contralateral loss of sensation on the body and upper extremity, and lower extremity if the damage involves the medial and midline zone. Damage to the primary motor and premotor/supplemental motor cortices results in **contralateral spastic hemiplegia** affecting the upper limb (lateral), the lower limb (medial and midline cortex), or the whole body (if internal capsule is included in the damage). Damage to Broca's area on the left (in all right-handed individuals and most left-handed individuals) results in **expressive aphasia**, whereas damage to Wernicke's area on the left results in **receptive aphasia**. Damage to the occipital zone on the banks of the calcarine fissure results in **contralateral blindness (hemianopia)**. Damage to the primary auditory cortex results in some diminished hearing (both sides, not just contralateral), with neglect on the contralateral side to simultaneously presented auditory stimuli. Damage to the frontal eye fields results in the inability to direct the eyes to the side opposite the lesion.

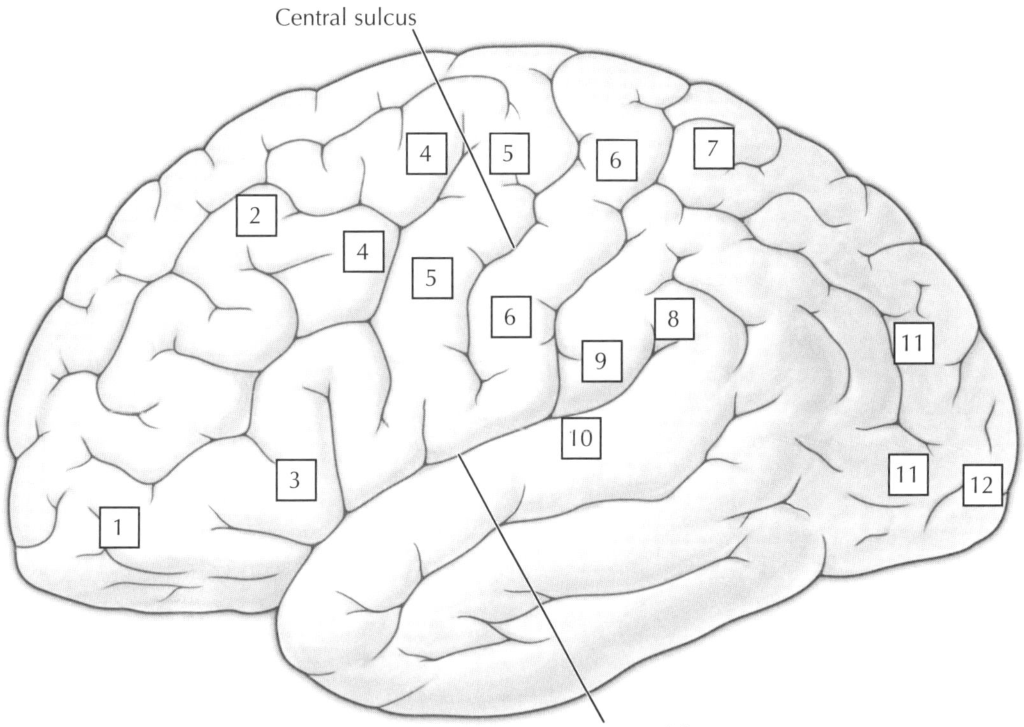

A. Lateral view of forebrain

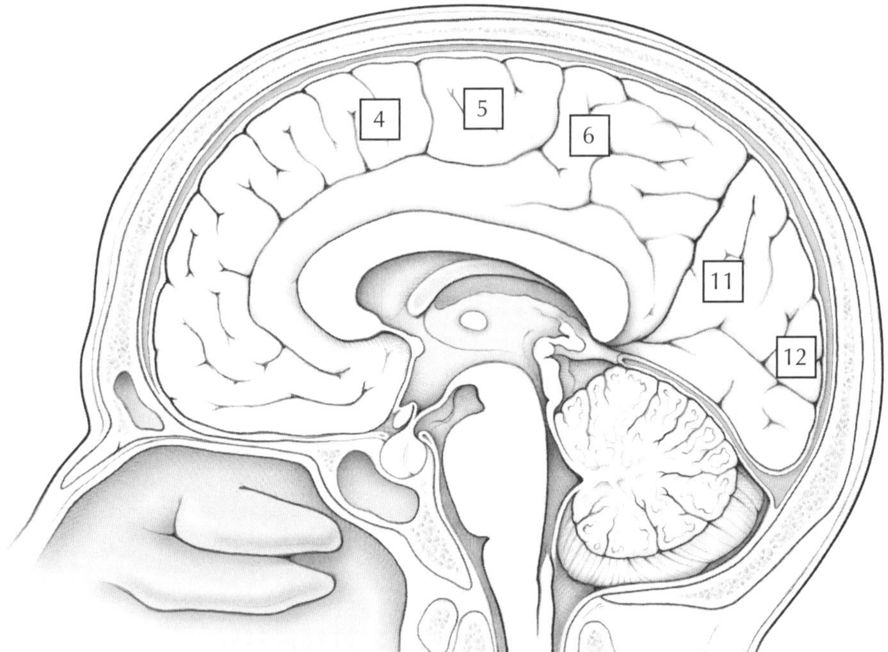

B. Medial (midsagittal) surface of the brain in situ

2 Midsagittal Surface of the Brain

The **midsagittal** view (lateral view along the midline) of the brain provides the layout of the entire **neuraxis,** including the **spinal cord**, **brainstem (medulla, pons, midbrain)**, **diencephalon**, and parts of the **telencephalon**. The spinal cord receives **sensory** input from the body and gives rise to **motor** and **autonomic** outflow to the body.

The brainstem receives sensory input from the head and neck, provides motor outflow to muscles of the head and neck, and provides parasympathetic preganglionic outflow for control of the thoracic and some abdominal viscera, salivary glands, lacrimal glands, the pupillary constrictor muscle, and the ciliary muscle for accommodation for near vision. These parasympathetic functions are accomplished through cranial nerves III, VII, IX, and X. The brainstem reticular formation is essential for consciousness and helps to alert the cortex. The **cerebellum** helps in regulating coordination and balance for motor regulation through the upper motor neurons of the brainstem and the cerebral cortex (through the thalamus).

The diencephalon consists of two major components, the **thalamus** and **hypothalamus**. The thalamus serves as the gateway to the cerebral cortex and helps to regulate input to the cortex (sensory, motor, and other types of cortex) and outflow from the cortex. The hypothalamus regulates visceral/autonomic functions of the body (through the brainstem and spinal cord), and neuroendocrine outflow (through both the **anterior and posterior pituitary glands**).

The telencephalon consists of the **basal ganglia**, **limbic forebrain**, **olfactory system**, and **cerebral cortex**. The basal ganglia interconnect with the thalamus and cerebral cortex and help the cortex to select automated and wanted patterns and subroutines of activity and to suppress unwanted patterns and subroutines of activity. The limbic forebrain provides emotional reactivity to external and internal stimuli and provides individuality of response. The olfactory system projects olfactory information into the limbic forebrain and provides rapid and appropriate responses to smell in the environment. The cerebral cortex provides a fine-grain analysis of the external and internal world, sophisticated and dexterous motor control, language function, the ability to look into the past and into the future, the ability to carry out executive functions, and is the source of intellect and cognitive understanding.

COLOR each region with a separate color.

- ☐ **1. Hypothalamus**
- ☐ **2. Thalamus**
- ☐ **3. Cerebral cortex**
- ☐ **4. Cerebellum (color one lobe)**
- ☐ **5. Spinal cord**
- ☐ **6. Medulla oblongata**
- ☐ **7. Pons**
- ☐ **8. Midbrain (mesencephalon)**
- ☐ **9. Pituitary gland**

Clinical Note

Spinal cord lesions usually involve somatosensory loss of pain sensation contralateral to the side of input; loss of fine, discriminative sensation ipsilateral to the side of input; motor deficits in the body (with changes in strength, tone, reflexes) ipsilateral to the side of the lesion; and sometimes autonomic changes in the sympathetic division (such as **Horner syndrome**) or the pelvic parasympathetic division (altered bowel, bladder, or reproductive system).

Brainstem lesions frequently involve specific dysfunction of cranial nerves III–XII. This may be accompanied by loss of somatosensory and somatic motor functions and by cerebellar dysfunction (ipsilateral). A large lesion in the brainstem that damages the reticular formation often results in coma and death.

Forebrain lesions are often accompanied by motor and sensory deficits on the opposite side of the body, and sometimes lower **contralateral facial palsy**. Damage to other sensory functions, such as vision, some auditory activities, or olfaction (from damage to the olfactory bulb or tract), may occur. Lesions on the left side may be accompanied by **expressive (frontal, Broca's area) aphasia**, or **receptive (posterior, Wernicke's area) aphasia**. Large lesions in the hemispheres may result in cognitive dysfunction. Damage to specific regions of the basal ganglia can produce movement disorders. Damage to the hippocampal formation (especially bilateral) leads to severe loss of short-term memory, confusion, and disorientation. Limbic lesions may result in emotional changes, fear and anxiety, compulsive disorders (from nucleus accumbens involvement), and other dysfunction.

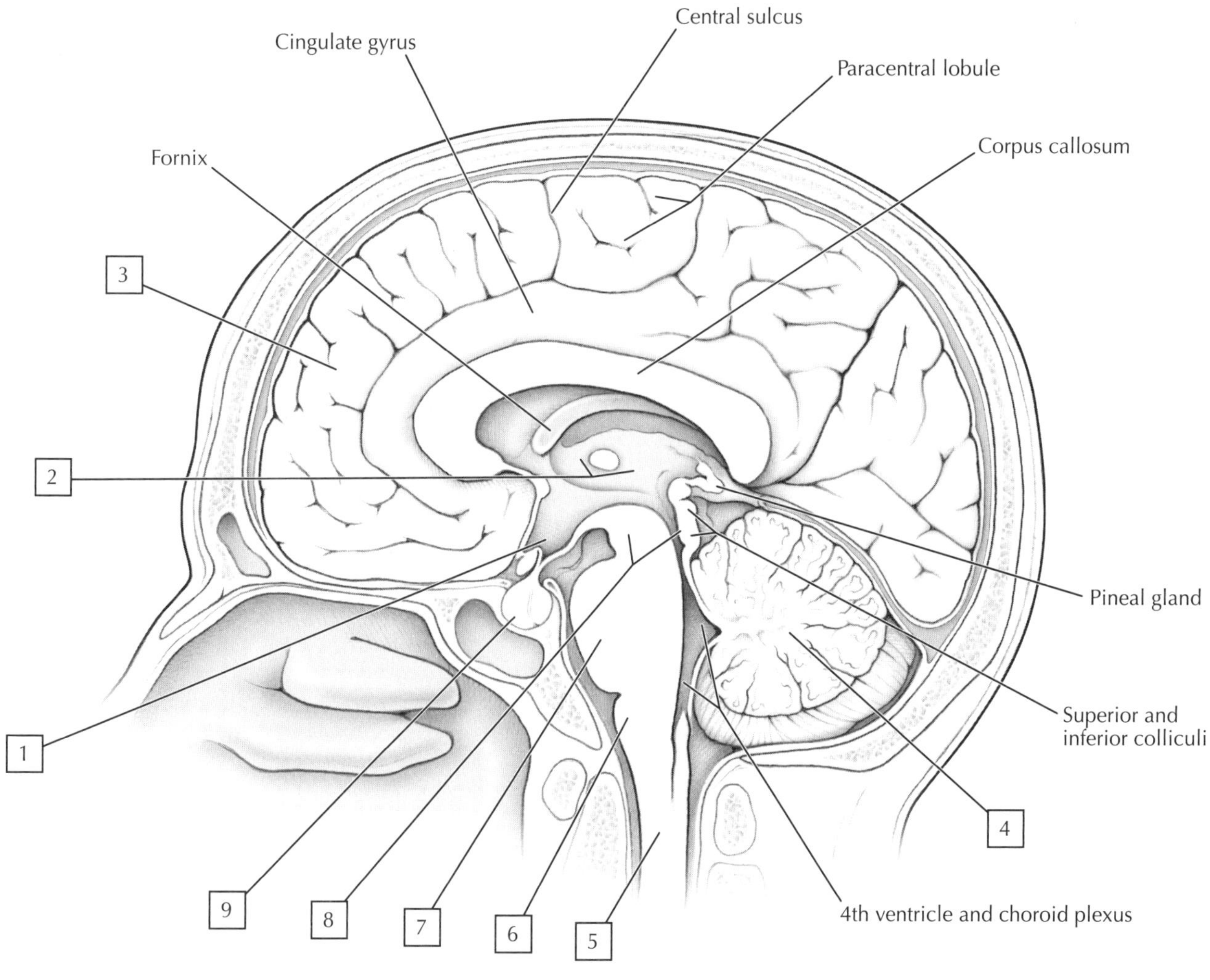
Central sulcus
Cingulate gyrus
Paracentral lobule
Corpus callosum
Fornix
3
2
Pineal gland
Superior and inferior colliculi
1
4
9
8
7
6
5
4th ventricle and choroid plexus

2 Basal Surface of the Brain

A view of the **basal surface of the brain**, with the brainstem and cerebellum removed, reveals the underside of the **temporal lobe**. These structures include the **primary olfactory cortex (uncus)**, the **parahippocampal gyrus** (overlying the **hippocampus**), and **periamygdaloid cortex** (adjacent to the subcortical **amygdala**). The undersurface of the **occipital lobe** is visible, with **primary visual cortex** and **visual association cortex**. Regions of the **thalamus** are visible, including the **pulvinar**, the **medial geniculate nucleus** (body), and the **lateral geniculate nucleus** (body). In the **hypothalamic region**, the **mammillary bodies**; the **optic nerve, chiasm, and tract**; and the **pituitary gland** are visible. The **olfactory bulb and tract** travel along the medial, inferior surface of the frontal lobe. In the cut cross section of the midbrain, produced by removing the brainstem and the cerebellum, the **cerebral peduncles** are prominent, representing the caudal continuation of the posterior limb and genu of the internal capsule. The **substantia nigra** (with pigmented dopamine neurons) and the **red nucleus** (origin of the rubrospinal tract) are also seen.

COLOR each of the following structures with a separate color.

- ☐ 1. **Olfactory bulb and tract**
- ☐ 2. **Pituitary gland**
- ☐ 3. **Primary olfactory cortex (uncus)**
- ☐ 4. **Mammillary bodies**
- ☐ 5. **Cerebral peduncle**
- ☐ 6. **Substantia nigra**
- ☐ 7. **Visual association cortex**
- ☐ 8. **Primary visual cortex**
- ☐ 9. **Parahippocampal gyrus**
- ☐ 10. **Periamygdaloid cortex**

Clinical Note

The cerebral peduncle is a caudal continuation of the posterior limb and genu of the internal capsule. The posterior limb carries corticospinal tract axons, corticorubral and corticoreticular axons, and cortical connections to subcortical sensory structures and pontine nuclei (to convey motor plans to the cerebellum). The genu carries corticobulbar tract axons, from the lateral-most region of the precentral and premotor cortex to the motor cranial nerve nuclei. Damage to the cerebral peduncle on one side has much the same clinical effect as damage to the posterior limb and genu of the internal capsule with regard to motor function. The clinical result is a **contralateral hemiplegia** with hypertonus, hyperreflexia, and some pathological reflexes (plantar extensor response), and a **contralateral drooping lower face** (due to loss of cortical control over the portion of the facial nerve motor nucleus supplying the lower muscles of facial expression, CNN VII). A difference is seen with sensory dysfunction. Sensory axons from the somatosensory ascending pathways from the ventral posterolateral (somatosensory) and ventral posteromedial (trigeminal, facial) thalamic nuclei travel in the posterior limb of the internal capsule, entering it at the level of the thalamus, but not in the cerebral peduncle (which is in the midbrain, not the diencephalon).

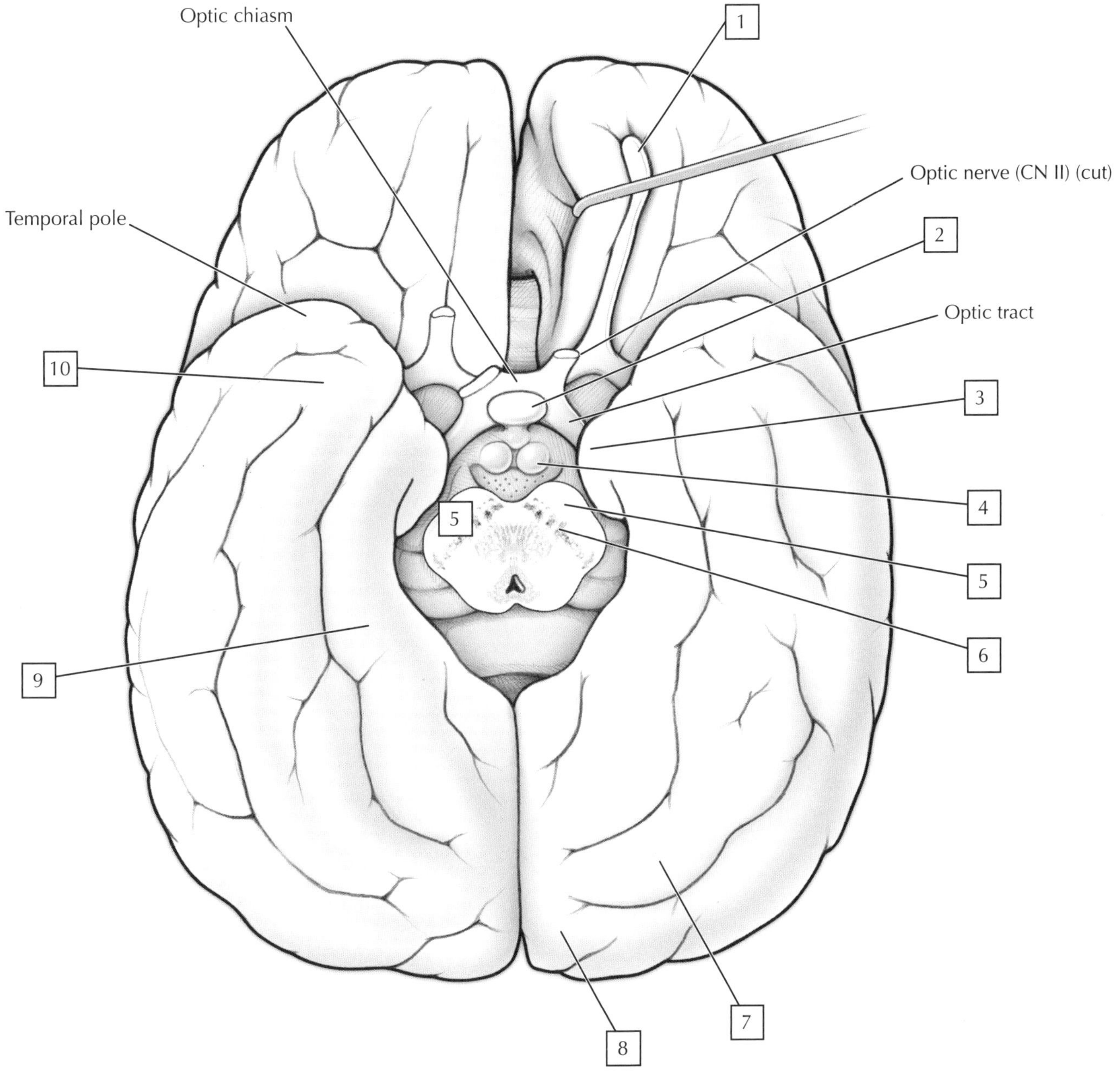
Optic chiasm
1
Optic nerve (CN II) (cut)
Temporal pole
2
Optic tract
10
3
4
5
5
6
9
7
8

2 Axial and Midsagittal Views of the Central Nervous System

The **nervous system** consists of the **central nervous system (CNS)** and the **peripheral nervous system (PNS)**. The CNS is made up of the **brain** and **spinal cord**. The brain is subdivided into the **brainstem** (**medulla**, **pons**, **midbrain**, and associated **cerebellum**) and **forebrain** (**diencephalon** and **telencephalon**). The principal components of the diencephalon are the **thalamus** and **hypothalamus**. The principal components of the telencephalon are the **basal ganglia**, the **limbic forebrain** structures, the **cerebral cortex**, and the **olfactory system**. The PNS consists of the input to, and output from, the CNS. This includes the primary **sensory** axons, ganglion cells, and sensory receptors; the **lower motor neuron** axons and their connections with skeletal muscles; and the **autonomic** preganglionic axons, ganglion cells, and postganglionic connections to smooth muscle, cardiac muscle, secretory glands, metabolic organs, and immunocytes in lymphoid organs.

Standard radiographs of the brain and spinal cord do not provide good depiction of detailed neural structures. To see neuroanatomical details, **magnetic resonance imaging (MRI)** is done. MRI uses short bursts (radiofrequency pulse) of electromagnetic waves that are absorbed by protons in the tissue being imaged. During the pulse, the protons are aligned because of the higher energy state. After the pulse, during the relaxation phase, the protons resume their unaligned state. The intervals between pulses and between collection times establish the parameters for contrast in the resultant image. **T1-weighted images** provide excellent viewing of detailed anatomy; the ventricles appear dark. **T2-weighted images** are used for observing pathology; the ventricles appear white.

COLOR the following components of the CNS with a different color for each component.

☐ 1. **Spinal Cord**

Brainstem

☐ 2. **Medulla**

☐ 3. **Cerebellum**

☐ 4. **Pons**

☐ 5. **Midbrain (and colliculi)**

Diencephalon

☐ 6. **Hypothalamus**

☐ 7. **Thalamus**

Telencephalon

☐ 8. **Cortically related white matter (corpus callosum, internal capsule)**

☐ 9. **Limbic forebrain (hippocampal formation and fornix, cingulate cortex)**

☐ 10. **Basal ganglia (caudate nucleus, putamen, globus pallidus)**

Ventricular System

☐ 11. **Lateral ventricle**

Clinical Note

The internal capsule is a key structure, both anatomically and functionally. Anatomically, it is an important landmark in both axial and coronal sections. In the axial section the internal capsule is shaped like a medially pointing V. Medial to the anterior limb is the head and body of the caudate nucleus (part of the basal ganglia). Medial to the posterior limb is the thalamus. Lateral to the V is the globus pallidus, and lateral to that, the putamen, both components of the basal ganglia.

Functionally, the internal capsule is the main "superhighway" into and out of the cortex. It carries axons of all of the sensory systems (except the olfactory system) from the thalamus to the appropriate zones of cerebral cortex. It carries all of the motor outflow from the cortex to the lower motor neurons of the spinal cord (corticospinal tract) and brainstem (corticobulbar tract). It also carries connections to the cerebellum (through the pontine nuclei) and to the basal ganglia. There are reciprocal connections between all major specific thalamic nuclei and their zones of cortical projections. Damage to the internal capsule, a frequent occurrence in strokes involving the middle cerebral artery, results in **contralateral hemiplegia** (increased tone and reflexes, and pathological reflexes) and **contralateral central facial palsy** (drooping lower face), as well as contralateral loss of somatic sensation.

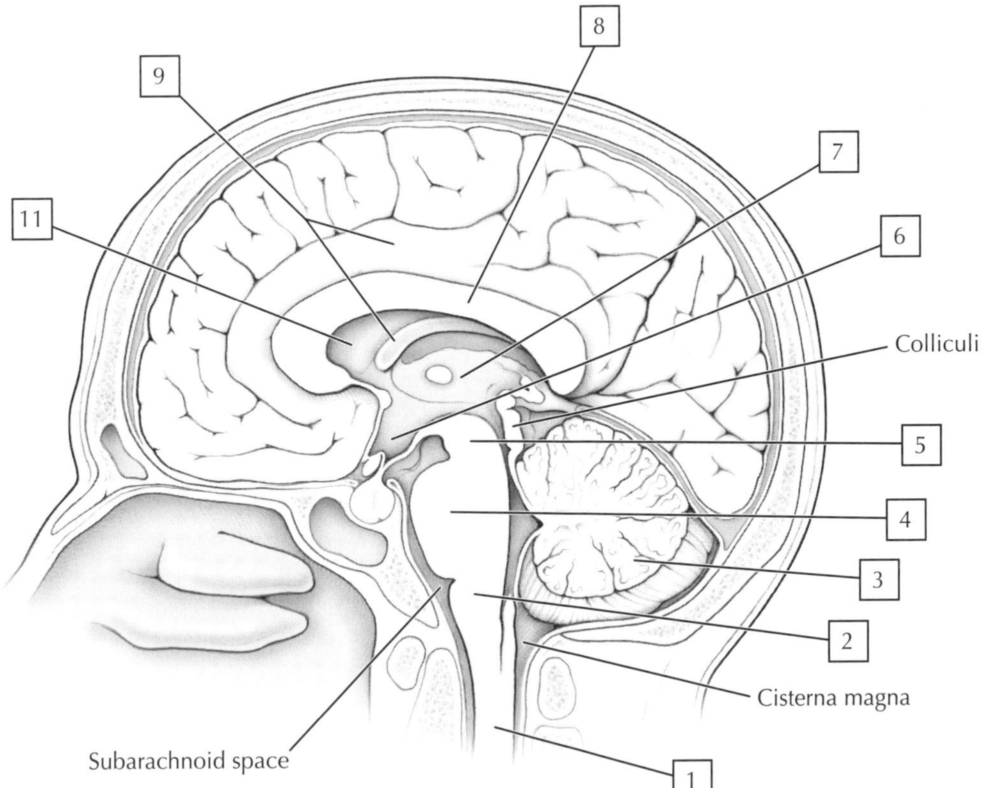

A. Sagittal view

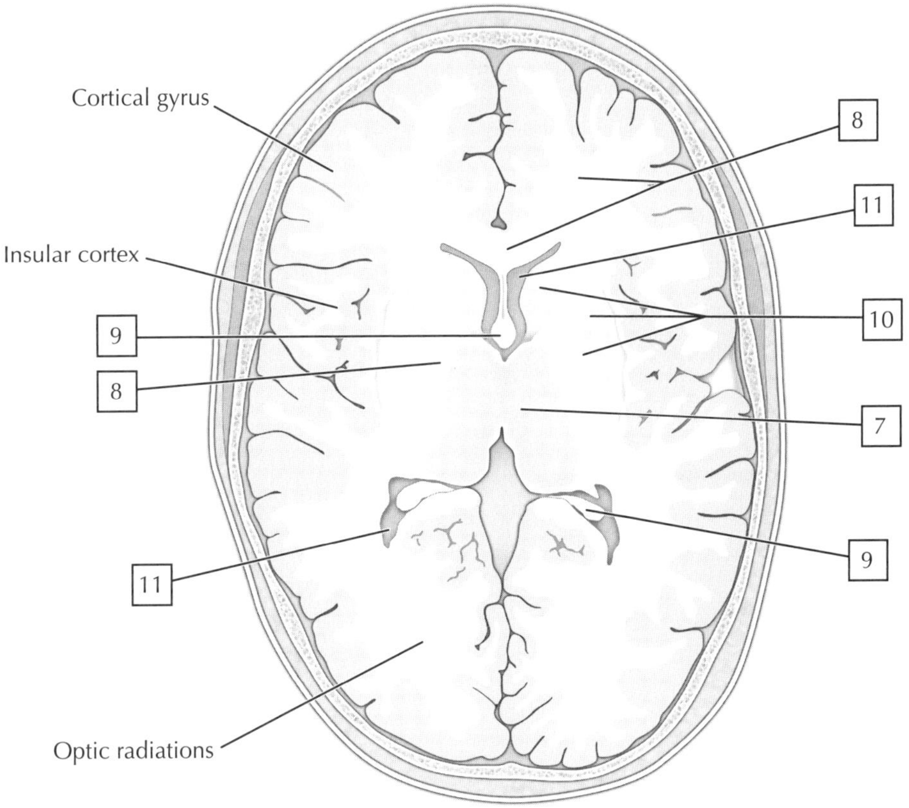

B. Axial view

2 Horizontal (Axial) Brain Sections Showing the Basal Ganglia

The basal ganglia are a collection of telencephalic nuclei (**caudate nucleus**, **putamen**, and **globus pallidus**) and their associated tracts, and some subtelencephalic nuclei (substantia nigra, subthalamus) that interconnect with one or more of the telencephalic components. The caudate nucleus and putamen are similar in nuclear composition and connectivity (e.g., they both receive dopaminergic input from the substantia nigra pars compacta); in humans, these two nuclei are split anatomically by the intervening presence of the **anterior limb of the internal capsule**, whereas in other species these two nuclei are united as the "caudoputamen." The globus pallidus has larger neurons and acts as the major output element for the telencephalic basal ganglia. The basal ganglia share loops of circuitry with the thalamus and associated cortical regions and assist the cortex in selecting automated and wanted subroutines of activity and suppressing unwanted subroutines of activity. The loops of basal ganglia–related circuitry include a motor loop, a limbic loop, a cognitive loop, and an oculomotor loop.

For anatomical landmarks, the upper illustration reveals, from lateral to medial: temporal lobe, lateral fissure, insular cortex, extreme capsule, claustrum, external capsule, putamen, external segment of the globus pallidus, internal segment of the **globus pallidus**, **genu** and **posterior limb of the internal capsule**, and **thalamus**. Enumerate these structures as the major anatomical landmarks of an axial section through the telencephalic basal ganglia.

COLOR each of the following structures with a separate color.

- ☐ 1. **Caudate nucleus (head)**
- ☐ 2. **Anterior limb (internal capsule)**
- ☐ 3. **Genu (internal capsule)**
- ☐ 4. **Posterior limb (internal capsule)**
- ☐ 5. **Putamen**
- ☐ 6. **Globus pallidus**
- ☐ 7. **Thalamus**
- ☐ 8. **Caudate nucleus (tail)**
- ☐ 9. **Occipital (posterior) horn of the lateral ventricle**

Clinical Note

When the basal ganglia are damaged, whether through physical lesions, neural degeneration, or disruption of a major neurotransmitter input (e.g., dopamine), the circuitry is disrupted between the thalamus, the cortex, and the basal ganglia. The most conspicuous of the systems to show clinical dysfunction with basal ganglia lesions is the motor system, resulting in movement disorders. With **Parkinson disease**, caused by the degeneration of dopaminergic neurons in the substantia nigra, pars compacta, and the subsequent loss of dopaminergic input to the caudate nucleus and the putamen, the patient demonstrates a resting tremor, muscular rigidity (through all ranges of motion), bradykinesia (difficulty initiating or stopping movement), and postural instability. With **Huntington chorea**, neurons in the caudate nucleus (and other structures) degenerate, resulting in choreiform movements (brisk, dance-like), emotional dysfunction, and cognitive decline. Other basal ganglia disorders may cause **athetosis** (slow, writhing movements), **spasmatic torticollis** (involuntary neck rotational movements), **dystonia**, and **hemiballismus** (flinging movements). Treatment approaches include pharmacological agents (e.g., dopamine replacement with SINEMET [L-dopa plus carbidopa]), deep brain stimulation, and, in some cases, surgical ablative procedures.

Horizontal (Axial) Brain Sections Showing the Basal Ganglia

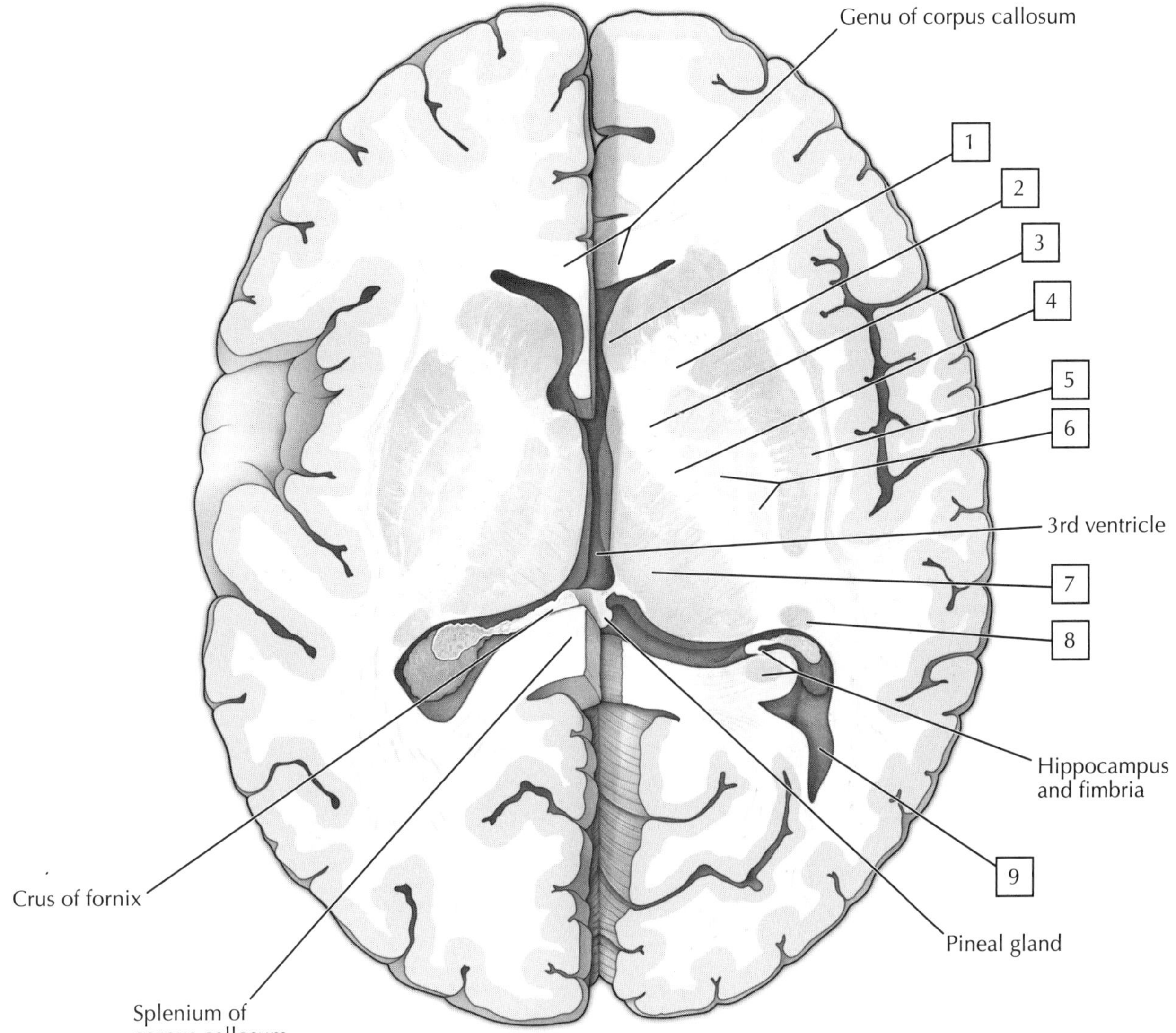

A. Axial sections showing the basal ganglia

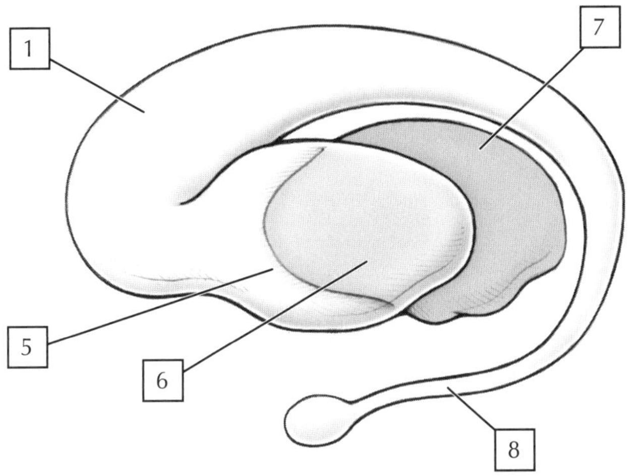

B. Schematic 3D depiction of the basal ganglia (lateral view)

2 Major Limbic Forebrain Structures

The **limbic system** was named for a ring of structures (**hippocampal formation**, **amygdala**, **cingulate cortex**, **septal nuclei**, **uncus**, **habenula**, etc.) that surround the thalamus and are associated with both cortical and subcortical structures to regulate emotional reactivity and behavior and to provide individuality of response to external and internal stimuli and events. Nauta subdivided limbic structures into the limbic forebrain and the limbic midbrain. These limbic structures interact with cortical circuitry and hypothalamic/brainstem structures to achieve tasks associated with emotional responsiveness and related behavior, motivational and reward behavior, consolidation of short-term memory, and environmentally appropriate and situationally appropriate (individualized responses) regulation of visceral/autonomic and neuroendocrine responses, along with the motor components to carry out the appropriate behaviors. Some limbic forebrain structures are arranged in a C-shaped configuration, including the hippocampal formation (**hippocampus** with **dentate gyrus**, **parahippocampal gyrus**, subiculum, entorhinal cortex and the **fornix**), and the amygdala and associated **stria terminalis.**

COLOR each of the following structures with a separate color.

- ☐ 1. **Habenula**
- ☐ 2. **Stria terminalis**
- ☐ 3. **Fornix**
- ☐ 4. **Cingulate cortex**
- ☐ 5. **Septal nuclei**
- ☐ 6. **Amygdala (amygdaloid nuclei)**
- ☐ 7. **Uncus (primary olfactory cortex)**
- ☐ 8. **Parahippocampal gyrus**
- ☐ 9. **Hippocampus**
- ☐ 10. **Dentate gyrus**

Clinical Note

The nuclei of the amygdala assess external and internal stimuli, and provide an emotional context for these inputs. Information is processed by amygdaloid nuclei from multiple cortical regions and provides emotional context, particularly for fear responses, both generalized fear and specific fear. Bilateral damage to the amygdala results in a loss of fear responses, as well as loss of the ability to sense fear on the face of other individuals.

The hippocampal formation processes extensive information from the temporal lobe, subiculum, and entorhinal cortex and sends connections through the fornix to the hypothalamus and septal nuclei, with subsequent connections through the thalamus to the cingulate cortex. The hippocampal formation is particularly vulnerable to **ischemic damage** (especially the CA1 sector). Damage results in the inability to consolidate new information into long-term memory traces, leading to severe forgetfulness, disorientation, and confusion, despite the retention of some long-term memory traces already laid down.

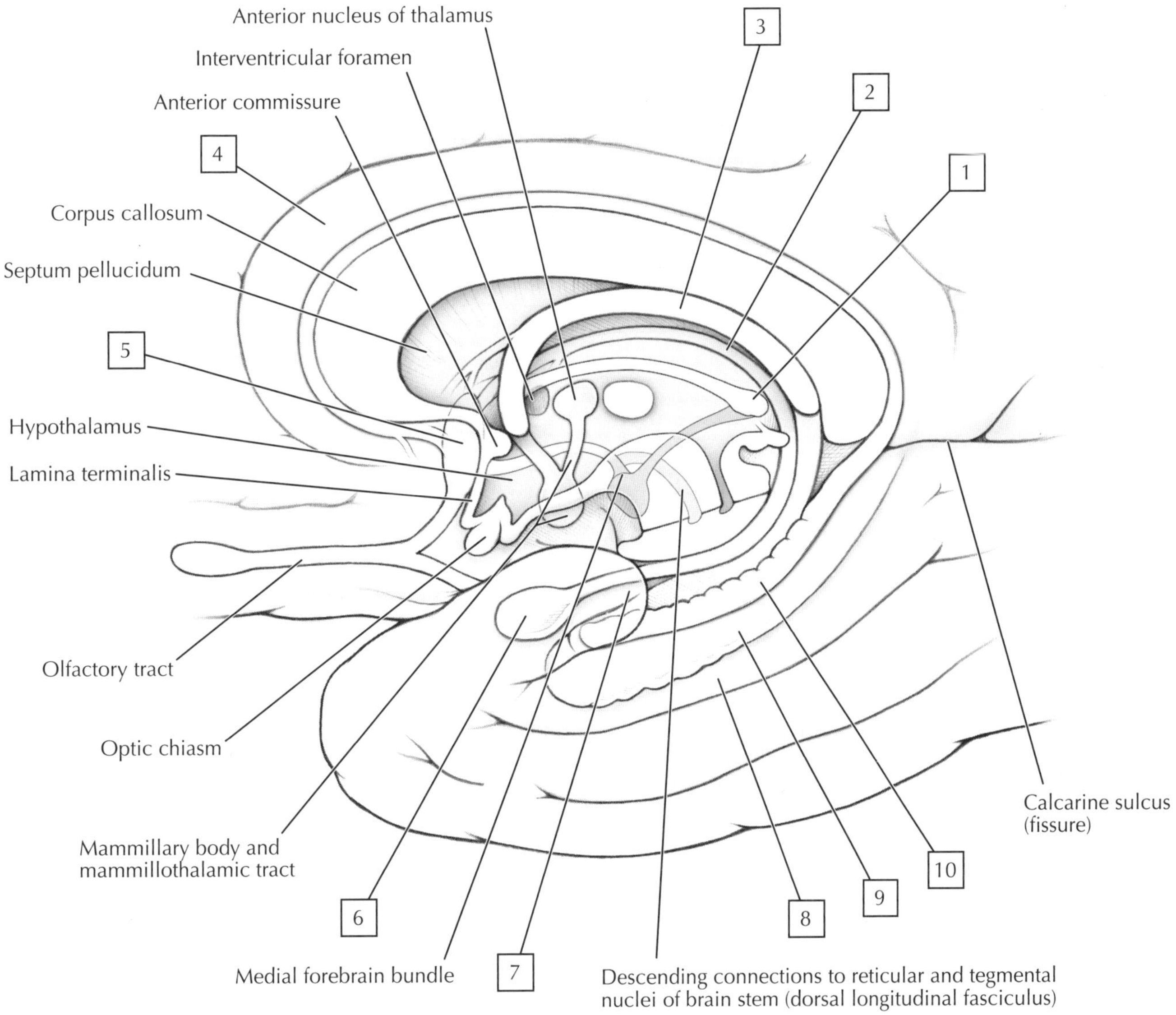
Anterior nucleus of thalamus
Interventricular foramen
Anterior commissure
4
Corpus callosum
Septum pellucidum
5
Hypothalamus
Lamina terminalis
Olfactory tract
Optic chiasm
Mammillary body and mammillothalamic tract
6
Medial forebrain bundle
7
3
2
1
Calcarine sulcus (fissure)
10
9
8
Descending connections to reticular and tegmental nuclei of brain stem (dorsal longitudinal fasciculus)

Chapter 3 Brainstem, Cerebellum, and Spinal Cord

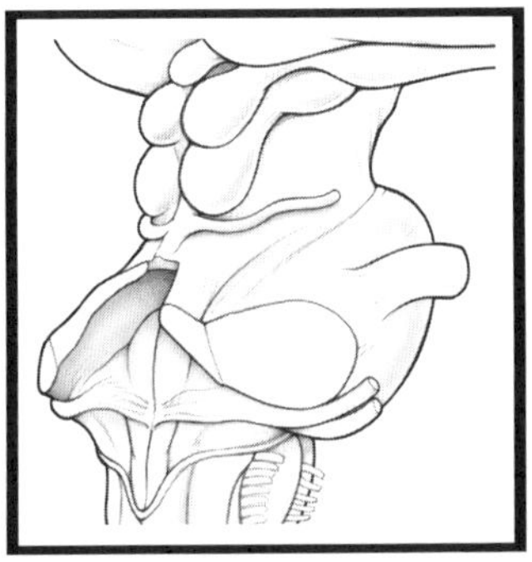
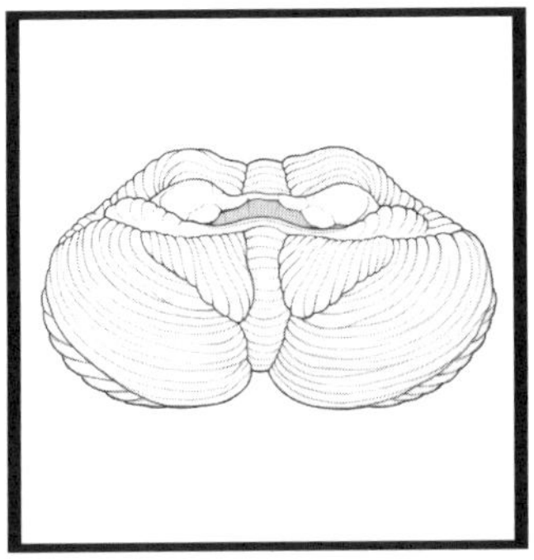
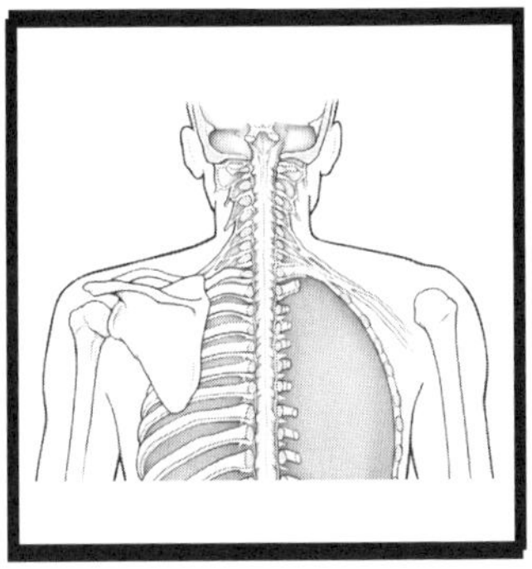
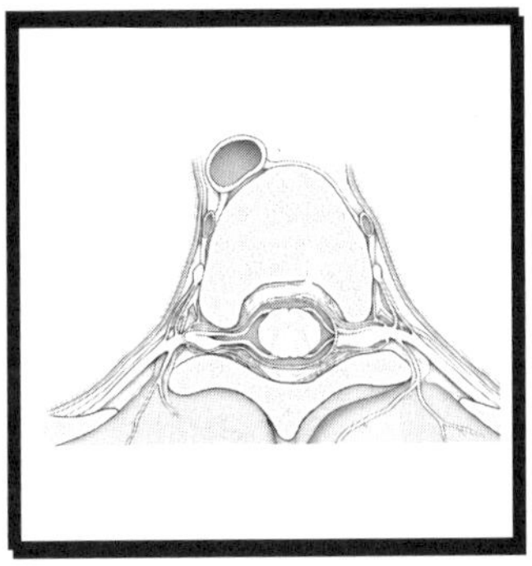

3 Brainstem Surface Anatomy: Posterolateral View

This view of the **brainstem** looks down on the posterior and lateral surfaces, with the entire telencephalon, most of the diencephalon, and the cerebellum removed. The three **cerebellar peduncles** (**inferior**, **middle**, and **superior**), which carry information into and out of the cerebellum, are sectioned. The **dorsal roots** carry input to the **spinal cord**, and the sensory components of the **cranial nerves** (**CNs**; e.g., **trigeminal**, **vestibulocochlear**, **facial**) carry input to the brainstem. **Tubercles, eminences, and trigones** on the floor of the fourth ventricle are named for nuclei just beneath them. The facial colliculus is an elevation on the dorsal surface of the pons under which the abducens nucleus and the looping fibers of the facial nerve are found. On the dorsal surface of the medulla, the **gracile and cuneate tubercles** are the protrusions under which the nuclei gracilis and cuneatus are found, processing epicritic information (fine discriminative touch, joint position sense, vibratory sensation). The **superior and inferior colliculi** form the dorsal surface of the midbrain, and process visual and auditory information, respectively. The **lateral and medial geniculate nuclei** (bodies) are located in the caudal and lateral margins of the **thalamus** and process visual and auditory information, respectively.

COLOR each of the following structures with a separate color.

- ☐ 1. **Superior colliculus**
- ☐ 2. **Inferior colliculus**
- ☐ 3. **Facial colliculus**
- ☐ 4. **Cuneate tubercle**
- ☐ 5. **Gracile tubercle**
- ☐ 6. **Dorsal roots of the spinal cord**
- ☐ 7. **Inferior cerebellar peduncle**
- ☐ 8. **Middle cerebellar peduncle**
- ☐ 9. **Superior cerebellar peduncle**
- ☐ 10. **Trigeminal nerve (CN V)**
- ☐ 11. **Medial geniculate body (nucleus) of the thalamus**
- ☐ 12. **Lateral geniculate body (nucleus) of the thalamus**

Clinical Note

Damage to the gracile and cuneate tubercles on the floor of the fourth ventricle would disrupt the ascending flow of epicritic information into the medial lemniscus and then to the ventral posterolateral thalamus and primary sensory cortex. Damage to the facial colliculus on the floor of the fourth ventricle would result in paralysis of ipsilateral lateral gaze (abducens; cranial nerve nucleus [CNN] VI) and medial gaze (damage to CNN VI interneurons whose axons travel in the medial longitudinal fasciculus (MLF) and regulate medial gaze via the oculomotor nucleus (CN III), which is clinically manifested as diplopia (double vision), and ipsilateral facial paralysis from disruption of the looping fibers of CN VII (facial).

The cerebellar peduncles interconnect the cerebellum with the spinal cord, brainstem, and thalamus. The inferior cerebellar peduncle interconnects the cerebellum mainly with the spinal cord, medulla, and pons. The middle cerebellar peduncle conveys cortical information, via the pontine nuclei in the basis pontis, to the cerebellum, informing it of cortical plans and activities. The superior cerebellar peduncle conveys output mainly to the red nucleus (rubrospinal tract) and nuclei ventral anterior and ventrolateral of the thalamus (regulating corticospinal outflow). Damage to the lateral hemispheres of the cerebellum and its associated peduncles results in **ipsilateral limb ataxia, mild hypotonus, dysmetria** (misjudgment of distance), decomposition of movements around several joints, an intention tremor, dysdiadochokinesia (inability to perform rapid alternating movements), and inability to dampen movements (rebound phenomena).

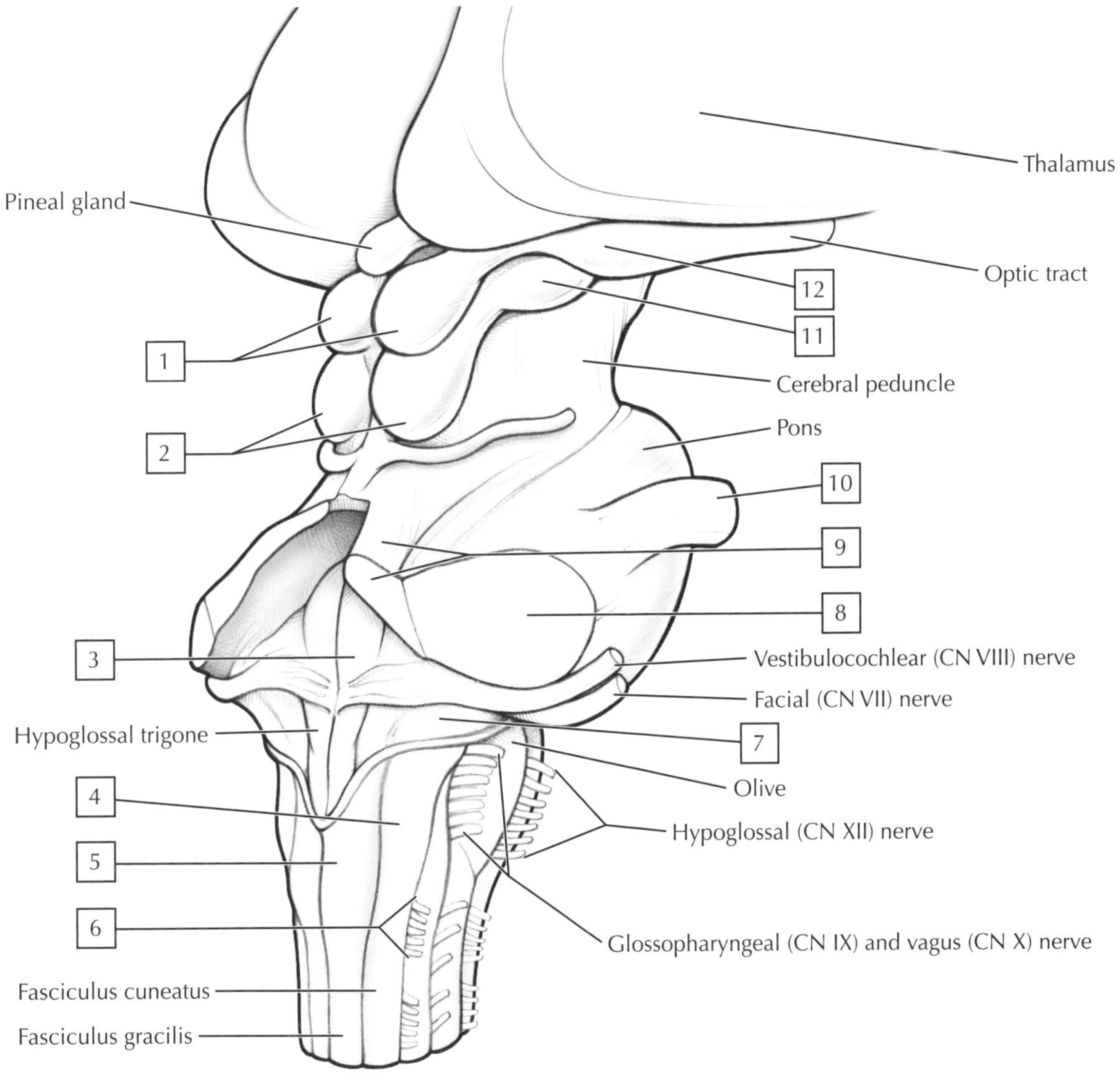
Thalamus
Pineal gland
Optic tract
12
11
1
Cerebral peduncle
2
Pons
10
9
8
3
Vestibulocochlear (CN VIII) nerve
Facial (CN VII) nerve
Hypoglossal trigone
7
Olive
4
Hypoglossal (CN XII) nerve
5
6
Glossopharyngeal (CN IX) and vagus (CN X) nerve
Fasciculus cuneatus
Fasciculus gracilis

Brainstem Surface Anatomy: Anterior View

The anterior (ventral) surface of the brainstem is characterized by the emergence of the **CNs**, except for CN IV, which emerges dorsally. These CNs convey sensory information from the **trigeminal system** and **special sense organs** into the central nervous system (CNS), and carry outflow from the brainstem motor systems to the muscles of the head and neck, and from the **cranial parasympathetic system**, via ganglia, to smooth muscles structures of the eye, to the salivary glands and lacrimal glands, and to cardiac muscle and smooth muscles of the thoracic and some abdominal viscera. Also conspicuous on the anterior surface of the brainstem are the anterior structures that contain the descending fibers of the corticospinal system (midbrain [cerebral peduncles], pons [basis pontis], and medulla [pyramids]). CNs I (**olfactory**) and II (**optic**) are CNS tracts, with axons myelinated by CNS glia (oligodendrocytes), not the peripheral supporting cells (Schwann cells) that myelinate peripheral axons of CNS III–XII.

CRANIAL NERVE SENSORY (S), MOTOR (M), AND AUTONOMIC (A) COMPONENTS	
CN I Olfactory	**S:** Olfaction (smell)
CN II Optic	**S:** Vision
CN III Oculomotor	**M:** To medial, inferior, and superior recti, inferior oblique, and levator palpebrae superioris muscles **A:** To ciliary muscle and pupillary constrictor muscle via the ciliary ganglion
CN IV Trochlear	**M:** To superior oblique muscle
CN V Trigeminal	**S:** To face, sinuses, teeth, general sensation to anterior two-thirds of oral cavity, tongue **M:** To muscles of mastication, tensor tympani muscle
CN VI Abducens	**M:** To lateral rectus muscle
CN VII Facial	**S:** Taste to anterior two-thirds of the tongue, soft palate **M:** To muscles of facial expression, stapedius muscle **A:** To submaxillary (submandibular) and sublingual salivary glands, and lacrimal glands via pterygopalatine and submandibular ganglia
CN VIII Vestibulocochlear	**S:** Linear and angular acceleration (balance and movement) and hearing
CN IX Glossopharyngeal	**S:** Taste to posterior one-third of tongue, general sensation to tonsil, pharynx, middle ear **M:** To stylopharyngeus muscle, pharyngeal musculature **A:** To parotid gland and nasal mucous glands via otic ganglion
CN X Vagus	**S:** To heart, lungs, bronchi, trachea, larynx, pharynx, gastrointestinal tract, small zone on external ear **M:** To pharynx, larynx musculature **A:** To heart, lungs, bronchi, proximal gastrointestinal tract via intramural ganglia
CN XI Accessory	**M:** To sternocleidomastoid muscle, upper two-thirds of trapezius muscle
CN XII Hypoglossal	**M:** To tongue muscles, strap muscles of the neck (via C nerve roots)

COLOR each of the following structures with a separate color.

- ☐ 1. **Olfactory tract (extending from the olfactory nerve)**
- ☐ 2. **Optic chiasm (site where the optic nerve traverses into the optic tract)**
- ☐ 3. **Oculomotor nerve (CN III)**
- ☐ 4. **Trochlear nerve (CN IV)**
- ☐ 5. **Trigeminal nerve (CN V)**
- ☐ 6. **Abducens nerve (CN VI)**
- ☐ 7. **Facial nerve (CN VII) (with nervus intermedius)**
- ☐ 8. **Vestibulocochlear nerve (CN VIII)**
- ☐ 9. **Glossopharyngeal nerve (CN IX)**
- ☐ 10. **Vagus nerve (CN X)**
- ☐ 11. **Hypoglossal nerve (CN XII)**
- ☐ 12. **Accessory nerve (CN XI)**

Clinical Note

CN II can be affected by demyelination in multiple sclerosis, a central demyelinating disease, resulting in ipsilateral optic neuritis, with loss of vision. For CNs III through XII, damage may occur from several causes. The brainstem lower motor neurons (LMNs) may be damaged by LMN disease (polio, bulbar palsy), mixed LMN–upper motor neuron diseases (amyotrophic lateral sclerosis), or brainstem vascular infarcts affecting vertebrobasilar blood supply to brainstem regions where the LMNs reside.
The CN axons are vulnerable to both central demyelinating diseases (e.g., multiple sclerosis) in the brainstem and peripheral demyelinating diseases (e.g., Guillain–Barré disease), tumors, compression, and diabetic neuropathies and other neuropathies. Sensory axons (CNs V, VII and nervus intermedius, VIII, IX, and X) are vulnerable to peripheral neuropathies, compression injury, demyelination, inflammation, tumors, and other insults. Injury or damage to CNS III, VII, IX, or X may result in parasympathetic dysfunction. CN III compression against the free edge of the tentorium cerebelli during transtentorial herniation may result in ipsilateral loss of pupillary constriction (fixed, dilated pupil), a key sign to look for in head injury, and loss of accommodation for near vision.

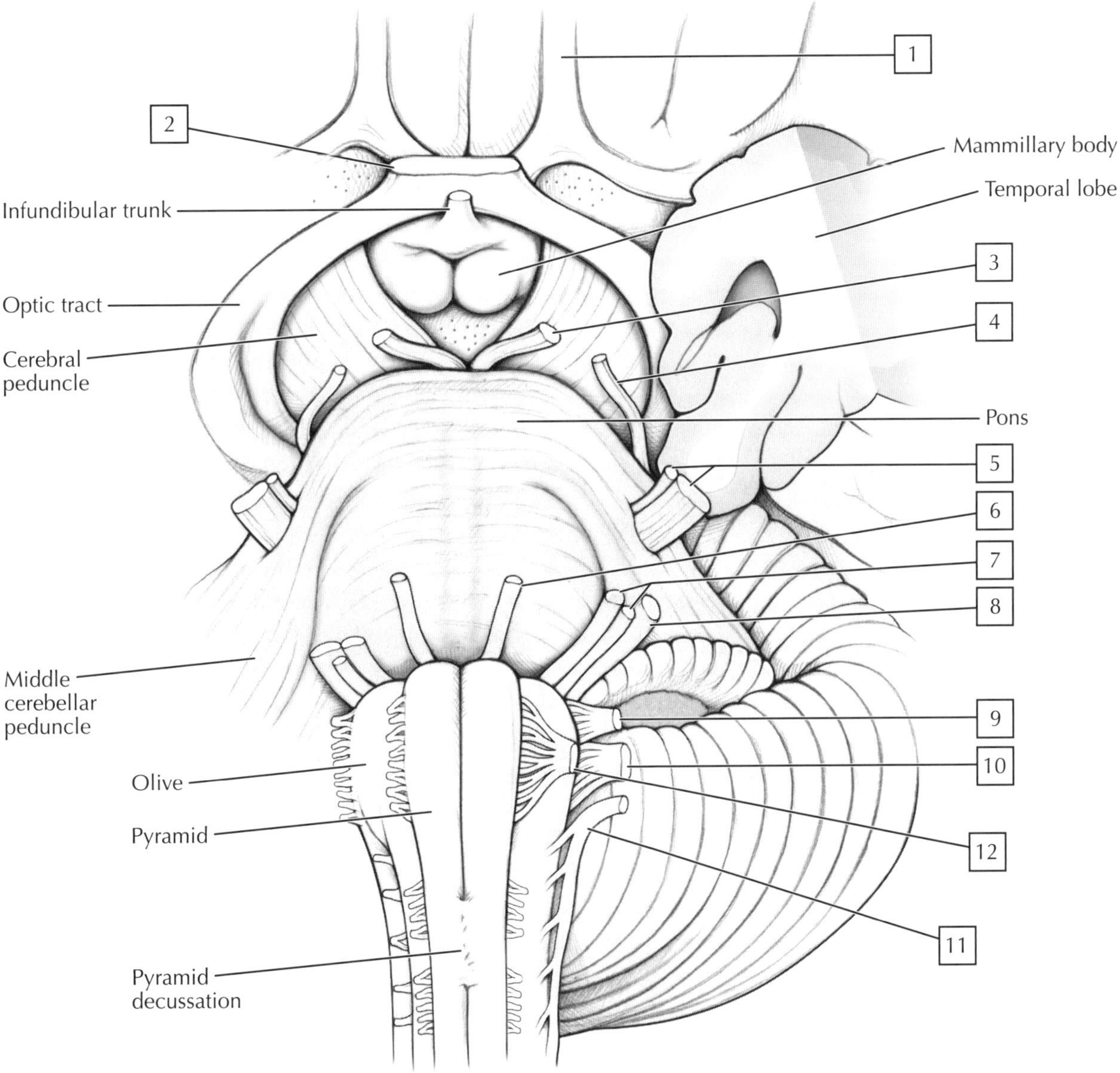
1
2
Mammillary body
Temporal lobe
Infundibular trunk
3
Optic tract
4
Cerebral peduncle
Pons
5
6
7
8
Middle cerebellar peduncle
9
10
Olive
Pyramid
12
11
Pyramid decussation

3 Cerebellar Anatomy

Illustrations **A** and **B** show the external features of the cerebellum (superior/dorsal and inferior/ventral surfaces, respectively). The superior view demonstrates the vertical organization of the cerebellum, with the **vermis**, **paravermis**, and **lateral hemispheres**. Each of these three regions is associated with specific deep nuclei and their respective upper motor neuronal systems.

REGION	DEEP CEREBELLAR NUCLEUS	UPPER MOTOR NEURONAL SYSTEM
Vermis	Fastigial nucleus Lateral vestibular nucleus	Lateral vestibulospinal tract and Reticulospinal tracts
Paravermis	Globose, emboliform nuclei	Rubrospinal tract (from red nucleus)
Lateral hemispheres	Dentate nucleus	Corticospinal tract (via ventrolateral nucleus of thalamus)

The inferior view shows the **anterior**, **middle**, and **flocculonodular lobes** of the cerebellum, traditional anatomical divisions with well-derived syndromes derived from known lesions. The three **cerebellar peduncles** (**inferior**, **middle**, **superior**) are sectioned to better view the inferior surface. These cerebellar peduncles convey inputs and outputs to and from the cerebellum.

Illustration **C** demonstrates the internal anatomy of the cerebellum, including the **deep nuclei** (**fastigial**, **globose**, **emboliform**, **dentate**) and the superior cerebellar peduncle.

COLOR each of the following structures with a separate color.

- ☐ 1. **Vermis (superior and inferior)**
- ☐ 2. **Paravermis**
- ☐ 3. **Lateral cerebellar hemispheres**
- ☐ 4. **Anterior lobe**
- ☐ 5. **Middle lobe**
- ☐ 6. **Superior cerebellar peduncle**
- ☐ 7. **Middle cerebellar peduncle**
- ☐ 8. **Inferior cerebellar peduncle**
- ☐ 9. **Flocculonodular lobe**
- ☐ 10. **Fastigial nucleus**
- ☐ 11. **Globose and emboliform nuclei**
- ☐ 12. **Dentate nucleus**

Clinical Note

The anterior lobe and vermis receive input from the body, particularly from the limbs, via the spinocerebellar tracts. The anterior lobe helps to coordinate the lower limbs via the lateral vestibular nucleus; damage results in a wide-based, ataxic, stiff-legged **gait.**

The middle cerebellar lobe (especially the lateral hemispheres) receives input from the body, input from the cerebral cortex via the pontine nuclei, and inputs from other sensory systems. Damage results in the classic cerebellar syndrome of **staggering gait, limb ataxia, dysmetria, dysdiadochokinesia, mild hypotonia, dysarthria**, and **oculomotor dysfunction**. The affected individual cannot perform tandem walking, finger-to-nose testing, heel-to-shin testing, or gait testing, nor can they produce coherent speech patterns, important components of classic field sobriety testing.

The flocculonodular lobe, consisting of the flocculi and the midline nodulus, is closely connected with the vestibular nuclei and influences basic tone, head movement, and eye movement. Selective damage can result in **impaired visual tracking**, **nystagmus**, **vertigo**, and **loss of balance from uncoordinated control of axial (not distal) musculature**. This syndrome is sometimes seen in children with medulloblastoma.

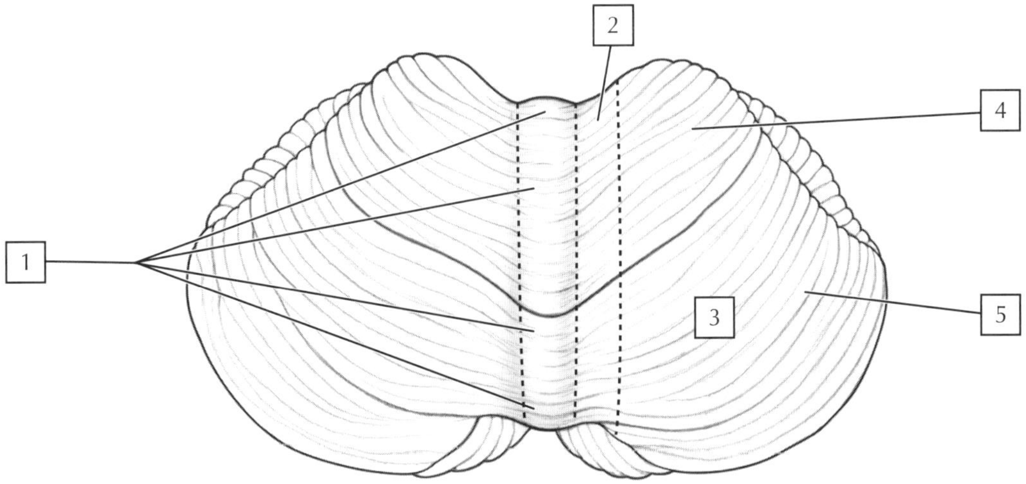

A. Superior surface

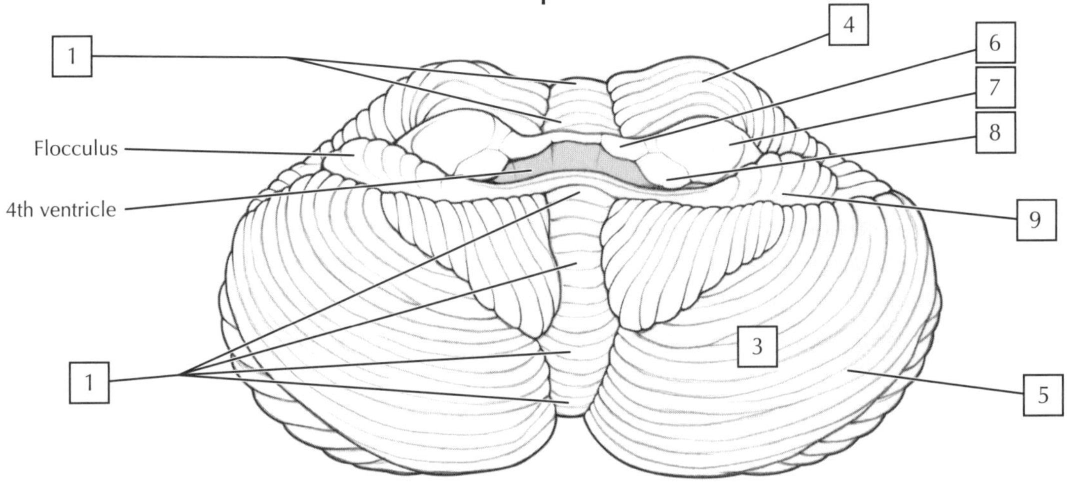

B. Inferior surface

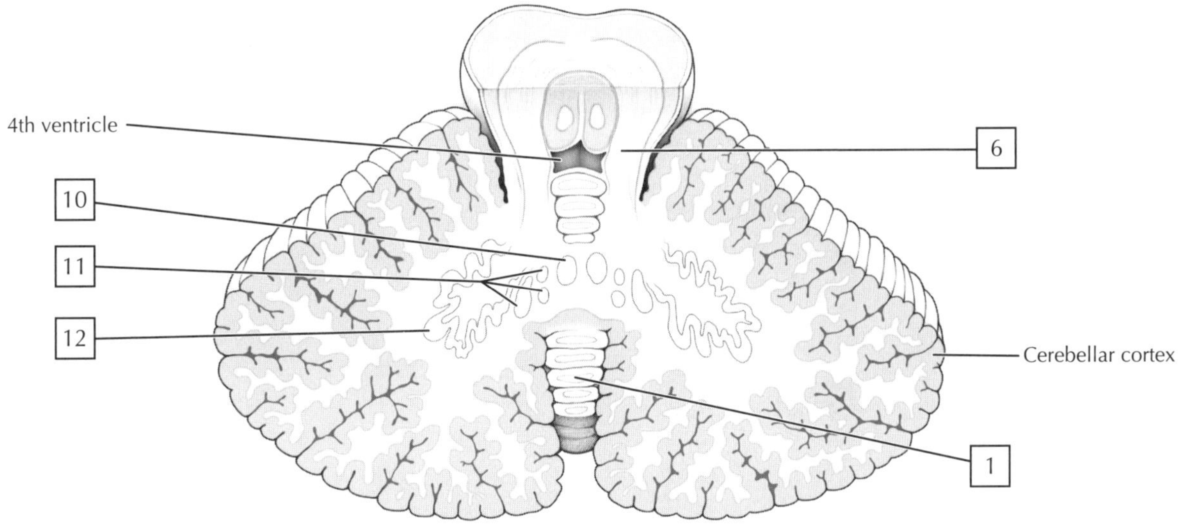

C. Section in plane of superior cerebellar peduncle

3 Spinal Cord Gross Anatomy: Posterior View

The **spinal cord** is protected in the **spinal canal** of the vertebrae of the vertebral column. In the illustration on the right of the spinal cord in situ, the posterior portions of the vertebrae have been removed. The spinal cord shows two regions of enlargement, the **cervical and lumbosacral enlargements**, corresponding to the increased input and output related to the limbs. The upper cervical spinal cord is continuous rostrally with the medulla through the **foramen magnum**. In development, the growth of the vertebral column outstrips the longitudinal growth of the spinal cord; hence, the spinal cord ends (at the conus medullaris) under the region of the **L1 vertebral body**. The **nerve roots** (**dorsal/posterior** [sensory]; **ventral/anterior** [motor, autonomic]) exit laterally from each spinal cord segment through the intervertebral foramina and traverse the subarachnoid space. For more caudal spinal cord segments, those nerve roots have a long course through the subarachnoid space, forming a horsetail-like accumulation of nerve roots, the **cauda equina**, located in an enlarged cistern of subarachnoid space, the **lumbar cistern**. This cistern is the best site for withdrawal of cerebrospinal fluid samples via a lumbar puncture. The **filum terminale** anchors the spinal cord caudally to the coccyx, and the **denticulate ligaments** (extensions of **pia mater**) anchor the spinal cord laterally to the other meninges (**dura mater**, **arachnoid mater**). These meninges surround the spinal cord and portions of the nerve roots where they exit through the intervertebral foramina.

COLOR each of the following structures with a separate color.

- ☐ 1. **Cervical enlargement (spina cord)**
- ☐ 2. **Dura mater**
- ☐ 3. **Lumbosacral enlargement (spinal cord)**
- ☐ 4. **Conus medullaris**
- ☐ 5. **Cauda equina**
- ☐ 6. **Filum terminale**
- ☐ 7. **Foramen magnum**
- ☐ 8. **Lumbar cistern**
- ☐ 9. **Dorsal root**
- ☐ 10. **Denticulate ligaments**

Clinical Note

The lumbar cistern is an important site for straightforward access to samples of cerebrospinal fluid. The cerebrospinal fluid flows from the ventricular system of the brain into the subarachnoid space; its composition is an important component of the analysis of neurological conditions such as infections, hemorrhages, inflammatory conditions, degenerative disorders, and other neurological disorders. The cerebrospinal fluid analysis includes pressure, color and appearance, viscosity, presence of red cells and white cells, cellularity, protein content, and glucose content.

The intervertebral foramina are sites of emergence of dorsal and ventral roots, on course to unite and form spinal nerves. The nucleus pulposus of intervertebral discs may herniate through the disc capsule and may impinge on dorsal roots (usually causing initial radiating pain) and/or ventral roots (causing motor dysfunction in innervated muscles). The resultant lesion is called a **radiculopathy**. A herniated disc (especially cervical) also may extend and impinge on the spinal cord, resulting in **myelopathy**, damaging descending motor tracts (corticospinal, rubrospinal), spinocerebellar tracts, and protopathic (pain and temperature) tracts (spinothalamic/spinoreticular). The most common sites of **disc herniation** are L5–S1 and L4–L5 in the lumbar region, and C6–C7, C5–C6, and C4–C5 in the cervical region.

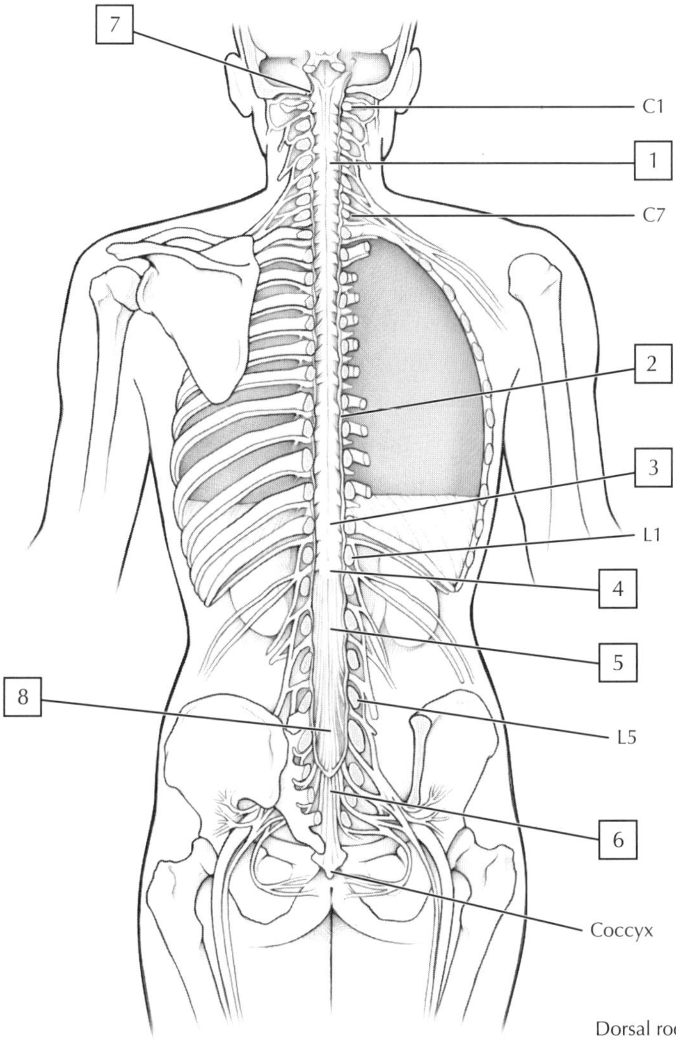

A. Spinal cord gross anatomy *in situ*

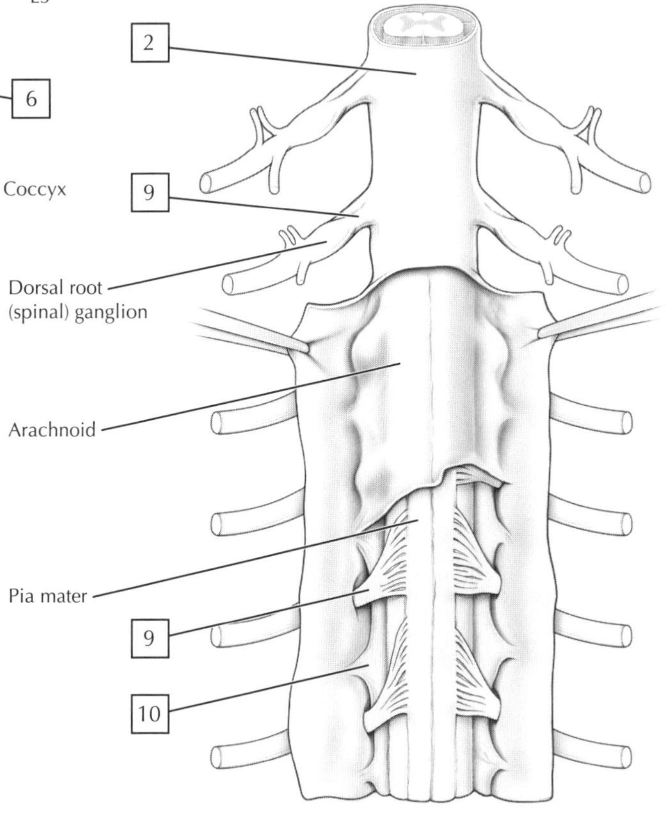

B. Meninges and spinal roots

3 Spinal Cord Cross-Sectional Anatomy *in situ*

In a cross-sectional view, the spinal cord sits within the spinal canal formed by the vertebrae (shown are the **vertebral body**, **spinous process**, and **transverse processes**). The spinal cord and proximal nerve roots are surrounded by three **meninges**, the **pia mater** (adheres to every contour of tissue), the **arachnoid mater** (extends over the sulci), and the tough membranous **dura mater** (helps to protect the cord). The **epidural space** contains fat (unlike the skull, where the epidural space is a potential space, containing meningeal arteries) and is the site for regional anesthesia for some childbirths and some spinal procedures. The subdural space is a potential space into which a bleed may occur. The **subarachnoid space** contains cerebrospinal fluid and helps to bathe and protect the spinal cord from injury. The **dorsal root** is associated with the **dorsal root ganglion** (contains the primary sensory cell bodies); it unites with the **ventral root** (contains lower motor neuron [LMN] axons and preganglionic autonomic axons) to form a **spinal nerve**. The spinal nerve branches into a **ventral ramus** (intercostal nerve) and a **dorsal ramus**. The spinal nerve also gives rise to the **white ramus communicans** (distal) with myelinated preganglionic sympathetic axons, which terminate in the sympathetic chain ganglion, and the **gray ramus communicans** (proximal) with unmyelinated postganglionic sympathetic axons. The spinal cord ends at the level of the L1 vertebral body. At lumbar vertebral levels, the spinal canal still contains the dura mater and arachnoid mater, with a large subarachnoid space (**lumbar cistern**) containing long nerve roots (**cauda equina**) extending toward their appropriate intervertebral foramina. The **filum terminale** anchors the spinal cord to the coccyx.

COLOR each of the following structures with a separate color.

- ☐ **1. Vertebral body**
- ☐ **2. Epidural space with fat**
- ☐ **3. Dura mater**
- ☐ **4. Subarachnoid space**
- ☐ **5. Spinous process**
- ☐ **6. Dorsal ramus of spinal nerve**
- ☐ **7. Dorsal root ganglion**
- ☐ **8. Dorsal root**
- ☐ **9. Ventral root**
- ☐ **10. White and gray rami communicans**
- ☐ **11. Cauda equina**
- ☐ **12. Filum terminale**

Clinical Note

The dorsal and ventral roots at each level unite to form a spinal nerve. Those nerve roots may be subject to damage from an impinging herniated nucleus pulposus (disc), with conspicuous radiating pain, and sometimes motor dysfunction. The nerve roots and peripheral nerves also may be subject to acute, inflammatory autoimmune demyelinating conditions (polyradiculopathy, Guillain–Barré syndrome). In many cases, an autoimmune response to Campylobacter jejuni from an enteric infection triggers the acute inflammatory response, resulting in progressive symmetrical weakness that may result in total paralysis, including loss of control of respiratory muscles. The damage to sensory components may result in paresthesias (numbness and tingling, painful sensations) in the distal extremities. The patient often recovers, but some patients may have residual deficits.

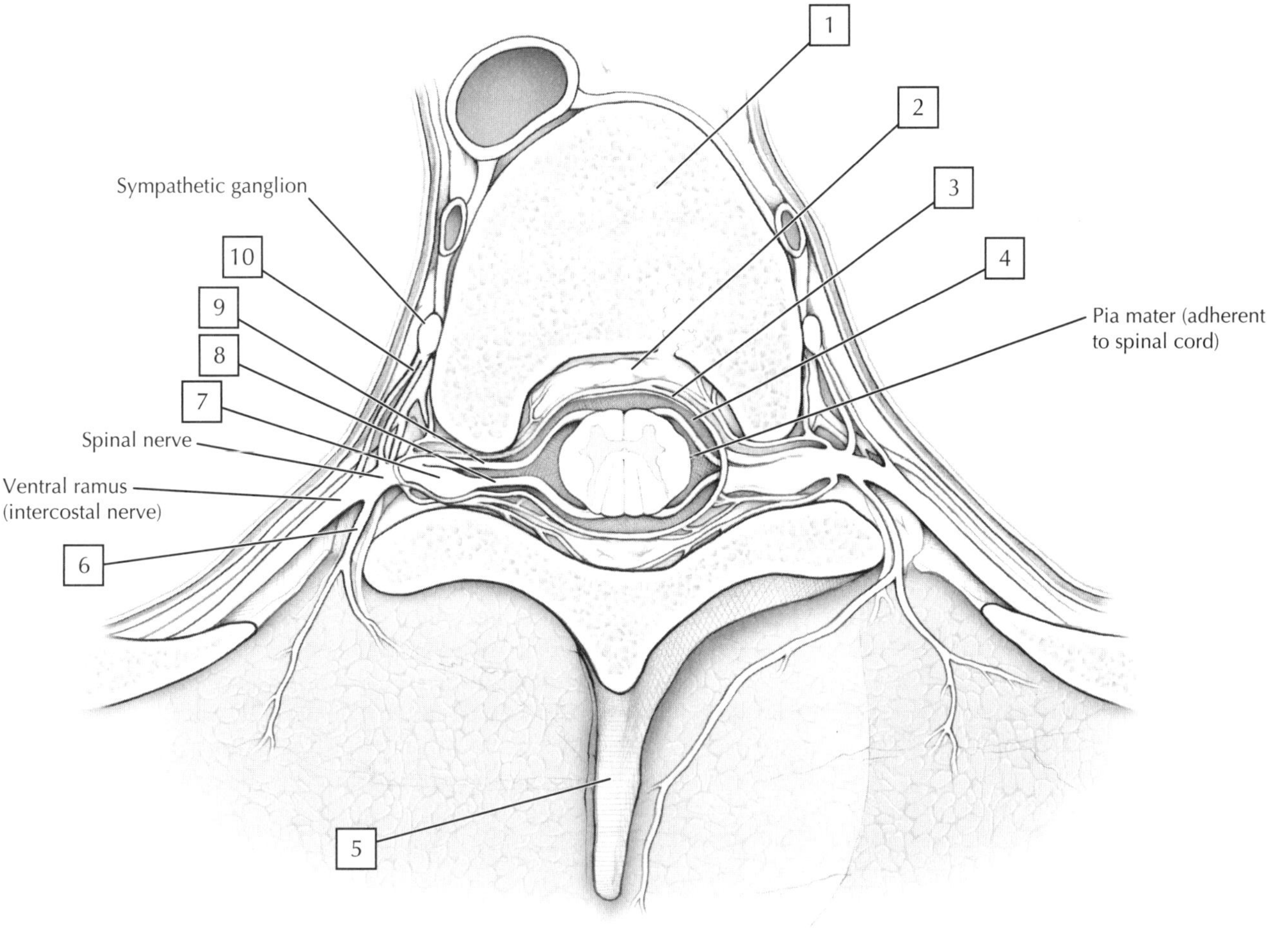

A. Section through thoracic vertebra

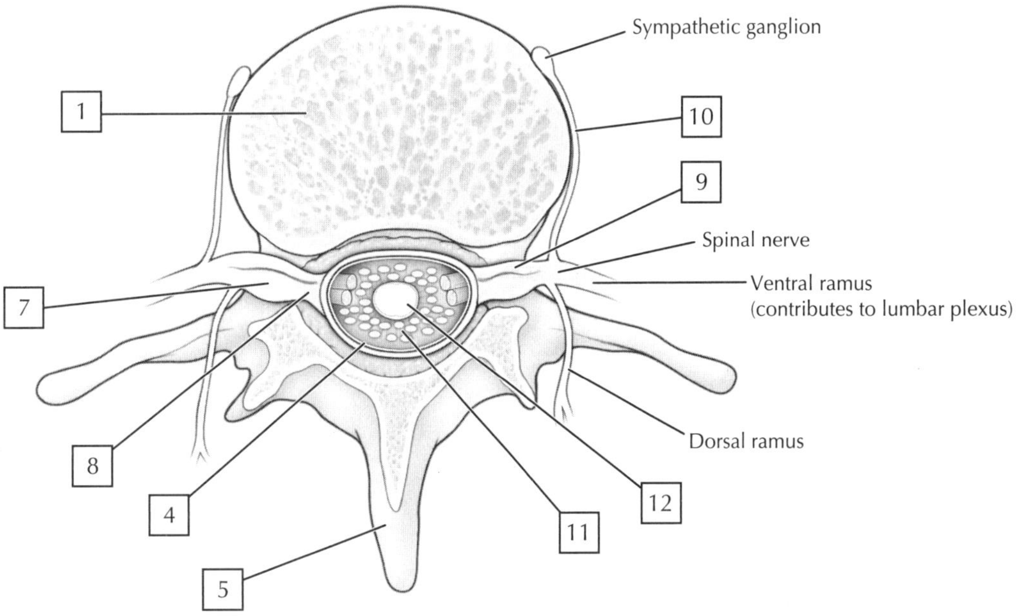

B. Section through lumbar vertebra

Spinal Cord White Matter and Gray Matter

The spinal cord has two zones of enlargement, the **cervical enlargement** and the **lumbosacral enlargement**, brought about by the increased sensory information from the limbs and the increased motor innervation of muscles supplying the limbs. The **white matter** (axons) is located in the outer regions of the spinal cord, and the **gray matter** (cell bodies) is found centrally in a butterfly-like pattern (or H pattern). The amount of white matter decreases progressively from rostral to caudal due to caudal-to-rostral addition of sensory information and due to rostral-to-caudal termination of descending motor information. The white matter is subdivided into **funiculi** (**dorsal, lateral,** and **ventral**); each funiculus contains several tracts or fasciculi. The gray matter is subdivided into a **dorsal horn**, **ventral horn**, and **intermediate gray region.**

The dorsal horn processes sensory information. The ventral horn contains the LMNs and processes motor information. The intermediate gray processes integrated information, and from T1–L2 contains a lateral horn (intermediolateral cell column) in which preganglionic sympathetic neurons are found. The dorsal funiculus conveys epicritic information (fine discriminative touch, vibratory sensation, joint position sense) in **fasciculi gracilis** (lower body) and **cuneatus** (upper body). The lateral funiculus conveys descending motor information **(lateral corticospinal tract, rubrospinal tract)** in the dorsal portion, descending autonomic information, ascending protopathic (pain and temperature) sensory information (**spinothalamic** and **spinoreticular tracts**) in the ventrolateral portion, and ascending spinocerebellar information (at the outer margin of the lateral funiculus). The ventral funiculus conveys motor information (**reticulospinal** and **vestibulospinal tracts**) related to basic tone and posture, and a small component (anterior) of the corticospinal system.

COLOR each of the following structures with a separate color.

- ☐ 1. **Dorsal funiculi**
- ☐ 2. **Cervical enlargement (gray matter)**
- ☐ 3. **Lateral funiculi**
- ☐ 4. **Ventral funiculi**
- ☐ 5. **Dorsal horn**
- ☐ 6. **Intermediate gray**
- ☐ 7. **Ventral horn**
- ☐ 8. **Lumbosacral enlargement (gray matter)**
- ☐ 9. **Spinothalamic tract and spinoreticular tract**
- ☐ 10. **Fasciculus cuneatus**
- ☐ 11. **Fasciculus gracilis**
- ☐ 12. **Lateral corticospinal tract**
- ☐ 13. **Rubrospinal tract**
- ☐ 14. **Reticulospinal tracts**
- ☐ 15. **Vestibulospinal tracts**

Clinical Note

White matter and gray matter are subject to damage from a variety of causes. LMNs may be damaged by degeneration from polio or neurodegenerative diseases such as amyotrophic lateral sclerosis, resulting in flaccid paralysis, loss of tone, and loss of reflexes. Selected interneuronal populations in the dorsal horn may undergo cell death (apoptosis) from continuous insult by glutamate toxicity in chronic pain syndromes, preventing the dampening of ongoing pain processing or generation.

Damage to the dorsal funiculus may occur in pernicious anemia or combined systems degeneration, resulting in paresthesias in the feet and legs (sometimes also arms and hands), sensory ataxia with a broad-based gait and loss of fine discriminative touch, vibratory sensation, and joint position sense.

Damage to the lateral funiculus (from vascular damage, disc impingement [myelopathy], syringomyelia, combined systems degeneration, other axonal degenerative disorders, or a mass lesion) may result in ipsilateral spastic paraparesis/paraplegia with increased tone, increased muscle stretch reflexes (spasticity), and plantar extensor responses from loss of corticospinal and rubrospinal influences. Damage to the spinothalamic tract and spinoreticular tract (system) may result in loss of pain and temperature sensation below the level of the lesion on the contralateral side of the body (these protopathic systems are already crossed).

A. Sections through spinal cord at various levels

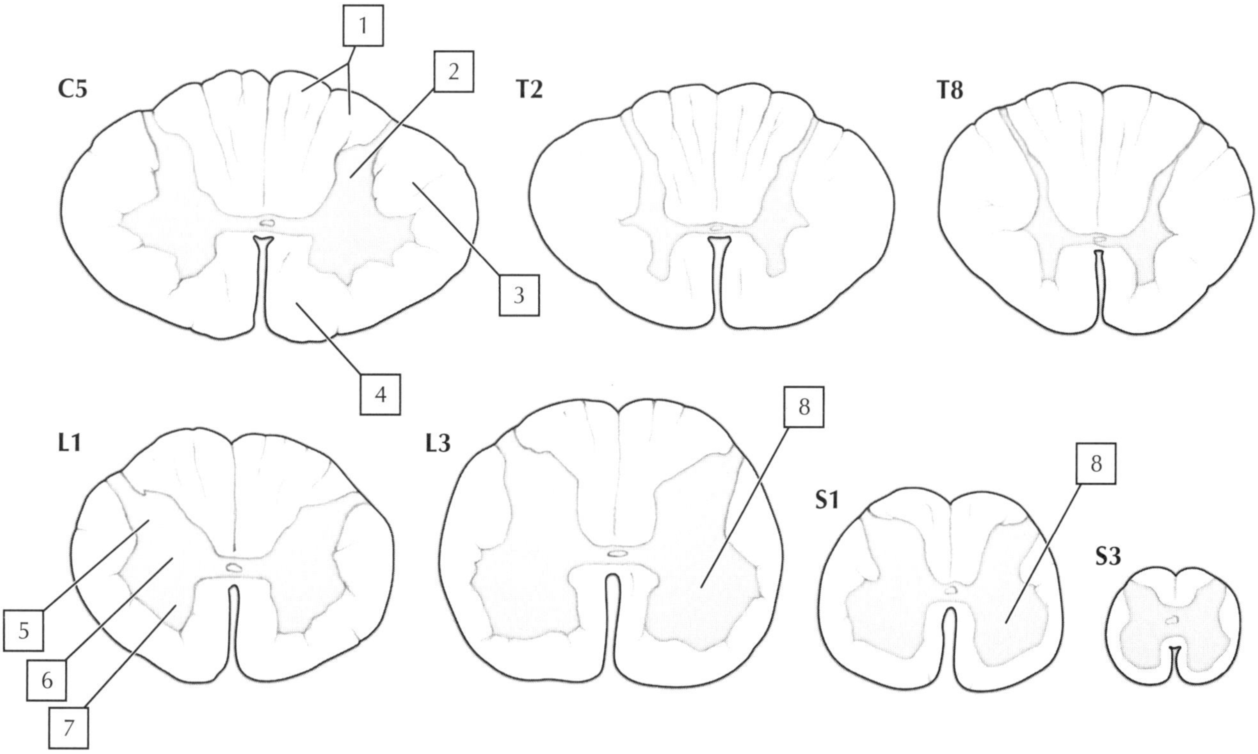

B. Principal fiber tracts of spinal cord (composite)

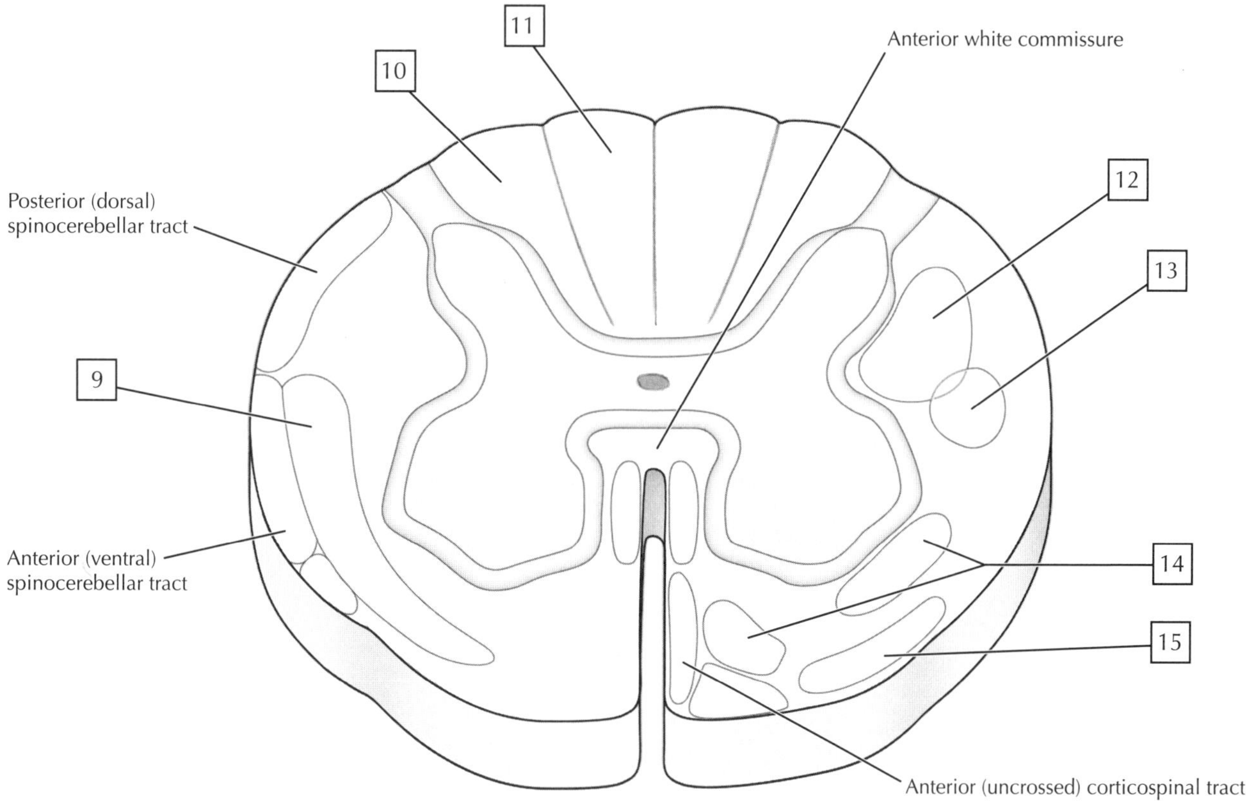

Chapter 4 Ventricles, Cerebrospinal Fluid, and Vasculature

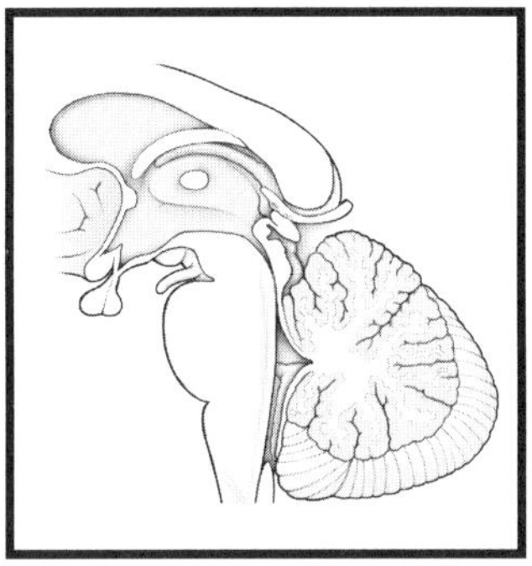

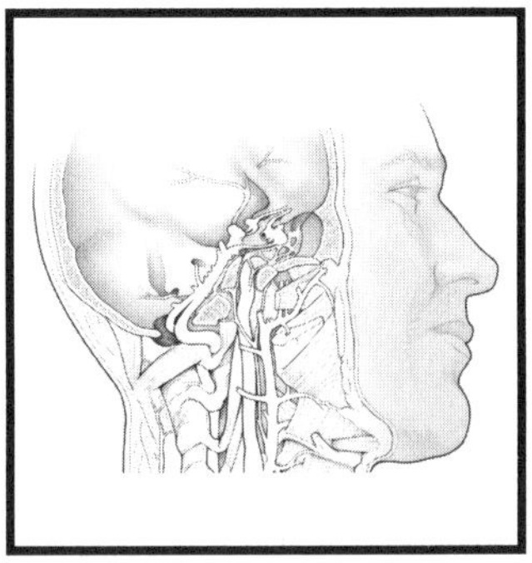

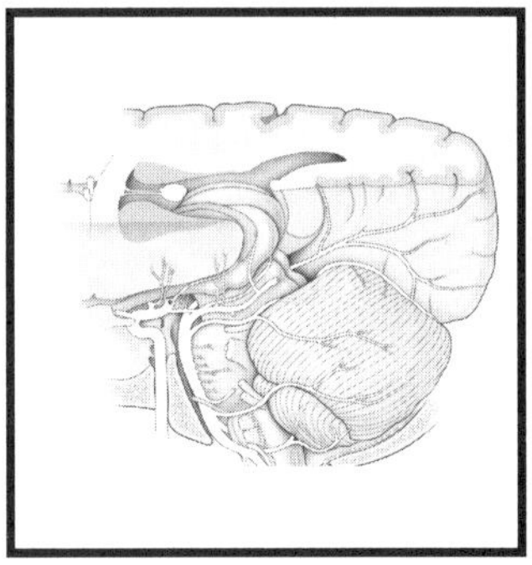

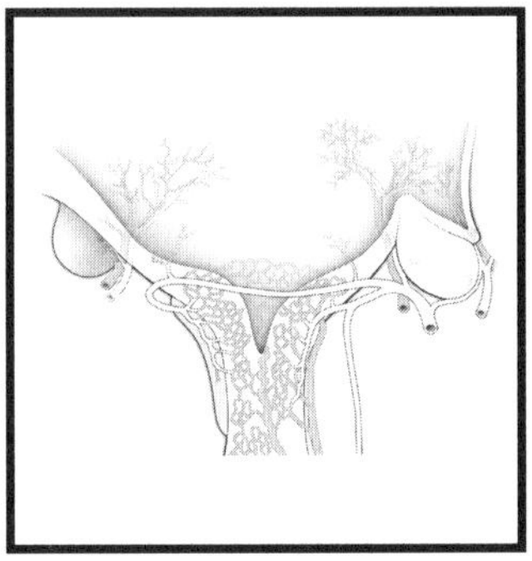

4 Ventricular System

The **ventricular system** is a fluid-filled set of cavities in the central nervous system (CNS) filled with cerebrospinal fluid (CSF). This system is derived from the expansion of the central canal of the neural tube. The **third ventricle** (present in the diencephalon), **cerebral aqueduct** (present in the midbrain), and the **fourth ventricle** (present in the pons and medulla) are derived from the differential neuronal growth and neural tube folding during development. The **lateral ventricles** are massive extensions of the rostral portion of the neural tube, taking the form of C-shaped paired structures sweeping from the frontal pole around the occipital pole and down into the temporal lobe. The lateral ventricles interconnect with the third ventricle through the **interventricular foramen of Monro**. The lateral, third, and fourth ventricles possess the **choroid plexus**, which provides an ultrafiltrate of blood for formation of the CSF. The CSF flows from rostral to caudal, exiting the ventricular system through the **medial foramen of Magendie** and the **lateral foramena of Luschka** in the caudal medulla. The CSF then circulates through the **subarachnoid space**, providing a cushioning for the CNS (brain and spinal cord). The CSF is absorbed through one-way valves, the **arachnoid granulations**, into the venous sinuses of the brain, which drain venous blood and CSF into the systemic venous circulation. Anatomically, it appears that there is a vestige of the ependymal of the central canal in the adult spinal cord, but that central canal does not carry CSF in normal circumstances. Cavitation of the central canal may occur in adults, producing a syrinx (syringomyelia), with subsequent damage to the anterior white commissure (bilateral segmental loss of pain and temperature sensation), possibly expanding to include LMN damage and other structural involvement in the spinal cord.

COLOR the following structures, using a separate color for each structure.

- ☐ 1. **Anterior horn of left lateral ventricle**
- ☐ 2. **Body of left lateral ventricle**
- ☐ 3. **Temporal horn of left lateral ventricle**
- ☐ 4. **Occipital horn of left lateral ventricle**
- ☐ 5. **Cerebral aqueduct of Sylvius**
- ☐ 6. **4th ventricle**
- ☐ 7. **Median aperture (foramen of Magendie)**
- ☐ 8. **3rd ventricle**
- ☐ 9. **Interventricular foramen of Monro**

Clinical Note

The C-shaped lateral ventricles serve as landmarks on imaging studies to reveal the integrity of surrounding structures and the anatomical conformation of the ventricular system. In Huntington disease, in which the caudate nucleus is degenerated, the anterior pole of the lateral ventricle is broadened medially to reflect the flattened head of the caudate nucleus. Midline shifts, presence of an impinging tumor, or expanded ventricles in hydrocephalus are also visible in imaging studies. The narrowest portion of the ventricular system, the cerebral aqueduct, is a site of potential blockage of flow of the CSF (atresia in development), resulting in an expansion of the upstream third ventricle and lateral ventricles (internal hydrocephalus). The exit routes from the ventricular system at the foramina of Magendie and Luschka are also sites at which blockage of CSF flow may occur, resulting in internal hydrocephalus throughout the ventricular system. The arachnoid granulations may be blocked in diseases such as acute purulent meningitis, resulting in increased intracranial pressure and external hydrocephalus. The production and absorption of CSF must exactly balance for CSF pressure to remain constant and normal. CSF may be sampled from the lumbar cistern with a lumbar puncture; the resultant analysis of pressure, electrolytes, cellularity, glucose, protein, pH, and other chemical parameters provides valuable information about the state of the nervous system, all of which are essential for accurate neurological diagnosis.

Internal hydrocephalus—increased intracranial pressure with expansion of the ventricles above the level of the block.

External hydrocephalus—increased intracranial pressure in the ventricular system and the subarachnoid spaces.

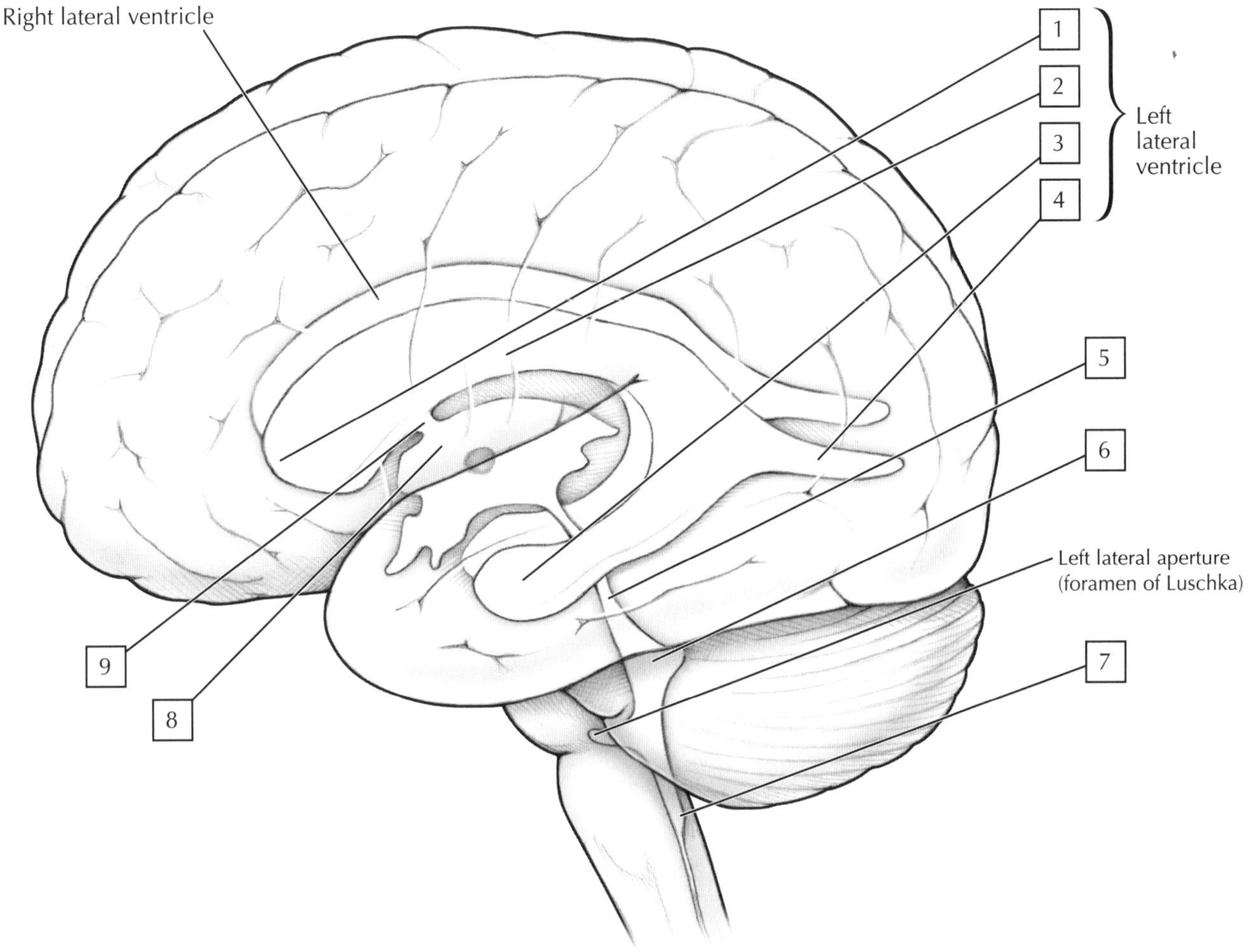

CSF Composition

	CSF	Blood plasma
Na^+ (mEq/L)	140–145	135–147
K^+ (mEq/L)	3	3.5–5.0
Cl^- (mEq/L)	115–120	95–105
HCO_3^- (mEq/L)	20	22–28
Glucose (mg/dL)	50–75	70–110
Protein (g/dL)	0.05–0.07	6.0–7.8
pH	7.3	7.35–7.45

4 Midsagittal View of the Ventricular System

A midsagittal view demonstrates structural features of the ventricular system. The **fourth ventricle** is rhomboid shaped (in the rhombencephalon, consisting of the medulla and pons), peaked toward the central zone and tapering at either end. The fourth ventricle extends laterally, forming lateral recesses, from which CSF escapes into the subarachnoid space. Caudally, the fourth ventricle tapers into the median aperture, the **foramen of Magendie**. The rostral end of the fourth ventricle tapers into the **cerebral aqueduct**, traveling through the central zone of the midbrain central (periaqueductal) gray. The aqueduct opens rostrally into a shallow midline vertical expanse of the ventricular system, the third ventricle, bordering the medial-most zones of the hypothalamus and **thalamus** and communicating with the lateral ventricles via the **interventricular foramen of Monro**. The roof of the third ventricle and the roof of the fourth ventricle contain **choroid plexus**, a source (along with the choroid plexus of the lateral ventricles) of secretion of the CSF. At the rostral end of the third ventricle is the rostral termination of the original neural tube, the **lamina terminalis.**

The roof and dorsolateral walls of the fourth ventricle are adjacent to the zone where the deep cerebellar nuclei and regions of the **cerebellum** are found. The floor of the fourth ventricle is composed of the upper portion of the brainstem tegmentum, including the tubercles, eminences, **colliculi** (e.g., facial colliculus), and areas associated with cranial nerve (CN) nuclei and their connections. On the floor of the fourth ventricle, laterally, is the **sulcus limitans**, the developmental landmark separating the alar plate (mainly sensory) above from the basal plate (mainly motor and autonomic) below. That separation of the sensory components laterally and motor and autonomic components medially is retained in the adult **medulla** and **pons**.

COLOR the following structures, using a separate color for each structure.

☐ 1. **Choroid plexus of the 3rd ventricle**
☐ 2. **Interventricular foramen of Monro**
☐ 3. **Thalamus**
☐ 4. **Lamina terminalis**
☐ 5. **Superior and inferior colliculi**
☐ 6. **Pons**
☐ 7. **4th ventricle**
☐ 8. **Tonsil of the cerebellum**
☐ 9. **Median aperture of Magendie**
☐ 10. **Cerebral aqueduct (of Sylvius)**
☐ 11. **Choroid plexus of the 4th ventricle**

Clinical Note

The choroid plexus is the source of production of the CSF from the lateral, third, and fourth ventricles. Production and absorption of CSF must be exactly balanced; even subtle differences can lead to alterations in intracranial pressure. Several pathological situations can lead to increased intracranial pressure and hydrocephalus. The most common source is outflow obstruction, either at the cerebral aqueduct or medullary foramina of Luschka and Magendie (internal hydrocephalus) or at the arachnoid granulations protruding into the dural sinuses (external hydrocephalus). On occasion, the choroid plexus may be subject to inflammation or a papilloma, resulting in hypersecretion of CSF, or alternatively may be damaged by trauma, radiation, meningitis, or other insults, resulting in hyposecretion of CSF. Diminished secretion of CSF is accompanied by a persistent headache.

Increased intracranial pressure in the posterior fossa, or the herniation of the cerebellar tonsils into the foramen magnum, may obstruct the outflow of CSF into the subarachnoid space.

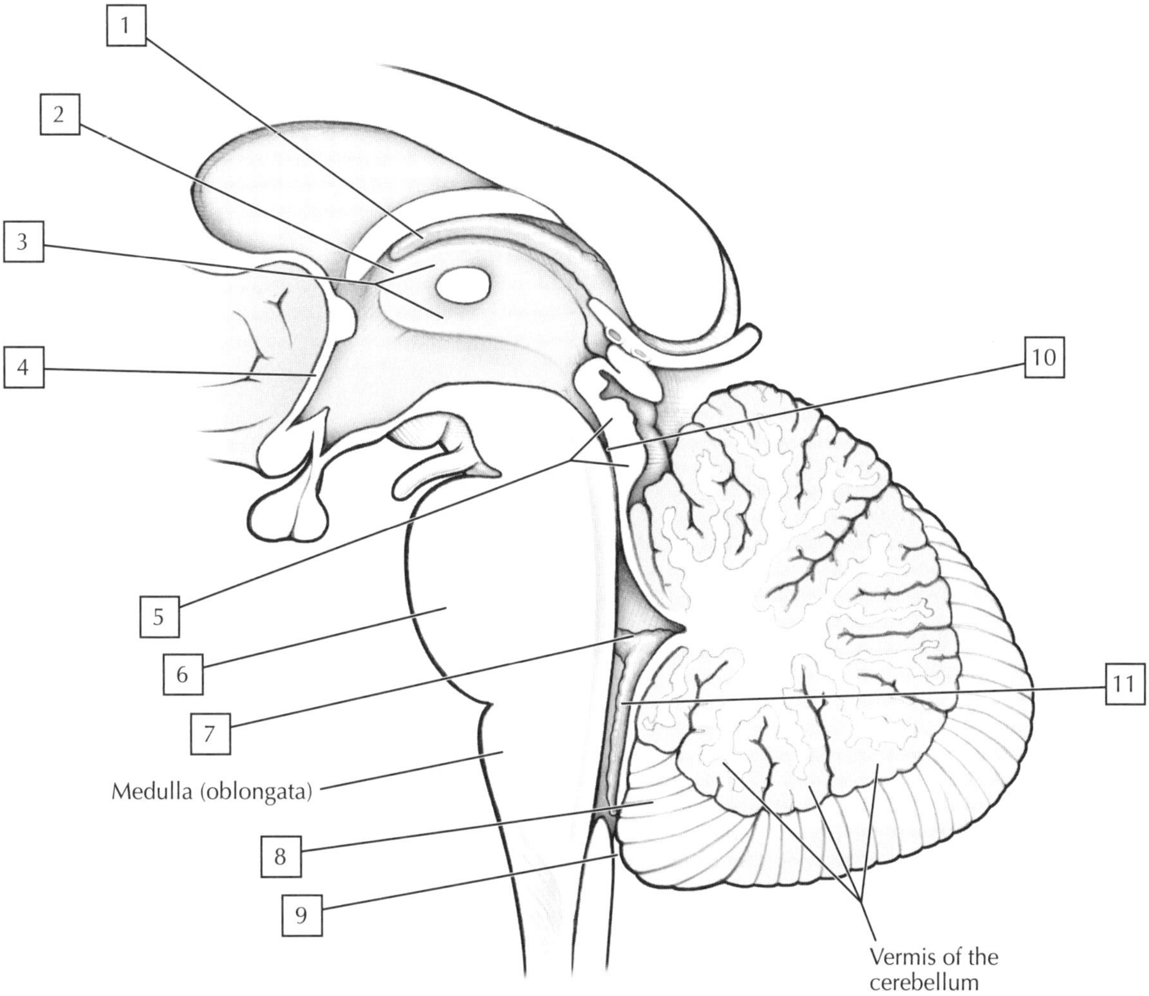
1
2
3
4
5
6
7
Medulla (oblongata)
8
9
10
11
Vermis of the cerebellum

4 Circulation of the Cerebrospinal Fluid

The **cerebrospinal fluid (CSF)** is secreted from the **choroid plexus** in the lateral, third, and fourth ventricles and flows in a rostral-to-caudal direction. The CSF helps to provide protection and buoyancy to central neural tissue and may also serve to convey molecular signals (e.g., prostaglandins, interleukins) from one CNS site to another, especially in the region of the hypothalamus. CSF exits through foramina in the fourth ventricle (Luschka and Magendie) into the **subarachnoid space**. Expanded regions of subarachnoid space are named **cisterns**. At the caudal end of the spinal cord, the **lumbar cistern**, with its nerve roots forming the cauda equina, provides an excellent site for sampling CSF. The **cisterna magna**, at the junction of the posterior cerebellum and the dorsal brainstem, is an enlarged cistern of CSF. Other cisterns visible on imaging include the **prepontine cistern**, the **interpeduncular cistern**, the **chiasmatic cistern**, and the **cistern of the great cerebral vein (of Galen).** The terminal point of CSF flow is the **arachnoid granulations**, which act as one-way valves to allow the escape of CSF into the dural sinuses and finally into the venous drainage from the brain (internal jugular vein).

Bridging veins and arteries are found in the subarachnoid space, especially in close apposition to the dural sinuses, such as the **superior sagittal sinus**.

COLOR each of the following structures, using a separate color for each structure.

- ☐ 1. **Bridging veins**
- ☐ 2. **Choroid plexus of the lateral ventricle**
- ☐ 3. **Superior sagittal sinus**
- ☐ 4. **Subarachnoid space**
- ☐ 5. **Arachnoid granulations**
- ☐ 6. **Cistern of the great cerebral vein (of Galen)**
- ☐ 7. **Cisterna magna**
- ☐ 8. **Choroid plexus of the 4th ventricle**
- ☐ 9. **Prepontine cistern**
- ☐ 10. **Interpeduncular cistern**
- ☐ 11. **Choroid plexus of the 3rd ventricle**
- ☐ 12. **Chiasmatic cistern**

Clinical Note

The flow of CSF from its initial secretion by the choroid plexus, its circulation through the internal ventricular system, its flow into the subarachnoid space, and back into the venous drainage of the brain through the arachnoid granulations, especially into the superior sagittal sinus, provides a precisely balanced fluid system to cushion and protect the CNS, including the optic nerve (which is a CNS tract). Any imbalance between production and absorption has significant clinical consequences with intracranial pressure.

Both veins and arteries traverse the subarachnoid space. The **bridging veins** extend through the subarachnoid space to drain venous blood into the venous sinuses. Trauma, or rapid torsional movements of the head, may cause a tear in bridging veins at the site where they enter the venous sinus. In elderly patients, where some degree of cerebral shrinkage may have occurred, the cranial contents may be more mobile and more subject to tearing movements. The resultant venous blood from the torn bridging vein can dissect the dura from the underlying arachnoid, producing a subdural hematoma. This happens more often in elderly patients but can also happen in young individuals during severe trauma. The resultant hematoma acts as a space-occupying mass, may pull fluid into the site of the bleed (edema), and can cause increased intracranial pressure and herniation of the brain, leading to major neurological damage and even death.

Cerebral arteries traveling in the subarachnoid space are subject to the presence of Berry aneurysms, weaknesses in the vessel wall that may rupture and cause a subarachnoid hemorrhage. This will result in "the worst headache of my life," irritation of the meninges, and possibly coma and even death.

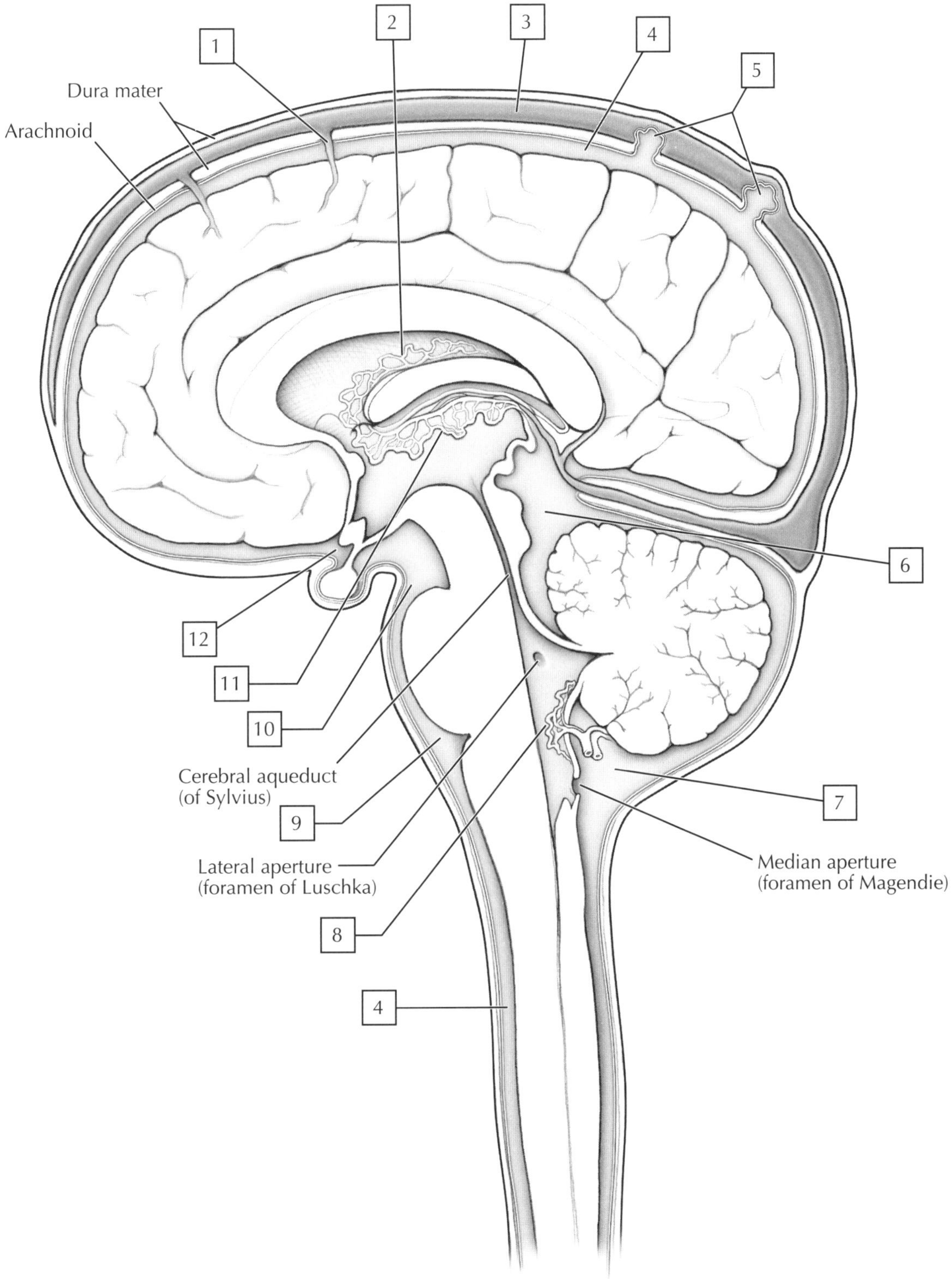
1
2
3
4
5
Dura mater
Arachnoid
6
7
12
11
10
Cerebral aqueduct
(of Sylvius)
9
Lateral aperture
(foramen of Luschka)
8
4
Median aperture
(foramen of Magendie)

4 Arterial Supply to the Brain and Meninges

The blood supply to the brain derives from the paired **internal carotid arteries** and the paired **vertebral arteries.** The **left common carotid artery** branches from the arch of the aorta, and the **right common carotid artery** branches from the brachiocephalic trunk; these common carotid arteries branch into the **internal carotid arteries** and the **external carotid arteries**. The internal carotid circulation is called the **anterior circulation** and supplies most of the forebrain (except for the occipital lobe and inferior portion of the temporal lobe) with blood. The middle meningeal artery, a branch of the external carotid artery, and other meningeal arteries supply the meninges with blood. The paired **vertebral arteries** branch from the **subclavian arteries**, ascend to the brainstem, and unite to form the **basilar artery** at the base of the pons; this **vertebrobasilar circulation** is called the **posterior circulation**, supplying the occipital lobe and the inferior portion of the temporal lobe. The internal carotid arteries give rise to the **anterior cerebral arteries (ACAs)** and the **middle cerebral arteries (MCAs)**, whereas the basilar artery gives rise to the paired **posterior cerebral arteries (PCAs)**. The vertebrobasilar system also supplies the brainstem, cerebellum, and rostral spinal cord with blood **(anterior spinal artery [ASA])**. The vertebral arteries and the basilar artery give rise to paramedian, short circumferential, and long circumferential branches, which supply specific anatomical territories of the brainstem and cerebellum.

Most of the major arteries supplying blood to the brain are end arteries, with few anastomotic interconnections. At the base of the rostral brainstem and diencephalon is the **circle of Willis**, an apparent circle composed of the paired ACAs, MCAs, and PCAs, the paired **posterior communicating arteries**, and the **anterior communicating artery**. In actuality, the circle of Willis does not usually provide robust flow between the anterior and posterior circulations. Therefore major occlusions of brain arteries usually produce downstream ischemic damage. Because the brain requires disproportionate amounts of oxygen and glucose for aerobic metabolism, the tolerance of brain tissue for ischemia is highly limited, and damage can ensue within minutes of an ischemic state.

COLOR each of the following structures, using a separate color for each structure.

- ☐ 1. **Right external carotid artery**
- ☐ 2. **Anterior cerebral arteries**
- ☐ 3. **Anterior communicating artery**
- ☐ 4. **Posterior communicating arteries**
- ☐ 5. **Middle meningeal artery**
- ☐ 6. **Posterior cerebral arteries**
- ☐ 7. **Basilar artery**
- ☐ 8. **Right internal carotid artery**
- ☐ 9. **Vertebral arteries**
- ☐ 10. **Right common carotid artery**
- ☐ 11. **Middle cerebral arteries**
- ☐ 12. **Anterior spinal artery**
- ☐ 13. **Circle of Willis (*dotted*)**

Clinical Note

The internal carotid arteries branch from the common carotid artery; this bifurcation represents a zone of turbulence, where atherosclerotic plaques commonly occur, leading to potential downstream ischemia in the territory of the MCA and ACA (termed a *stroke*). Treatment options for significant atherosclerotic plaquing include medical treatment, carotid endarterectomy (removal of the atherosclerotic plaques), and placement of a carotid stent. Any arterial site of tortuous bends may enhance turbulent flow and increase the likelihood of atherosclerosis. The internal carotid artery passes through the cavernous sinus and may form carotid-cavernous fistulae, resulting in damage to the extraocular cranial nerves (CNs) and the trigeminal ophthalmic division (CN V1), which also pass through the cavernous sinus. The first branch of the internal carotid artery is the **ophthalmic artery** (giving rise to the **central retinal artery**), a common site where **transient ischemic attacks**, forerunners of a potential full-blown stroke, may occur. A tear in the **middle meningeal artery** from a skull fracture can precipitate an epidural bleed, arterial in nature, which may become a space-occupying lesion with possible increased intracranial pressure and brain herniation.

Note: The ophthalmic, maxillary, and mandibular divisions of CN V are denoted by CN V1, CN V2, and CN V3, respectively.

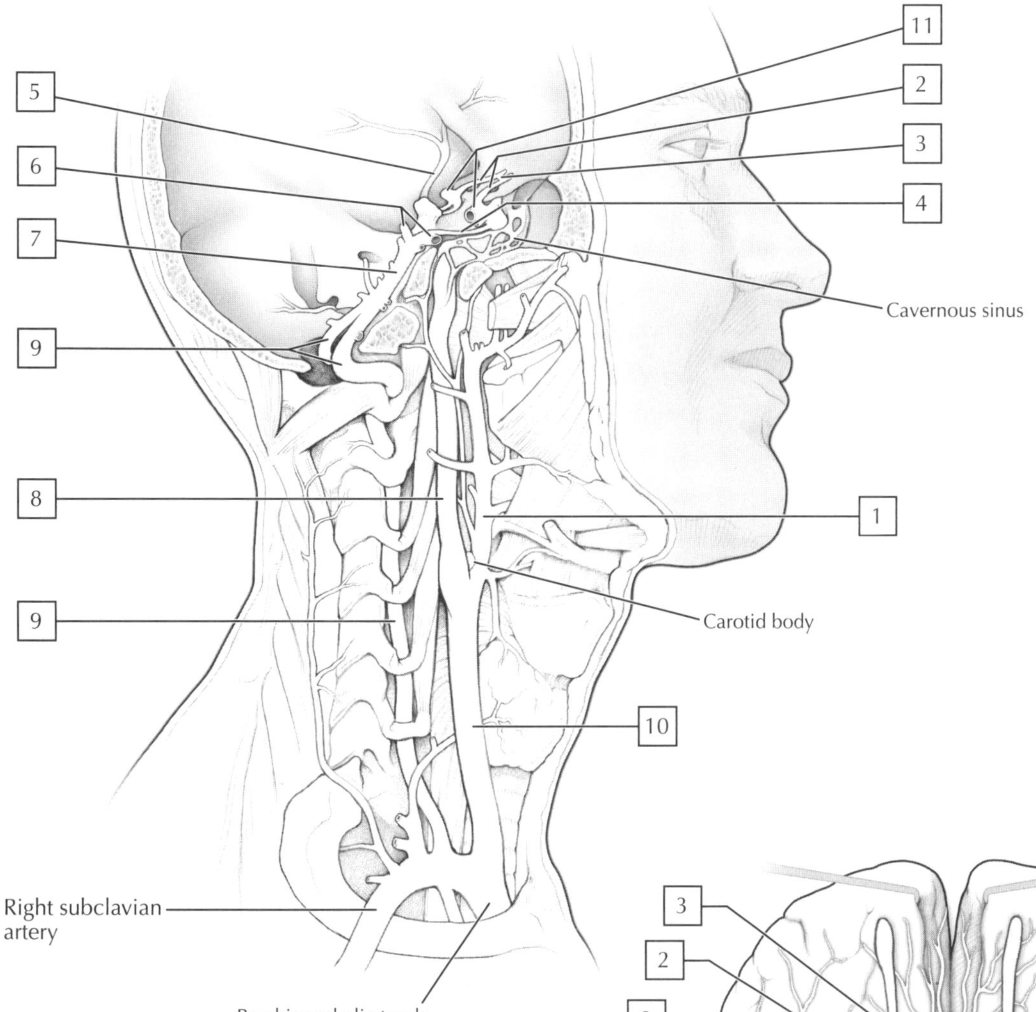

A. Arteries to brain and meninges—lateral view

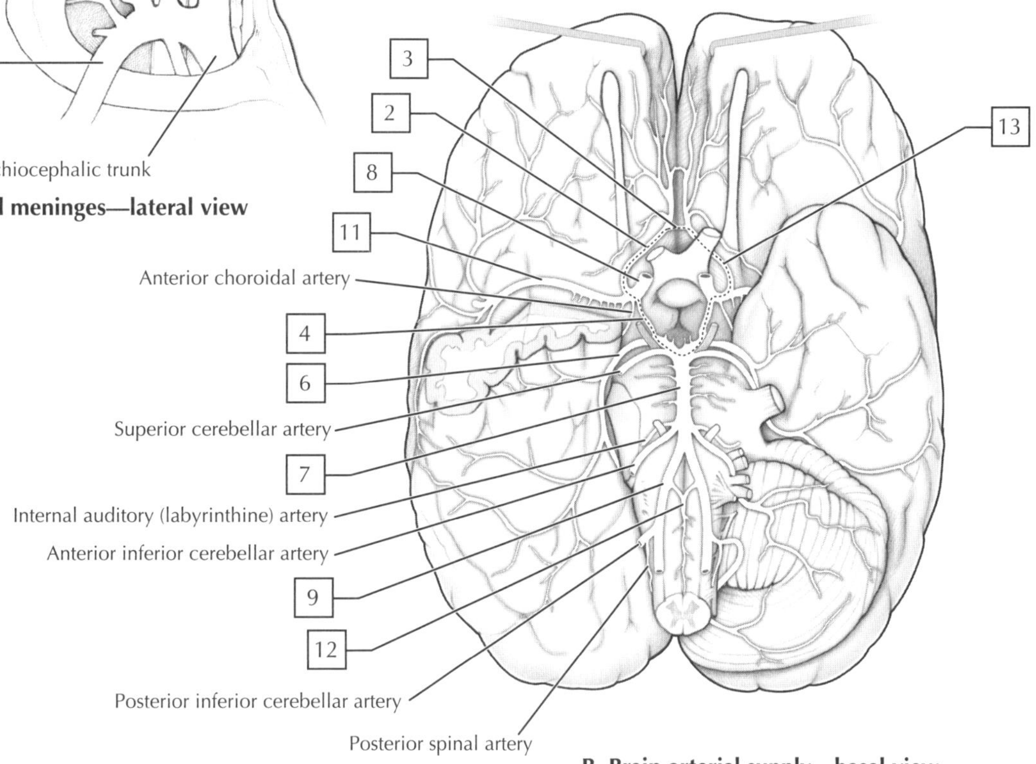

B. Brain arterial supply—basal view

4 Arterial Distribution to the Brain: Circle of Willis, Choroidal Arteries, and Lenticulostriate Arteries

The anterior circulation (**MCAs** and **ACAs**) and the posterior circulation (**PCAs**) join together at the **circle of Willis**, interconnected by the paired **posterior communicating arteries**. The **anterior communicating artery** interconnects the paired ACAs. Although this arrangement appears to provide interconnection for blood flow between the anterior and posterior circulation, this circle of Willis is only patent for such purposes in approximately 20% of the population.

The **choroidal arteries** provide arterial branches to parts of the midbrain, diencephalon, and telencephalon. The **anterior choroidal artery** arises from the **internal carotid artery** just proximal to its branching to form the MCA and the ACA. The anterior choroidal artery supplies the **choroid plexus** of the lateral and third ventricles, forebrain structures (part of the internal capsule, globus pallidus, tail of the caudate nucleus, part of the hippocampal formation, and the amygdala), diencephalic structures (optic chiasm and tract, part of the lateral geniculate nucleus), and midbrain structures (part of the cerebral peduncle, red nucleus, and substantia nigra).

The **posterior choroidal arteries** are branches of the PCAs; they traverse the foramen of Monro and supply the choroid plexus of the lateral ventricles. The medial branches (**medial posterior choroidal artery**) run beneath the splenium of the corpus callosum and supply the choroid plexus of the third ventricle, the midbrain tegmentum, the posterior thalamus, and the pineal gland. The lateral branches (**lateral posterior choroidal artery**) supply the choroid plexus of the lateral ventricle, parts of the basal ganglia (posterior part of the caudate nucleus), pulvinar, parts of the posterior thalamus, the fornix, and sometimes parts of the hippocampus, parahippocampal gyrus, and medial temporal lobe.

The **lenticulostriate arteries** are small, penetrating arteries arising from the proximal MCA; they supply the **posterior limb of the internal capsule**, parts of the basal ganglia (lateral putamen, globus pallidus, and parts of the head and body of the caudate nucleus), and the external capsule.

COLOR the following structures, using a separate color for each structure.

- ☐ 1. **Anterior communicating artery**
- ☐ 2. **Anterior cerebral artery**
- ☐ 3. **Middle cerebral artery**
- ☐ 4. **Posterior communicating arteries**
- ☐ 5. **Anterior choroidal artery**
- ☐ 6. **Medial posterior choroidal artery**
- ☐ 7. **Lateral posterior choroidal artery**
- ☐ 8. **Choroid plexus of the lateral ventricle**
- ☐ 9. **Posterior cerebral artery**
- ☐ 10. **Lenticulostriate arteries**
- ☐ 11. **Internal carotid artery**
- ☐ 12. **Internal capsule**

Clinical Note

Occlusion of the anterior choroidal artery most significantly affects the blood supply to the posterior limb of the internal capsule, the thalamus, and the optic chiasm and tract. The resultant damage includes contralateral hemiplegia (upper motor neuron syndrome with hyperreflexia and hypertonus), contralateral diminished sensation, and contralateral homonymous hemianopia.

A medial posterior choroidal artery infarct rarely occurs in isolation and is usually accompanied by vascular damage to an array of other branches of the PCA.

An infarct in the lateral posterior choroidal artery is seen occasionally. The main functional deficit is usually a contralateral visual field deficit, quadrantanopia or hemianopia, due to involvement of the lateral geniculate nucleus. Additional problems may include a hemisensory deficit, hemineglect, aphasia, and memory disturbance due to hippocampal and temporal lobe involvement. Damage in the lateral posterior choroidal artery is usually not severe and is often transient.

An infarct in the lenticulostriate arteries, branches of the MCA, often results in contralateral hemiplegia and contralateral sensory deficit. Language may be affected (medial temporal lobe involvement on the left), and a contralateral upper quadrantanopia may occur (Meyer loop involvement in the temporal lobe). Involvement of lenticulostriate arteries in occlusive vascular disease is often a classic component of an MCA stroke.

Arterial Distribution to the Brain: Circle of Willis, Choroidal Arteries, and Lenticulostriate Arteries

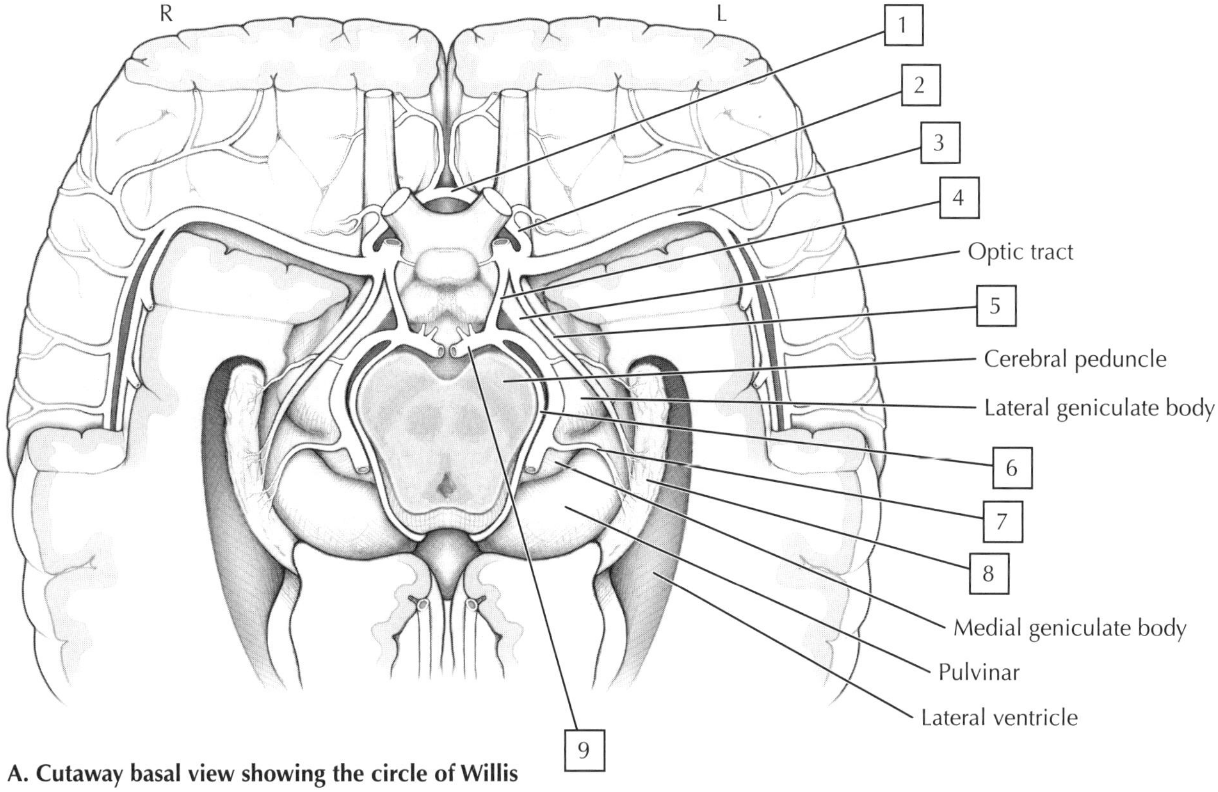

A. Cutaway basal view showing the circle of Willis

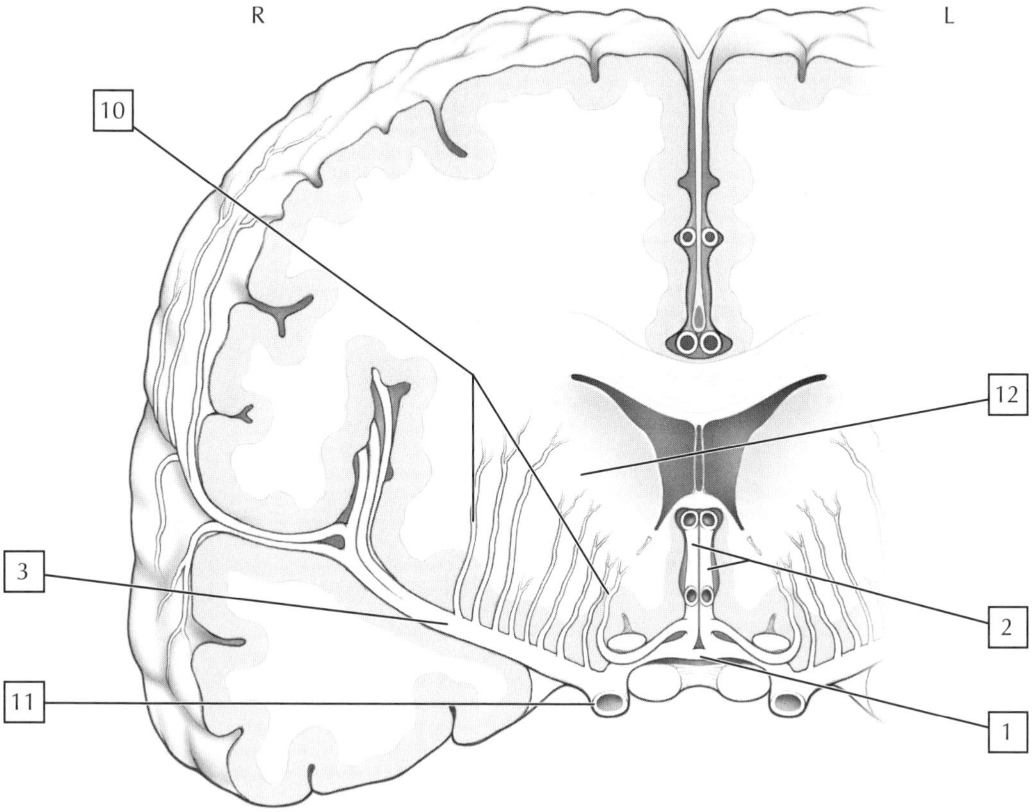

B. Coronal section through the head of the caudate nucleus

4 Arterial Distribution to the Brain: The Cerebral Arteries

The cerebral arteries are the end-artery distribution of the anterior and posterior circulations. The **internal carotid artery** branches into the **ACA** and the **MCA.** The end branch of the **vertebrobasilar system** is the **PCAs.** The MCA emerges from the **lateral fissure** and sends many branches into discrete regions along the surface of the convexity of the frontal and parietal lobes (separated by the **central sulcus**), and the anterior and medial portions of the temporal lobe. End branch infarcts can result in contralateral deficits of the motor and sensory systems, affecting mainly the upper extremity and the facial region. Deeper branches of the MCA distribute into the internal capsule and the basal ganglia; deeper or more extensive infarcts may affect all descending axons and ascending sensory axons in the posterior limb of the internal capsule, resulting in contralateral hemiplegia and contralateral loss of sensation.

The ACA distributes blood to the midline regions of the frontal and parietal lobes, particularly the cortical sites (such as the **paracentral lobule**) representing motor and sensory processing from the contralateral lower extremity. End branch infarcts will affect the lower contralateral extremity.

The PCA distributes blood to the **occipital lobe** and the **inferior surface of the temporal lobe**. End branch infarcts, especially those branches that run in the **calcarine fissure**, will affect mainly the visual fields, resulting in a contralateral hemianopia.

Clinical Note

The MCA, with its many cortical branches and penetrating branches, provides widespread regions of the convexity of the hemisphere and deeper structures of the forebrain with arterial blood. This arterial system is a very common site of vascular infarcts and insults, known as *strokes*. The early warning of a pending stroke may be a transient ischemic attack, a brief period of a frank neurological deficit (such as fleeting blindness) attributable to occlusion of a branch of the proximal internal carotid artery or the MCA. Strokes involving the MCA fall into several categories: (1) **atherosclerotic strokes** (approximately one-third); (2) **embolic strokes** (approximately one-third); (3) **lacunar infarcts** in small distal arteries (approximately 20%); (4) **cerebral hemorrhages** (approximately 10%); and (5) **ruptured aneurysms** (often from an artery in the circle of Willis) and arteriovenous malformations (a small percent).

The lacunar infarcts are small (a few microns to 2 cm in diameter) and occur in small, penetrating arteries, often those supplying the internal capsule, the putamen and caudate nucleus, the thalamus, the pons, and regions of cerebral white matter. These lacunar infarcts usually are associated with atherosclerotic disease accompanying diabetes and/or hypertension. Because these are small circumscribed vascular lesions, the symptoms will reflect the exact location and distribution of the involved artery.

COLOR the following structures, using a separate color for each structure.

- ☐ 1. **Internal carotid artery**
- ☐ 2. **Anterior cerebral artery**
- ☐ 3. **Middle cerebral artery**
- ☐ 4. **Central sulcus**
- ☐ 5. **Lateral fissure**
- ☐ 6. **Paracentral lobule**
- ☐ 7. **Posterior cerebral artery**
- ☐ 8. **Occipital lobe**
- ☐ 9. **Calcarine fissure (sulcus)**
- ☐ 10. **Inferior surface of the temporal lobe**

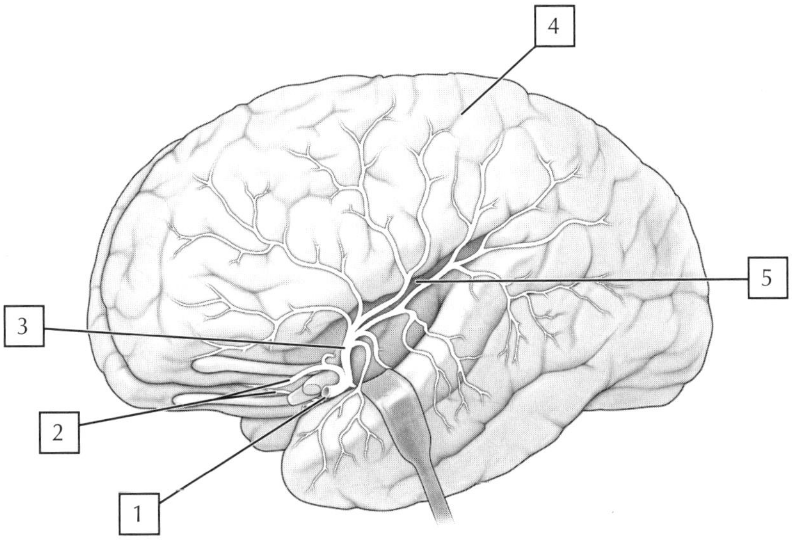

A. Lateral view with lateral fissure opened

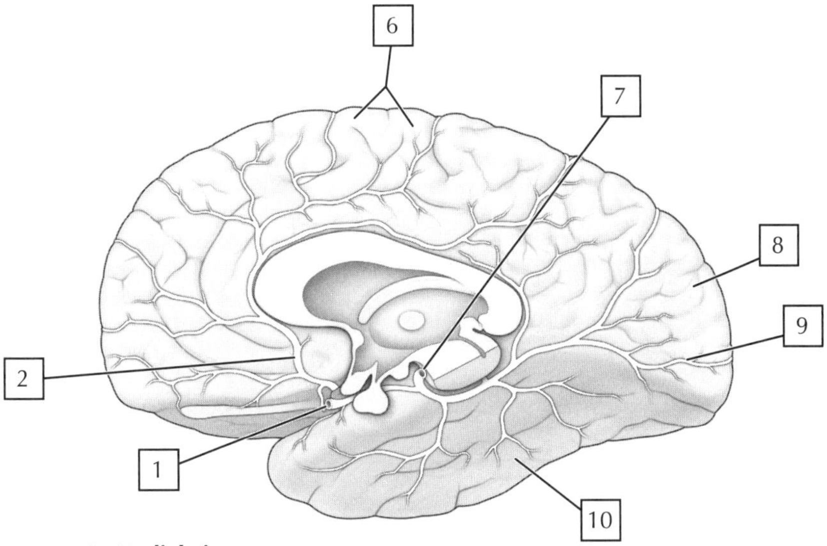

B. Medial view

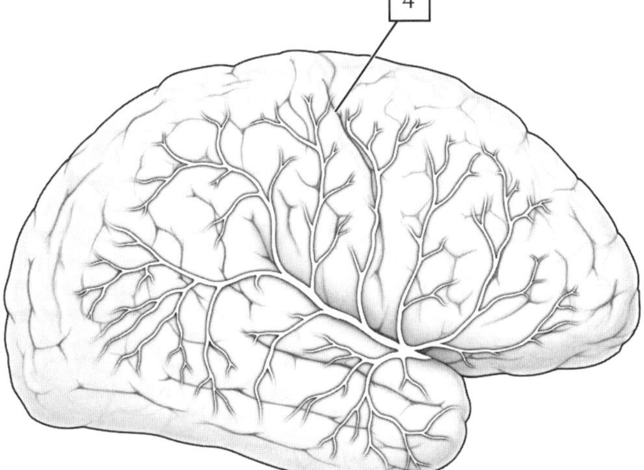

C. Lateral view with lateral fissure closed

4 Arterial Distribution to the Brain: The Vertebrobasilar System

The **vertebral arteries** arise from the subclavian arteries and ascend toward the brain. They make a hairpin turn, penetrate the dura, and travel along the anterior surface of the medulla, sending penetrating paramedian arteries and circumferential (short and long) arteries to supply the **medulla**. The vertebral arteries unite at the rostral end of the medulla to form the single **basilar artery**, which runs rostrally in the basilar groove of the pons. Similar branches from the basilar artery supply the **pons** with arterial blood. The end branches of the basilar artery are the paired **PCAs**, which loop posteriorly to supply the occipital lobe and the inferior surface of the temporal lobe. The PCA also gives rise to many penetrating branches, such as the **posterior choroidal arteries**, which supply components of the forebrain and midbrain with blood.

The paramedian penetrating branches of the vertebral artery and basilar artery supply a wedge-shaped zone of tissue that often includes CNs (ipsilaterally), and the corticospinal/upper motor system (regulating contralateral lower motor neurons and associated musculature); hence an infarct results in an "alternating hemiplegia" with ipsilateral CN deficits and contralateral upper motor neuron deficits. Some of the major **circumferential arteries** include, from caudal to rostral, the **posterior inferior cerebellar artery**, the **anterior inferior cerebellar artery**, the **internal auditory (labyrinthine) artery**, and the **superior cerebellar artery**. The caudal portion of the vertebral arteries gives rise to paired short branches, which unite to form the **anterior spinal artery (ASA)**, running along the anterior median fissure, and the paired **posterior spinal arteries (PSAs)**, running along the medial region of the dorsal root entry zone. These arteries functionally supply the cervical spinal cord with blood.

Clinical Note

The paramedian penetrating arteries from the vertebral artery and basilar artery supply a medial wedge of tissue in the medulla or pons with blood. An infarct results in ipsilateral CN damage and contralateral motor and sensory changes in the body. In the medulla, such a syndrome results in an ipsilateral CN XII lesion, with weakness and wasting of ipsilateral tongue muscles, contralateral hemiparesis in the body (from damage to descending upper motor axons of the corticospinal system), and a contralateral loss of fine discriminative touch, vibratory sensation, and joint position sense (epicritic sensory modalities) in the body (from damage to the medial lemniscus), with sparing of the entire protopathic system for pain and temperature sensation (spinothalamic/spinoreticular system, located laterally).

Damage to a circumferential artery results in a seemingly confusing array of symptoms, unless the detailed anatomy of the arterial distribution is considered. An infarct in the posterior inferior cerebellar artery (lateral medullary syndrome, Wallenberg syndrome) results in (1) loss of pain and temperature sensation in the ipsilateral face (descending nucleus and tract of CN V) and the contralateral body (spinothalamic/spinoreticular system); (2) dysphagia and dysarthria (ipsilateral nucleus ambiguus); (3) ataxia and falling to the ipsilateral side (inferior cerebellar peduncle and its tracts); (4) vertigo with nausea, vomiting, and nystagmus (ipsilateral vestibular nuclei); and (5) ipsilateral Horner syndrome (ptosis, miosis, hemianhidrosis) from damage to the descending fibers in the lateral medulla controlling the T1–T2 intermediolateral sympathetic preganglionic outflow to the superior cervical ganglion.

COLOR the following structures, using a separate color for each structure.

- ☐ 1. **Superior cerebellar artery**
- ☐ 2. **Basilar artery**
- ☐ 3. **Pons**
- ☐ 4. **Internal auditory (labyrinthine) artery**
- ☐ 5. **Anterior inferior cerebellar artery**
- ☐ 6. **Medulla**
- ☐ 7. **Posterior inferior cerebellar artery**
- ☐ 8. **Vertebral artery**
- ☐ 9. **Anterior spinal artery**
- ☐ 10. **Posterior spinal artery**
- ☐ 11. **Posterior cerebral artery**
- ☐ 12. **Posterior (lateral) choroidal artery**

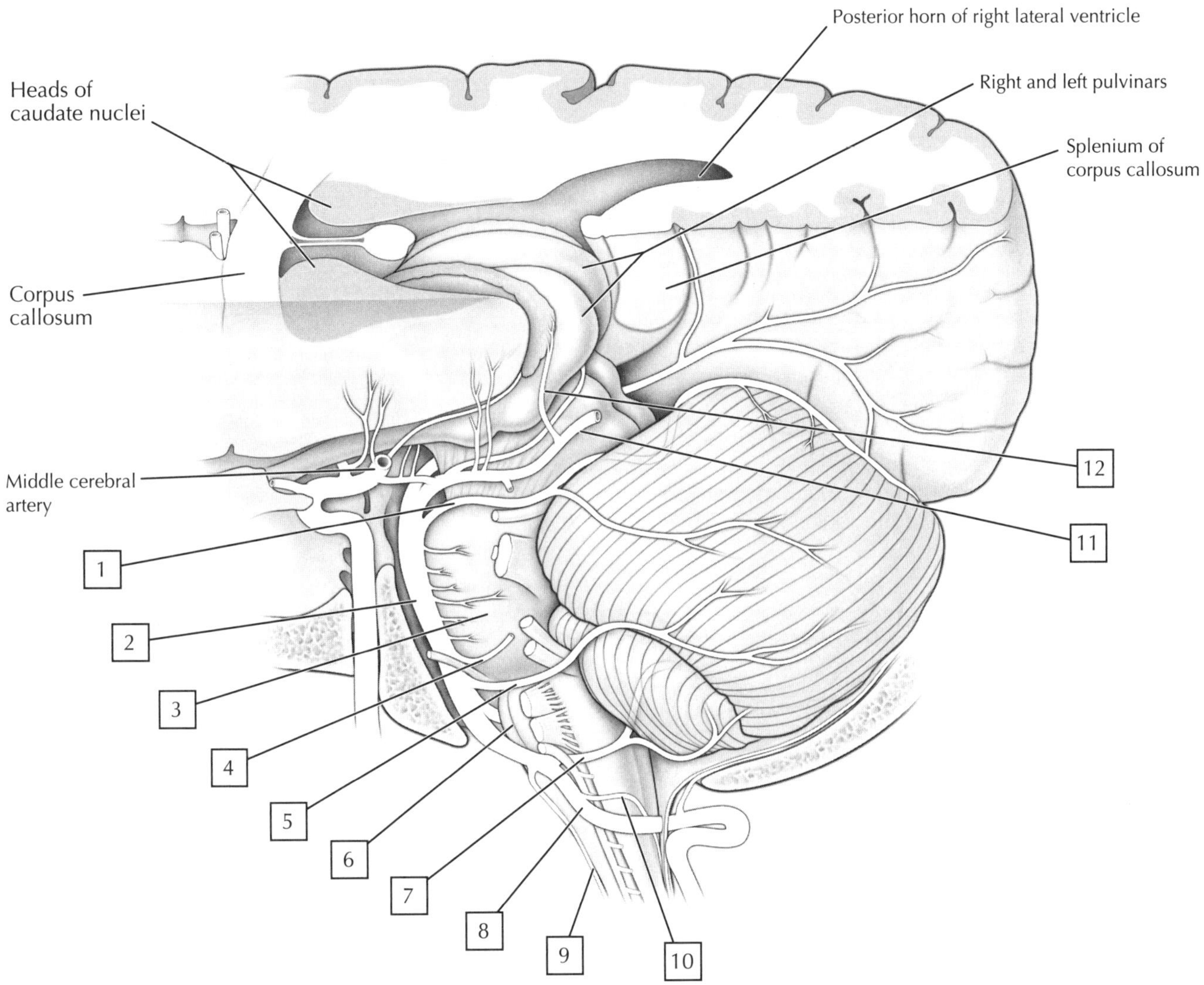
Posterior horn of right lateral ventricle
Heads of caudate nuclei
Right and left pulvinars
Splenium of corpus callosum
Corpus callosum
Middle cerebral artery
12
11
1
2
3
4
5
6
7
8
9
10

4 Blood Supply to the Hypothalamus and Pituitary Gland

The blood supply to the **hypothalamus** derives from many penetrating branches from vessels of the circle of Willis, including the ACA and the posterior communicating artery (PCA), and from the internal carotid artery (ICA). The **superior hypophyseal artery (anterior and posterior branches)** derived from the internal carotid artery (or sometimes the posterior communicating artery) also provides some arterial blood supply to the hypothalamus. There are numerous and variable anastomotic vascular channels among these small, penetrating arterial branches.

The superior hypophyseal arteries also supply the **infundibular stalk** and anastomose with branches of the **inferior hypophyseal arteries**, derived from the ICA. This primary hypophyseal portal system arises from small arterioles and a **primary plexus of the hypophyseal portal system**. These capillaries coalesce into **long hypophyseal veins**, which give rise to a **secondary hypophyseal plexus**, with a second set of capillaries. This portal vascular system allows neurons in the hypothalamus, which produce releasing factors and inhibitory factors for the secretion of anterior pituitary hormones from **the anterior pituitary gland (adenohypophysis)**, to secrete these factors into a private portal system that delivers them to cells in the anterior pituitary in extraordinarily high concentrations, far higher than found in the general circulation. Anterior pituitary hormones are then secreted into the efferent venous flow, which empties into the general circulation through the **cavernous sinus**.

Blood supply to the **posterior pituitary gland (neurohypophysis)** derives from the medial and lateral branches of the inferior hypophyseal artery, which then branches into a regular, single capillary plexus, into which the posterior pituitary hormones, oxytocin and (arginine) vasopressin are secreted. These hormones continue into the general circulation through the efferent veins via the cavernous sinus. This vascular arrangement is not a portal vascular system.

Clinical Note

The hypophyseal portal system of the anterior pituitary is only one of three such systems in the body (others are the hepatic portal system and the adrenal portal system). This vascular arrangement permits exquisite control of the secretion of anterior pituitary hormones by neurons of the hypothalamus that produce and excrete releasing factors and inhibitory factors. This arrangement also allows peripheral feedback from target organ hormones back on the anterior pituicytes and releasing factor/inhibitory factor-producing hypothalamic neurons. As an example, corticotropin-releasing factor (hormone) is secreted from hypothalamic neurons into the hypophyseal portal system to regulate the secretion of adrenocorticotropic hormone (ACTH) from pituicytes. Vasopressin also aids in the regulation of the secretion of ACTH. ACTH is secreted into the general circulation. It acts on cortical cells of the adrenal cortex, which release cortisol and other corticosteroids (called *glucocorticoids*) into the general circulation. Glucocorticoids then provide feedback to both the pituicytes in the anterior pituitary secreting ACTH and the hypothalamic releasing factor and inhibitory factor neurons of the hypothalamus secreting corticotropin releasing factor. This system is called the **hypothalamic–pituitary–adrenal axis**. The glucocorticoids also are secreted into the adrenal portal system, where they provide high concentrations in proximity to the adrenal medullary chromaffin cells. These portally delivered glucocorticoids induce phenylethanolamine *N*-methyl transferase (PNMT), an enzyme that induces the synthesis of epinephrine from norepinephrine, providing an additional major stress hormone component of the sympatho-adrenal system.

The glucocorticoids help to regulate glucose metabolism, insulin secretion, adipose distribution, some immune responses, and many other functions.

COLOR the following structures, using a separate color for each structure.

- ☐ **1. Hypothalamus**
- ☐ **2. Primary plexus of the hypophyseal portal system**
- ☐ **3. Long hypophyseal portal veins**
- ☐ **4. Posterior pituitary lobe (neurohypophysis)**
- ☐ **5. Posterior pituitary capillary plexus**
- ☐ **6. Inferior hypophyseal artery**
- ☐ **7. Secondary plexus of the hypophyseal portal system**
- ☐ **8. Anterior pituitary gland (adenohypophysis)**
- ☐ **9. Infundibular stalk**
- ☐ **10. Superior hypophyseal artery branches**
- ☐ **11. Cavernous sinus**

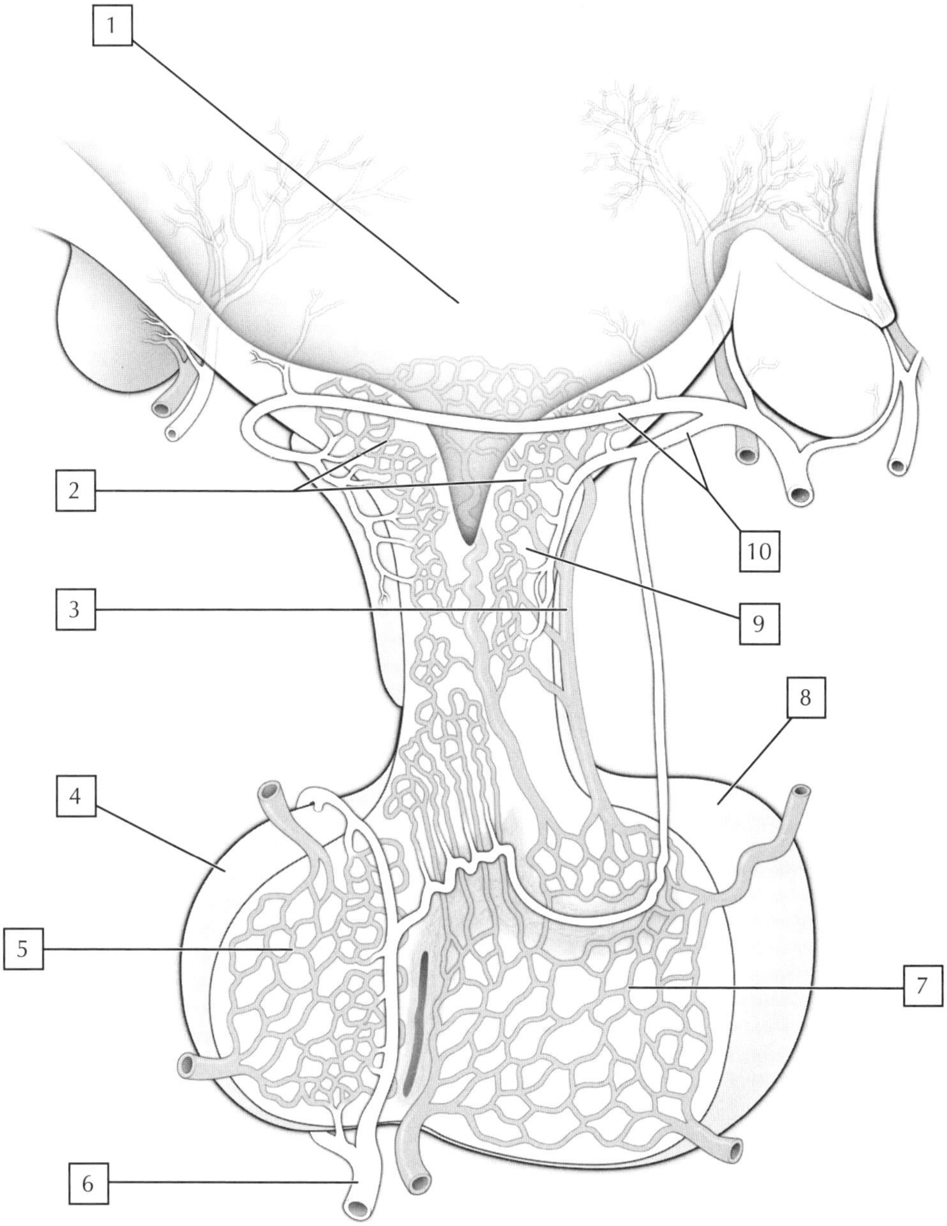
1
2
3
4
5
6
7
8
9
10

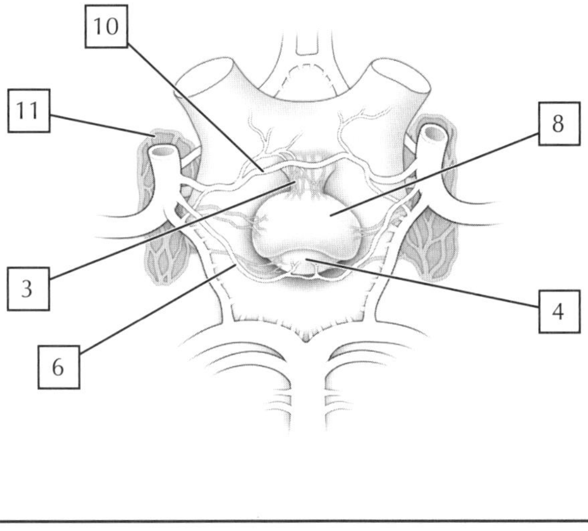
10
11
8
3
4
6

4 Arterial Blood Supply to the Spinal Cord

The major blood supply to the spinal cord arises from branches of the **vertebral arteries**, the **ASA** and the paired **PSAs**, via penetrating branches and a **pial plexus**. The ASA travels at the ventral (anterior) midline of the spinal cord in the anterior median fissure and sends alternating **central branches** into the left and right sides of the spinal cord. The PSAs travel in the **zone medial to the dorsal root entry** and form tortuous plexuses along the entire longitudinal length of the spinal cord. Both the ASA and the PSAs appear to form a full channel for delivery of arterial blood to the entire spinal cord, but the flow from the vertebral arteries into these systems is not sufficient to keep the entire spinal cord fully supplied; it only provides adequate arterial blood flow to the cervical spinal cord. For the rest of the spinal cord, blood flow derived from the aorta travels through the **intercostal arteries** and **radicular arteries**, which extensively anastomose with the spinal arterial systems. There is often one major lumbar **anterior radicular artery (artery of Adamkiewicz)** that provides extensive arterial blood to the spinal cord.

The ASA supplies the anterior two-thirds of the spinal cord, while the PSAs supply the posterior one-third of the spinal cord. In cross section, the inner core (zone) of the spinal cord is provided with blood by the central branches, a middle zone is supplied by both the central branches and branches from the pial plexus, and the outer circumferential zone is supplied by the pial plexus.

COLOR the following structures, using a separate color for each structure.

- ☐ 1. **Anterior spinal artery**
- ☐ 2. **Vertebral arteries**
- ☐ 3. **Anterior radicular artery (artery of Adamkiewicz)**
- ☐ 4. **Intercostal arteries**
- ☐ 5. **Posterior spinal arteries**
- ☐ 6. **Radicular arteries**
- ☐ 7. **Central branches of the spinal arteries**
- ☐ 8. **Pial arterial plexus**
- ☐ 9. **Zone medial to the dorsal root entry zone**
- ☐ 10. **Spinal cord zone supplied by branches from the pial plexus**
- ☐ 11. **Spinal cord zone supplied by central branches and branches from the pial plexus**
- ☐ 12. **Spinal cord zone supplied by central branches**

Clinical Note

The ASA provides alternating central branches into successive longitudinal levels of the spinal cord. If an infarct in this artery occurs, it will likely affect the central branch on one side. Initially, there will be sharp radiating leg pain, accompanied by flaccid paralysis in the affected ipsilateral limb(s). If the infarct is bilateral, the flaccid paralysis will be found in a pattern of paraplegia or quadriplegia. As this acute spinal shock phase resolves over subsequent days/weeks, the paralysis will resolve to lower motor neuronal damage to the neurons of the anterior horn deprived of blood, and an upper motor neuronal pattern for musculature below the level of the lesion, with hypertonus, hyperreflexia, and plantar extensor responses in affected legs (due to damage to the descending lateral corticospinal tract and rubrospinal tract). Bladder, bowel, and erectile function are also affected due to damage to descending control fibers traveling in the lateral funiculus, and will resolve to a status of spastic bladder, reflex bowel contractions, and erectile dysfunction, respectively, if paraplegia or quadriplegia are present. Pain and temperature sensation will be absent as a result of damage to the blood supply to the spinothalamic/spinoreticular system (protopathic somatosensory system). If the ASA damage occurs above the T1 spinal cord level, then Horner syndrome (ptosis, miosis, anhidrosis) also will be seen on the affected side.

A PSA infarct will result in loss of epicritic sensation (fine, discriminative touch, vibratory sensation, joint position sense) below the level of the lesion on the affected side(s) due to loss of function in axons of the dorsal funiculus.

A. Anterior longitudinal view

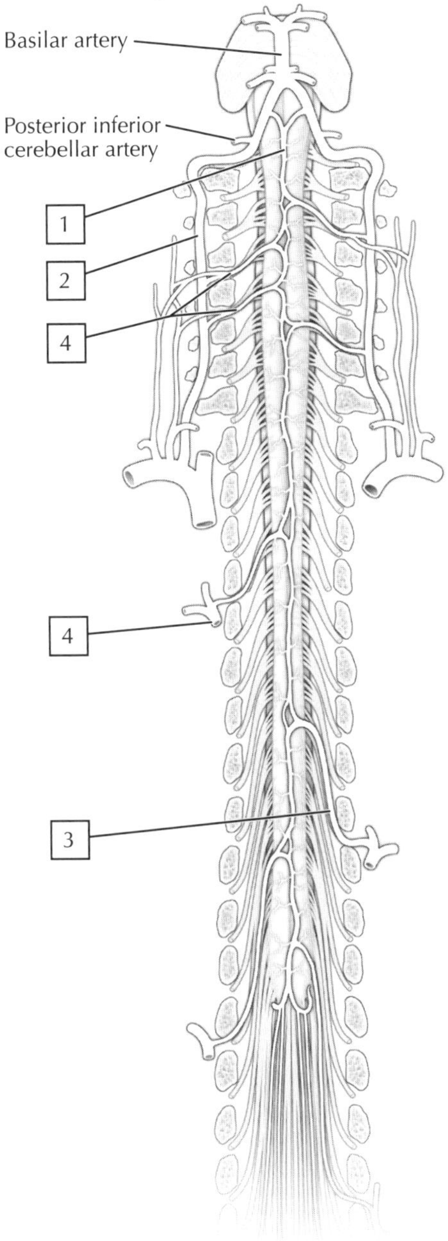

B. Posterior longitudinal view

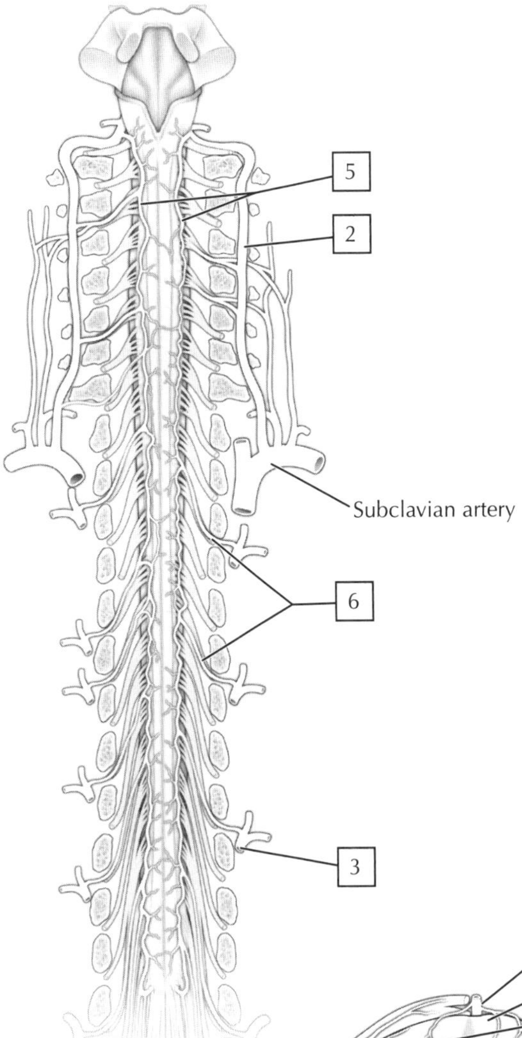

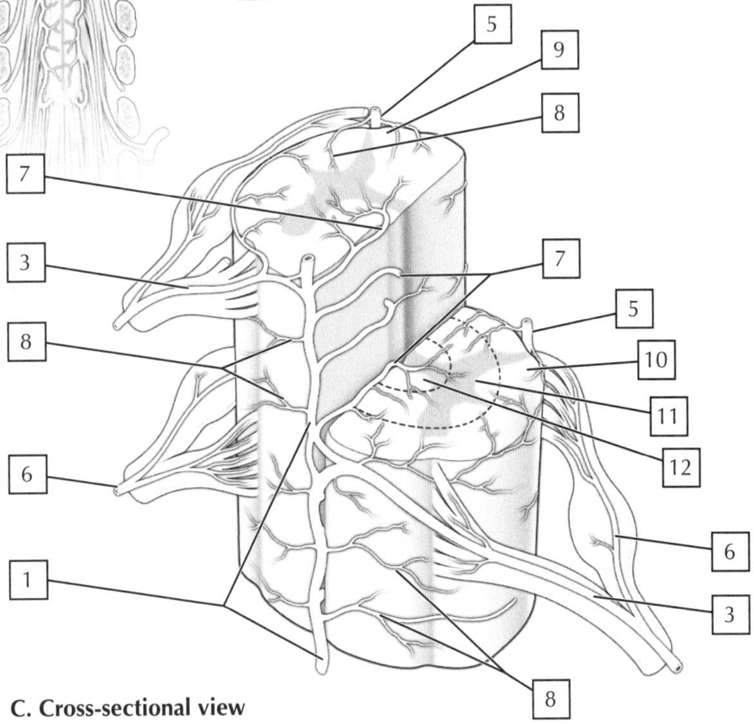

C. Cross-sectional view

4 Venous Drainage of the Brain and Venous Sinuses

Venous drainage of the brain takes place through a network of venules and veins, emptying into the dural sinuses that drain into the **internal jugular vein**. From the brain arteries and arterioles, a very fine, thin-walled capillary network in brain tissue allows for rapid transfer of oxygen and glucose into the regions of high demand for neuronal activity (a basis for functional imaging). The **cerebral veins** empty into the dural sinuses by traversing the subarachnoid space. The dural sinuses are thick-walled channels formed from a split of the inner and outer layers of **dura**. The veins drain into these dural sinuses; if severe trauma occurs, these cerebral veins can tear from their entrance zones into the dural sinuses, resulting in venous blood dissecting the dural membrane from the underlying arachnoid membrane. The resultant subdural hematoma may be acute (from severe trauma, especially in a young person) or chronic (in some elderly patients, even with nonsevere head trauma, where the bridging veins have more free space to traverse due to gradual loss of brain mass). Arachnoid granulations from the subarachnoid space, with their one-way valves, drain the CSF into the venous sinuses.

The **falx cerebri** and **tentorium cerebelli** are tough, fused layers of dura that separate the anterior, middle, and posterior fossae from each other. The layers of dura split to form dural sinuses in outer (**superior sagittal sinus**) and inner (**inferior sagittal sinus**) midline regions, draining blood from superficial and deep regions of the brain, respectively. The **great cerebral vein of Galen** and the **straight sinus** merge with the **transverse sinus** and **sigmoid sinus** to drain deeper regions and posterior zones of the brain into the **confluence of sinuses**, ultimately draining into the internal jugular vein.

COLOR the following structures, using a separate color for each structure.

- ☐ 1. **Falx cerebri**
- ☐ 2. **Cavernous sinus**
- ☐ 3. **Tentorium cerebelli**
- ☐ 4. **Straight sinus**
- ☐ 5. **Confluence of sinuses**
- ☐ 6. **Superior sagittal sinus**
- ☐ 7. **Great cerebral vein of Galen**
- ☐ 8. **Transverse sinus**
- ☐ 9. **Sigmoid sinus**
- ☐ 10. **Inferior sagittal sinus**
- ☐ 11. **Dura**
- ☐ 12. **Cerebral veins**
- ☐ 13. **Internal jugular vein**

Clinical Note

Venous thrombosis may occur with infections. Cavernous sinus thrombosis can be a sequela of paranasal or middle ear infections or a furuncle in the facial region. The resultant thrombosis causes pain, headache, ipsilateral visual loss, palsies of the extraocular nerves (CNs III, IV, VI) with exophthalmos (protrusion of the eyeball), or ophthalmic nerve (CN V1) dysfunction. The lesion can expand to the **cavernous sinus** of the other side, or expand to other venous sinuses, and can even result in hemiparesis. Venous thrombosis of the transverse sinus may lead to damage of ipsilateral CNs IX, X, XI.

Venous sinus thrombosis also may occur following dehydration, cancer, polycythemia vera, other hypercoagulability syndromes, or inflammatory conditions.

General symptoms of venous thrombosis include severe headache, nausea and vomiting, weakness, sensory loss, sometimes aphasia, and possibly coma.

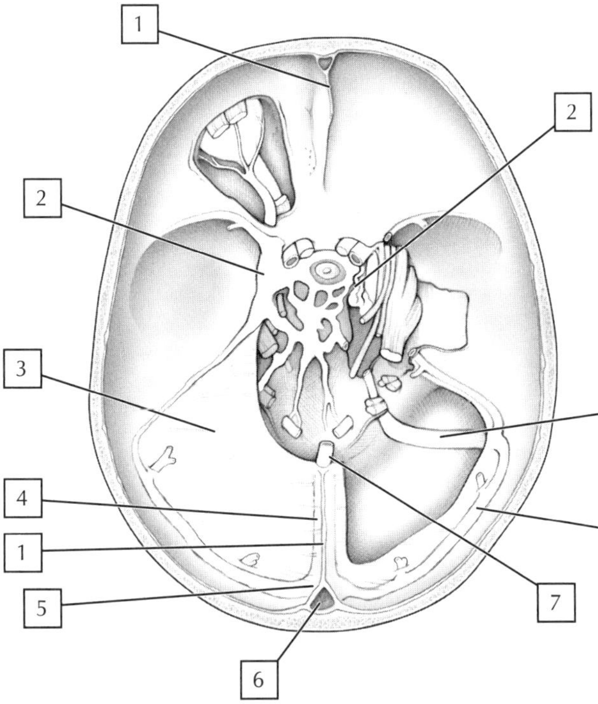

A. Venous sinuses—axial view

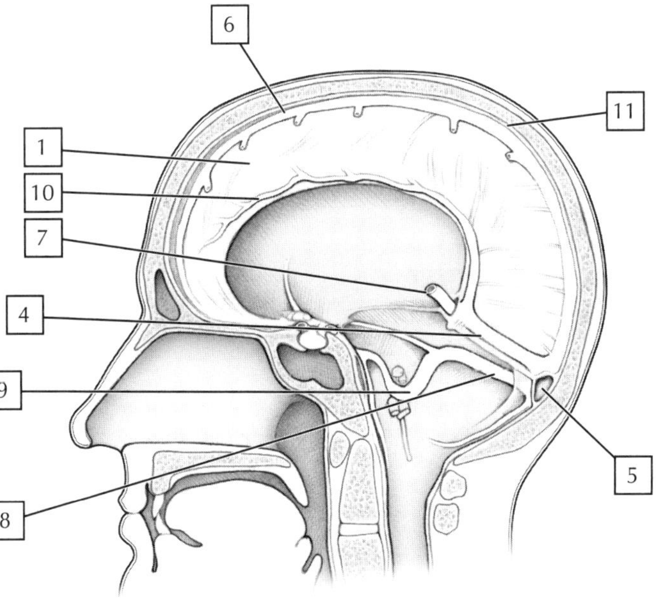

B. Venous sinuses—sagittal view

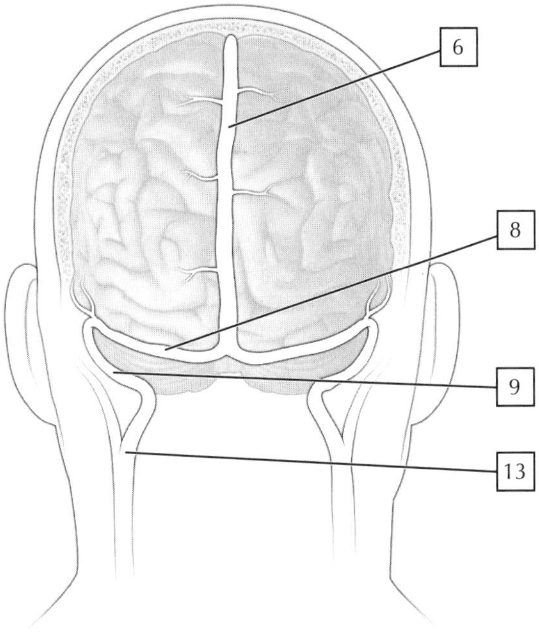

C. Venous sinuses—posterior view

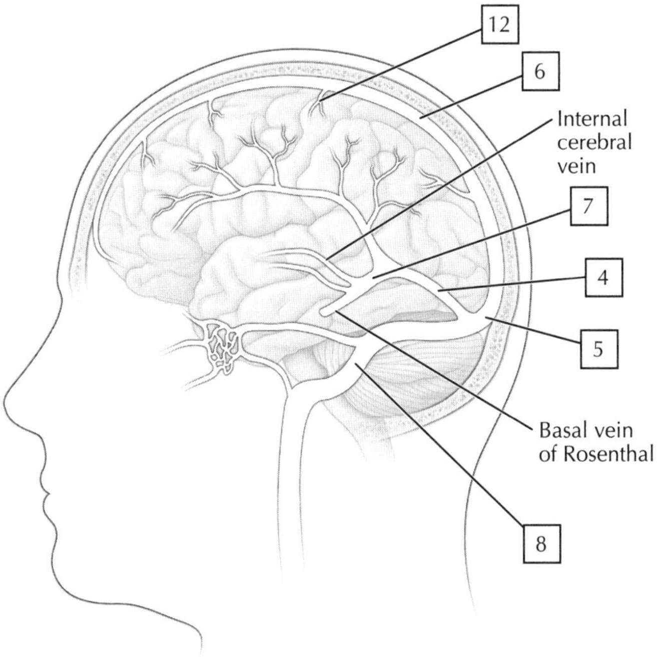

D. Venous sinuses—lateral view

SECTION I REVIEW QUESTIONS

1. For each of the following descriptors, indicate which structure is involved.

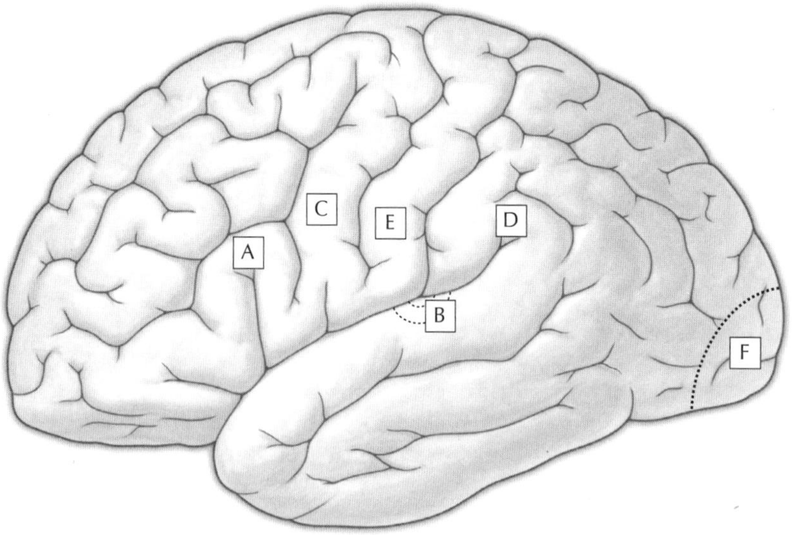

(1) ____________________

(2) ____________________

(3) ____________________

(4) ____________________

(5) ____________________

(6) ____________________

(1) A tumor affecting this area will result in aphasia affecting language expression.
(2) A stroke affecting this region will result in contralateral loss of sensation in the upper body.
(3) A tumor encroaching on this region will result in contralateral spastic paralysis, especially involving the upper extremity.
(4) Damage to this area from the presence of an abscess will result in contralateral neglect of simultaneously presented auditory stimuli.
(5) A major arterial ischemic event affecting this site will result in contralateral hemianopia.
(6) Damage to this region will result in the patient being unable to understand spoken language.

2. Match the following region on the diagram with the description of its role or involvement.

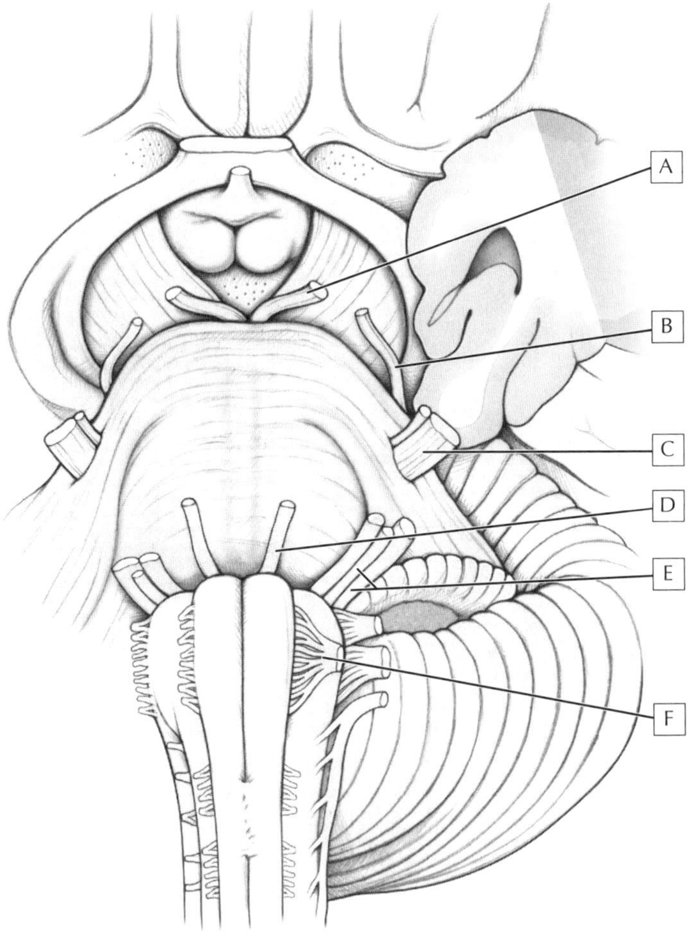

(1) ______________________

(2) ______________________

(3) ______________________

(4) ______________________

(5) ______________________

(6) ______________________

(1) Damage to this nerve will result in difficulty looking in and down on the affected side.
(2) Damage to this site will result in ipsilateral tinnitus and vertigo.
(3) Pressure from a hematoma in the forebrain will compress this nerve, resulting in an ipsilateral fixed and dilated pupil.
(4) Damage to this nerve will lead to paralysis of the ipsilateral muscles of mastication and loss of sensation on the ipsilateral side of the face.
(5) Damage to this nerve will result in protrusion of the tongue to the damaged side.
(6) Damage to this nerve will result in the inability to look laterally with the ipsilateral eye.

3. Match the region of the spinal cord with a description of its role or activity.

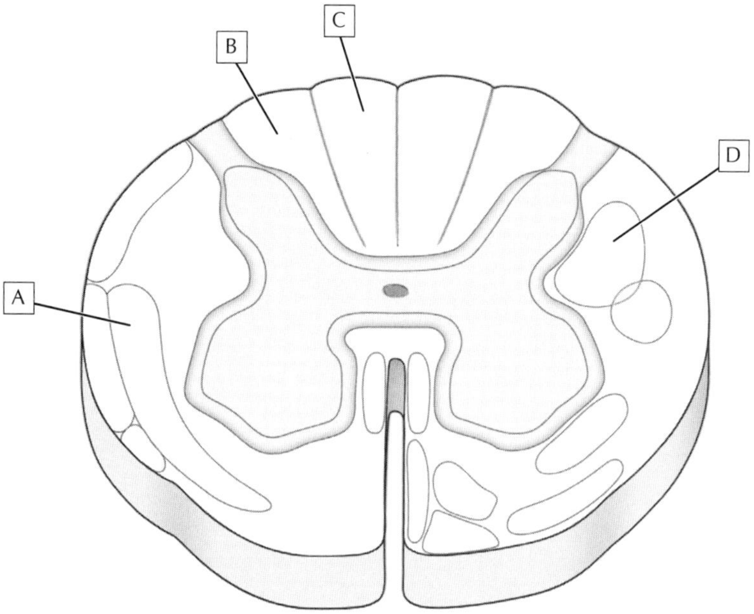

(1) ____________________

(2) ____________________

(3) ____________________

(4) ____________________

(1) Carries vibratory sensation from the ipsilateral foot
(2) Carries joint position sense from the ipsilateral hand, wrist, and elbow
(3) Carries pain and temperature sensation from the contralateral limb
(4) Carries cortical control over ipsilateral lower motor neuron activation

4. Which of the following substances or structures is most likely to be retrogradely transported in a lower motor neuron's axon back to the cell body?
   A. Synthetic enzyme acetylcholine transferase
   B. Viruses and toxins
   C. Microtubules and neurofilaments
   D. Calmodulin
   E. Synaptic vesicles

5. An elderly patient experiences cerebrovascular ischemic damage, resulting in spastic paresis of his contralateral leg and loss of sensation in that leg. The artery most likely damaged is:
   A. Middle cerebral
   B. Posterior cerebral
   C. Anterior cerebral
   D. Lenticulostriate small arteries
   E. Vertebral artery

6. Neurodegenerative diseases affecting the basal ganglia will most likely result in:
   A. Aphasias and agnosias
   B. Contralateral hemiplegia
   C. Perceptual disorders
   D. Movement disorders
   E. Memory disorders

7. Which of the following regions is most likely to process information that is interpreted according to emotional context and fear responses?
   A. Amygdala
   B. Nucleus accumbens
   C. Hippocampal formation
   D. Superior parietal lobule (cortex)
   E. Basal ganglia

8. Occlusion of what artery will result in right spastic hemiplegia, right hemianesthesia, and expressive aphasia?
   A. Left middle cerebral
   B. Left anterior cerebral
   C. Right middle cerebral
   D. Right anterior cerebral
   E. Basilar

9. Which neuron type has no dendrites extending from the cell body and no synapses on the cell body?

   ____

10. Where is the action potential first initiated in a lower motor neuron? ____________________

11. What cell is most likely to secrete inflammatory cytokines into the local brain microenvironment? ____________________

   ____

12. What type of pathology is most likely found at the circle of Willis? ______________________

13. What type of cerebral hemorrhage is most likely to result in blood in the cerebrospinal fluid? ______________________

14. What major white matter pathway carries both the corticospinal tract and sensory information from the opposite side of the body? ______________________

15. What components of the cerebellum are considered to be the "vestibulocerebellum"? ______________________

16. At what site in the ventricular system is a blockage most likely to result in internal hydrocephalus? ______________________

17. Occlusion of what artery is most likely to result in loss of pain and temperature sensation in the ipsilateral face and the contralateral body? ______________________

18. What ion channel is present only at the nodes of Ranvier that permits reinitiation of the action potential? ______________________

19. Match:
    A. Resting potential
    B. Graded potential
    C. Action potential

1. Results from a differentially permeable membrane due to diffusion and separation of positive/negative charges	_____
2. Travels along the axonal membrane at a constant velocity	_____
3. Depends on excitatory and inhibitory activity of ligand-gated ion channels	_____
4. Occurs when the rapid influx of Na^+ ions cannot be countered by the efflux of K^+ ions	_____
5. Dissipates from the point of origin over both time and space	_____

20. Match:
    A. Astrocytes
    B. Oligodendroglia
    C. Microglia

1. Insulate and separate synaptic sites in the CNS	_____
2. Can become activated, phagocytose debris, and release inflammatory mediators	_____
3. Can replicate and try to repair damage in multiple sclerosis	_____
4. Can send endfoot processes to blood vessels and the pial membrane	_____
5. Can produce scar tissue in the brain following a penetrating injury	_____

21. Match:
    A. Bridging veins
    B. Arteries of the circle of Willis
    C. Arachnoid granulations
    D. Subdural space
    E. Epidural space
    F. Dura mater

1. This structure acts as a one-way valve for absorption of CSF into a dural sinus	_____
2. This structure splits into an inner and outer lay and contains venous blood	_____
3. A skull fracture can tear a meningeal artery, permitting blood to accumulate here	_____
4. These structures extend from the brain to empty into the dural sinuses	_____
5. Torn bridging veins from head trauma can result in blood accumulating here	_____
6. Berry aneurysms often are due to weakness in the wall of this structure	_____

22. Match:
    A. Middle cerebral artery
    B. Anterior cerebral artery
    C. Posterior cerebral artery
    D. Basilar artery paramedian branch
    E. Posterior inferior cerebellar artery

1. Gives rise to lenticulostriate arteries, known as the "arteries of stroke"	_____
2. A stroke here results in contralateral motor weakness and contralateral loss of epicritic sensation in the lower extremity	_____
3. A stroke here results in an ipsilateral cranial nerve lesion and a contralateral upper motor neuron lesion	_____
4. A stroke here gives rise to a loss of pain and temperature sensation on the ipsilateral face and the contralateral body	_____
5. A stroke in this artery results in a contralateral visual deficit	_____
6. A stroke in this artery can result in contralateral hemiparesis and drooping contralateral facial muscles	_____
7. This artery branches from the vertebral artery	_____

23. At what site on a pyramidal cell in the motor cortex would an incoming axon, releasing an excitatory neurotransmitter, have the greatest likelihood of provoking an action potential in the axon?
    A. At the axon hillock
    B. At a large dendrite branching from the cell body
    C. At the distal axon terminal associated with the axon
    D. At an incoming excitatory axon terminal synapsing on the cell body near the emergence of the axon
    E. At a distal pyramidal cell dendrite

24. Which of the following cells is most likely to release proinflammatory cytokines into the local microenvironment?
    A. Protoplasmic astrocyte
    B. Oligodendrocyte
    C. Vascular endothelial cell
    D. Activated microglial cell
    E. Pituicyte in the anterior pituitary gland

25. Which of the following substances or structures is most likely to be retrogradely transported in a lower motor neuron's axon back to the cell body?
    A. Synthetic enzyme acetylcholine transferase
    B. Viruses and toxins
    C. Microtubules and neurofilaments
    D. Calmodulin
    E. Synaptic vesicles

26. Following a gastrointestinal illness, a 45-year-old man awakens and discovers weakness in his lower extremities. Over a few hours, this weakness progresses proximally and also involves the upper extremities. The neurological examination shows loss of movement of the limbs, loss of tone, and loss of muscle stretch reflexes in the affected muscles. If you were to exam this patient with a conduction velocity study, what type of fiber would mostly likely show a loss of conduction?
    A. Postganglionic sympathetic fibers innervating the vasculature
    B. Ia afferent fibers from the affected muscles
    C. Large diameter axons in the pyramidal tract
    D. Nociceptive axons carrying pain information from the affected muscles
    E. Axons carrying information about warmth and cold from the extremities

27. Which of the following neurotransmitters is synthesized and posttranslationally processed in the cell body?
    A. Norepinephrine
    B. Glutamate
    C. Acetylcholine
    D. Serotonin
    E. Beta endorphin

28. What is found in the superior sagittal sinus only in pathological circumstances?
    A. Arterial blood
    B. Venous blood
    C. Cerebrospinal fluid
    D. Protruding arachnoid granulations
    E. Channels from bridging veins

29. Which major white matter pathway carries both the corticospinal tract and sensory information from the opposite side of the body?
    A. Posterior limb of the internal capsule
    B. Corpus callosum
    C. Anterior commissure
    D. Cerebral peduncle
    E. Dorsal columns of the spinal cord

30. At what site is a herniated disc (nucleus pulposus) most likely to produce both a radiculopathy (radiating pain) and a myelopathy (spinal cord involvement)?
    A. Cervical spine (C5–6)
    B. Lumbar spine (L4–5)
    C. Sacral spine (S1–2)
    D. Conus medullaris
    E. Cauda equina

31. At what site in the ventricular system is a blockage most likely to result in internal hydrocephalus?
    A. Aqueduct
    B. Interventricular foramen of Monro
    C. Foramen of Magendie
    D. Third ventricle
    E. Arachnoid granulations in the dural sinuses

32. What major pathology is often found at the circle of Willis?
    A. Blocked recirculation of cerebral venous blood
    B. Occlusive vascular strokes
    C. Transient ischemic attacks
    D. Subdural hematomas
    E. Berry aneurysms

33. Damage to which artery is least likely to involve the somatic motor system to the body or its upper motor neuronal voluntary control?
    A. Middle cerebral
    B. Anterior spinal
    C. Anterior cerebral
    D. Paramedian branches of the vertebral and basilar arteries
    E. Posterior inferior cerebellar artery

ANSWER KEY

1.
   (1) A, Broca area
   (2) E, Lateral primary somatosensory cortex
   (3) C, Motor cortex
   (4) B, Auditory cortex
   (5) F, Primary visual cortex
   (6) D, Wernicke area
2.
   (1) B, Trochlear nerve (CN IV)
   (2) E, Vestibulocochlear nerve (CN VIII)
   (3) A, Oculomotor nerve (CN III)
   (4) C, Trigeminal nerve (CN V)
   (5) F, Hypoglossal nerve (CN XII)
   (6) D, Abducens nerve (CN VI)
3.
   (1) C, Fasciculus gracilis
   (2) B, Fasciculus cuneatus
   (3) A, Spinothalamic tract and spinoreticular tract
   (4) D, Lateral corticospinal tract
4. B
5. C
6. D
7. A
8. A
9. Dorsal root ganglion cell
10. Initial segment of the axon
11. Activated microglia
12. Berry aneurysm
13. Subarachnoid hemorrhage
14. Posterior limb of the internal capsule
15. Vermis and flocculonodular lobe
16. Aqueduct (of Sylvius)
17. Posterior inferior cerebellar artery (PICA) or vertebral artery
18. Sodium channel
19.
   (1) A
   (2) C
   (3) B
   (4) C
   (5) B
20.
   (1) A
   (2) C
   (3) B
   (4) A
   (5) A
21.
   (1) C
   (2) F
   (3) E
   (4) A
   (5) D
   (6) B
22.
   (1) A
   (2) B
   (3) D
   (4) E
   (5) C
   (6) A
   (7) E
23. A
24. D
25. B
26. B

27. E
28. A
29. A
30. A
31. A
32. E
33. E

Chapter 5 Peripheral Nervous System

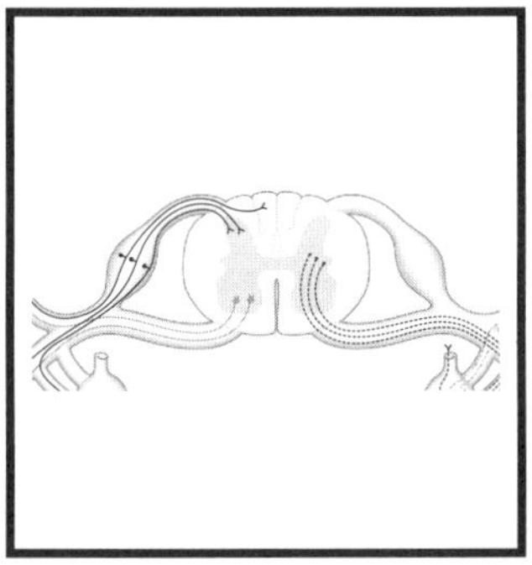

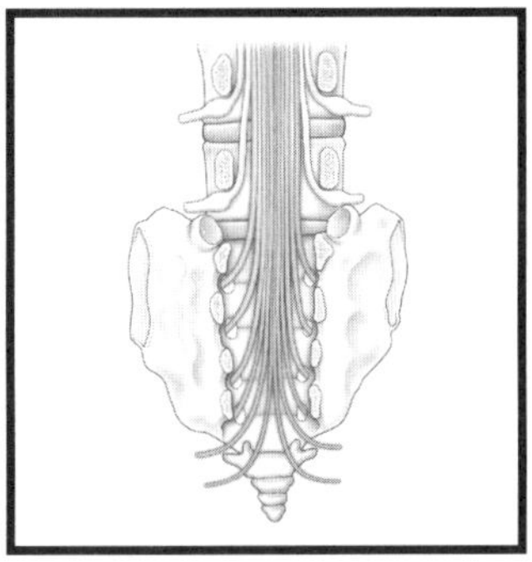

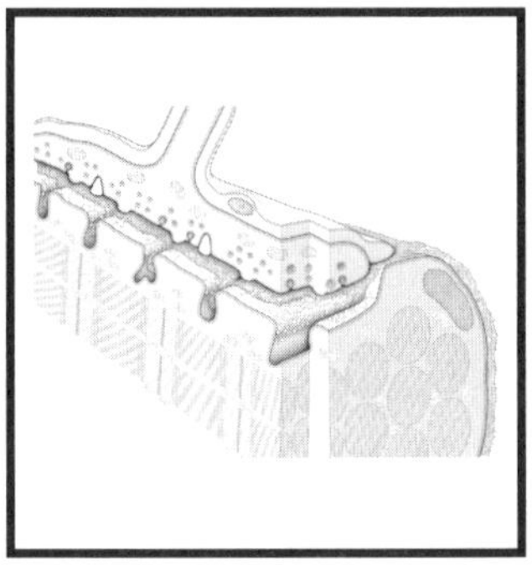

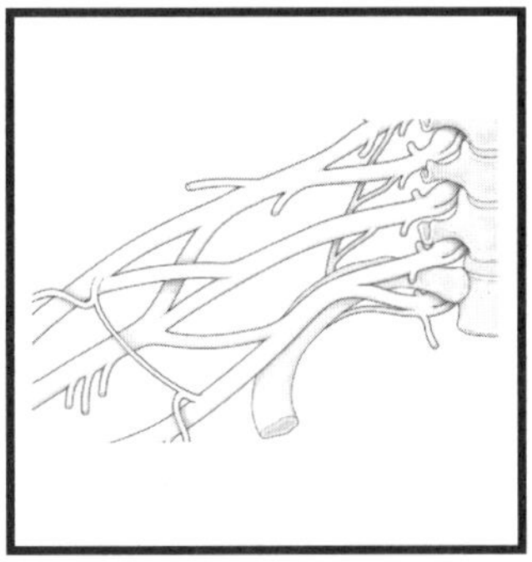

5 Spinal Cord With Sensory, Motor, and Autonomic Components of Peripheral Nerves

Peripheral nerves are made up of **afferent (sensory)** and **efferent (motor, autonomic)** components of the **peripheral nervous system,** and the related supportive tissues; the axons enter or exit the spinal cord via the **dorsal roots** (sensory) and **ventral roots** (motor, autonomic), and enter or exit the brain via the **cranial nerves**.

The sensory components of the **peripheral nervous system (PNS)** include the **dorsal root ganglia/cranial nerve ganglia,** the peripheral **axons,** and the associated **sensory receptors.** The sensory receptors are the transducing elements that respond to an adequate stimulus (e.g., nociception from **free nerve endings,** mechanical distortion from **encapsulated nerve endings,** such as vibratory stimuli from **Pacinian corpuscles**) and cause an action potential to fire in the adjacent initial segment of the primary sensory axon. The sensory receptor acts as a dendrite. The resultant action potential propagates proximally into the spinal cord dorsal horn via the dorsal root, or into the brainstem via cranial nerves; the action potential also can act distally, sometimes producing release of bioactive molecules at the site of initial receptor stimulation (e.g., substance P release at sites of initiation of nociception).

The motor components of the PNS include the **peripheral motor axons,** whose lower motor neuron (LMN) cell bodies are in the **spinal cord ventral horn** or **brainstem motor cranial nerve nuclei** and their **neuromuscular junctions** (motor end plates) terminating on the **skeletal muscle fibers.**

The autonomic components of the PNS include (1) the peripheral **preganglionic autonomic axons** from both sympathetic and parasympathetic nervous system, including those traveling in the **splanchnic nerves**; these preganglionic cell bodies are in the spinal cord (T1–L2 intermediolateral cell column in the **lateral horn** for the sympathetics, or **brainstem autonomic cranial nerve nuclei** and **intermediate gray neurons in the S2–S4** spinal cord level for the parasympathetics); (2) the autonomic ganglia on which they synapse (**sympathetic chain ganglia and collateral ganglia** for the sympathetic nervous system and **intramural ganglia** for the parasympathetic nervous system); (3) the **postganglionic axons**; and (4) the **autonomic target tissues** (cardiac muscle, smooth muscle, secretory glands, metabolic cells, and cells of the immune system) on which the neuroeffector junctions of the postganglionic axons synapse.

COLOR each of the following structures, using a separate color for each structure.

- ☐ **1. Dorsal horn of the spinal cord**
- ☐ **2. Dorsal root**
- ☐ **3. Dorsal root ganglion**
- ☐ **4. Pacinian corpuscle**
- ☐ **5. Skeletal muscle fibers with motor end plate**
- ☐ **6. Free nerve ending**
- ☐ **7. Ventral root**
- ☐ **8. Ventral horn of the spinal cord**
- ☐ **9. Collateral sympathetic ganglion**
- ☐ **10. Splanchnic nerve**
- ☐ **11. Sympathetic chain ganglion**
- ☐ **12. Lateral horn of the spinal cord**

Clinical Note

The sensory, motor, and autonomic neurons of the PNS have some components in the CNS. The central terminations of the primary sensory neurons are in the spinal cord and brainstem. The cell bodies and proximal axons of the motor neurons (LMNs) and preganglionic autonomic neurons are found in the spinal cord and brainstem. These central components are vulnerable to central neural disorders, and the proximal axons are vulnerable to central demyelination (e.g., multiple sclerosis). The peripheral axons are protected by Schwann cells and are vulnerable to peripheral neuropathies and peripheral demyelinating disorders (Guillain–Barré syndrome). A peripheral neuropathy can be a mononeuropathy (one nerve), a polyneuropathy (multiple nerves), a demyelinating neuropathy, a selective axonal neuropathy, a traumatic neuropathy, or others. Damage to peripheral sensory axons results in loss of sensory modalities (sensations) carried by those axons, or pain from pressure on the axons. Damage to peripheral motor axons results in loss of movement, strength, tone, and reflexes. Damage to peripheral autonomic components can result in selective loss of autonomic functions. Sensorimotor neuropathies, such as the autosomal dominant Charcot-Marie-Tooth disease, occur at an age between 5 and 25, produce weakness and wasting of muscles (motor component) starting in the legs, loss of sensation in the limbs (sensory component), and slowed conduction velocity. It is usually a slowly progressive demyelinating disease.

Spinal Cord With Sensory, Motor, and Autonomic Components of Peripheral Nerves

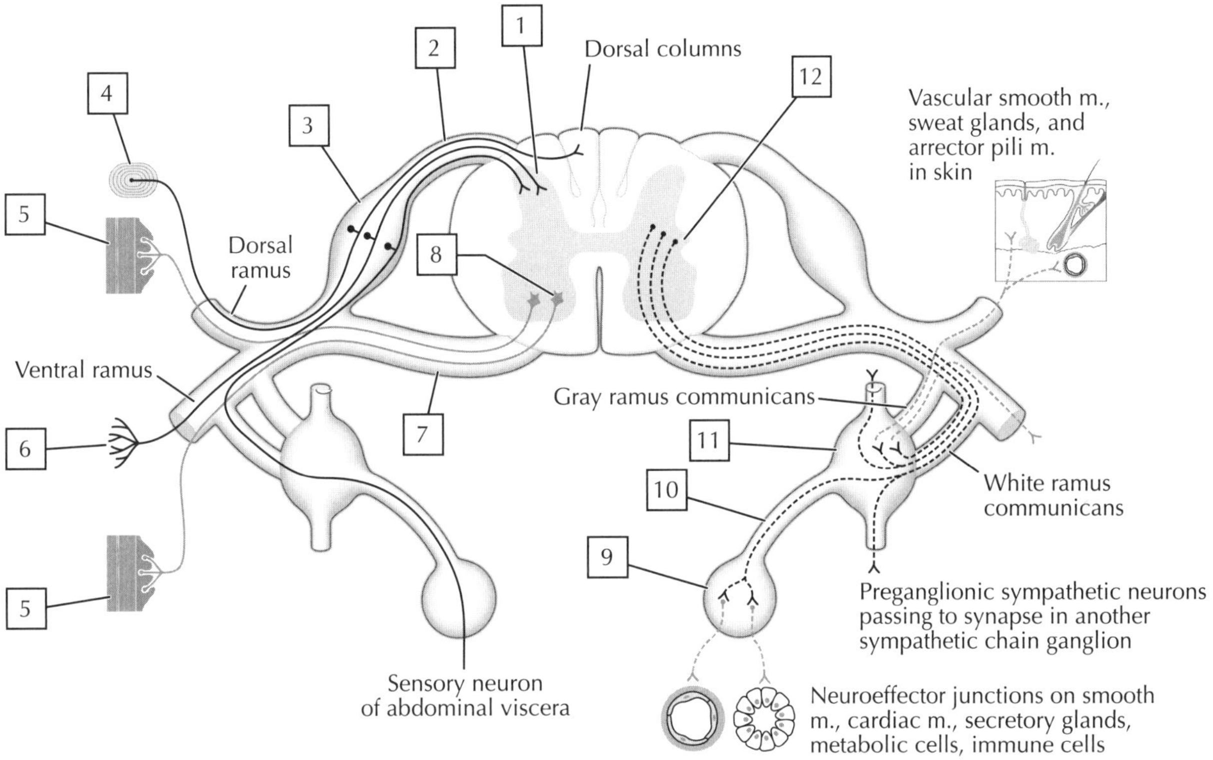

Sensory Motor Preganglionic sympathetic Postganglionic sympathetic

m., muscle.

5 Anatomy of a Peripheral Nerve

A **peripheral nerve** contains bundles of **myelinated and unmyelinated axons,** surrounded by protective connective tissue sheaths, along with small **blood vessels (vasa vasorum),** which run longitudinally with the nerve and its fascicles. Axons are organized into longitudinally oriented spiral arrays of **nerve fiber bundles,** present in a peripheral nerve as **fascicles.** Unmyelinated axons are surrounded by a **Schwann cell sheath of cytoplasm,** while myelinated axons are insulated by Schwann cell membrane wrappings called **myelin sheaths,** with one Schwann cell per intermodal site on a single axon. The **nodes (of Ranvier)** are bare spaces between the myelinated segments, which contain the sodium channels permitting initiation (and reinitiation) of the action potential.

The **endoneurium** is loose supportive connective tissue found among the axons within a fascicle. The **perineurium** enwraps fascicles of multiple axons, providing both support and a barrier function, the **blood–nerve barrier**, which is the nerve's equivalent of the blood-brain barrier. The **epineurium** is the tough external layer of supportive connective tissue that enwraps the entire nerve.

COLOR the following structures, using a separate color for each structure.

- ☐ 1. **Vasa nervorum (longitudinal vessels)**
- ☐ 2. **Epineurium (inner and outer layers)**
- ☐ 3. **Fascicles**
- ☐ 4. **Nerve fiber bundles in a fascicle**
- ☐ 5. **Perineurium**
- ☐ 6. **Axons in nerve fiber bundles in fascicles**
- ☐ 7. **Intact axons**
- ☐ 8. **Myelin sheath**
- ☐ 9. **Axons undergoing dissolution**
- ☐ 10. **Endoneurium**

Clinical Note

A peripheral nerve contains both myelinated and unmyelinated axons. Each type of axon can be damaged by specific neuropathies, such as leprosy for unmyelinated axons, and inflammatory demyelinating diseases such as **Guillain–Barré syndrome** for myelinated axons. Some chemical insults and some metabolic diseases such as diabetes and chronic alcoholism can damage both myelinated and unmyelinated axons together. Such neuropathies often appear as distal, symmetrical polyneuropathies, with the damage initially occurring distally, and then moving proximally.

If a peripheral nerve is subjected to pressure, traction, or trauma, all axons at the site can be damaged. In the case of the median nerve at the flexor retinaculum, repetitive movement can cause inflammation or decreased vascular flow to this segment of the median nerve, resulting in severe pain in the distribution of the nerve, and loss of sensory and motor functions distally. This compression neuropathy is called **carpal tunnel syndrome**. A crush injury or other physical trauma to a nerve results in localized disruption of the axons and supporting cells (Schwann cells), causing distal degeneration of the axons (called **Wallerian degeneration**). The axons and Schwann cells break up into globules and undergo **dissolution** and phagocytosis. The basement membrane remains intact, so if the proximal and distal ends of the damaged peripheral nerve are properly aligned or anastomosed, the proximal axons can slowly extend distally in an attempt to reach the target from which they had been separated by the injury. This is a slow, regenerative process, proceeding at approximately 1 mm/day, if successful. The cell bodies for the damaged axons undergo a process of damage repair, called **central chromatolysis**. Their Nissl substance (rough endoplasmic reticulum) distributes peripherally in the cell body; the genome shifts its protein synthesis away from neurotransmitter processes toward growth and repair. If the neuron can successfully extend its axonal process back to its target, the Schwann cells will replicate and remyelinate the reconnecting axons, but the internodal segment will remain shorter than before the injury, with slightly slowed conduction velocity.

A. Axonal anatomy

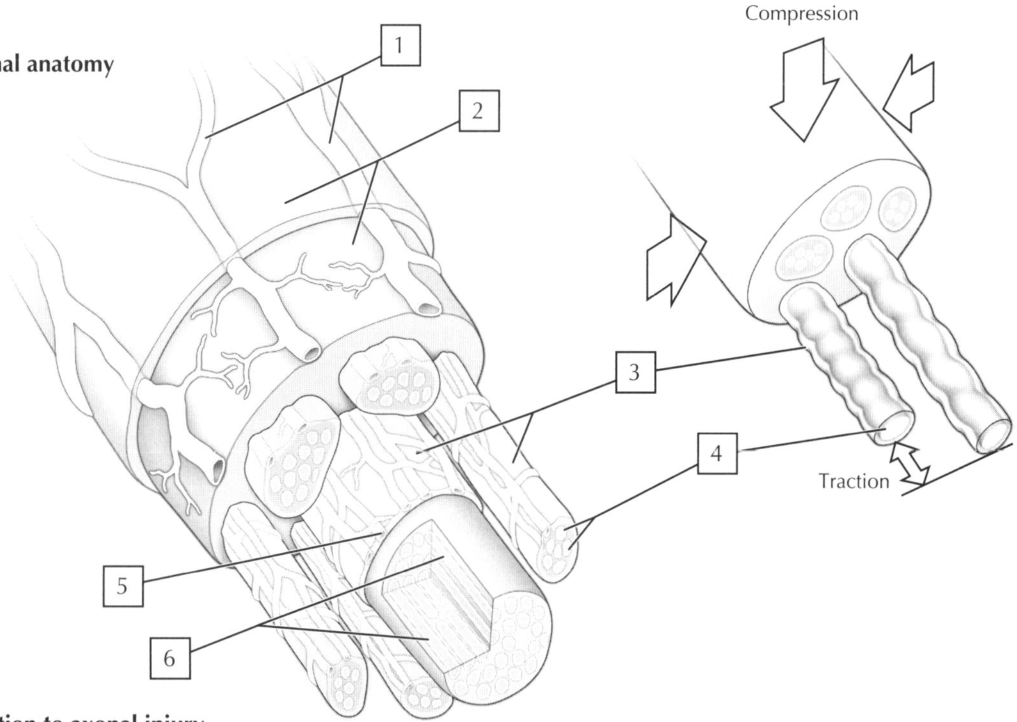

B. Reaction to axonal injury

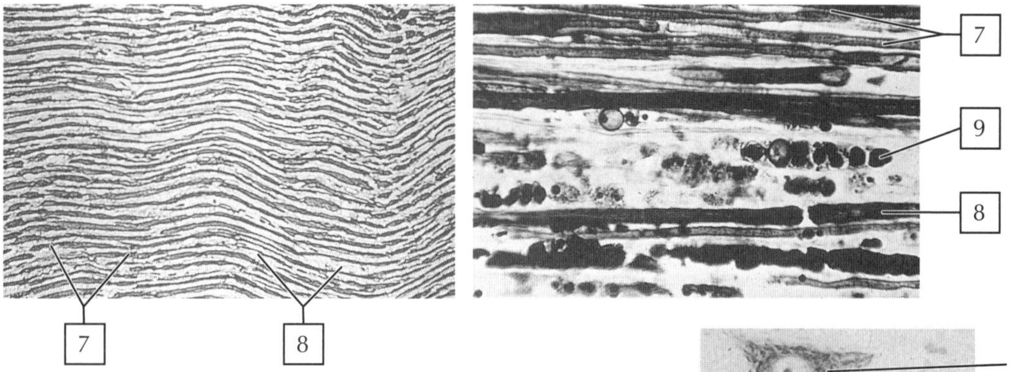

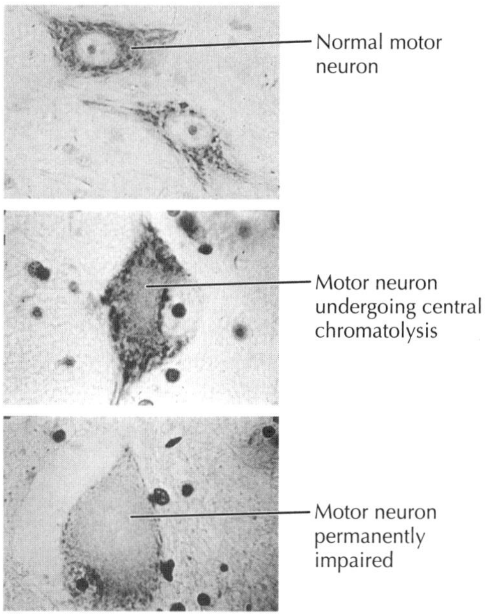

C. Sunderland classification of nerve injury

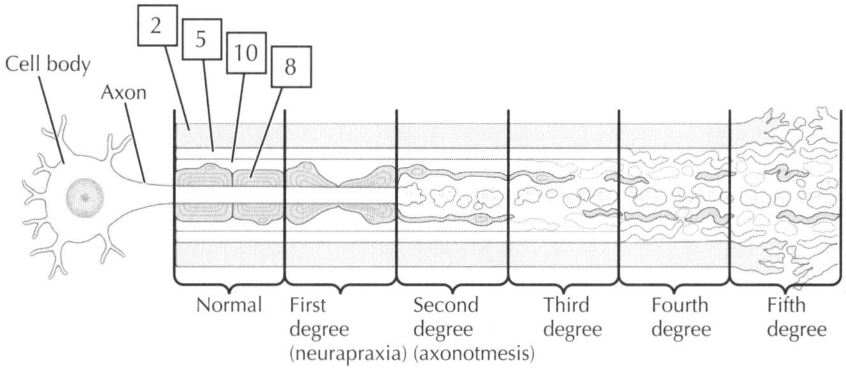

Classification of nerve injury by degree of involvement of various neural layers

5 Relationship of Spinal Nerve Roots to Vertebrae

At birth, the **spinal cord segments** are aligned vertically with the vertebrae, segment for segment. As the infant grows, the longitudinal growth of the vertebral column exceeds the longitudinal growth of the spinal cord, with the spinal cord remaining more rostral. The spinal cord demonstrates a **cervical enlargement** and a **lumbar (lumbosacral) enlargement,** representing the increasing motor and sensory supply required for the growing limbs. Consequently, the dorsal and ventral nerve roots must extend caudally to retain their appropriate relationship with the vertebral foramina with which they were originally associated. By adulthood, the caudal-most portion of the spinal cord, called the **conus medullaris,** is located under the **L1 vertebral body.** The caudally extending nerve roots travel in the **subarachnoid space,** bathed in cerebrospinal fluid, forming a loose collection of nerve roots called the **cauda equina.** This **lumbar cistern** (subarachnoid space) is the commonly used site for withdrawing cerebrospinal fluid from a lumbar puncture; the loose packing of nerve roots in the cauda equina prevents damage from the insertion of the needle for the lumbar puncture. The spinal cord is anchored to the coccyx by the **filum terminale,** a tough extension of pial membrane.

At both cervical and especially lumbar (L4–L5 and L5–S1) sites, intervertebral disks may herniate, with the **nucleus pulposus** of the disc extruding from the capsule and impinging on specific nerve roots, often producing radiating pain and perhaps motor dysfunction in areas of distribution of the root. In the cervical cord, the herniating disk may impinge on both the nerve roots (radiculopathy) and adjacent lateral spinal cord (myelopathy).

COLOR the following structures, using a separate color for each structure.

- ☐ 1. **Cervical enlargement of the spinal cord**
- ☐ 2. **Lumbar (lumbosacral) enlargement of the spinal cord**
- ☐ 3. **Conus medullaris**
- ☐ 4. **Cauda equina**
- ☐ 5. **Filum terminale**
- ☐ 6. **Nucleus pulposus of intervertebral disk**
- ☐ 7. **Nerve root compressed by herniating nucleus pulposus**
- ☐ 8. **Herniation of intervertebral disk**
- ☐ 9. **Capsule of intervertebral disk**

Clinical Note

The anatomical associations of the spinal cord leave sites of vulnerability for potential pathology. The location of the conus medullaris under the L1 vertebral body concentrates many vital structures in a single location that may be damaged by a spinal injury. If the conus medullaris is damaged, a classic **conus medullaris syndrome** may be seen. This is an incomplete spinal cord injury accompanied by bowel and bladder dysfunction, sexual dysfunction, severe back pain, possible weakness in the lower extremities but not total paralysis, and some numbness or paresthesias in the lower extremities.

Lumbar and sacral nerve roots may be compressed by the herniation of the nucleus pulposus from an intervertebral disk, most commonly occurring at L4–L5 and L5–S1. This is accompanied by **radiating pain** in the distribution of the nerve root, and possible numbness in the root distribution. Depending on the nerve root, there may be weakness, muscle atrophy, or reflex changes.

At a cervical level, a similar radiculopathy may be seen, with radiating pain, weakness, and other changes. In addition, the herniating nucleus pulposus may impinge on the lateral margin of the adjacent spinal cord, which may produce ipsilateral spasticity below the level of the lesion (damage to lateral corticospinal and rubrospinal tracts), contralateral loss of pain and temperature sensation below the level of the lesion (spinothalamic/spinoreticular system), initial ipsilateral ataxia and gait alterations (from initial impingement on the spinocerebellar tracts in the lateral funiculus), and, if the myelopathy is above the T1–T2 level, ipsilateral Horner syndrome (ptosis, miosis, and anhydrosis).

A. Spinal cord nerve root relationships

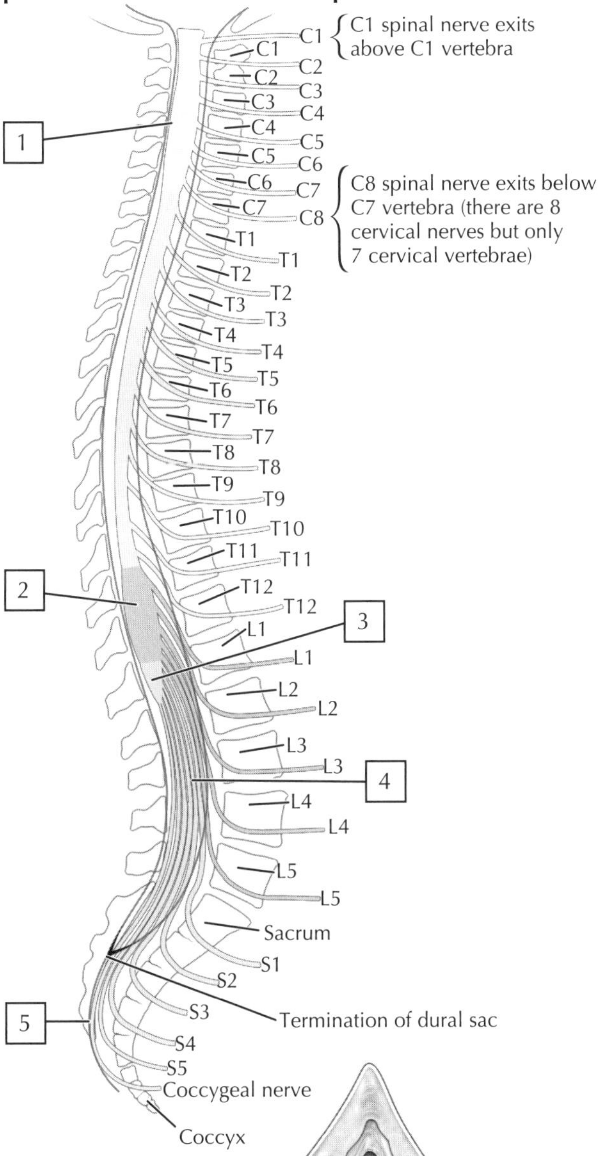

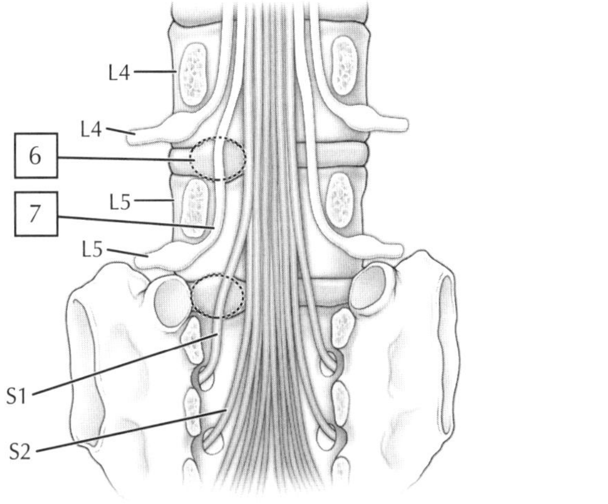

B. Lumbar disk protrusion does not usually affect the nerve exiting above the disk. Lateral protrusion at disk level L4–5 affects L5 spinal nerve, not L4 spinal nerve. Protrusion at disk level L5–S1 affects S1 spinal nerve, not L5 spinal nerve.

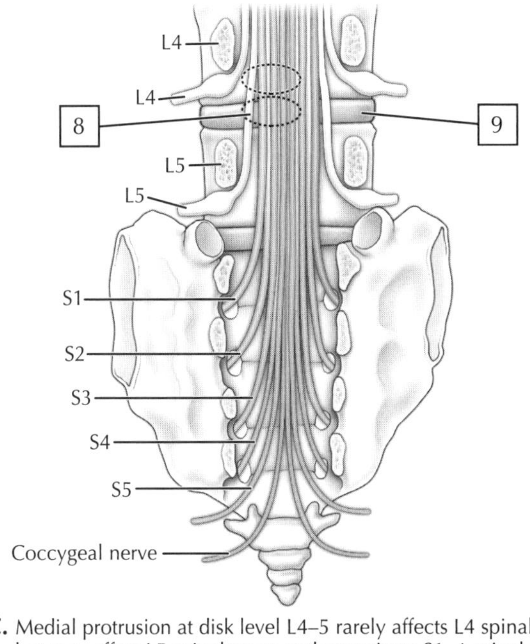

C. Medial protrusion at disk level L4–5 rarely affects L4 spinal nerve but may affect L5 spinal nerve and sometimes S1–4 spinal nerves.

E. Surgical exposure of lower lumbar disk herniation

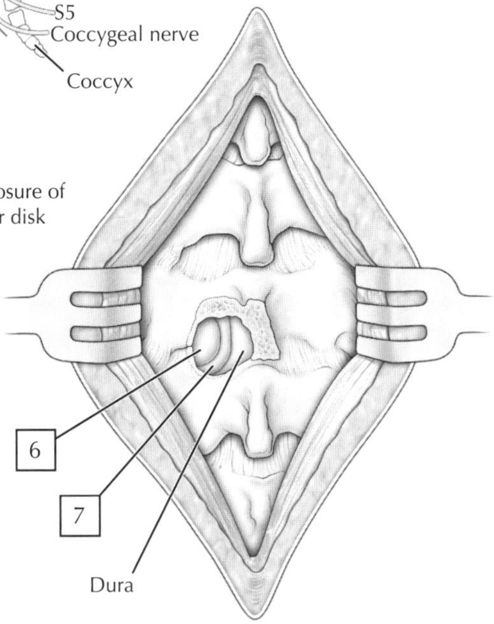

D. Cross section showing compression of nerve root

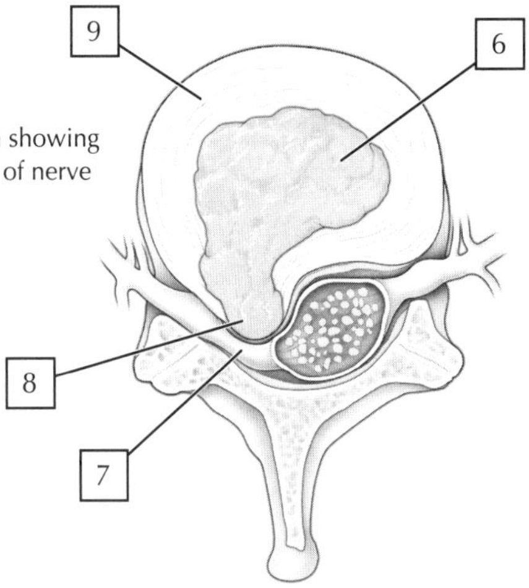

Sensory Channels: Reflex and Cerebellar

Sensory receptors transduce stimuli in the periphery into action potentials that travel along the primary sensory axons, destined for termination in the central nervous system. **Primary sensory unmyelinated and myelinated axons**, derived from **dorsal root ganglion primary sensory cell bodies**, send their information into three types of secondary sensory channels: (1) **reflex channels** through which information is directed monosynaptically or polysynaptically to the LMNs or preganglionic autonomic neurons; (2) **cerebellar channels** through which information is directed to the cerebellar deep nuclei and cerebellar cortex for the smoothing and coordinating of movement (a 2-neuron chain); and (3) **lemniscal channels** through which sensory information is brought to the cortex via the thalamus for conscious interpretation (at least a three-neuron chain).

Monosynaptic reflex channels direct **muscle spindle** primary sensory information from a muscle spindle via Ia afferents to LMNs, which in turn innervate **skeletal muscle fibers** in which those muscle spindles are found, resulting in the classic **muscle stretch reflex**. Polysynaptic reflex channels direct extensive sensory information (from **free nerve endings** and encapsulated nerve endings) via interneurons to LMNs to achieve many types of reflexes, such as the flexor reflex, Golgi tendon organ reflexes, recurrent inhibition, Renshaw inhibition, and others.

Cerebellar channels direct extensive information from muscles, joints, tendons, ligaments, and cutaneous sources (unconscious proprioception) to secondary sensory neurons, which send their connections to deep cerebellar nuclei and cerebellar cortex via the **spinocerebellar pathways;** there are four major spinocerebellar pathways derived from **secondary sensory neurons** in the spinal cord and caudal medulla, including the dorsal and ventral spinocerebellar tract (associated with the lower body, T6 and below) and the cuneocerebellar tract and rostral spinocerebellar tract for the upper body (above T6).

Lemniscal channels are addressed in the next plate (see Plate 5.5).

COLOR the following structures, using a separate color for each structure.

- ☐ 1. **Primary sensory cell body**
- ☐ 2. **Unmyelinated sensory axon**
- ☐ 3. **Myelinated sensory axon**
- ☐ 4. **Free nerve ending**
- ☐ 5. **Muscle spindle**
- ☐ 6. **Lower motor neuron**
- ☐ 7. **Skeletal muscle fibers**
- ☐ 8. **Spinocerebellar tract**
- ☐ 9. **Secondary sensory neurons of the spinocerebellar systems**

Clinical Note

Reflex channels provide moment-to-moment adjustments to motor activities through sensory inputs to the LMNs, either directly for muscle stretch reflexes or indirectly through interneurons for the other reflexes. If either the sensory inputs for reflexes or the motor outputs from the LMNs are damaged, the reflexes will no longer occur. In peripheral neuropathies, muscle stretch reflexes may be abolished, and muscle tone and movement are absent with motor axon damage or Ia afferent damage. Reflexes may also be altered from central nervous system damage. With a spinal cord injury, descending upper motor neuron (UMN) control over LMNs is lost, resulting in hyperresponsive and hyperreflexic muscle stretch reflexes as the LMNs become dominated by sensory input. Similarly, flexor reflex withdrawal responses may become hyperresponsive in the state of spasticity that follows spinal cord injury.

Cerebellar channels may also become damaged with injury to the spinocerebellar tracts at the lateral edge of the lateral funiculus of the spinal cord, with injury to the inferior cerebellar peduncle, or with degenerative disease that affects the spinocerebellar systems. As a result, an ataxic gait ensues, along with loss of coordination of upper extremity movements and the presence of classical cerebellar symptoms. If that damage extends inward to UMN tracts deeper in the lateral funiculus, a UMN lesion will occur, resulting in spasticity with hemiparesis below the level of the lesion, hypertonus, hyperreflexia, and pathological reflexes. UMN damage with spasticity masks the damage to the spinocerebellar systems.

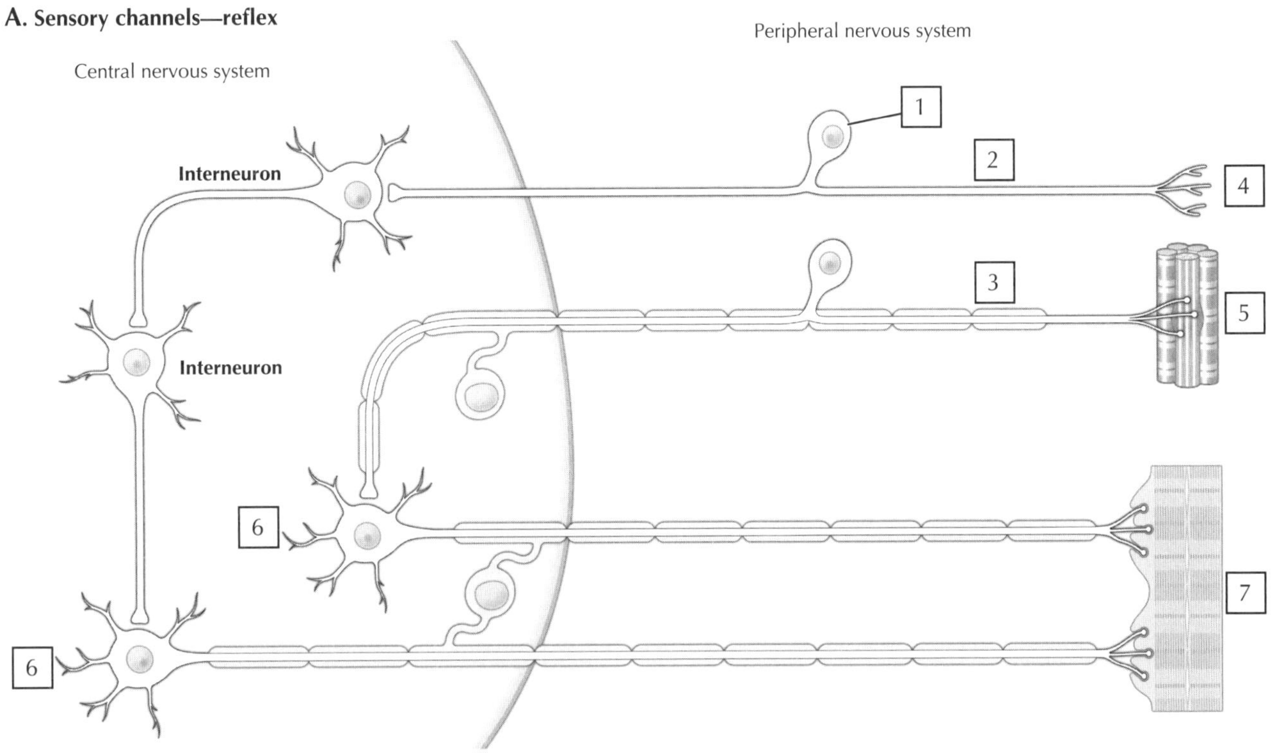
A. Sensory channels—reflex
Central nervous system
Peripheral nervous system
Interneuron
Interneuron
1
2
3
4
5
6
6
7

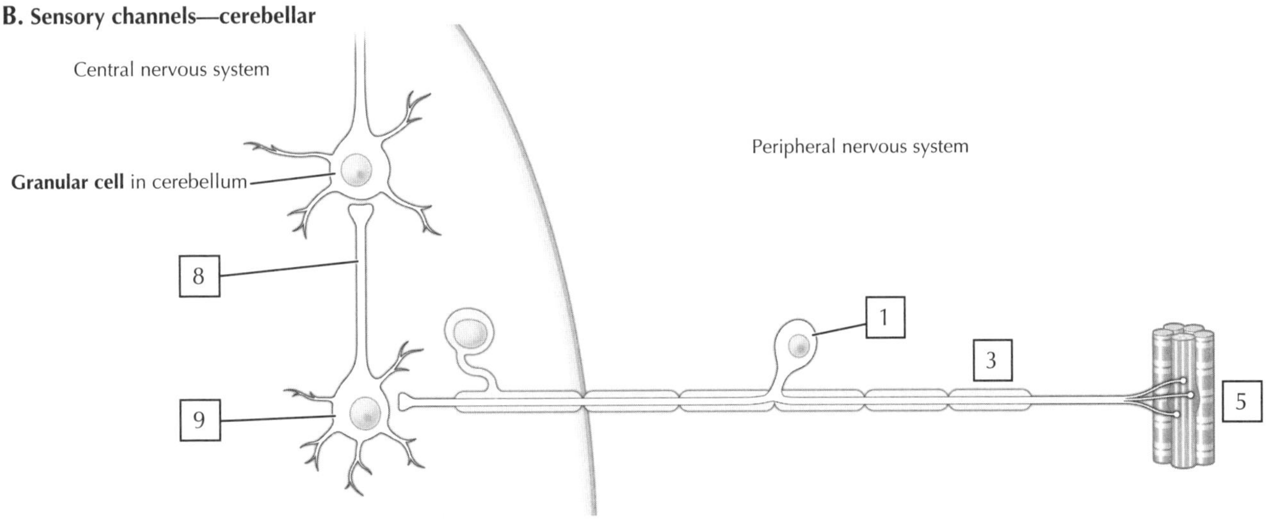
B. Sensory channels—cerebellar
Central nervous system
Peripheral nervous system
Granular cell in cerebellum
8
9
1
3
5

5 Sensory Channels: Lemniscal

Lemniscal channels are secondary sensory channels receiving specific sensory information from **primary sensory neurons; the secondary sensory neurons** carry complex sensory information to **specific nuclei in the thalamus**, which permit bidirectional communication with the **primary sensory cortex** to permit conscious interpretation. For interpretation of fine, discriminative touch, joint position sense (conscious proprioception), vibratory sensation, and other derived modalities, called **epicritic sensation or modalities,** the primary sensory receptors (encapsulated nerve endings such as **Pacinian corpuscles, Meissner corpuscles,** and others) initiate action potentials in the **primary sensory myelinated axons** (from **dorsal root ganglion** primary sensory neurons); these axons enter the spinal cord at the dorsal root entry zone, head rostrally in **fasciculi gracilis and cuneatus** in the dorsal funiculus, and terminate in the caudal medulla in the secondary sensory nuclei, **nucleus gracilis** (for information below T6) and **nucleus cuneatus** (for information from T6 and above). These nuclei send topographically organized information across the midline into the **medial lemniscus (ML)**, which terminates in the **ventral posterolateral (VPL) nucleus of the thalamus**. Nucleus VPL conveys information via the **posterior limb of the internal capsule** to the **primary sensory cortex** on the postcentral gyrus of the parietal lobe, topographically organized.

For interpretation of pain and temperature sensation, called **protopathic** modalities, **bare nerve endings** and some encapsulated nerve endings initiate action potentials, mainly in **primary sensory unmyelinated axons** and in some small, myelinated axons from primary sensory neurons. These axons terminate in the **dorsal horn of the spinal cord**. Some neurons of the dorsal horn (in lamina I and V) send axons across the midline in the **anterior white commissure** of the spinal cord and into the **spinothalamic tract** in the anterolateral white matter of the spinal cord. These axons ascend to the VPL nucleus of the thalamus and terminate in different regions of this nucleus than do epicritic axons of the ML. The protopathic information is then sent to the primary sensory cortex as well as to a small caudal parietal lobe region for the **secondary sensory cortex.** Some primary sensory protopathic axons terminate in a region of the dorsal horn called **substantia gelatinosa**, which sends the nociceptive information through a cascade of neurons in the spinal cord. Neurons in deeper layers of the dorsal horn send **crossed spinoreticular axons** through the anterior white commissure, and also uncrossed axons, into the **lateral reticular formation**, **parabrachial nuclei**, **periaqueductal gray**, and other brainstem regions. Some of this bilateral, potentially neuropathic pain information is channeled through **nonspecific nuclei of the thalamus** and activates regions of the limbic forebrain and extensive areas of the cerebral cortex. This type of pain processing engages circuitry for emotional connotation and severity of pain.

COLOR the following structures, using a separate color for each structure.

- ☐ **1. Primary sensory neurons (in dorsal root ganglion)**
- ☐ **2. Pacinian corpuscles**
- ☐ **3. Free (bare) nerve endings**
- ☐ **4. Fasciculi gracilis and cuneatus**
- ☐ **5. Nuclei gracilis and cuneatus**
- ☐ **6. Medial lemniscus**
- ☐ **7. Ventral posterolateral nucleus of the thalamus**
- ☐ **8. Primary sensory cortex**
- ☐ **9. Dorsal horn of the spinal cord**
- ☐ **10. Spinothalamic tract**

Clinical Note

In the spinal cord and caudal brainstem, the epicritic information (in the ML) and the protopathic information (in the spinothalamic/spinoreticular system) are located separately from each other. Thus a lesion in the dorsal column of the spinal cord or in the midline region of the medulla may result in loss of epicritic information but preservation of protopathic information.
A lesion in the lateral funiculus of the spinal cord, or in the lateral region of the brainstem (e.g., posterior inferior cerebellar artery syndrome) may result in loss of protopathic information with preservation of epicritic information. In the spinal cord, a hemisection lesion (Brown–Séquard lesion) will damage the fasciculi gracilis and cuneatus (causing ipsilateral loss of epicritic sensation below the level of the lesion) and the anterolateral funiculus on the same side (causing contralateral loss of protopathic sensation below the level of the lesion). The patient will report abnormal but different sensations on both sides of the body below the level of the lesion. These situations are referred to as dissociated sensory loss.

A. Sensory channels—lemniscal

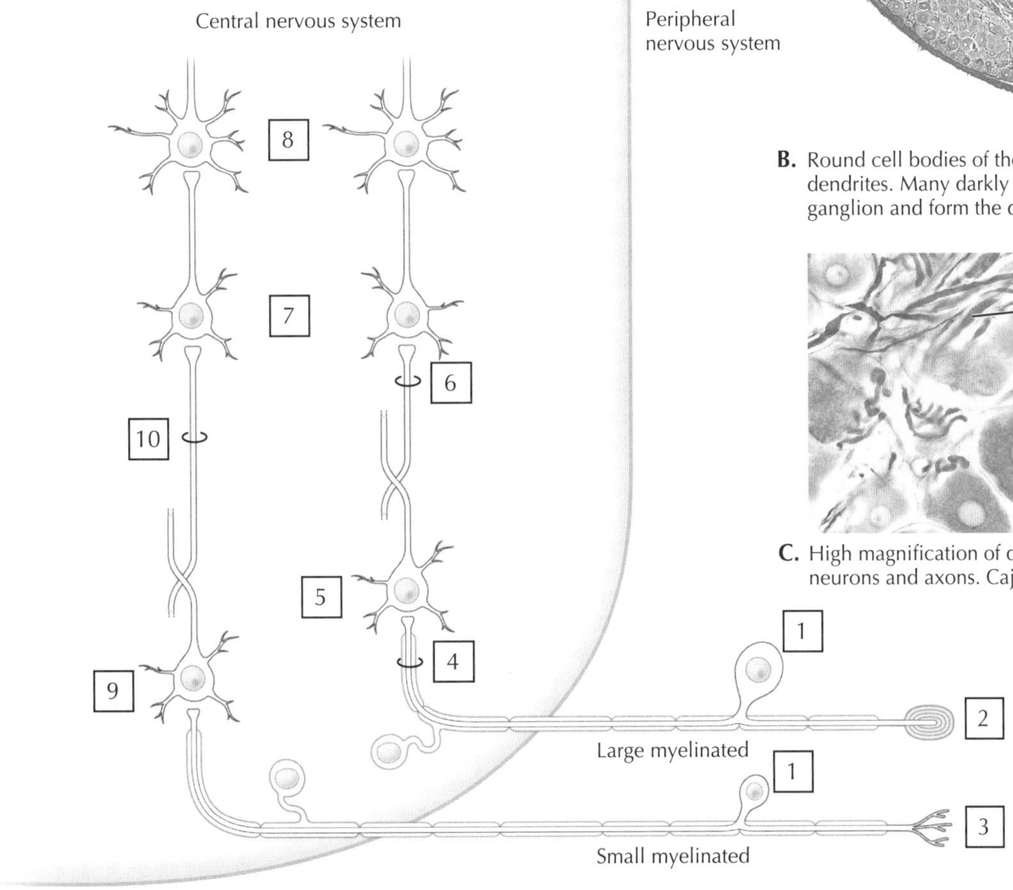

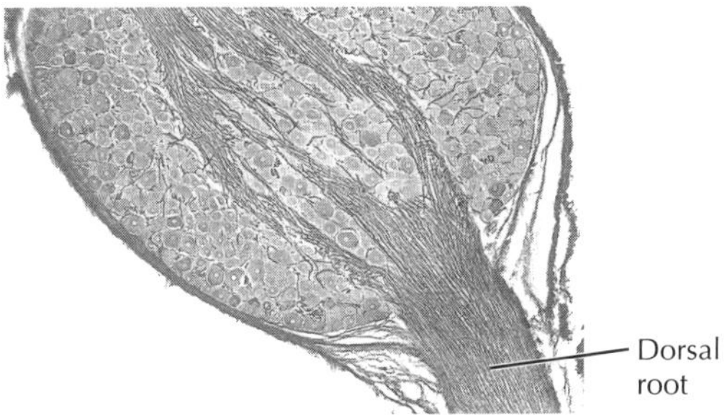

B. Round cell bodies of the dorsal root ganglion, devoid of dendrites. Many darkly stained axons course through the ganglion and form the dorsal root. Cajal stain (fiber stain).

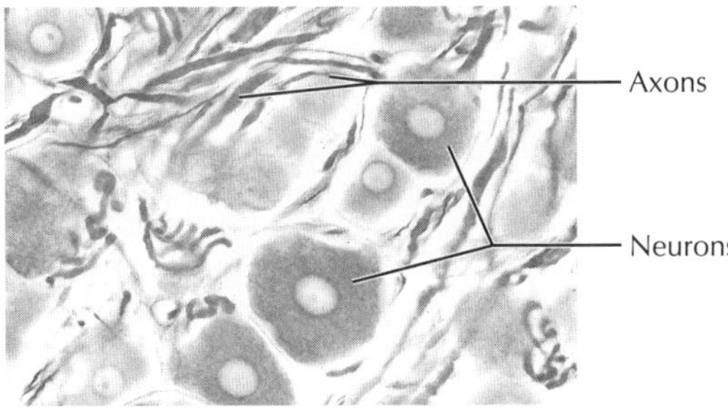

C. High magnification of dorsal root ganglion primary sensory neurons and axons. Cajal stain.

Motor Channels: Basic Organization of Lower and Upper Motor Neurons

LMNs are the neuronal final common pathway from the central nervous system to the skeletal muscles. LMNs are found in the anterior horn of the spinal cord and in motor cranial nerve nuclei in the brainstem. These LMNs send myelinated axons via the spinal and cranial nerves to supply groups of muscle fibers with cholinergic synapses, at neuromuscular junctions, thereby activating nicotinic receptors on the skeletal muscle fibers to initiate muscle action potentials and cause muscle contraction. Without the LMNs and their innervated muscle fibers (called a motor unit), there would be no movement or behavior. These LMNs are regulated by sensory inputs (direct from the muscle spindles, indirect from other sensory inputs) and by descending motor pathways called UMNs.

The Upper Motor Neurons Are Found in the Brainstem and in the Cerebral Cortex

UPPER MOTOR NEURONS	ACTION
Corticospinal tract	Controls fine hand movements
Rubrospinal tract	Influences upper extremity movements
Lateral vestibulospinal tract	Regulates powerful antigravity musculature
Pontine reticulospinal tract	Regulates extensor tone and posture
Medullary reticulospinal tract	Regulates flexor tone and posture
Medial vestibulospinal tract	Regulates neck movements related to position
Tectospinal tract	Regulates head and neck movements related to visual and auditory stimuli
Interstitiospinal tract	Regulates torsion movements of the trunk around a central axis

COLOR the following structures, using a separate color for each structure.

- ☐ **1. Skeletal muscle fibers**
- ☐ **2. Myelinated motor axon**
- ☐ **3. Lower motor neuron**
- ☐ **4. Interneuron**
- ☐ **5. Brainstem UMN cell group**
- ☐ **6. Brainstem UMN descending tract**
- ☐ **7. Cortical UMN**
- ☐ **8. Corticospinal tract**

Clinical Note

The UMNs provide the major regulation of the LMNs. Reflexes provide moment-to-moment adjustment of LMN activity from sensory inputs. Brainstem UMNs (**pontine and medullary reticulospinal tracts** and the **lateral vestibulospinal tract**) provide control over basic tone and posture, with the lateral vestibulospinal tract providing the most powerful drive over antigravity (extensor) tone. The **rubrospinal tract** helps to counter extensor predominance for the upper extremities by providing a flexor bias. The corticospinal tract provides fine motor control over the hand and fingers and allows skilled movements and tool use. The **tectospinal tract**, **medial vestibulospinal tract**, and **interstitiospinal tract** provide specialized control of head and neck movements and torsional trunk movements related to position and visual/auditory inputs.

The corticospinal tract descends through the posterior limb of the internal capsule (accompanied by corticorubral projections and other descending motor projections). In the spinal cord, the lateral corticospinal tract descends in the dorsal portion of the lateral funiculus, accompanied by the rubrospinal tract. Damage to this region disrupts both of these systems, resulting in ipsilateral spastic hemiplegia with hypertonus, hyperreflexia, and pathological movements. In the rare instances where the corticospinal tract is damaged in isolation (e.g., in the medullary pyramids with a paramedian arterial branch infarct), spasticity is not seen but there is loss of control of fine hand and finger movements. Damage to the corticospinal system in association with damage to the corticorubrospinal system is characterized by the typical "UMN syndrome." UMN damage can be caused by strokes, spinal injury, cerebral palsy, and other disorders.

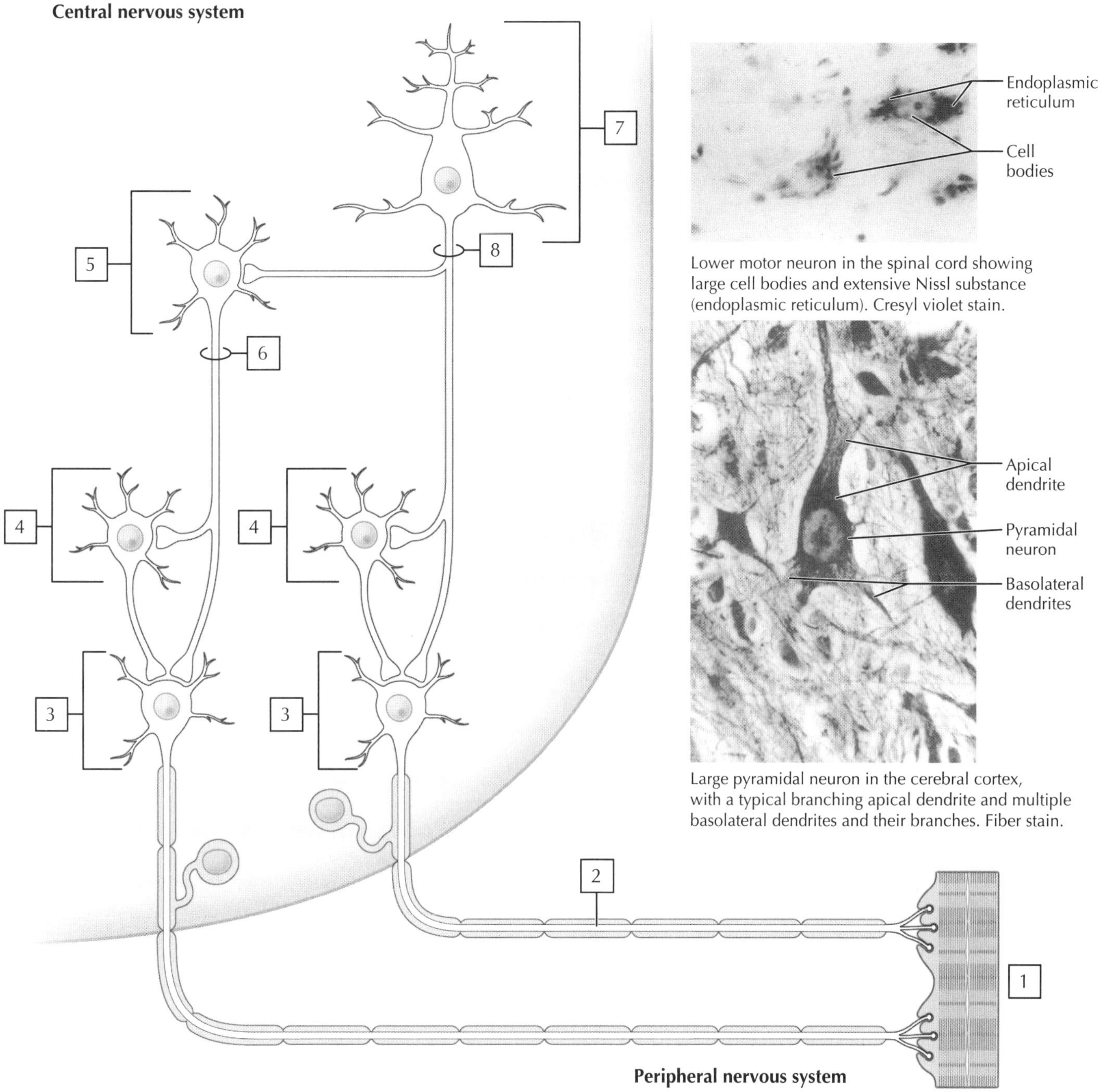

Lower motor neuron in the spinal cord showing large cell bodies and extensive Nissl substance (endoplasmic reticulum). Cresyl violet stain.

Large pyramidal neuron in the cerebral cortex, with a typical branching apical dendrite and multiple basolateral dendrites and their branches. Fiber stain.

Autonomic Channels

The final common pathway for the autonomic innervation of **effector tissue** (cardiac muscle, smooth muscle, secretory glands, metabolic cells, and cells of the immune system) consists of preganglionic autonomic neurons in the **T1–L2 intermediolateral cell column** in the lateral horn of the spinal cord **(sympathetics)**, the **S2–S4 intermediate gray of the spinal cord**, and specific **autonomic nuclei of the brainstem (parasympathetics)**. The preganglionic neurons send cholinergic axons to **ganglion cells** in the **sympathetic chain ganglia and collateral ganglia** (sympathetics) and to **intramural ganglia** (parasympathetics). The sympathetic ganglion cells send mainly noradrenergic projections to their effector tissue (possessing alpha and beta adrenoceptors), and parasympathetic ganglion cells send cholinergic projections to their effector tissue (possessing mainly muscarinic cholinergic receptors).

The preganglionic autonomic neurons are controlled by a complex array of **nuclei and centers from the brainstem** (e.g., nucleus solitarius, serotonergic raphe nuclei, noradrenergic and adrenergic central nuclei in the medulla and pons, parabrachial nuclei, opioid neuron groups, cardiovascular and respiratory centers, and others), **hypothalamus** (e.g., paraventricular nuclei, and anterior and posterior hypothalamic regions), and **limbic forebrain structures** (e.g., amygdaloid nuclei), all of which are extensively interconnected. These central regulatory zones over the preganglionic autonomic neurons are the equivalent of the UMNs for the motor system. Many of the regions of brainstem, hypothalamus, and limbic forebrain that control autonomic outflow and their related visceral regulatory functions also control the cells of origin for **posterior pituitary hormones** (oxytocin and vasopressin) and **anterior pituitary hormones** (via releasing factor and inhibitory factor neurons projecting to the median eminence and its **hypophyseal-portal system**). While some of these central regulatory connections to preganglionic autonomic neurons are precise and highly localized (e.g., cardiovascular and respiratory centers), many of the projections are more widespread and regulate the general state of sympathetic arousal (fight-or-flight) or parasympathetic activation (digestive and elimination functions, homeostatic, and reparative functions).

Preganglionic autonomic neurons also are subject to **sensory inputs** via the **dorsal root ganglion cells**, with appropriate reflex regulation through polysynaptic channels using **interneurons**.

COLOR the following structures, using a separate color for each structure.

- ☐ 1. **Limbic forebrain structures**
- ☐ 2. **Hypothalamus**
- ☐ 3. **Brainstem nuclei and centers for autonomic control**
- ☐ 4. **Preganglionic sympathetic neuron**
- ☐ 5. **Spinal cord interneuron**
- ☐ 6. **Sympathetic ganglion cell**
- ☐ 7. **Sensory neurons in the dorsal root ganglion**
- ☐ 8. **Autonomic target tissue (effector tissue)**
- ☐ 9. **Hypophyseal-portal system**
- ☐ 10. **Anterior pituitary hormones**

Clinical Note

Sympathetic activation provides an acute fight-or-flight response to perceived danger. Blood is diverted from the viscera to muscles, heart rate increases, respiration deepens, pupils dilate, and the body prepares for immediate response to the emergency. When the sympatho-adrenal axis remains chronically elevated, with chronically high output of epinephrine and norepinephrine, detrimental physiological effects ensue.

Metabolically and physiologically, these stress hormones can increase clotting and platelet aggregation, increase vascular endothelial cell damage contributing to atherosclerosis, increase production of free radicals, increase the likelihood of arrhythmias and cardiovascular events, increase glucose release from the liver and increase glycogenolysis, increase insulin and insulin-like growth factor-1 production, increase insulin resistance and decrease insulin sensitivity, and increase chronic production of inflammatory mediators such as interleukin (IL)-6, IL-1 beta, and C-reactive protein. These chronic alterations increase the risk for cardiovascular disease, strokes, type 2 diabetes, and many cancers.

Immunologically, these stress hormones also decrease natural killer cell activity and cell-mediated immunity, and increase the likelihood of metastases and recurrence in some cancers. Recent data have shown that patients who take a nonspecific beta-blocker, such as propranolol, experience fewer metastases (breast cancer, non–small cell lung cancer) and benefit from a considerable extension of survival with ovarian cancer. Thus the chronic state of activation of the sympathetic nervous system is of great physiological importance.

Clinically, sympathetic activation can be caused by physical (exercise), physiological (injury, surgery, pain), or emotional (stress, depression, isolation, posttraumatic stress) factors.

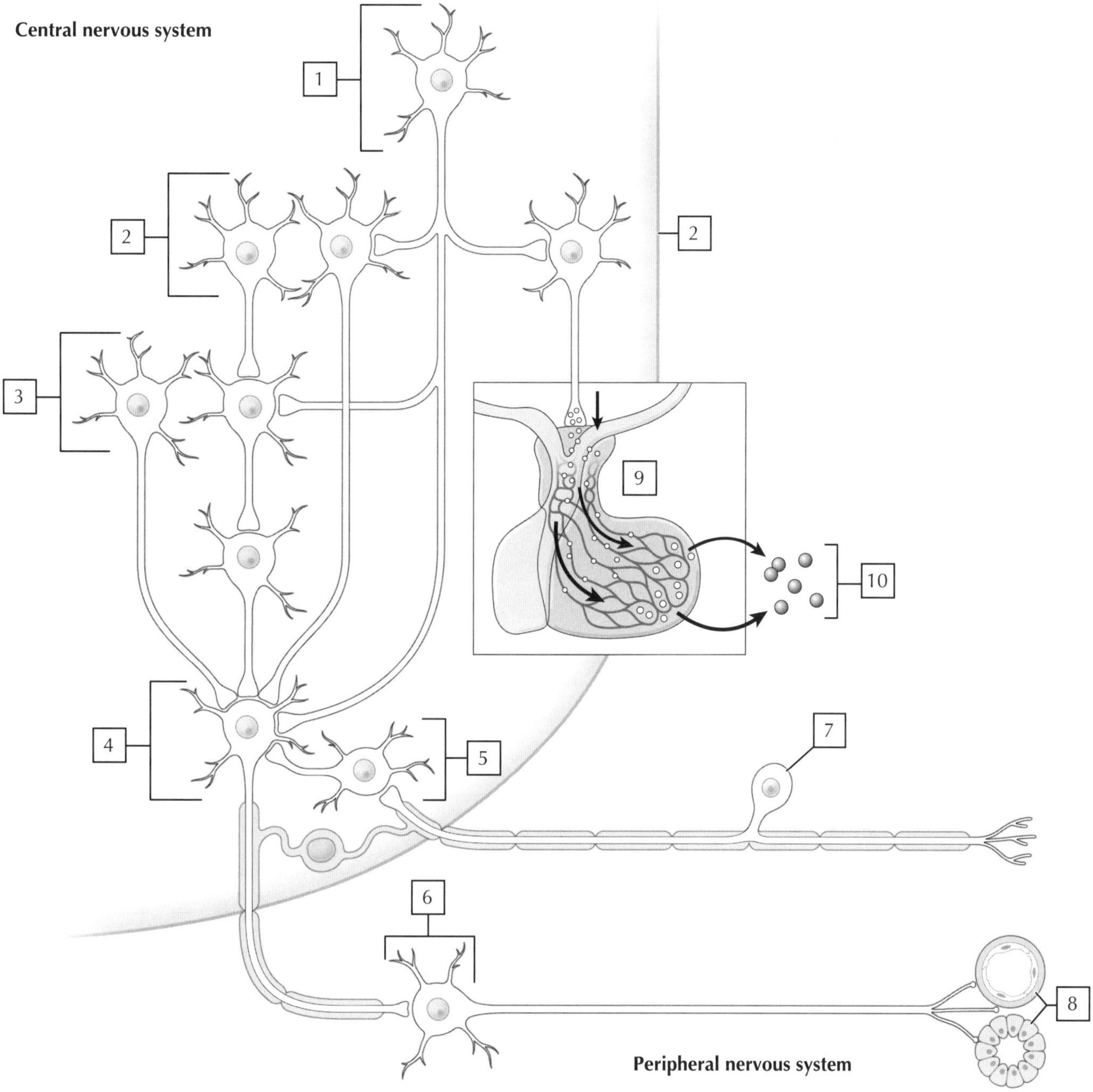
Central nervous system
1
2
2
3
9
10
4
5
7
6
8
Peripheral nervous system

Cutaneous Receptors

Cutaneous receptors are the transducing elements of the distal portion of primary sensory axons related to the skin and subcutaneous regions. They act as dendrites, and when a mechanical, thermal, or nociceptive stimulus depolarizes the sensory receptor to the point of reaching threshold, an action potential will be transduced at the immediately adjacent **initial segment of the distal axon.** This action potential will propagate toward the central nervous system proximally, and may also induce the release of bioactive molecules, such as substance P, from the distal portion of the axon and its sensory receptor at the site of the stimulus. Some receptors are thought to code for specific consciously perceived modalities (e.g., Pacinian corpuscles with vibratory sensation), but other perceived sensations may involve the interpretation of stimuli of multiple sensory receptors.

Sensory Receptors and Their Coded Modalities and Actions	
RECEPTORS	**CODED MODALITIES AND ACTIONS**
Bare (free) nerve endings	Nociception and thermal sensation
Pacinian corpuscles	Vibration, brief touch—rapidly adapting mechanoreceptors
Merkel disks	Maintained deformation, sustained touch on the skin—slowly adapting mechanoreceptors
Meissner corpuscles	Moving touch—rapidly adapting mechanoreceptors
Ruffini endings	Steady pressure applied to hairy skin—slowly adapting mechanoreceptor
Hair follicle receptors	Response to movement of hairs—rapidly adapting
Krause end bulbs	Possible thermoreceptor response

COLOR the following structures, using a separate color for each structure.

- ☐ 1. **Meissner corpuscle**
- ☐ 2. **Krause end bulb**
- ☐ 3. **Free nerve endings**
- ☐ 4. **Pacinian corpuscle**
- ☐ 5. **Merkel disk**
- ☐ 6. **Ruffini ending**
- ☐ 7. **Nerve plexus (receptors) around hair follicle**
- ☐ 8. **Initial segment of primary sensory axon associated with Merkel disk**
- ☐ 9. **Initial segment of primary sensory axon associated with Pacinian corpuscle**

Clinical Note

In the early days of research of primary sensory receptors, there were some investigators who thought specific anatomical sensory receptors coded mechanoreceptor, thermoreceptor, or nociceptor information that corresponded to conscious perception of specific sensations or modalities. While this applies in some situations, such as the association between activation of free nerve endings from unmyelinated C fibers and the perception of pain, or the rapid on–off stimulus of Pacinian corpuscles and the perception of vibratory sensation, there are many sensations (e.g., pleasurable stimulation of skin) that may involve the activation of many sensory receptor types in specific patterns.

In addition, some receptors may evoke responses in their primary sensory axons that participate in multiple sensory tasks and contribute to all three types of sensory channels. Some mechanoreceptors and nociceptors may evoke a flexor reflex withdrawal response through reflex channels. These same mechanoreceptors may contribute sensory information, along with stimuli from muscle spindles, tendons, ligaments, and joints, into spinocerebellar channels to keep the cerebellum informed about the state of stimulation in the periphery on a moment-to-moment basis. These same mechanoreceptors and their activated axons may contribute information into either protopathic or epicritic lemniscal channels that convey information through the medial lemniscus or the spinothalamic/spinoreticular system to the thalamus, and then to regions of the sensory cortex for conscious interpretation of these stimuli.

A. Glabrous skin

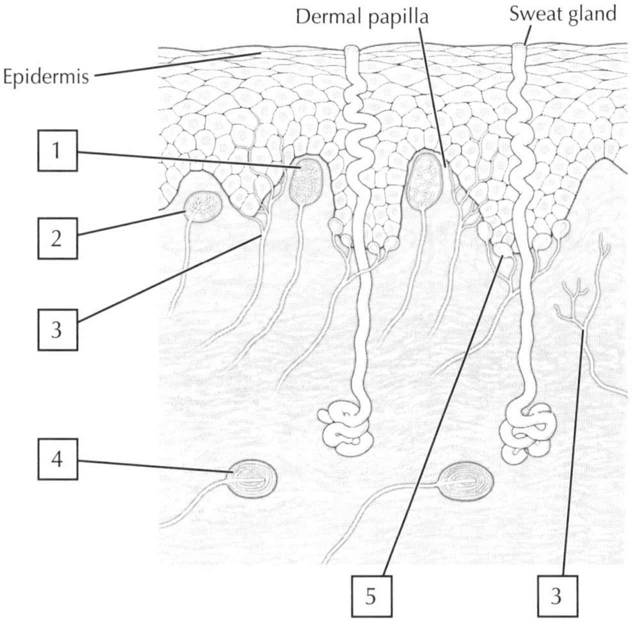

B. Hairy skin

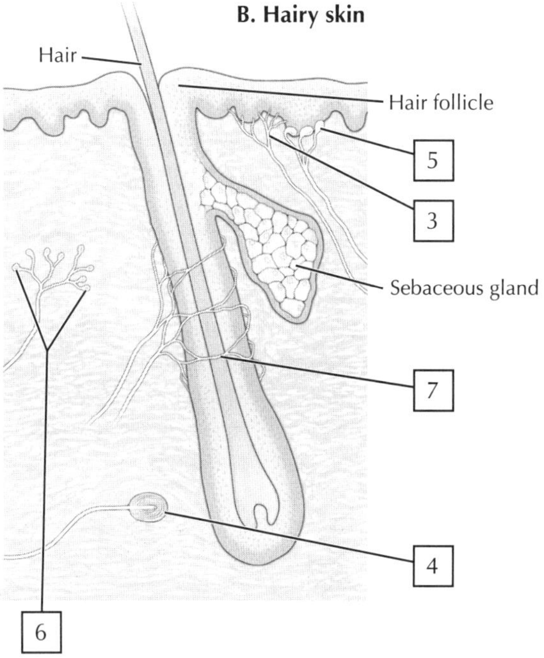

C. Detail of Merkel disk

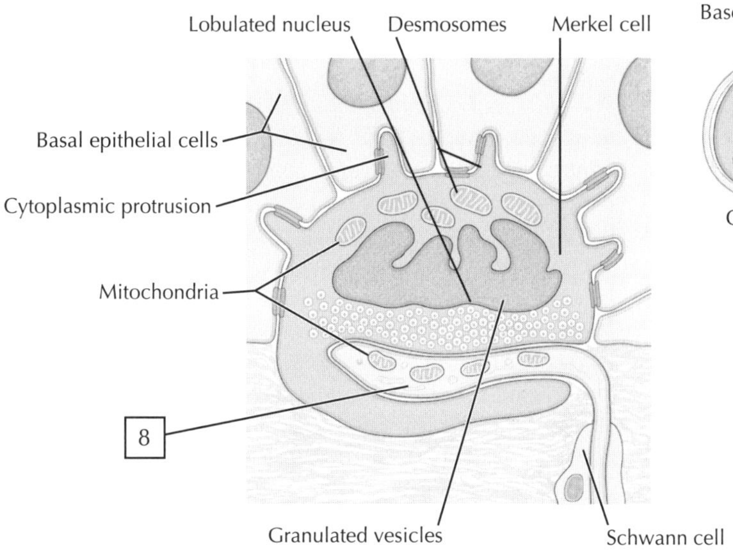

D. Detail of free nerve ending

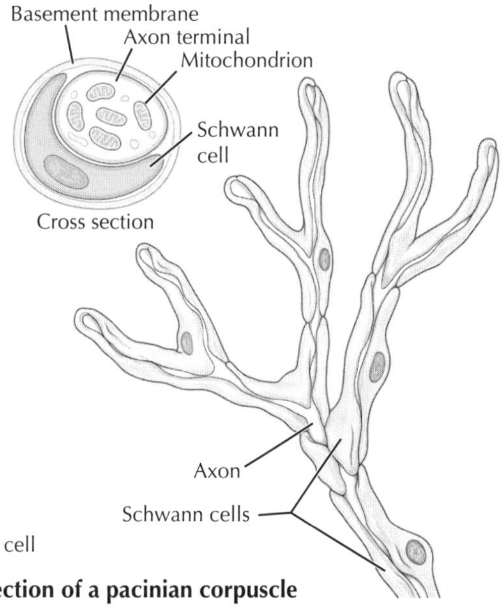

E. Histological cross section and longitudinal section of a pacinian corpuscle

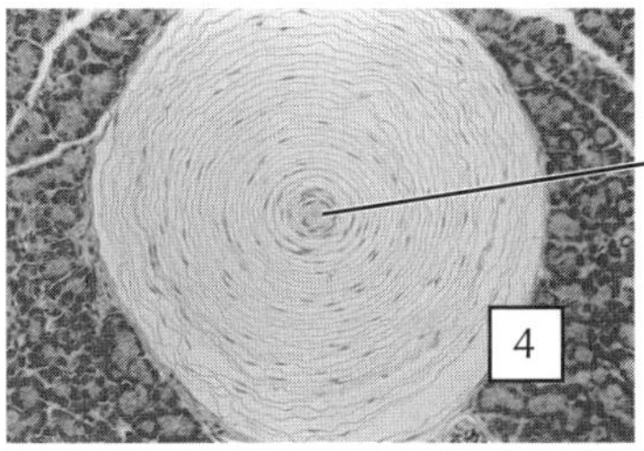

a. Cross section

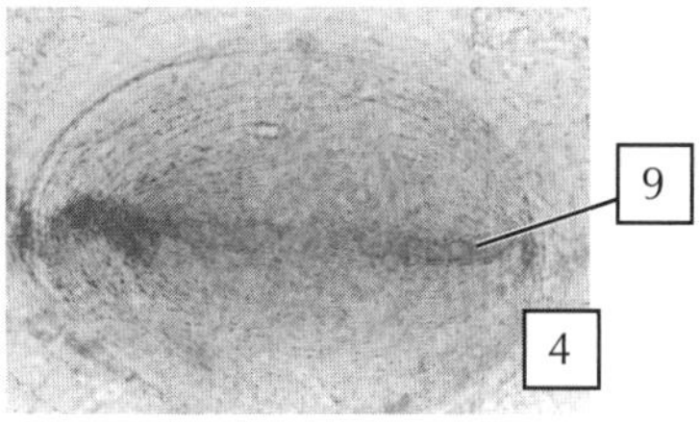

b. Pacinian corpuscle longitudinal section, enwrapped by layers of lamellae. Small supporting cells are interspersed among the lamellae.

5 Neuromuscular Junction, Autonomic Neuroeffector Junctions, and Neurotransmission

The **neuromuscular junction** is the site of contact between the efferent endings **(axon terminals)** of a LMN and the skeletal muscle fibers it innervates. The motor axon loses its myelin sheath and forms an expanded nerve ending in a trough on the muscle fibers, protected above by **Schwann cells;** the nerve ending contains **synaptic vesicles** with a dense accumulation of acetylcholine (ACh) molecules (**quantal content** of approximately 10,000/vesicle), which are released following a motor action potential by fusion with the **presynaptic membrane.** The ACh is released into the **synaptic cleft** and stimulates **ACh receptors** located on the **postsynaptic membrane,** which is thrown into **junctional folds**, which contains a high density of ACh receptors. The simultaneous release of a few hundred synaptic vesicle packets of ACh (**quantal release**) normally provides a sufficient stimulation of ACh receptor sites to raise the muscle membrane potential to threshold, induce a muscle action potential, and provoke a muscle contraction.

Autonomic neuroeffector junctions are sites of contact between the efferent endings of postganglionic autonomic neurons and their target tissues, including cardiac muscle, smooth muscle, secretory glands, metabolic cells, and cells of the immune system. The **postsynaptic sympathetic endings** form a string of beaded **varicosities** using norepinephrine as their neurotransmitter; **postsynaptic parasympathetic endings** also form varicosities releasing ACh. The varicosities associated with cardiac muscle, smooth muscle, and secretory glands do not form classic synapses with presynaptic and postsynaptic thickenings and standardized synaptic separation. These endings provide paracrine-like secretion of neurotransmitter from synaptic vesicles in the varicosity. The **sympathetic nerve terminals** in contact with liver cells and associated with cells of the immune system in the parenchyma of lymphoid organs can form appositions as close as 6 nm (closer than a standard synapse), also releasing norepinephrine as a paracrine secretion.

COLOR the following structures, using a separate color for each structure.

- ☐ 1. **Axon terminal at the neuromuscular junction**
- ☐ 2. **ACh receptor sites (nicotinic receptors)**
- ☐ 3. **Synaptic cleft**
- ☐ 4. **Postsynaptic membrane**
- ☐ 5. **Junctional folds of the muscle membrane**
- ☐ 6. **Schwann cell**
- ☐ 7. **Presynaptic membrane**
- ☐ 8. **Synaptic vesicles**
- ☐ 9. **Sympathetic nerve varicosities on smooth muscle cells**
- ☐ 10. **Sympathetic nerve varicosities on mucous cells of a salivary gland**
- ☐ 11. **Parasympathetic nerve varicosities on serious cells of a salivary gland**
- ☐ 12. **Sympathetic nerve terminals adjacent to T lymphocytes in the parenchyma of lymphoid tissue**

Clinical Note

The neuromuscular junctions permit a motor action potential to release enough ACh to evoke consistent and dependable contraction of the innervated muscle fibers (the **motor unit**). The number of muscle fibers supplied by a single LMN varies from just a few (extraocular muscles) to thousands (large muscles such as the quadriceps). If some LMNs are damaged or lost by LMN disease such as polio or a component of amyotrophic lateral sclerosis, adjacent LMNs may sprout to innervate the resultant denuded muscle fibers, thereby resulting in very large motor units.

The neuroeffector junctions permit selective or collective actions on effector target tissues of the autonomic nervous system. During a sympathetic fight-or-flight response, extensive activation of the sympathetic nerves results in increased heart rate and contractility, dilated pupil, glucose mobilization from the liver, increased respiration, diminished gastrointestinal (GI) and other visceral activity, and diversion of blood flow to the muscles. This evolved for short-term adaptability to threats and dangers. Chronic activation of the sympathetic nervous system can have highly detrimental long-term effects, including suppression of cell-mediated immune activity and natural killer response, insulin and glucose metabolic dysfunction, increased likelihood of cardiovascular and cerebrovascular disease, and other serious chronic problems.

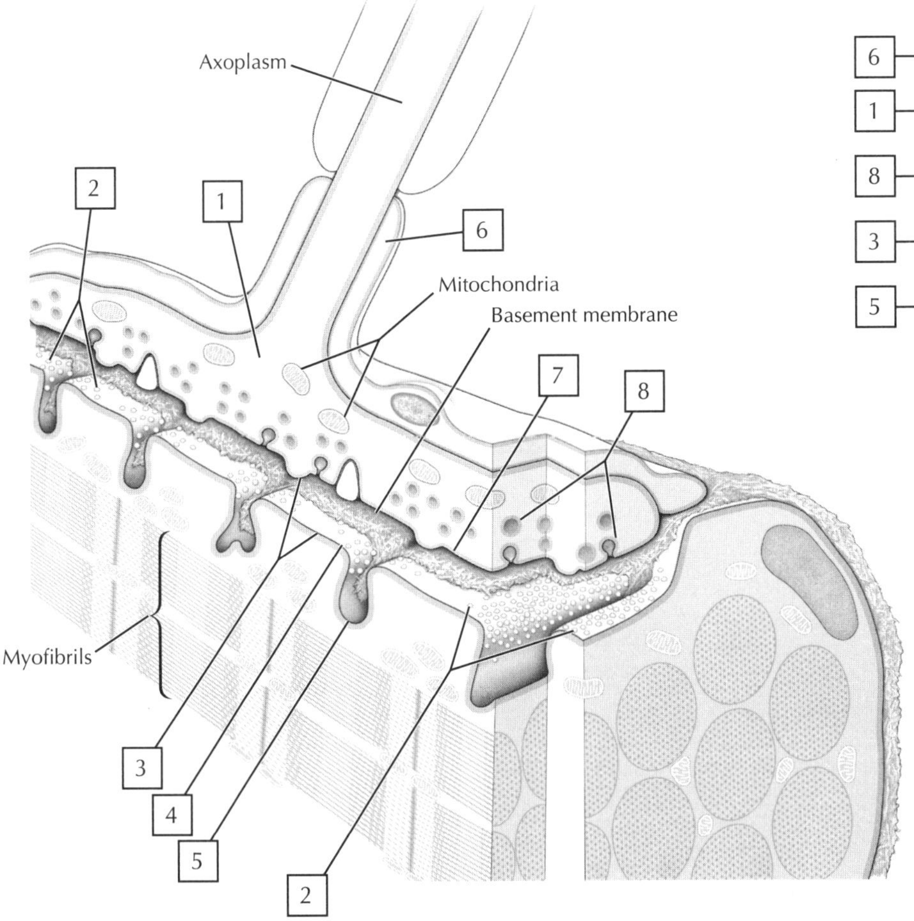

A. Longitudinal view of a neuromuscular junction

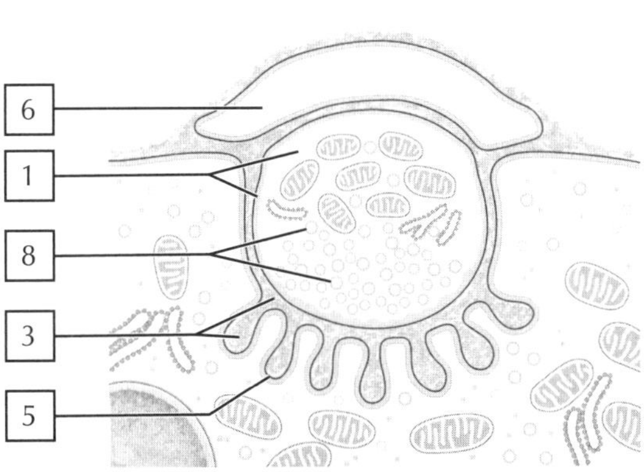

B. Synaptic trough (cross section)

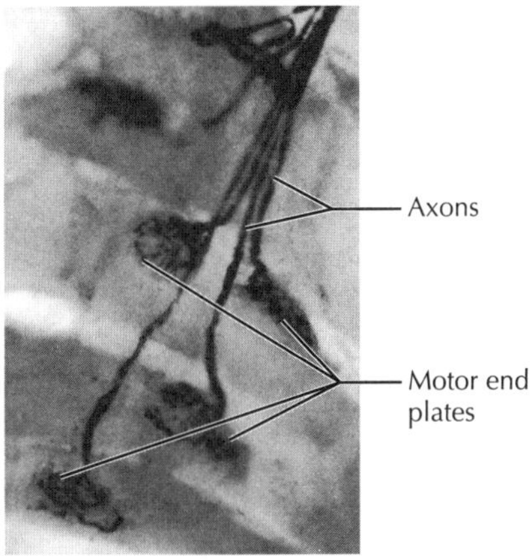

C. Histologic staining of motor end plates on skeletal muscle fibers

D. Smooth muscle

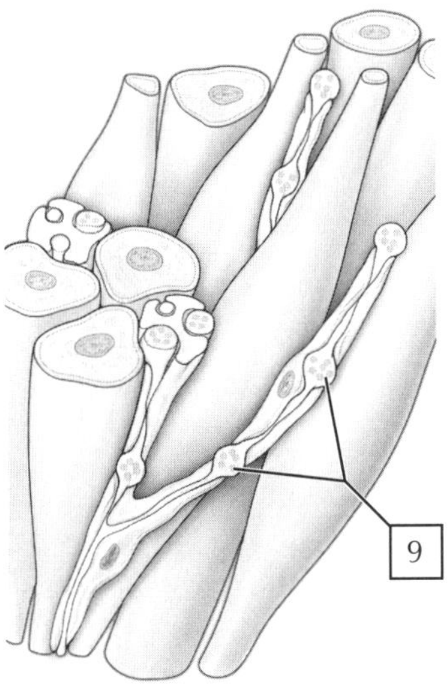

E. Gland (submandibular)

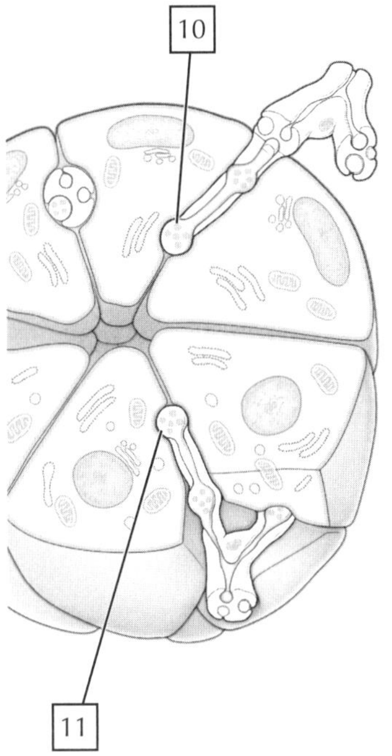

F. Lymphoid tissue (spleen)

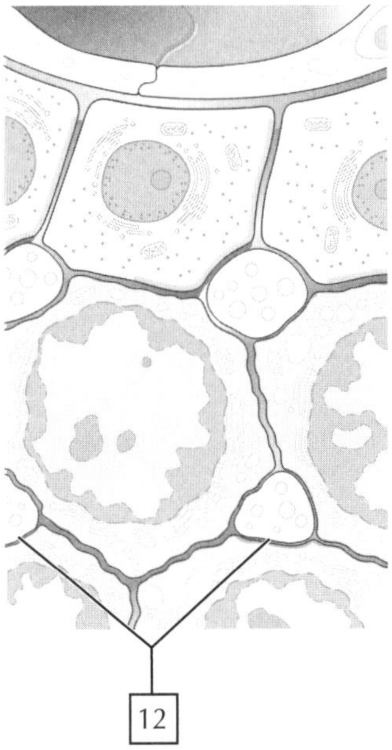

5 Brachial Plexus

The brachial plexus is formed by the **ventral roots of C5–C8,** with some contribution from **T1 and C4.** Sensory and sympathetic fibers also distribute with the brachial plexus. The roots give rise to three trunks, three ventral and three dorsal divisions, three cords, and many terminal branches, the peripheral nerves. Major peripheral nerves derived from the brachial plexus include the **musculocutaneous nerve** (C[4], C5, C6, C7) via the lateral cord; the **axillary nerve** (C5, C6 via the posterior cord), the **radial nerve** (C5, C6, C7, C8, T1 via the posterior cord); the **median nerve** (C[5], C6, C7, C8, T1 via the lateral and medial cords); and the **ulnar nerve** (C[7], C8, T1 via the medial cord).

COLOR the following structures, using a separate color for each structure.

- ☐ **1. C5 nerve roots**
- ☐ **2. C6 nerve roots**
- ☐ **3. C7 nerve roots**
- ☐ **4. C8 nerve roots**
- ☐ **5. T1 nerve roots**
- ☐ **6. Musculocutaneous nerve**
- ☐ **7. Axillary nerve**
- ☐ **8. Radial nerve**
- ☐ **9. Median nerve**
- ☐ **10. Ulnar nerve**

Clinical Note

The complex course of distribution of the nerve roots from C5–T1 through the brachial plexus, including the roots, trunks, dorsal and ventral divisions, cords, and finally the peripheral nerves, results in each peripheral nerve receiving contribution from two or more nerve roots, and each nerve root contributing to many peripheral nerves. The brachial plexus itself is vulnerable to injury, especially at birth (a superior plexus paralysis particularly affecting C5 and C6 contributions), which may lead to paresis of shoulder abduction and external rotation, and paresis of elbow flexion, with sparing of the hands. These impairments are brought about by damage to the motor supply to the deltoid, supraspinatus, infraspinatus, biceps, supinator, and brachioradialis muscles. The arm hangs down and is rotated medially, and the forearm is pronated. The upper plexus lesion also may result in sensory loss over the deltoid area, and the radial aspect of the forearm and hand.

Damage to the inferior brachial plexus (C8, T1) may occur because of pressure by a cervical rib. The motor consequences are paralysis of finger flexion and paralysis of all small muscles of the hand, resulting in a claw hand. This lesion also may produce an ulnar sensory loss, and possibly ipsilateral Horner syndrome.

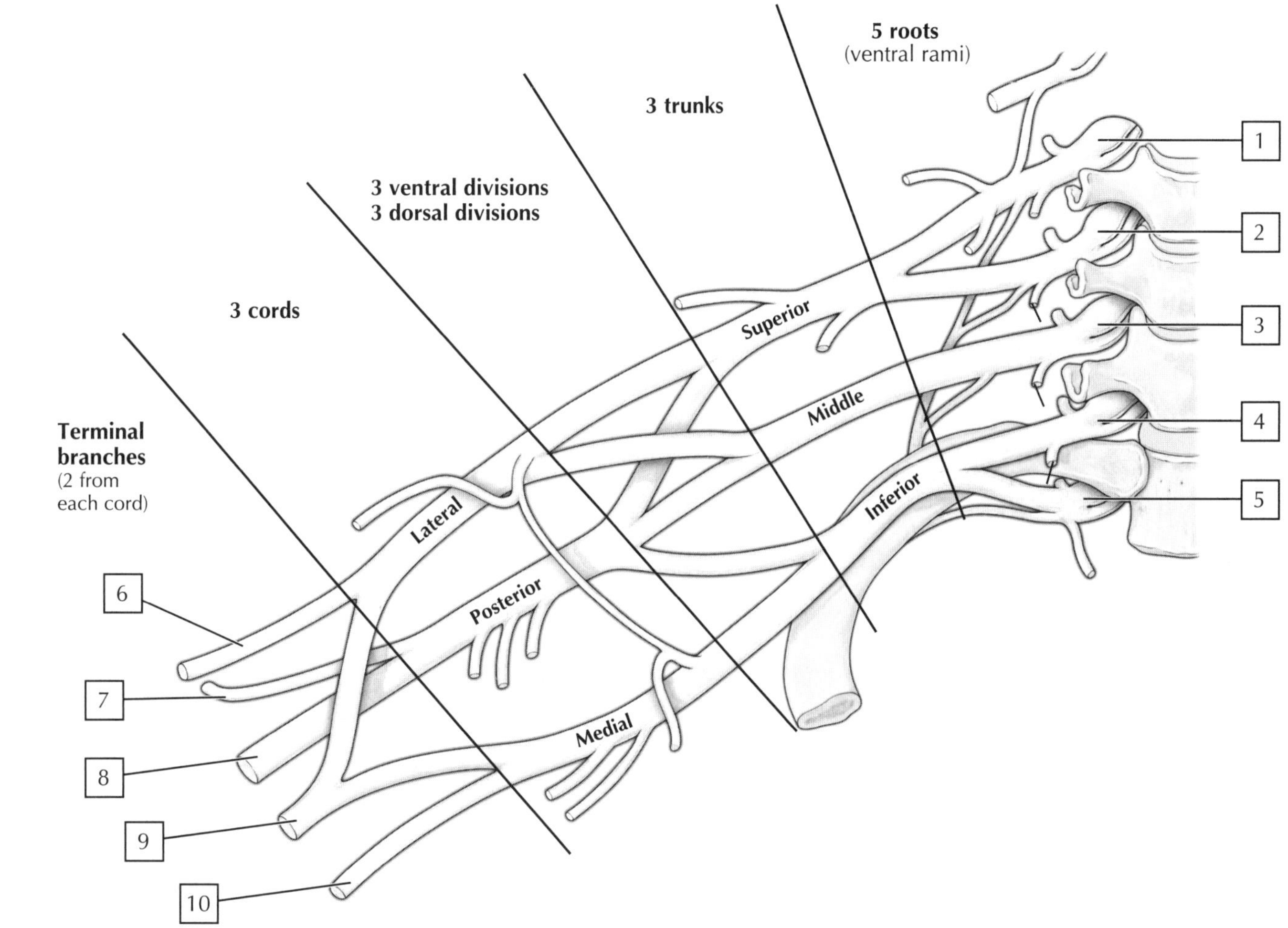
5 roots
(ventral rami)
3 trunks
3 ventral divisions
3 dorsal divisions
3 cords
Terminal
branches
(2 from
each cord)
Superior
Middle
Inferior
Lateral
Posterior
Medial
1
2
3
4
5
6
7
8
9
10

5 Dermatomal Distribution

A dermatome is the cutaneous area supplied by a single **dorsal root.** The cell bodies are in dorsal root ganglia, the distal axon is associated with sensory receptors, and the proximal axon enters the spinal cord and is associated with specific spinal cord segments. The **dermatomal maps** demonstrate the regions of the body associated with each dorsal root and its associated spinal level. For the trigeminal nerve distribution to the facial area, the three subdivisions (V1 **[ophthalmic]**; V2 **[maxillary];** and V3 **[mandibular]**) do not overlap, as do the spinal dermatomes. Thus a lesion of one trigeminal subdivision will result in total anesthesia of the region supplied.

LEVEL OF DERMATOMES	
C3	Clavicles
C5, C6, C7	Lateral parts of the upper limb
C8, T1	Medial sides of the upper limb
C6	Thumb
C6, C7, C8	Hand
C8	Ring and little fingers
T4	Level of nipples
T10	Level of umbilicus
T12	Inguinal or groin area
L1, L2, L3, L4	Anterior and inner surfaces of the lower limb
L4, L5, S1	Foot
L4	Medial side of the great toe
L5, S1, S2	Outer and posterior sides of the lower limb
S1	Lateral margin of the foot and little toe
S2, S3, S4	Perineum

COLOR the following structures, using a separate color for each dermatome.

- ☐ 1. **C5 dermatome**
- ☐ 2. **C6 dermatome**
- ☐ 3. **C7 dermatome**
- ☐ 4. **T1 dermatome**
- ☐ 5. **T4 dermatome**
- ☐ 6. **T10 dermatome**
- ☐ 7. **L4 dermatome**
- ☐ 8. **L5 dermatome**
- ☐ 9. **S1 dermatome**
- ☐ 10. **S2 dermatome**
- ☐ 11. **Ophthalmic zone of CN V**
- ☐ 12. **Mandibular zone of CN V**

Clinical Note

The territory supplied by a single dorsal root consists of the direct level of the dermatome, the level above, and the level below. Thus if a dorsal root is cut, the dermatomal region is not anesthetic (total loss of sensation); rather, it is hypoesthetic (diminished sensation). This is unlike damage to a peripheral nerve, where the territory supplied by that nerve loses all sensation following a lesion. If a dermatomal region is anesthetic because of dorsal root damage, it would require damage to three consecutive dorsal roots.

However, if a dorsal root is subjected to pressure, irritation from a bone spicule or herniated disk, or by an inflammatory process, that irritative focus causes radiating pain in the distribution of the dermatome. With classical herniated disk problems (C5–C6, C6–C7, L4–L5, L5–S1), a key symptom is radiating pain, sometimes very severe; the localization of that pain provides diagnostic information about where the problem is located. Knowledge of the dermatomes is critically important in distinguishing between nerve root damage (radiculopathies) and peripheral nerve problems (neuropathies). For example, shingles (postherpetic neuralgia) will show a nerve root distribution, not a peripheral nerve distribution.

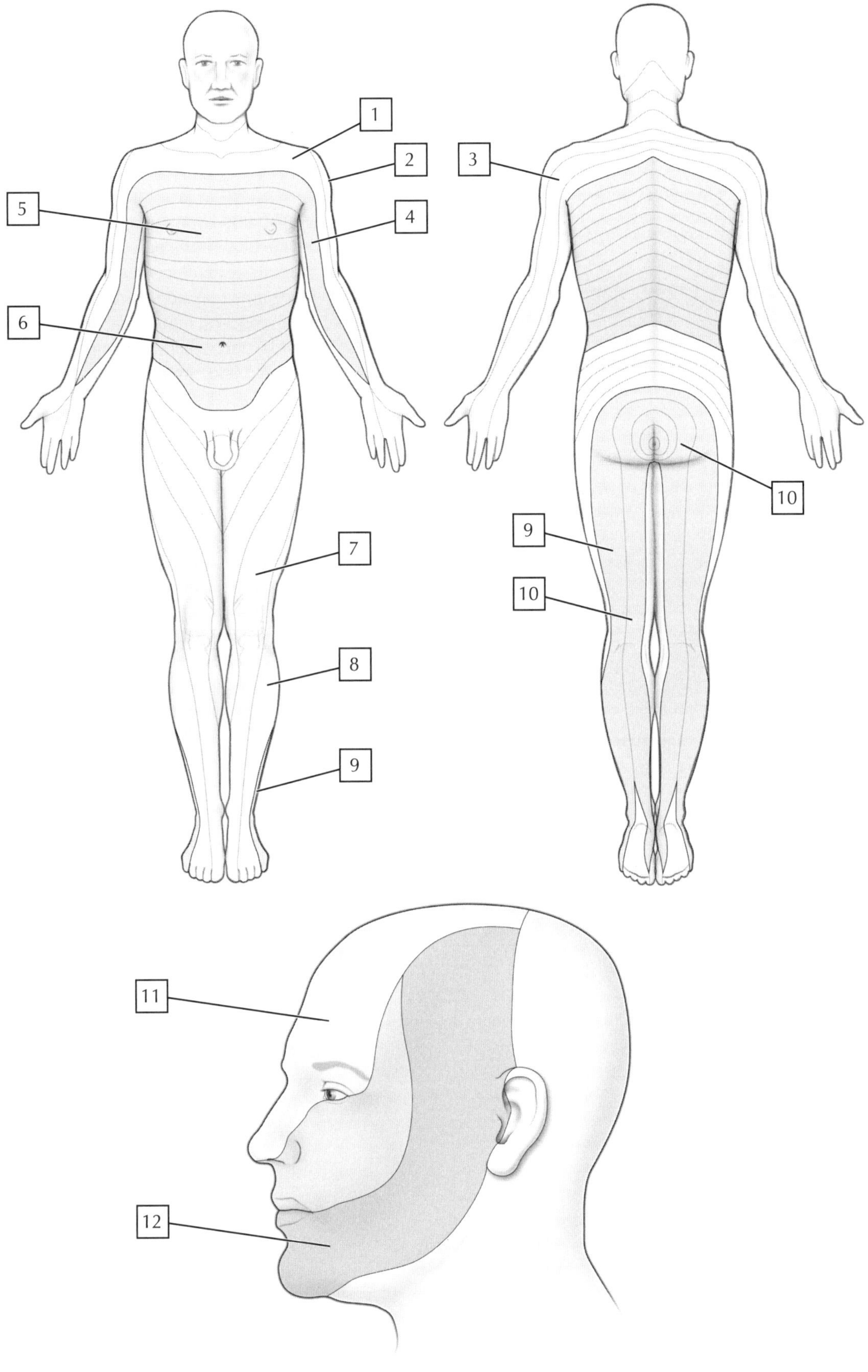
1
2
3
4
5
6
7
8
9
10
11
12

5 Cutaneous Distribution of Peripheral Nerves

Specific peripheral nerves are derived from nerve roots, with sensory, motor, and autonomic components sorted and recombined through specific plexuses, such as the brachial plexus, lumbar plexus, sacral plexus, and coccygeal plexus. Sensory axons, derived from the dorsal root ganglion cells, distribute their peripheral (distal) axons and associated sensory receptors to specific cutaneous regions of the body. The territory of distribution of a peripheral nerve may be composed of multiple dorsal root contributions (e.g., median nerve, C5–T1).

Major Peripheral Nerves and Their Nerve Root Contributions	
PERIPHERAL NERVE	**NERVE ROOT CONTRIBUTION**
Supraclavicular	C3, C4
Axillary	C5, C6
Lateral antebrachial cutaneous	C5–C7
Medial antebrachial cutaneous	C8, T1
Radial	C5–T1
Ulnar	C8, T1
Median	C5–T1
Iliohypogastric	L1
Ilioinguinal	L1
Genitofemoral	L1, L2
Femoral	L2–L4
Common fibular (peroneal)	L4–S2
Sural	S1, S2

COLOR the following structures, using a separate color for each structure.

☐ 1. **Cutaneous territory of supraclavicular nerve**
☐ 2. **Cutaneous territory of axillary nerve**
☐ 3. **Cutaneous territory of lateral antebrachial cutaneous nerve**
☐ 4. **Cutaneous territory of radial nerve**
☐ 5. **Cutaneous territory of ulnar nerve**
☐ 6. **Cutaneous territory of median nerve**
☐ 7. **Cutaneous territory of iliohypogastric nerve**
☐ 8. **Cutaneous territory of genitofemoral nerve**
☐ 9. **Cutaneous territory of femoral nerve**
☐ 10. **Cutaneous territory of common fibular (peroneal) nerve**
☐ 11. **Cutaneous territory of sural nerve**

Clinical Note

Structural insult or damage to a peripheral nerve results in a total loss of all sensation, epicritic and protopathic, in the cutaneous territory of that peripheral nerve. Peripheral nerve territories do not overlap with each other. This is in contrast to nerve root distribution, where there is overlap of approximately three dermatomes for each sensory nerve root. Peripheral neuropathies often are polyneuropathies, with multiple nerves affected; the metabolic neuropathies (type 2 diabetes, alcoholic, toxic neuropathies) often appear as distal symmetrical sensory losses. The sensory loss in these polyneuropathies may involve epicritic sensation, protopathic sensation, or both; paresthesias and painful sensations may sometimes occur. Pressure or entrapment of a peripheral nerve may lead to painful sensations and paresthesias in the cutaneous territory of that peripheral nerve (e.g., median nerve entrapment in carpel tunnel syndrome, lateral femoral cutaneous nerve compression with lateral thigh pain and paresthesias).

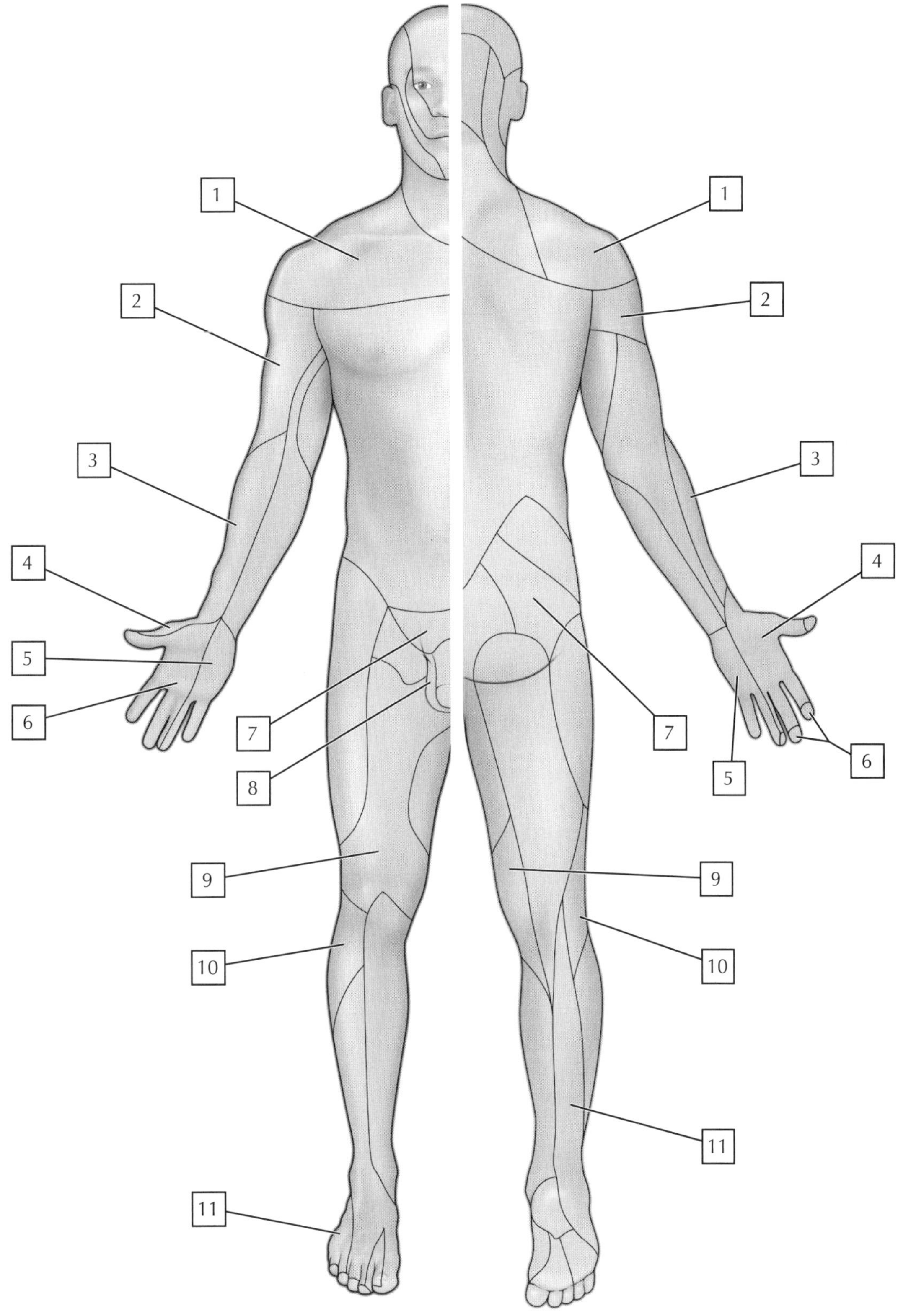
1
1
2
2
3
3
4
4
5
6
7
8
7
5
6
9
9
10
10
11
11

5 Cholinergic and Adrenergic Distribution to Motor and Autonomic Structures

All **LMNs** use acetylcholine (ACh) as their neurotransmitter at neuromuscular junctions on **skeletal muscle;** the ACh stimulates nicotinic (N) receptors on the muscle membrane.

All **preganglionic axons** from neurons of both the **sympathetic and parasympathetic nervous systems** use ACh as their neurotransmitter, stimulating N receptors on the ganglion cells (**sympathetic chain ganglia and collateral ganglia** for sympathetic nervous system, and **intramural ganglia** for parasympathetic nervous system) for the fast response; additional muscarinic (M) and dopamine receptors on the ganglion cells mediate longer-term excitability. **Preganglionic sympathetic axons** to **adrenal medullary chromaffin cells** use ACh as their neurotransmitter, stimulating N receptors on the chromaffin cells.

Postganglionic sympathetic axons use mainly norepinephrine (NE), with or without additional neuropeptides such as neuropeptide Y, as their neurotransmitter, stimulating **alpha or beta receptor subtypes** on their effector tissues. The sympathetic postganglionic axons to sweat glands use ACh as their neurotransmitter. **Postganglionic parasympathetic axons** use ACh as their neurotransmitter, stimulating mainly **M receptors** on their target tissues.

Clinical Note

Clinical use of cholinergic and adrenergic agents depends on a comprehensive knowledge of the distribution and actions of ACh on nicotinic and muscarinic receptors, and the distribution and actions of NE on alpha and beta receptors. In the heart, beta 1 receptors increase the force and rate of contraction, increase cardiac output, and dilate coronary arteries; M2 receptors decrease the force and rate of contraction and decrease cardiac output. In the bladder and ureters, alpha 1 receptors cause contraction. In the blood vessels, alpha 2 receptors cause constriction. In the liver, beta 2 receptors cause glycogenolysis. In the pancreas, beta 2 receptors stimulate insulin release, and alpha 2 receptors inhibit insulin release. In the immune system, beta receptor stimulation inhibits cell-mediated immunity and natural killer cell activity; use of a nonspecific beta blocker decreases metastases in several types of cancer, but cardiospecific beta blockers have no beneficial effect.

In myasthenia gravis, an autoantibody blocks the cholinergic nicotinic receptors at the neuromuscular junction leading to rapid muscle fatiguability.

COLOR the following structures, using a separate color for each structure. For synapses, use a colored arrow to point to it.

- ☐ **1. Lower motor neuron**
- ☐ **2. Cholinergic synapse on skeletal muscle fiber**
- ☐ **3. Sympathetic preganglionic neurons**
- ☐ **4. Preganglionic cholinergic synapses on sympathetic chain ganglion and collateral ganglion**
- ☐ **5. Postganglionic noradrenergic synapse stimulating alpha and beta receptors on target tissues**
- ☐ **6. Preganglionic cholinergic synapse on adrenal medullary chromaffin cells**
- ☐ **7. Parasympathetic preganglionic neuron**
- ☐ **8. Parasympathetic preganglionic cholinergic synapse on intramural ganglion**
- ☐ **9. Postganglionic parasympathetic cholinergic synapse stimulating M receptors on target tissues**

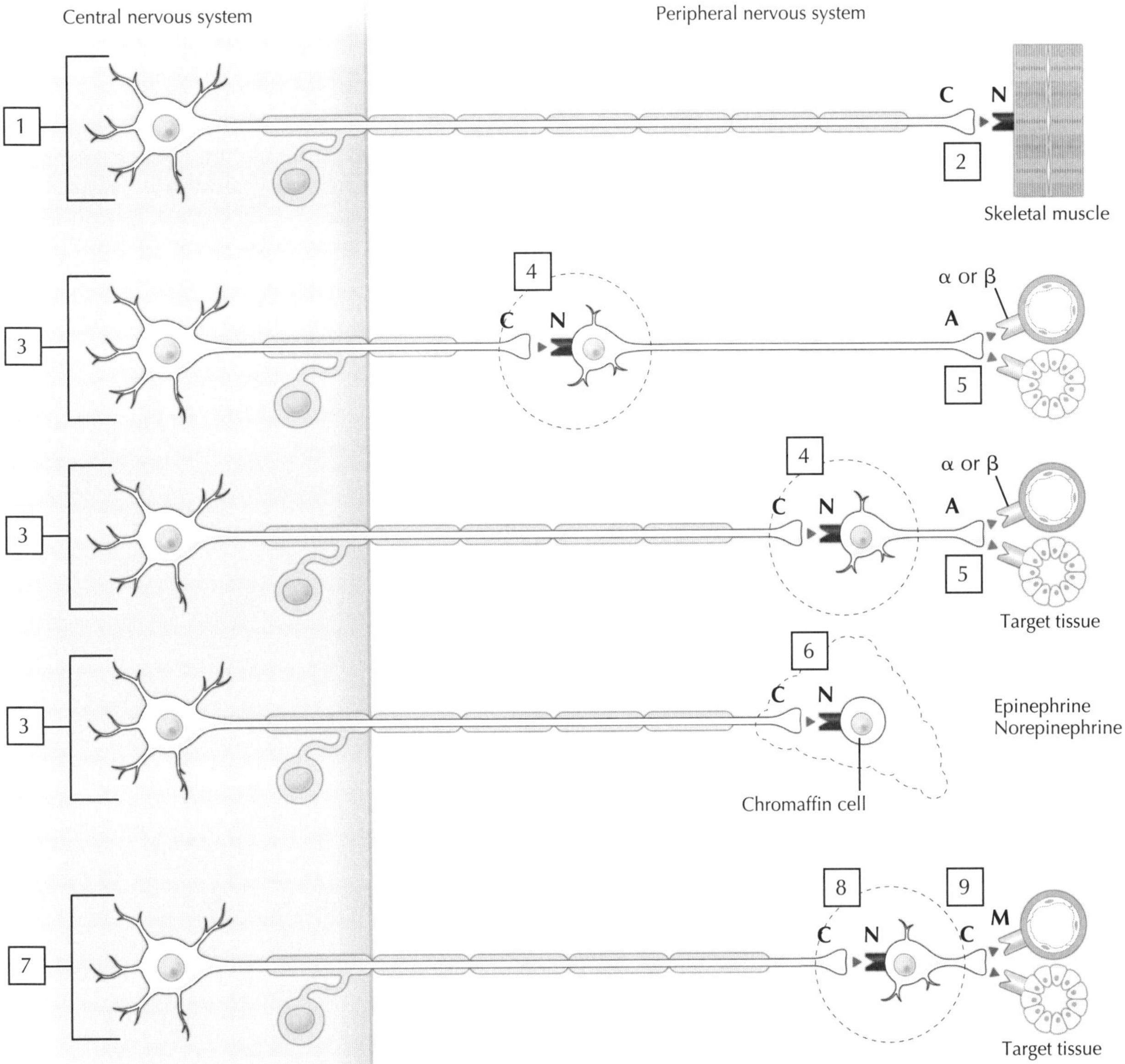

Synapses	Receptors	
A Adrenergic	α or β	Alpha or beta adrenergic
C Cholinergic	**N**	Nicotinic
	M	Muscarinic

Autonomic Distribution to the Head and Neck

Autonomic distribution to the head and neck arises from three parasympathetic nuclei in the brainstem and from the sympathetic **T1–T2 intermediolateral cell column** in the spinal cord. For the parasympathetic system, the **nucleus of Edinger–Westphal** in the midbrain sends cholinergic axons through **CN III** to the **ciliary ganglion**. The ciliary ganglion sends cholinergic axons to supply the pupillary constrictor muscle and the ciliary muscle for accommodation to near vision. The **superior salivatory nucleus** in the pons sends cholinergic axons through **CN VII** to the **pterygopalatine ganglion** and the **submandibular ganglion.** The pterygopalatine ganglion sends cholinergic axons to innervate the lacrimal glands and nasal mucosal glands, and the submandibular ganglion sends cholinergic axons to innervate the submandibular (submaxillary) and sublingual salivary glands. The **inferior salivatory nucleus** in the medulla sends cholinergic axons through **CN IX** to the otic ganglion. The otic ganglion sends cholinergic axons to innervate the parotid salivary gland.

For the sympathetic nervous system, the **neurons of the intermediolateral cell column** (lateral funiculus) at levels T1 and T2 send cholinergic axons through the ventral roots to the **superior cervical ganglion**. The superior cervical ganglion sends noradrenergic axons to innervate the pupillary dilator muscle, and the sweat glands and vascular smooth muscle in the head and neck.

Clinical Note

The aperture of the pupil is regulated by the opposing actions of the pupillary constrictor muscle (innervated by axons from the ciliary ganglion, a parasympathetic structure) and the pupillary dilator muscle (innervated by axons of the superior cervical ganglion, a sympathetic structure). If CN III is damaged, as often happens with increased intracranial pressure and transtentorial herniation that compresses the CN III nerve against the free edge of the tentorium cerebelli, the innervation of the pupillary constrictor is dysfunctional. This removal of ciliary ganglion influence results in a fixed (unresponsive), dilated pupil (from unopposed action of the dilator muscle) and loss of accommodation to near vision. This fixed, dilated pupil is a key diagnostic sign of impending transtentorial herniation following a head injury, a major intracranial bleed, cerebral edema, or a space-occupying lesion.

If the sympathetic supply to the pupil is disrupted (**Horner syndrome**) from damage in the descending brainstem and spinal central sympathetic axons, from T1–T2 intermediolateral cell column or related axonal damage, or from superior cervical ganglion damage, the result will be an ipsilateral constricted pupil (miosis), ptosis (dysfunction of Müller's muscle), and anhydrosis (loss of sweating).

COLOR the following structures, using a separate color for each structure.

- ☐ 1. **Nucleus of Edinger–Westphal**
- ☐ 2. **CN III**
- ☐ 3. **Ciliary ganglion**
- ☐ 4. **Superior salivatory nucleus**
- ☐ 5. **CN VII**
- ☐ 6. **Pterygopalatine ganglion**
- ☐ 7. **Submandibular ganglion**
- ☐ 8. **Inferior salivatory nucleus**
- ☐ 9. **CN IX**
- ☐ 10. **Otic ganglion**
- ☐ 11. **Neuron in T1–T2 intermediolateral cell column**
- ☐ 12. **Superior cervical ganglion**

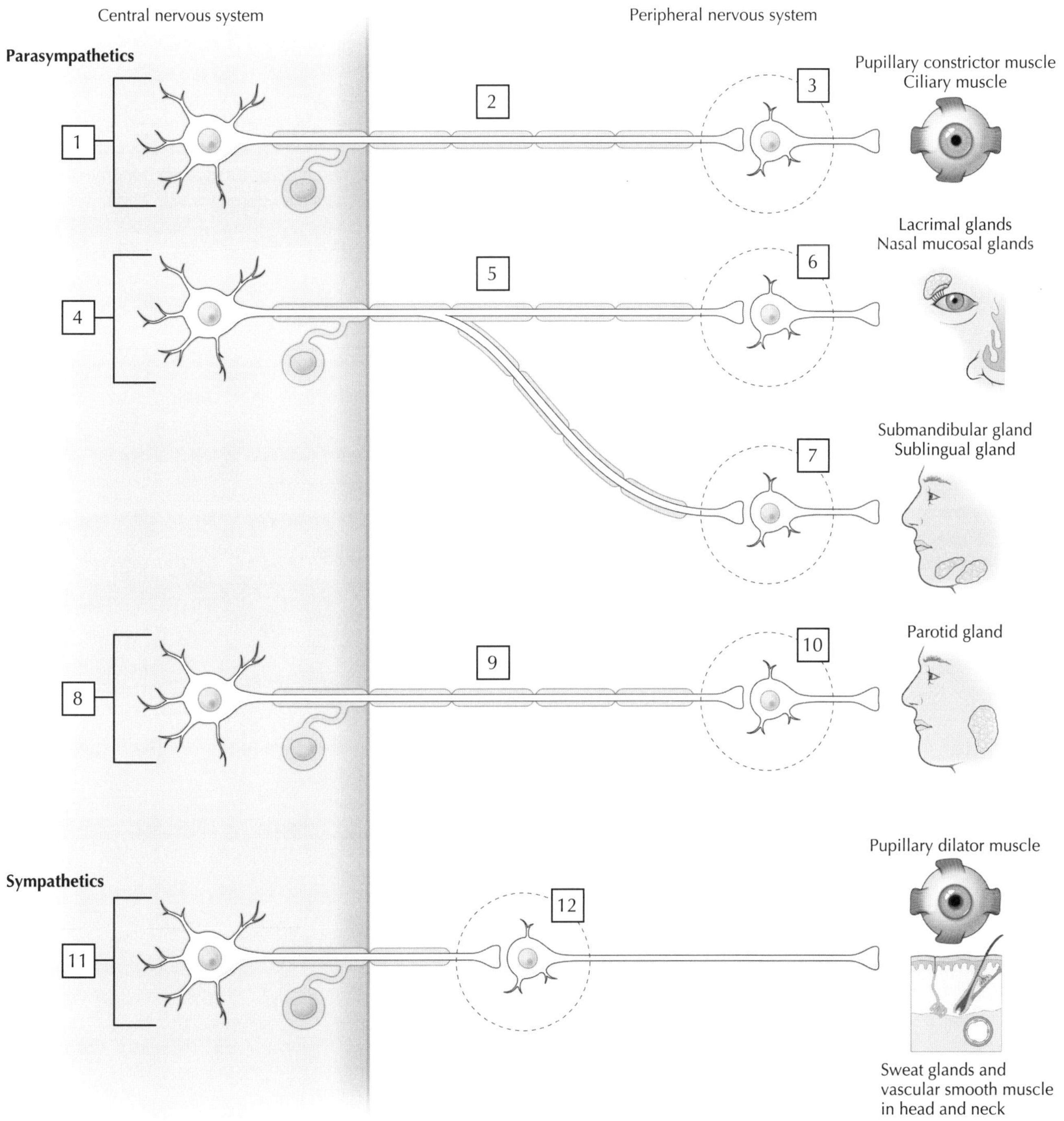
Central nervous system
Peripheral nervous system
Parasympathetics
1
2
3
Pupillary constrictor muscle
Ciliary muscle
4
5
6
Lacrimal glands
Nasal mucosal glands
7
Submandibular gland
Sublingual gland
8
9
10
Parotid gland
Sympathetics
11
12
Pupillary dilator muscle
Sweat glands and
vascular smooth muscle
in head and neck

Enteric Nervous System

The GI tract is innervated by both parasympathetic and sympathetic neural components, affecting smooth muscle contraction and peristalsis, secretion, immune reactivity, and other activities. Neurons in the **intermediolateral cell column at levels T5–L2** send axons, some through **splanchnic nerves**, to the **celiac ganglion**, **superior mesenteric ganglion**, and **inferior mesenteric** ganglion; these ganglia send noradrenergic axons into the **myenteric plexus, submucosal plexus,** and into the **mucosa**. Neurons in the **dorsal (motor) nucleus of CN X (vagus)** and parasympathetic neurons in the **S2–S4 intermediate gray** send axons to **intramural ganglia**; these ganglia supply the same structures. Classically, the parasympathetic system activates GI activity, and the sympathetic system slows GI activity.

The GI system also contains a large pool of neurons, the **enteric nervous system,** which are independent of sympathetic or parasympathetic control. In the absence of enteric neurons, the sympathetic and parasympathetic inputs cannot coordinate control of GI activity. There are approximately 100 million enteric neurons, found mainly in the **submucosal plexus (Meissner)** and **myenteric plexus (Auerbach plexus),** providing neural regulation of both the small and large intestines. The enteric neurons regulate peristaltic responses through **longitudinal and circular smooth muscle** (which can proceed without autonomic input), pacemaker activities, and automated secretory processes. The myenteric plexus controls mainly motility, and the submucosal plexus controls mainly fluid secretion and absorption. The enteric nervous system uses at least 20 distinct neurotransmitters; ACh and substance P (SP) are excitatory to smooth muscle, and vasoactive intestinal polypeptide (VIP) and nitric oxide (NO) are inhibitory. Extrinsic inputs from the autonomic nerves help to coordinate these enteric processes.

Clinical Note

For optimal functioning of the GI tract, both the enteric neuronal network and the autonomic input from the sympathetics and parasympathetics must work in a coordinated fashion. A complex array of endocrine, paracrine, and neurocrine mediators must work in concert. If there is damage to the extrinsic innervation of the GI tract from a neuropathy (e.g., **diabetic neuropathy**), a disorder of motility may result, with either diarrhea or constipation.

The enteric neurons derive from the neural crest. If these neural crest components fail to migrate properly to the colon, a disorder called **chronic megacolon** (**Hirschsprung's disease**) ensues. The intrinsic circuitry for peristalsis, pacemaker activity, and other GI activities cannot occur, and autonomic actions cannot compensate. Peristalsis is absent and intestinal obstruction will ensue.

Some commonly used narcotic analgesics will block gut constriction and peristalsis, resulting in severe constipation.

COLOR the following structures, using a separate color for each structure.

- ☐ **1. Dorsal (motor) nucleus of CN X (vagus)**
- ☐ **2. CN X (vagus nerve)**
- ☐ **3. Intermediolateral cell column of the spinal cord**
- ☐ **4. Celiac ganglion**
- ☐ **5. Superior mesenteric ganglion**
- ☐ **6. Inferior mesenteric ganglion**
- ☐ **7. Splanchnic nerve**
- ☐ **8. Longitudinal smooth muscle**
- ☐ **9. Myenteric plexus**
- ☐ **10. Circular smooth muscle**
- ☐ **11. Submucosal plexus**
- ☐ **12. Mucosa**

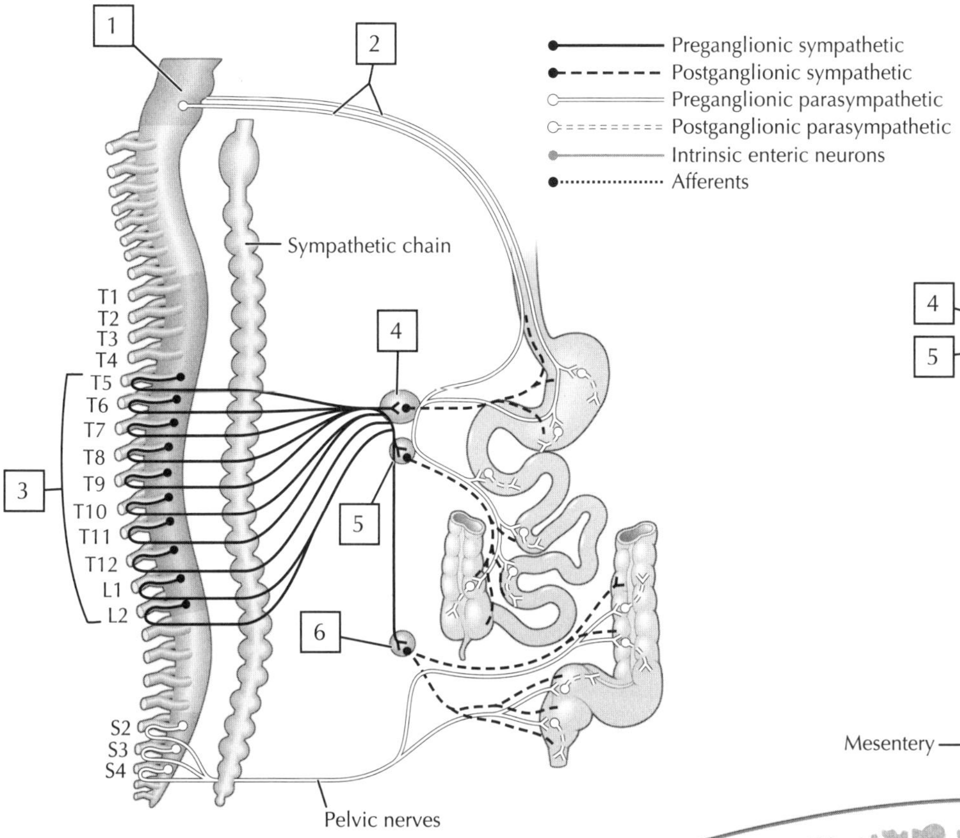

A. Autonomic innervation of the gastrointestinal tract

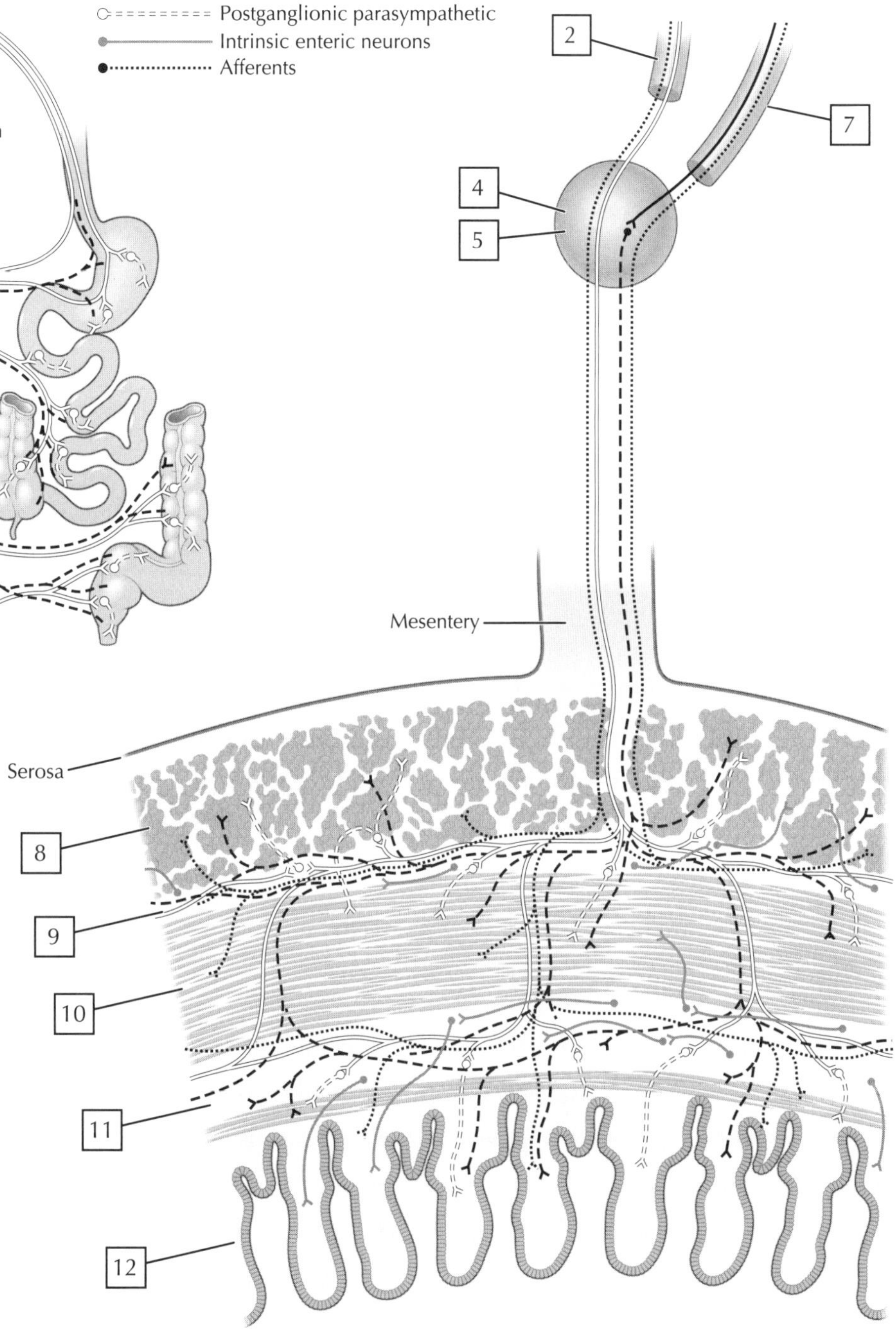

B. Enteric nervous system

Chapter 6 Spinal Cord

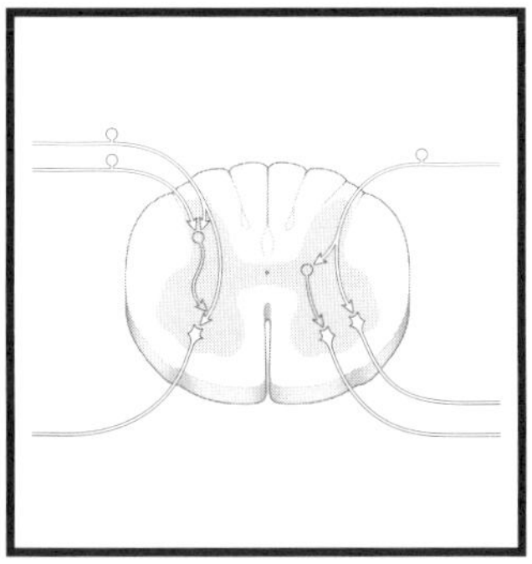

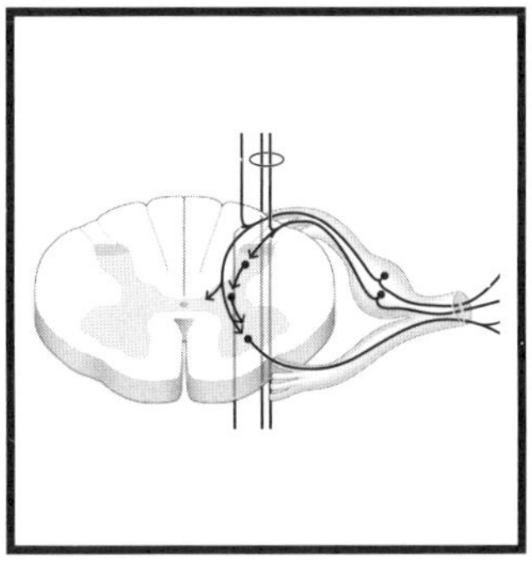

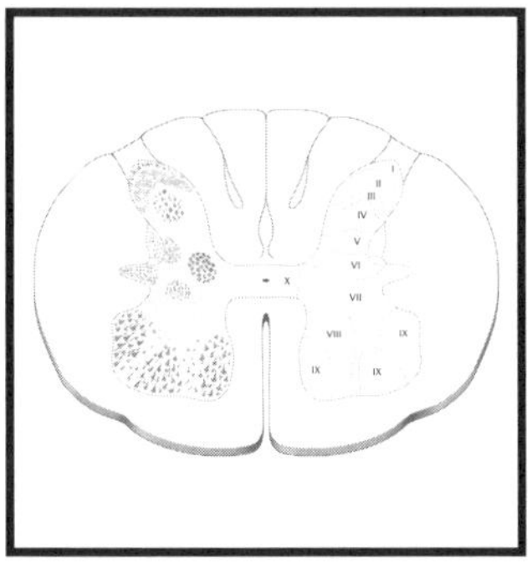

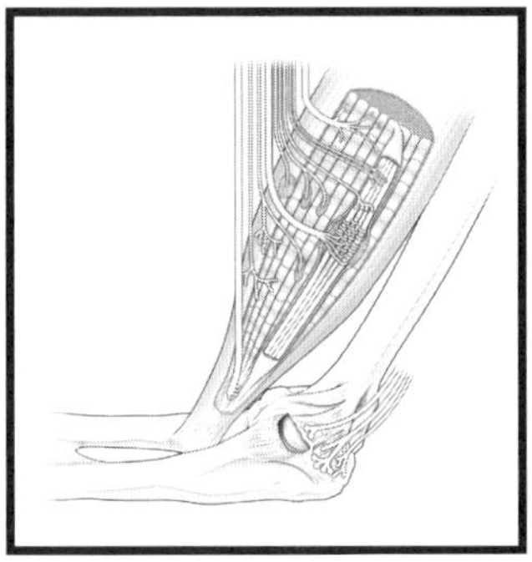

6 Cytoarchitecture of the Spinal Cord Gray Matter

The gray matter of the spinal cord is found in the interior of the spinal cord in a butterfly pattern or H pattern, in contrast to the cerebral cortex and cerebellum, where the gray matter is found on the outside. The gray matter has a different configuration at each level; there are cervical and lumbosacral enlargements, reflecting extensive inputs and outputs from the limbs. The thoracic gray matter is relatively sparse. This illustration is a schematized cross section of the spinal cord representing all levels. The gray matter is configured into a **dorsal (posterior) horn,** a **ventral (anterior) horn,** and in the T1–L2 regions, a **lateral horn,** reflecting the presence of the intermediolateral cell column of preganglionic sympathetic neurons. In general, the dorsal horn carries out sensory processing, and the ventral horn carries out motor processing.

The gray matter is organized into some specific neuronal clusters (nuclei), but many regions contain intermixed populations of neurons. The **marginal zone** (lamina I), **substantia gelatinosa** (lamina II), and **nucleus proprius** (deeper region of the dorsal horn) receive sensory input for processing of reflex information and lemniscal information for pain and temperature sensation (both acute and chronic). **Nucleus dorsalis (of Clarke)** and other regions receive information for spinocerebellar channels and processing. The **intermediolateral cell column** (T1–L2) is the site of preganglionic sympathetic neurons, and the **intermediomedial cell column** (S2–S4) is the site of preganglionic parasympathetic neurons. The anterior horn cells **(lower motor neurons)** are found in clusters in the ventral (anterior) horn, with topographical organization; **motor neurons supplying distal limb musculature** are found laterally, those **supplying the proximal limb musculature** are found centrally, and those **supplying the trunk musculature** are found medially.

Clinical Note

In the spinal cord, many functional populations of neurons are intermixed. Discrete nuclei subserving specific functions are few. This led investigators to seek alternative neuronal classifications in the spinal cord. Rexed subdivided the gray matter into 10 laminae. The dorsal horn laminae are used frequently for describing pain processing, and knowledge of the laminae and their functional processing is helpful in neurological diagnosis. Primary sensory input for "fast" pain and temperature processing (e.g., pin prick and general warm and cold temperature detection, as done in a neurological examination) terminates in laminae I and V; neurons in these laminae then send axons across the midline in the anterior white commissure to ascend in the ventrolateral white matter as the spinothalamic tract. This tract terminates in regions of the ventral posterolateral (VPL) nucleus of the thalamus, which projects to the sensory cortex (SI and SII). Primary sensory input conveying slow, chronic, agonizing pain terminates in the substantia gelatinosa (lamina II and some in lamina III); these neurons send a cascade of connections through the other laminae deeper in the dorsal horn, and to lamina VII. These neurons in lamina VII send both contralateral and ipsilateral connections through the ventrolateral white matter as the spinoreticular system. The spinoreticular system and spinothalamic tract travel together as they move rostrally. The spinoreticular system sends connections into the brainstem lateral reticular formation, parabrachial nuclei, periaqueductal gray, and nonspecific regions of the thalamus. This nociceptive information terminates in many regions of the cerebral cortex and has interconnections with limbic forebrain structures, which provide emotional context for chronic and severe pain.

COLOR the following structures, using a separate color for each structure.

- ☐ 1. **Dorsal (posterior) horn**
- ☐ 2. **Lateral horn**
- ☐ 3. **Ventral (anterior) horn**
- ☐ 4. **Lower motor neurons supplying trunk musculature**
- ☐ 5. **Lower motor neurons supplying proximal limb musculature**
- ☐ 6. **Lower motor neurons supplying distal limb musculature**
- ☐ 7. **Intermediomedial cell column**
- ☐ 8. **Intermediolateral cell column**
- ☐ 9. **Nucleus dorsalis (of Clarke)**
- ☐ 10. **Nucleus proprius**
- ☐ 11. **Substantia gelatinosa**
- ☐ 12. **Marginal zone**

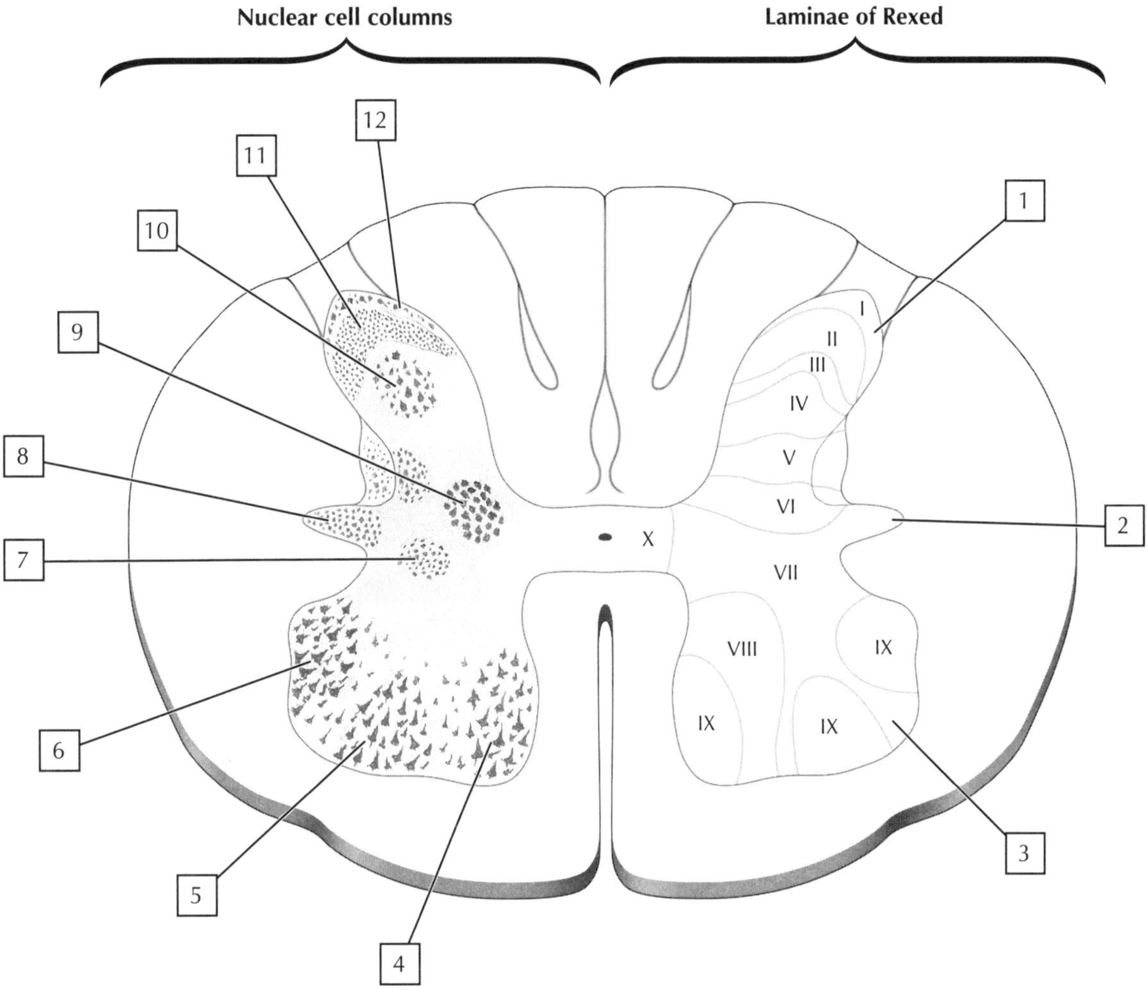

Nuclear cell columns
Laminae of Rexed
12
11
10
9
8
7
6
5
4
1
2
3
I
II
III
IV
V
VI
X
VII
VIII
IX
IX
IX

Spinal Cord Histological Cross Sections

These histological cross sections at C7, T7, L4, and S2 demonstrate major gray matter components and white matter components (tracts, fasciculi) characteristic for these levels. All levels contain dorsal horn nuclei (e.g., **substantia gelatinosa, nucleus proprius**) or lamina, reflecting the extensive sensory processing of protopathic sensory information at every level, both "fast" pain and temperature, and slow, chronic, agonizing pain; these neurons send ascending protopathic information via the **spinothalamic/spinoreticular pathways** in the **anterolateral funiculus.** Axons carrying epicritic sensation (fine, discriminative touch, vibratory sensation, joint position sense) enter the spinal cord at the dorsal root entry zone, enter the ipsilateral dorsal funiculus, and ascend into the medulla to terminate in nuclei gracilis (lower body) and cuneatus (upper body). Every level also contains **lower motor neurons** (LMNs) **in the anterior horn** whose axons exit via the ventral roots and terminate as motor end plates on skeletal muscle fibers. The large volume of gray matter associated with the limbs results in a cervical enlargement and lumbosacral enlargement. The **lateral horn** is found in levels T1 to L2, due to the presence of preganglionic sympathetic neurons in the **intermediolateral cell column**. Some levels contain clusters of neurons (e.g., **nucleus dorsalis of Clarke** [C8–L2]) and dorsal horn border cells that receive unconscious proprioceptive information and project axons through spinocerebellar tracts (e.g., **dorsal and ventral spinocerebellar tracts,** respectively) to the cerebellum. S2–S4 levels contain preganglionic parasympathetic neurons of the **intermediomedial cell column**.

The spinal cord tracts of clinical significance include the dorsal column tracts **(fasciculi gracilis and cuneatus)**; the anterolateral white matter tracts (the **spinothalamic and spinoreticular** system); and the dorsolateral white matter tracts (the **lateral corticospinal tract** and the rubrospinal tract).

COLOR the following structures, using a separate color for each structure.

- ☐ 1. **Anterior horn with lower motor neurons**
- ☐ 2. **Nucleus proprius**
- ☐ 3. **Substantia gelatinosa**
- ☐ 4. **Fasciculus gracilis**
- ☐ 5. **Fasciculus cuneatus**
- ☐ 6. **Lateral corticospinal tract**
- ☐ 7. **Dorsal spinocerebellar tract**
- ☐ 8. **Spinothalamic/spinoreticular tracts (system)**
- ☐ 9. **Ventral spinocerebellar tract**
- ☐ 10. **Nucleus dorsalis (of Clarke)**
- ☐ 11. **Lateral horn with intermediolateral cell column**
- ☐ 12. **Sacral parasympathetic nucleus (intermediomedial cell column)**

Clinical Note

Spinal cord cytoarchitecture (gray matter structures) and myeloarchitecture (tracts) provide an anatomical basis for explaining functional deficits seen with various spinal cord disorders and damage. For gray matter structures, LMNs are conspicuously present in the ventral (anterior) horn. Damage to LMNs results in flaccid paralysis of the formerly innervated skeletal muscle fibers, with loss of tone, movement, and reflexes. Damage to the ventral roots also results in the same clinical picture for affected muscle fibers.

For white matter structures, lesions that involve fasciculus gracilis and/or cuneatus result in the ipsilateral loss of epicritic sensation (fine, discriminative touch, vibratory sensation, joint position sense) below the level of the lesion. Below T6, there is only fasciculus gracilis; at levels above T6, both fasciculi gracilis and cuneatus are present. Lesions that involve the ventrolateral funiculus will damage fibers of the crossed spinothalamic/spinoreticular tracts (systems), with contralateral loss of pain and temperature sensation below the level of the lesion. In the long term, chronic pain manages to ascend to higher levels through the reticular formation, other brainstem nuclei, nonspecific thalamus, and many cortical regions. Lesions that involve the dorsolateral portion of the lateral funiculus result in ipsilateral loss of upper motor neuronal control of LMNs below the level of the lesion. This results in spastic paresis, with hypertonus, hyperreflexia, and some pathological reflexes such as clonus and the plantar extensor response.

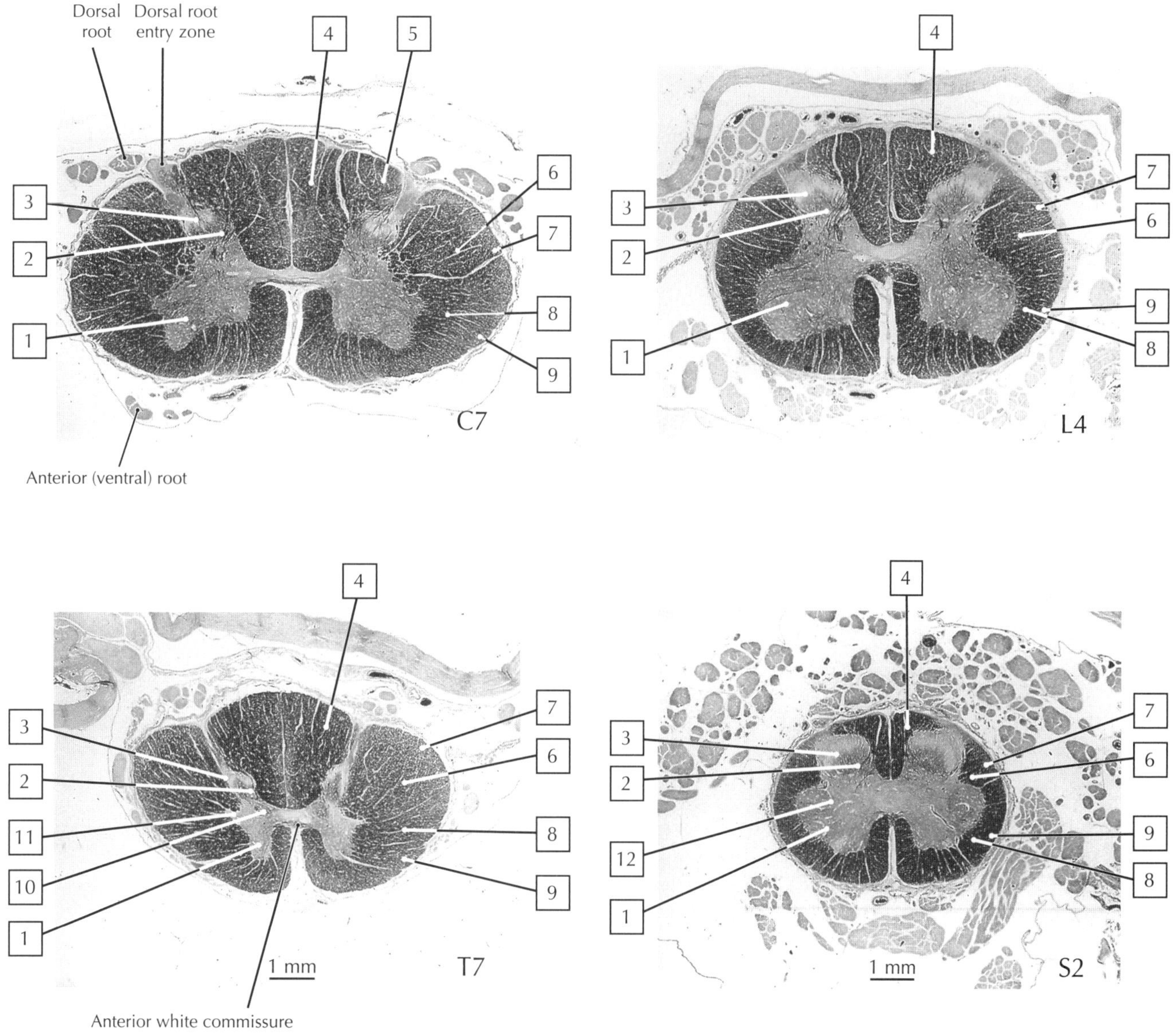

From Praxinos G, Mai JK (2004) The Human Nervous System, *2nd ed, Philadelphia: Elsevier; Fig. 7.22.*

6 Spinal Cord Syndromes

The spinal cord may be damaged by trauma, vascular lesions, inflammatory injuries, and other conditions such as myelopathy accompanying radiculopathy. A full spinal cord crush injury or severing will result in total loss of sensory processing below the level of the lesion, spastic paralysis below the level of the lesion (**lateral corticospinal tract** and **rubrospinal tract**) accompanied by LMN dysfunction at the level of a trauma or crush injury that destroys LMNs, and autonomic dysfunction below the level of the lesion (e.g., bowel, bladder, and reproductive organ dysfunction and, if above T1, Horner syndrome).

A spinal cord hemisection **(Brown–Séquard lesion)** results in ipsilateral epicritic sensory loss, contralateral protopathic loss **(spinothalamic/spinoreticular tracts)**, and ipsilateral spastic paresis below the level of the lesion, along with ipsilateral Horner syndrome if the lesion is above T1.

A **dorsal (posterior) column lesion** results in bilateral loss of epicritic sensation below the level of the lesion.

Anterior spinal artery syndrome results in bilateral spastic paresis below the level of the lesion, LMN damage at the level of the arterial lesion, bilateral loss of protopathic sensation at and below the level of the lesion, with preservation of epicritic sensation.

Central cord syndrome results in bilateral flaccid paralysis at the level of the lesion, and bilateral spastic paresis and bilateral loss of protopathic sensation below the level of the lesion, affecting mainly the upper extremities. Some loss of epicritic sensation may occur.

COLOR the following structures, using a separate color for each structure.

- ☐ 1. **Dorsal (posterior) columns**
- ☐ 2. **Lateral corticospinal tract**
- ☐ 3. **Spinothalamic/spinoreticular system (tracts)**
- ☐ 4. **Dorsal (posterior) column syndrome**
- ☐ 5. **Brown–Séquard syndrome (lateral cord hemisection)**
- ☐ 6. **Anterior spinal artery syndrome**
- ☐ 7. **Central cord syndrome**

Clinical Note

A syndrome not described in this illustration is a spinal cord myelopathy that affects the lateral funiculus from either inflammatory disease or the impingement of a herniated nucleus pulposus from a disk problem. A lesion impinging on the lateral funiculus may begin as ataxia and clumsiness due to damage of the dorsal and ventral spinocerebellar tracts at the lateral edge of the lateral funiculus. Deeper impingement affecting the lateral corticospinal tract and rubrospinal tract results in ipsilateral spastic hemiparesis with hypertonus, hyperreflexia, and pathological reflexes, which will overshadow the spinocerebellar symptoms. If the damage includes the ventrolateral funiculus, protopathic sensation will be diminished or lost on the contralateral side below the level of the lesion.

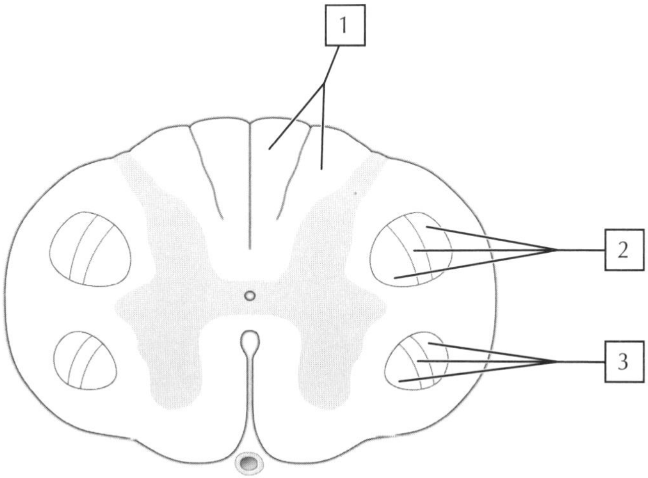

A. Localization of major white matter tracts

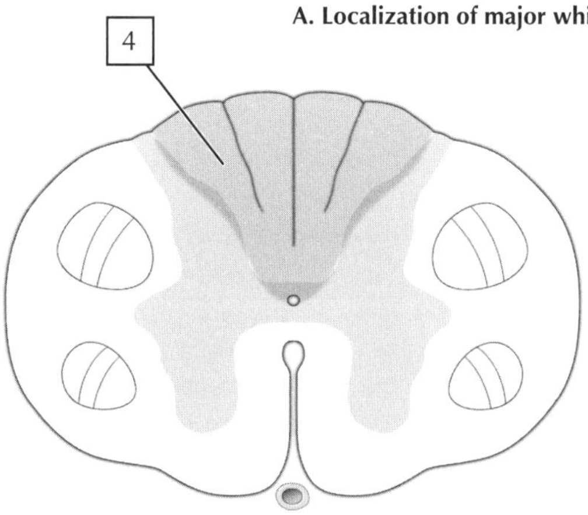

B. Posterior column syndrome (uncommon)
Loss of position sense below lesion

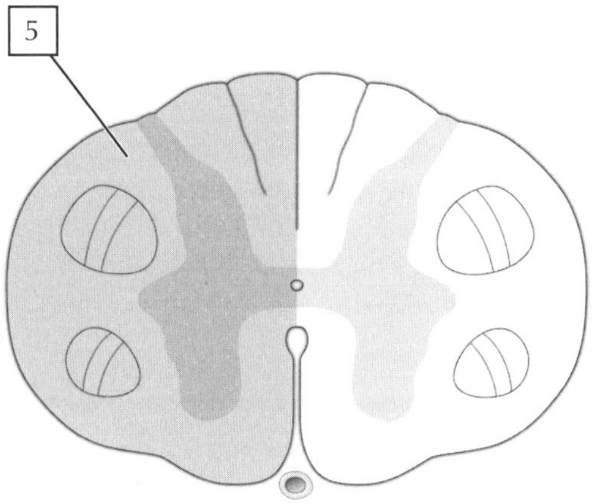

C. Brown-Séquard syndrome (lateral cord hemisection)
Ipsilateral paralysis and loss of position sense; contralateral analgesia

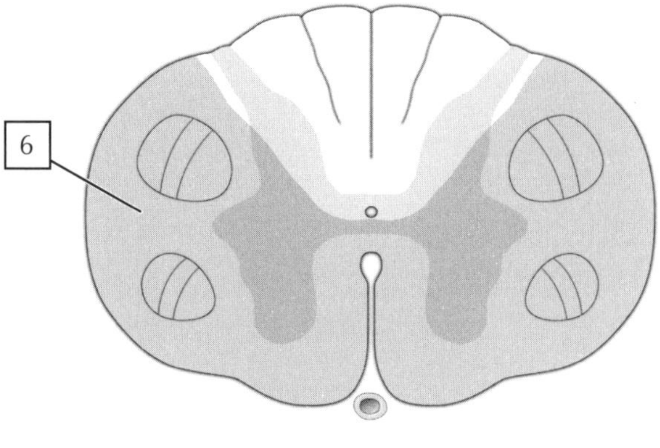

D. Anterior spinal artery syndrome
Bilateral paralysis and dissociated sensory loss below lesion (analgesia but preserved position sense)

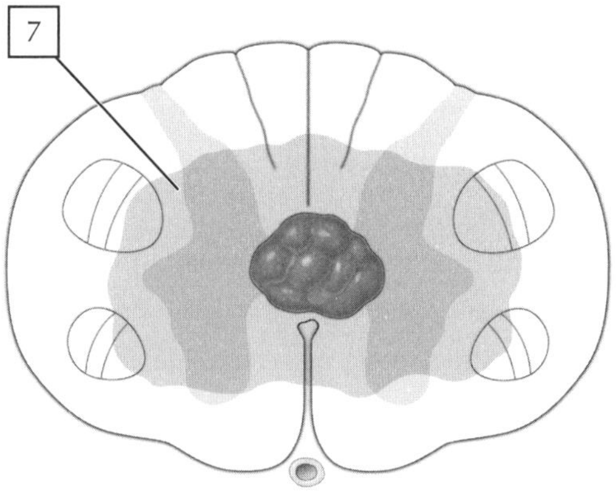

E. Central cord syndrome
Parts of three main tracts involved on both sides; upper limbs more affected than lower limbs

6 Spinal Cord Lower Motor Neuron Organization and Control

LMNs, including both alpha-LMNs (to extrafusal motor fibers) and gamma-LMNs (to intrafusal motor fibers in muscle spindles), are topographically organized both by spinal cord segment (reflecting the myotomes) and by location within the ventral horn at each level. **LMNs for trunk musculature** are found medially, **for proximal limb musculature** are found centrally, and **for distal limb musculature** are found laterally, in the anterior horn.

LMNs from many spinal cord levels on both sides are interconnected by interneuronal networks that are needed for coordination of motor movements, particularly represented by flexor reflexes. Sensory information enters the dorsal horn, terminates on many subsets of **dorsal horn interneurons,** and extends to appropriate LMNs and their immediate pre-LMN interneurons, to achieve appropriate motor responses through **polysynaptic reflexes** such as the **flexor reflexes.** Sensory inputs for muscle stretch reflexes originate from **Ia afferents (proprioceptive fibers)** from muscle spindles, enter the spinal cord through the dorsal roots (cell bodies in **dorsal root ganglia**), and terminate directly on **alpha-LMNs**. These alpha-LMNs send axons through the **ventral roots** to terminate on **skeletal muscle fibers** associated with the original stretch.

Superimposed on this complex array of LMNs and their interneuronal networks are the descending pathways from upper motor neurons (UMNs) in the brainstem (lateral vestibulospinal tract, medullary and pontine reticulospinal tracts, and rubrospinal tract) and cerebral cortex (lateral and anterior corticospinal tracts). The regulatory control of LMNs from these tracts is directed to both the alpha-LMNs and the gamma-LMNs, called alpha-gamma coactivation.

COLOR the following structures, using a separate color for each structure.

- ☐ 1. **Dorsal horn interneurons**
- ☐ 2. **Ia afferents (proprioceptive fibers)**
- ☐ 3. **Axons for polysynaptic reflexes**
- ☐ 4. **Dorsal root ganglion**
- ☐ 5. **Ventral roots**
- ☐ 6. **Flexor reflex interneurons**
- ☐ 7. **Alpha motor neurons (LMNs)**
- ☐ 8. **Skeletal muscle fibers**
- ☐ 9. **LMNs for proximal upper limb musculature**
- ☐ 10. **LMNs for distal upper limb musculature**
- ☐ 11. **LMNs for proximal lower limb musculature**
- ☐ 12. **LMNs for distal lower limb musculature**

Clinical Note

LMNs are critical components of all movement and behavior requiring muscle activity. The LMNs are the "final common pathway" for all motor activity, according to the British neurophysiologist Sir Charles Sherrington. The LMNs are in the company of a host of interneurons, some of them associated with specific LMNs, and many of them interconnected with other interneurons that can help to regulate groups of interneurons. Many of these interneurons are subject to regulation from sensory input, UMNs, or both. One special sensory input, from Ia afferents from muscle spindles, is the only direct sensory input synapsing on LMNs without intervention of interneurons, except for reciprocal inhibition. This is the monosynaptic muscle stretch reflex. All other sensory inputs to LMNs occur through polysynaptic reflexes. Many of these polysynaptic channels have a flexor bias to overcome the powerful extensor antigravity tone of musculature, especially limb musculature. These include recurrent inhibition and Renshaw cell bias. Superimposed on these local interneuronal circuits are descending upper motor neuronal channels, most of which terminate on interneurons. Only the corticospinal tract has significant direct synapses on LMNs, and that holds for only approximately 10% of the corticospinal connections.

If the upper motor neuronal descending connections are damaged, as occurs with a stroke (in the cortex, internal capsule, cerebral peduncle), a brainstem lesion, increased intracranial pressure and cerebral edema, or herniation, this releases the spinal cord interneuronal pools from descending influence. Clinically, this results in hyperresponsiveness of sensory-evoked reflex motor responses, including increased muscle stretch reflexes and increased reactivity to nociceptive reflexes and flexor reflexes. Sensory stimuli below the level of a spinal cord lesion may result in an exaggerated and conspicuous flexion-crossed extension reflex, normally not seen in an intact individual.

A. Lower motor neuron organization and control

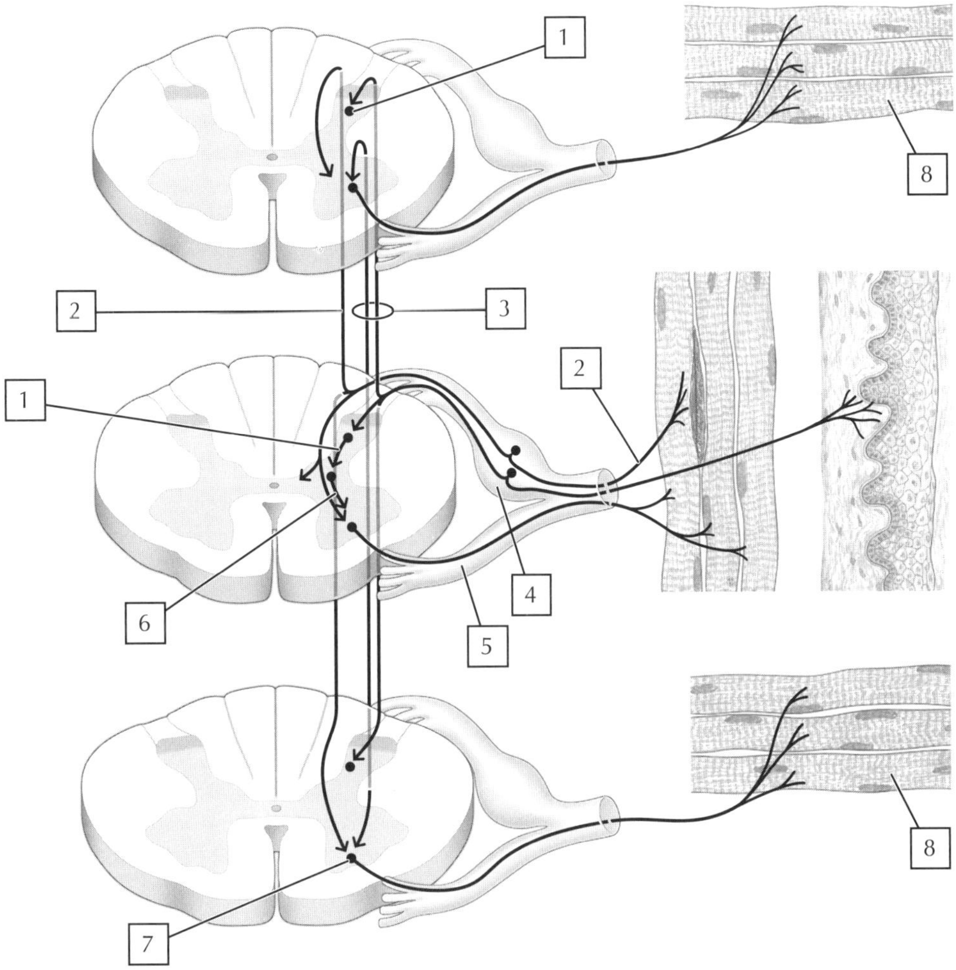

B. Schematic representation of motor neurons

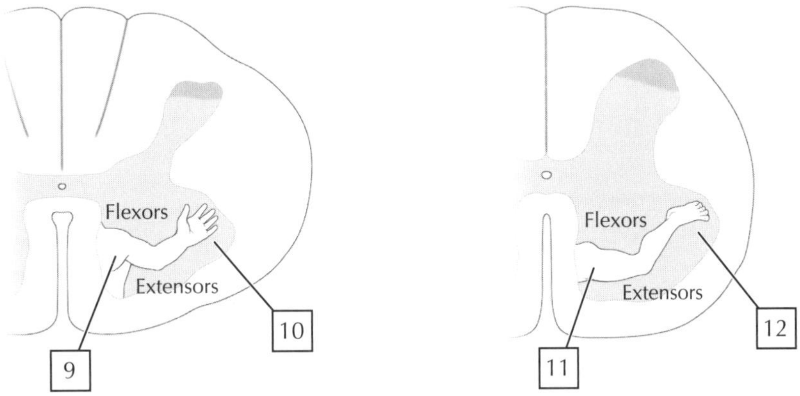

6 Spinal Somatic Reflex Pathways

Many pools of interneurons elicit specific responses directed toward LMNs. For muscle stretch reflexes, **Ia afferents from muscle spindles in extensor muscles** directly synapse on **extensor LMNs** in the ipsilateral LMN pool to the same (homonymous) muscle. **Ia afferents from muscle spindles in flexor muscles** terminate on inhibitory interneurons that provide **axoaxonic presynaptic inhibition** on the extensor response. There also is reciprocal inhibition, whereby Ia afferents for a muscle stretch reflex stimulate the appropriate **LMN flexor or extensor response**, and inhibit the antagonist response. The Golgi tendon organ response from **Ib afferents associated with force exerted on tendons**, when activated by high-threshold stretch on the tendon, sends axons to inhibitory interneurons that inhibit the homonymous LMNs associated with that tendon through an inhibitory synapse, releasing the stretch on the tendon. When LMNs send action potentials to the homonymous muscle, collaterals in the ventral horn synapse on **Renshaw cells**, which enhance flexor movements and inhibit extensor movements, via interneurons that favor flexor activity. Flexor (withdrawal) reflexes are specific to appropriate responses from **nociceptive stimuli (fibers)** that potentially threaten harm. These **flexor reflex interneurons** allow specific and generalized responses (e.g., removal of a hand from a hot burner, or a comprehensive full-body response from stepping on a tack) through large collections of interneuronal pools, interconnected to provide appropriate protective responses.

Clinical Note

A host of reflex responses are present in the spinal cord that help to maintain appropriate tone and activity in muscle movement and achievement of behavior. Muscle stretch reflexes help to maintain homeostasis of muscle contraction, helping to support contraction or relaxation of specific muscle fibers to keep the whole muscle in an appropriate state of contraction, often set by UMNs. This response demonstrates both reciprocal inhibition and axoaxonal regulation. Ib afferents from Golgi tendon organs can be activated as a high-threshold response when a state of muscle contraction threatens to damage the muscle; this tendon organ response inhibits the homonymous muscle as a protective response. Superimposed on these responses is a bias (Renshaw cells) toward flexor movements; most skilled dexterous movements are flexor movements, requiring a bias toward inhibiting the powerful extensor antigravity muscles and enhancing skilled flexor movements, such as those driven by direct corticospinal regulation.

These many afferent fibers, in addition to participating in reflex regulation, also send connections (Ia afferents, Ib afferents, unmyelinated, and myelinated proprioceptive fibers) to secondary sensory nuclei in the cerebellar pathways (e.g., dorsal nucleus of Clarke, dorsal horn border cells, external [lateral, accessory] cuneate nucleus, central dorsal horn cells), providing unconscious proprioceptive information to the cerebellum about the status of individual muscle fibers, whole muscle activity, tendons, ligaments, joints, and cutaneous sources.

COLOR the following structures, using a separate color for each structure.

- ☐ 1. **Ia afferent from muscle spindle in extensor muscle**
- ☐ 2. **Ia afferent from muscle spindle in flexor muscle**
- ☐ 3. **Axoaxonic presynaptic inhibition synapse**
- ☐ 4. **LMN axons to extensor muscles**
- ☐ 5. **Extensor LMN**
- ☐ 6. **LMN axons to flexor muscles**
- ☐ 7. **Renshaw cell**
- ☐ 8. **Ib afferent from a Golgi tendon organ from a flexor muscle**
- ☐ 9. **Nociceptive fibers**
- ☐ 10. **Flexor reflex interneurons**

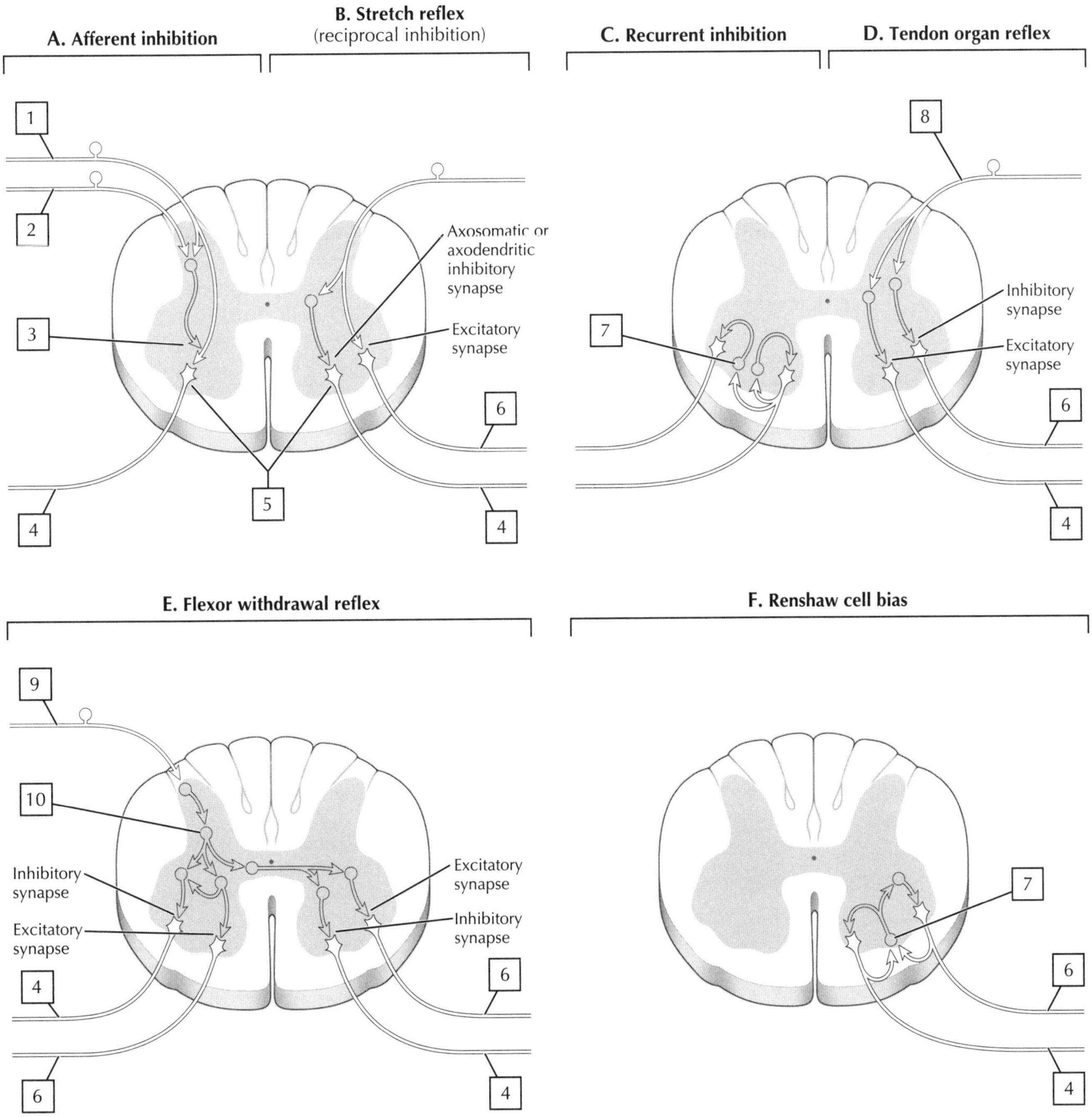
A. Afferent inhibition
B. Stretch reflex
(reciprocal inhibition)
C. Recurrent inhibition
D. Tendon organ reflex
1
2
3
4
5
6
7
8
Axosomatic or
axodendritic
inhibitory
synapse
Excitatory
synapse
Inhibitory
synapse
Excitatory
synapse
E. Flexor withdrawal reflex
F. Renshaw cell bias
9
10
Inhibitory
synapse
Excitatory
synapse
Excitatory
synapse
Inhibitory
synapse

6 Muscle and Joint Receptors and Muscle Spindles

Muscle spindles are complex receptors with both sensory and motor components, intended to keep skeletal muscle fibers in an appropriate state of contraction, especially driven by UMNs, both in static positions and during contractions. Muscle spindles are receptors organized in parallel with skeletal muscle fibers. A spindle has small intrafusal muscle fibers, including **nuclear bag fibers** and **nuclear chain fibers.** The **intrafusal fibers are innervated by gamma motor neurons** in the spinal cord. **Alpha motor neurons innervate extrafusal skeletal muscle fibers. Ia afferent fibers (annulospiral endings)** enwrap nuclear bag fibers, and respond to both the static length of the bag fiber and the rate of change (velocity) of the bag fiber. **Group II afferent fibers (flower spray endings)** enwrap nuclear chain fibers and respond to the static length of chain fibers. **Group Ib fibers (from Golgi tendon organs** in the tendon) respond to stretch of the whole muscle, representing the force generated by that muscle. **Joint receptors** innervate many regions of the joint and its capsule and respond to both static and dynamic actions, some reacting to all ranges of motion, and some reacting to extremes of motion.

COLOR the following structures, using a separate color for each structure.

- ☐ 1. **Alpha motor neurons to extrafusal skeletal muscle fibers**
- ☐ 2. **Gamma motor neurons to intrafusal muscle fibers in the muscle spindle**
- ☐ 3. **Ia afferent fibers from annulospiral endings**
- ☐ 4. **Group II fibers from flower spray endings**
- ☐ 5. **Ib afferent fibers from Golgi tendon organs in tendons**
- ☐ 6. **Joint receptors**
- ☐ 7. **Nuclear bag fibers**
- ☐ 8. **Nuclear chain fibers**
- ☐ 9. **Intrafusal muscle fibers**

Clinical Note

The muscle spindle is a critical structure in maintaining muscle contraction and allowing proper movement through both sensory control and UMN control. The muscle spindle is attached in parallel with extrafusal skeletal muscle fibers. The intrafusal muscle fibers (nuclear chain and nuclear bag fibers) are innervated by gamma-LMNs, and the skeletal extrafusal muscle fibers are innervated by alpha motor neurons. The nuclear chain fibers have sensory innervation from group II fibers and report muscle length to the central nervous system. The nuclear bag fibers have sensory innervation from Ia fibers and report both muscle length and velocity to the central nervous system. These Ia afferents have some direct connections to alpha-LMNs associated with the extrafusal muscle fibers, activated during a muscle stretch reflex.

The muscle stretch reflex occurs when passive stretch causes the intrafusal fibers of the muscle spindle to stretch. This activates the Ia afferents, which send action potentials to activate the synapse on alpha-LMNs, resulting in contraction in the skeletal muscle that was stretched. This restores homeostasis. A challenge for the muscle stretch reflex is that it must function in its dynamic range of sensitivity at all ranges of muscle contraction, from relaxation to maximal contraction. The gamma-LMNs cause contraction of the intrafusal muscle fibers associated with the nuclear chain fibers and nuclear bag fibers, keeping them in their dynamic range of sensitivity at all states of contraction of the skeletal muscle fiber. This is achieved by the UMNs activating both the alpha-LMNs and the gamma-LMNs simultaneously, called alpha-gamma coactivation. If gamma-LMNs were not coactivated, there would be no muscle stretch reflex, resulting in hyporeflexia or areflexia. If gamma-LMNs were driven to a greater extent than alpha-LMNs (which may occur in spasticity), then the muscle spindle response is on a hair trigger, and passive stretch will result in a vigorous response (hyperreflexia).

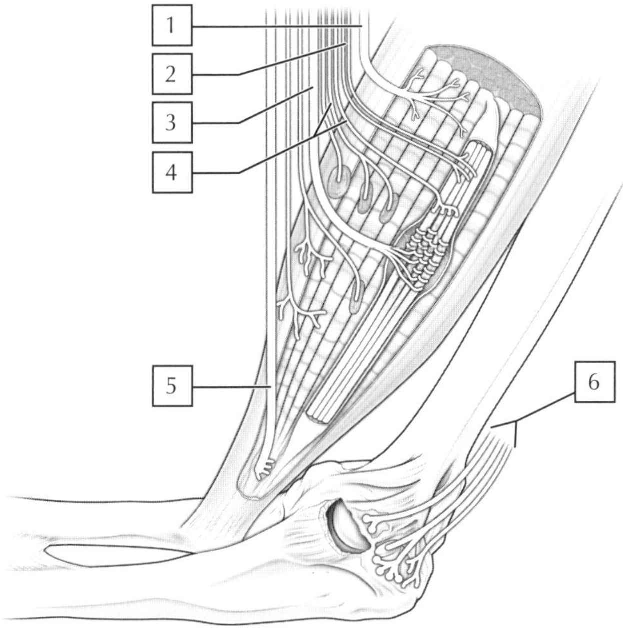

Muscle spindle within whole muscle

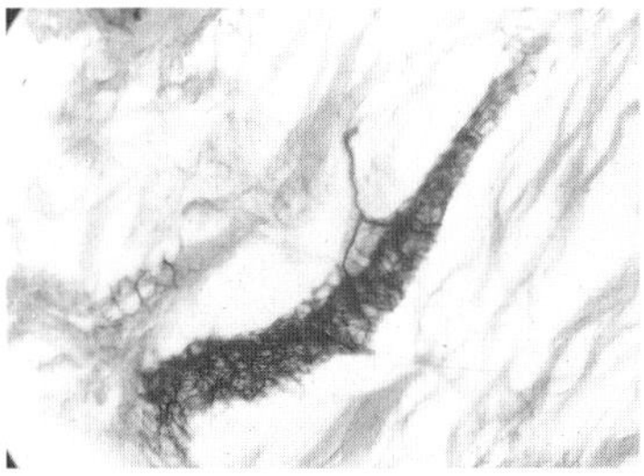

Type III joint receptor (Golgi-like) in a knee ligament. These receptors are high-threshold, slowly adapting, active at far ranges of movement. Fiber stain.

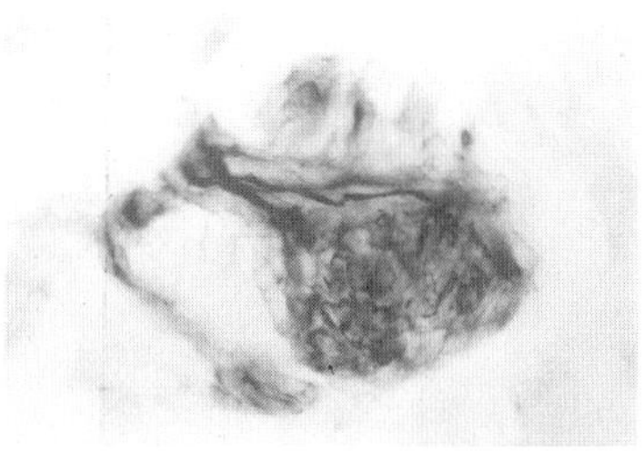

Type I receptor in a joint capsule. These receptors are low-threshold, slowly adapting, usually active at all ranges of movement and positions of the joint. Fiber stain.

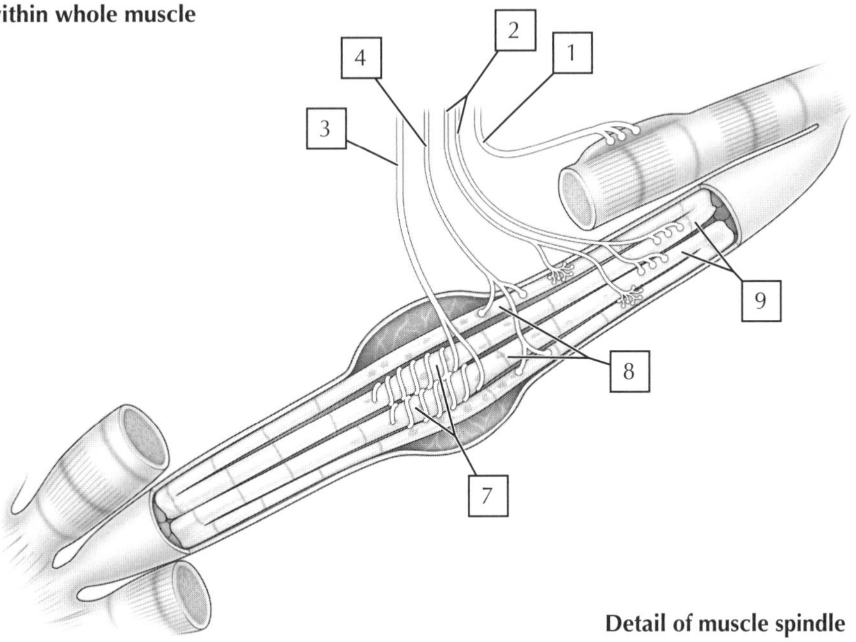

Detail of muscle spindle

Chapter 7 Brainstem and Cerebellum

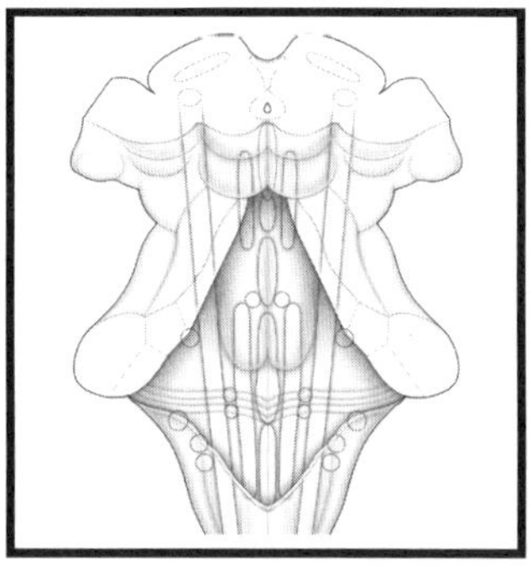
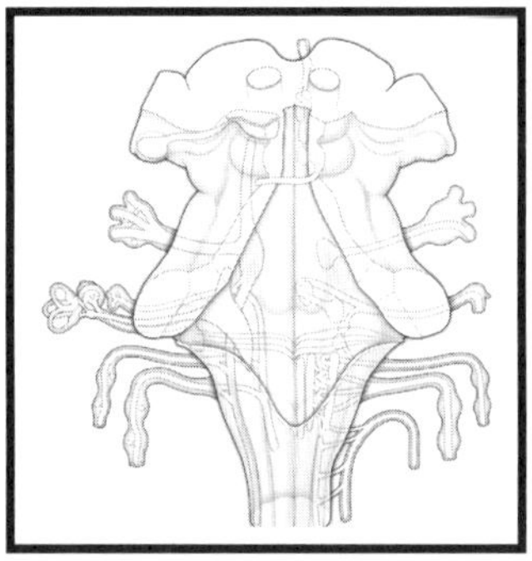
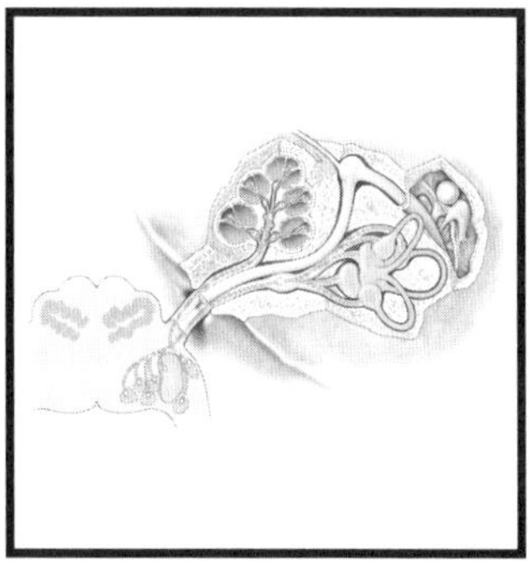
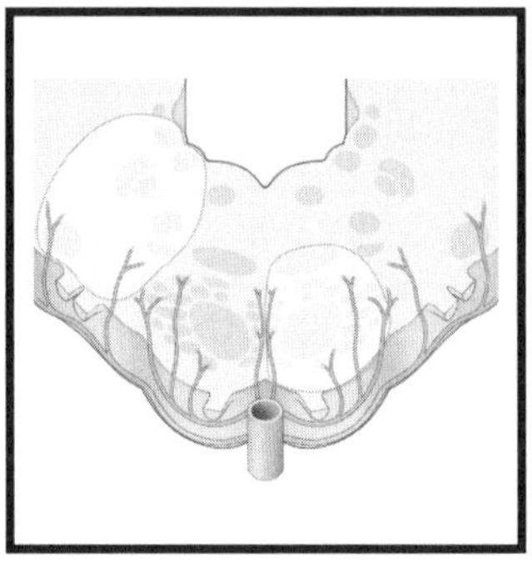

7 Cranial Nerves

The cranial nerves (CNs) provide the sensory inputs and the motor and parasympathetic outputs for the brainstem and forebrain, similar to the spinal nerves providing sensory inputs and motor and autonomic outputs for the spinal cord. **Cranial nerve (CN) I** and **CN II** are actually central nervous system (CNS) tracts, whose axons are myelinated by oligodendrocytes. **CN III–XII** are peripheral nerves, whose peripheral axons are myelinated by Schwann cells.

SENSORY CRANIAL NERVE COMPONENTS	
CN I: Olfactory	Olfaction
CN II: Optic	Vision
CN V: Trigeminal	Face, sinuses, teeth, general sensation to anterior 2/3 of the oral cavity and tongue
CN VII: Facial (N. Intermedius)	Taste to the anterior 2/3 of the tongue and soft palate
CN VIII: Vestibulocochlear	Hearing and balance (linear acceleration or gravity, and angular acceleration or movement)
CN IX: Glossopharyngeal	Taste to posterior 1/3 of the tongue, general sensation to tonsil, pharynx, and the middle ear
CN X: Vagus	Heart, lungs, bronchi, trachea, larynx, pharynx, gastrointestinal (GI) tract to the descending colon, a component of the external ear
MOTOR CRANIAL NERVE COMPONENTS	
CN III: Oculomotor	Medial, inferior, and superior rectus muscles; inferior oblique; levator palpebrae superioris
CN IV: Trochlear	Superior oblique muscle
CN VI: Abducens	Lateral rectus muscle
CN V: Trigeminal V3 Mandibular division	Muscles of mastication, tensor tympani
CN VII: Facial	Muscles of facial expression, stapedius
CN IX: Glossopharyngeal	Stylopharyngeus, pharyngeal muscles
CN X: Vagus	Pharyngeal and laryngeal muscles
CN XI: Accessory	Sternocleidomastoid, upper 2/3 of trapezius
CN XII: Hypoglossal	Intrinsic muscles of the tongue, intrahyoid muscles
PARASYMPATHETIC (AUTONOMIC) CRANIAL NERVE COMPONENTS	
CN III: Oculomotor	Ciliary muscle and pupillary constrictor muscle via the ciliary ganglion
CN VII: Facial (N. Intermedius)	Submandibular (submaxillary), sublingual, lacrimal glands and nasal mucosa via the pterygopalatine and submandibular ganglia
CN IX: Glossopharyngeal	Parotid gland via the otic ganglion
CN X: Vagus	Heart, lung, bronchi, GI tract via intramural ganglia

COLOR the following structures, using a separate color for each structure.

- ☐ **1. Olfactory nerve**
- ☐ **2. Optic nerve**
- ☐ **3. Oculomotor nerve**
- ☐ **4. Trochlear nerve**
- ☐ **5. Trigeminal nerve**
- ☐ **6. Abducens nerve**
- ☐ **7. Facial nerve with nervus intermedius**
- ☐ **8. Vestibulocochlear nerve**
- ☐ **9. Glossopharyngeal nerve**
- ☐ **10. Vagus nerve**
- ☐ **11. Accessory nerve**
- ☐ **12. Hypoglossal nerve**

Clinical Note

The site of CN entrance or exit from the brainstem is critical to understanding vulnerability of individual CNs to specific pathology. CN II is subject to demyelination and optic neuritis in multiple sclerosis. CN III may be compressed against the tentorium cerebelli during transtentorial herniation, causing a fixed, dilated pupil. CN VIII is the site of an acoustic Schwannoma, resulting in hearing loss and vertigo. Exiting fibers of CN XII may be damaged by a paramedian infarct in the medulla, resulting in paralysis and atrophy of the ipsilateral tongue musculature.

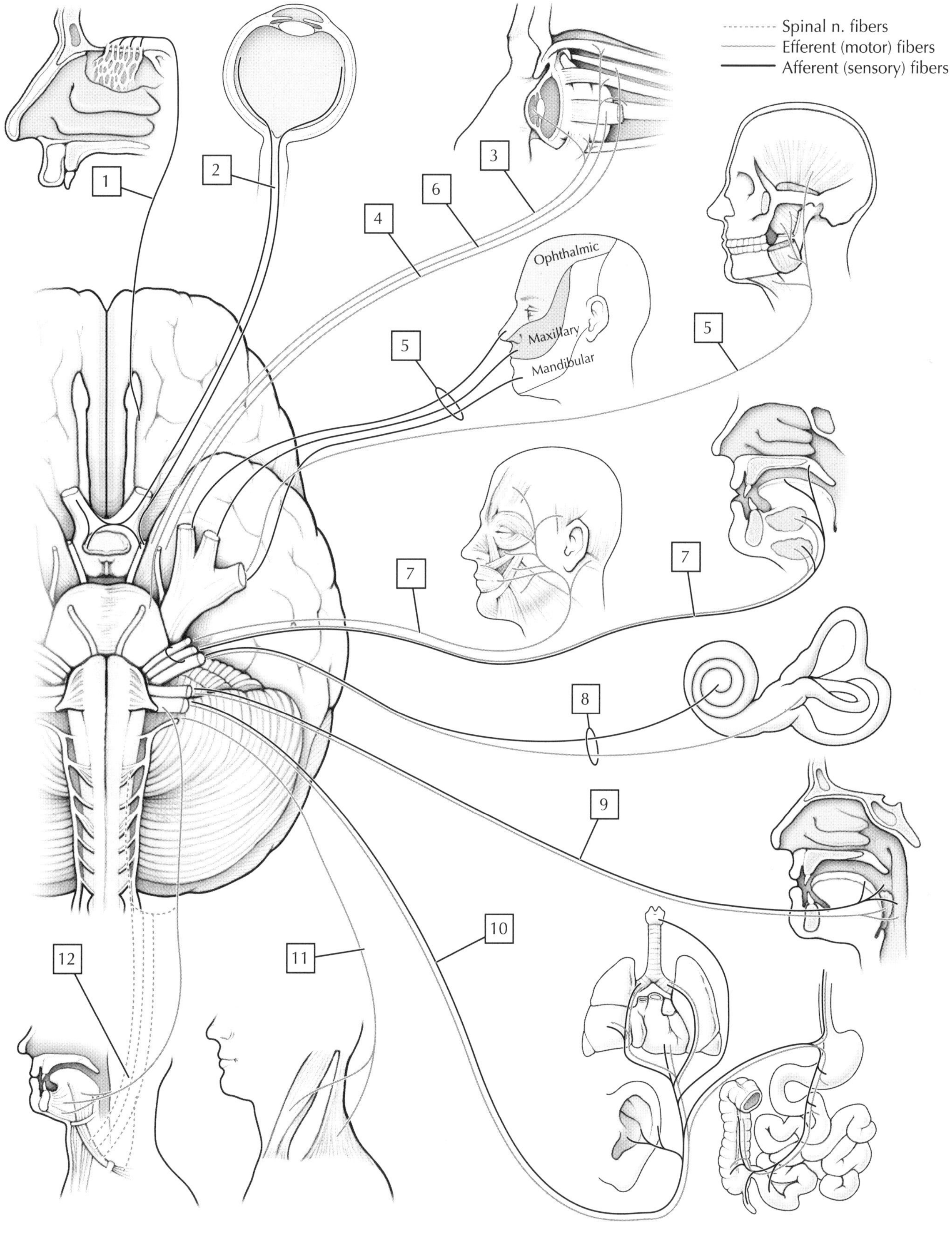
Spinal n. fibers
Efferent (motor) fibers
Afferent (sensory) fibers
1
2
3
6
4
Ophthalmic
Maxillary
Mandibular
5
5
7
7
8
9
10
11
12

7 Cranial Nerves and Their Nuclei: Schematic View From Above

CN nuclei are associated with the sensory, motor, and autonomic components of the CNs. They are found throughout the brainstem, in the upper cervical spinal cord, and in the caudal diencephalon.

MOTOR CRANIAL NERVE NUCLEI	ASSOCIATED CRANIAL NERVE
Oculomotor nucleus	CN III
Trochlear nucleus	CN IV
Motor nucleus of V (trigeminal)	CN V
Abducens nucleus	CN VI
Facial nucleus	CN VII
Nucleus ambiguus	CN IX and CN X
Spinal accessory nucleus	CN XI
Hypoglossal nucleus	CN XII
SENSORY CRANIAL NERVE NUCLEI	**ASSOCIATED CRANIAL NERVE**
Superior colliculus	CN II
Lateral geniculate nucleus (body)	CN II
Mesencephalic nucleus of V	CN V
Principal (main, chief) sensory nucleus of V	CN V
Descending (spinal) nucleus of V	CN V
Dorsal and ventral cochlear nuclei	CN VIII
Vestibular nuclei (medial, lateral, inferior, superior)	CN VIII
Nucleus of the solitary tract (solitarius)	CN VII, CN IX, CN X
AUTONOMIC CRANIAL NERVE NUCLEI	**ASSOCIATED CRANIAL NERVE**
Nucleus of Edinger–Westphal	CN III
Superior salivatory nucleus	CN VII
Inferior salivatory nucleus	CN IX
Dorsal (motor) nucleus of the vagus nerve	CN X

COLOR the following structures, using a separate color for each structure.

- ☐ 1. **Superior colliculus**
- ☐ 2. **Lateral geniculate nucleus (body)**
- ☐ 3. **Mesencephalic nucleus of CN V**
- ☐ 4. **Principal (main, chief) sensory nucleus of CN V**
- ☐ 5. **Dorsal and ventral cochlear nuclei**
- ☐ 6. **Vestibular nuclei**
- ☐ 7. **Descending (spinal) nucleus of CN V**
- ☐ 8. **Nucleus of the solitary tract (solitarius)**
- ☐ 9. **Dorsal (motor) nucleus of the vagus nerve (CN X)**
- ☐ 10. **Inferior salivatory nucleus**
- ☐ 11. **Superior salivatory nucleus**
- ☐ 12. **Nucleus of Edinger–Westphal**

Clinical Note

The sensory, motor, and parasympathetic CN nuclei are CNS components. Therefore these nuclei are subject to damage from vascular infarcts, inflammatory processes, tumors, trauma, and other disorders of the CNS, resulting in sensory, motor, and/or parasympathetic dysfunction specific for the modality carried by the CN. For example, a brainstem infarct from occlusion of the posterior inferior cerebellar artery (PICA) or the vertebral artery, known as *lateral medullary syndrome* or *Wallenberg syndrome*, damages the blood flow to descending nucleus and tract of V, nucleus ambiguus, inferior cerebellar peduncle, vestibular nuclei, descending sympathetic brainstem axons, and the ascending spinothalamic/spinoreticular tracts (system). Knowledge of the precise anatomical location of these nuclei and tracts, and the functional consequences of their damage, is essential for proper neurological evaluation and differential diagnosis.

Cranial Nerves and Their Nuclei: Schematic View From Above

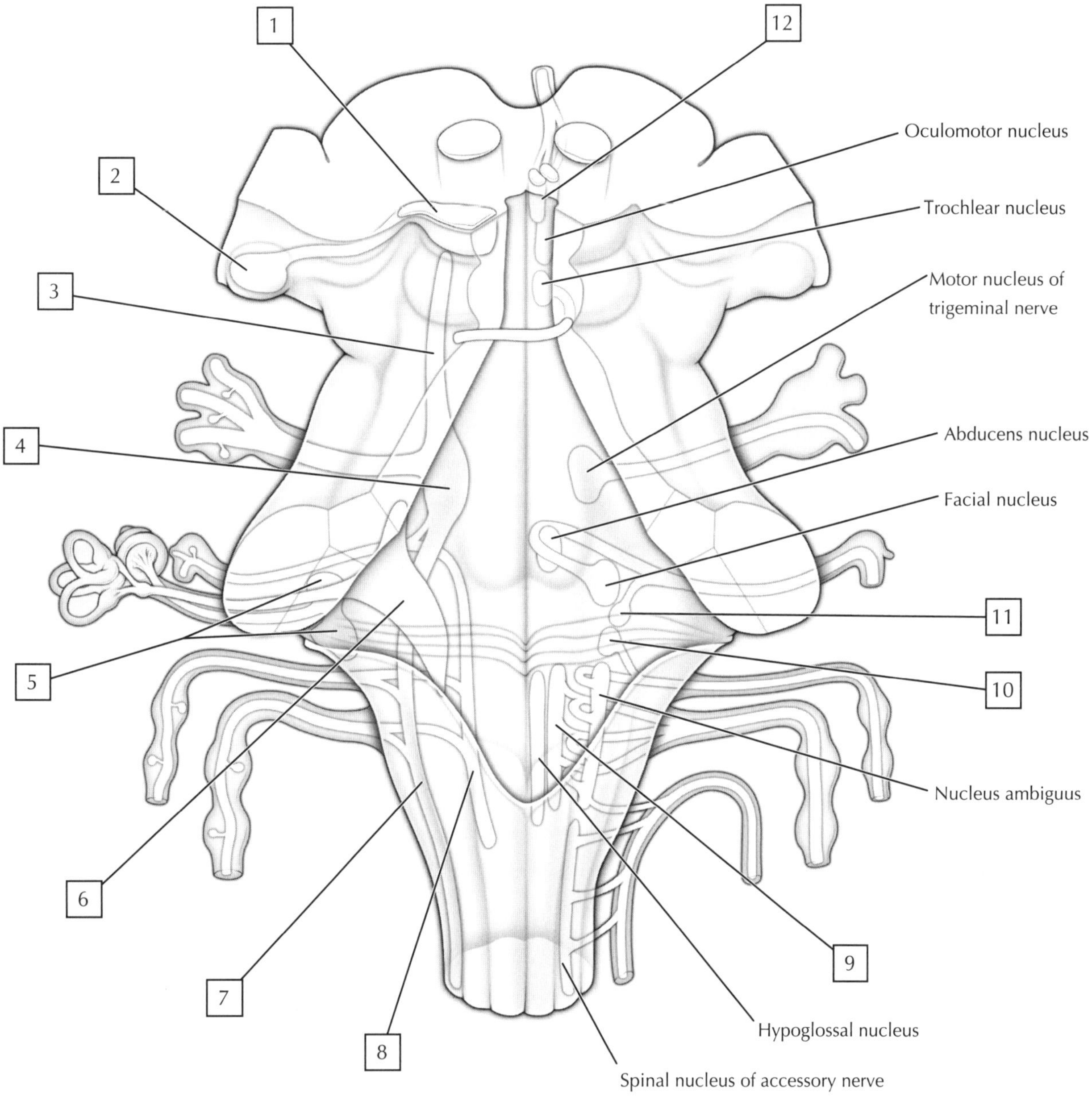

Vestibulocochlear Nerve (CN VIII)

The **vestibulocochlear nerve** has two components: the **vestibular nerve** and the **cochlear nerve.** The vestibular nerve arises from axons whose cell bodies (bipolar neurons) are located in the **vestibular ganglion (Scarpa ganglion).** The peripheral axons innervate hair cells in the **utricle** and **saccule** that respond to linear acceleration (gravity) and low-frequency vibration, respectively, and innervate hair cells in the ampullae **of the semicircular ducts (superior, lateral, and posterior)** that respond to angular acceleration (movement). These components provide coordination and equilibration of position, and movement of the head and neck. The central axons terminate in the **vestibular nuclei (medial, lateral, superior, and inferior),** which help to control the tone of body musculature, the tone and position of neck musculature, and the regulation of eye movements with respect to gravity and body movement.

The cochlear nerve arises from axons whose cell bodies (bipolar neurons) are located in the **cochlear ganglion (spiral ganglion).** The peripheral axons innervate hair cells that lie along the cochlear duct in the organ of Corti. These hair cells are stimulated by differential movement of the tectorial membrane with respect to the rather rigidly fixed organ of Corti, based on fluid movements through the scala vestibuli and scala tympani, precipitated by the ossicles transmitting movement against the oval window. The central portion of the axons terminate in the **cochlear nuclei (dorsal and ventral)** and transmit information about sound through a complex array of brainstem nuclei to the medial geniculate nucleus (body) of the thalamus, which sends axons to the auditory cortex on the transverse gyrus of Heschl, located on the temporal lobe right at the margin of the lateral fissure.

COLOR the following structures, using a separate color for each structure.

- ☐ 1. **Cochlear ganglion (spiral ganglion)**
- ☐ 2. **Cochlear nerve**
- ☐ 3. **Vestibulocochlear nerve (CN VIII)**
- ☐ 4. **Vestibular nuclei**
- ☐ 5. **Cochlear nuclei**
- ☐ 6. **Vestibular nerve**
- ☐ 7. **Vestibular ganglion (Scarpa ganglion)**
- ☐ 8. **Saccule**
- ☐ 9. **Ampulla of the posterior semicircular duct**
- ☐ 10. **Utricle**
- ☐ 11. **Ampulla of the lateral semicircular duct**
- ☐ 12. **Ampulla of the superior semicircular duct**

Clinical Note

The vestibulocochlear nerve enters the brainstem at the ventrolateral margin at the junction of the medulla and the pons, known as the cerebellopontine angle. At this site, Schwann cell tumors, called *acoustic Schwannomas*, may arise, usually from the vestibular portion of CN VIII but rapidly involving the cochlear division of CN VIII as well. Vestibular symptoms often begin as vertigo, dizziness, unsteadiness, spatial disorientation, and nausea. Auditory symptoms often begin as tinnitus, and as the nerve is further compromised, ipsilateral loss of hearing can lead to deafness and inability to localize sound. An acoustic Schwannoma may also involve the facial nerve, producing ipsilateral facial palsy. If the tumor is not removed, it can expand rostrally to involve CN V, or caudally to involve CNs IX and X. The tumor also may impinge on the cerebellum and adjacent brainstem. The acoustic Schwannoma is not a malignant tumor and remains localized and encapsulated. It is amenable to surgical removal, a procedure which on some occasions removes the entire Schwannoma and is curative.

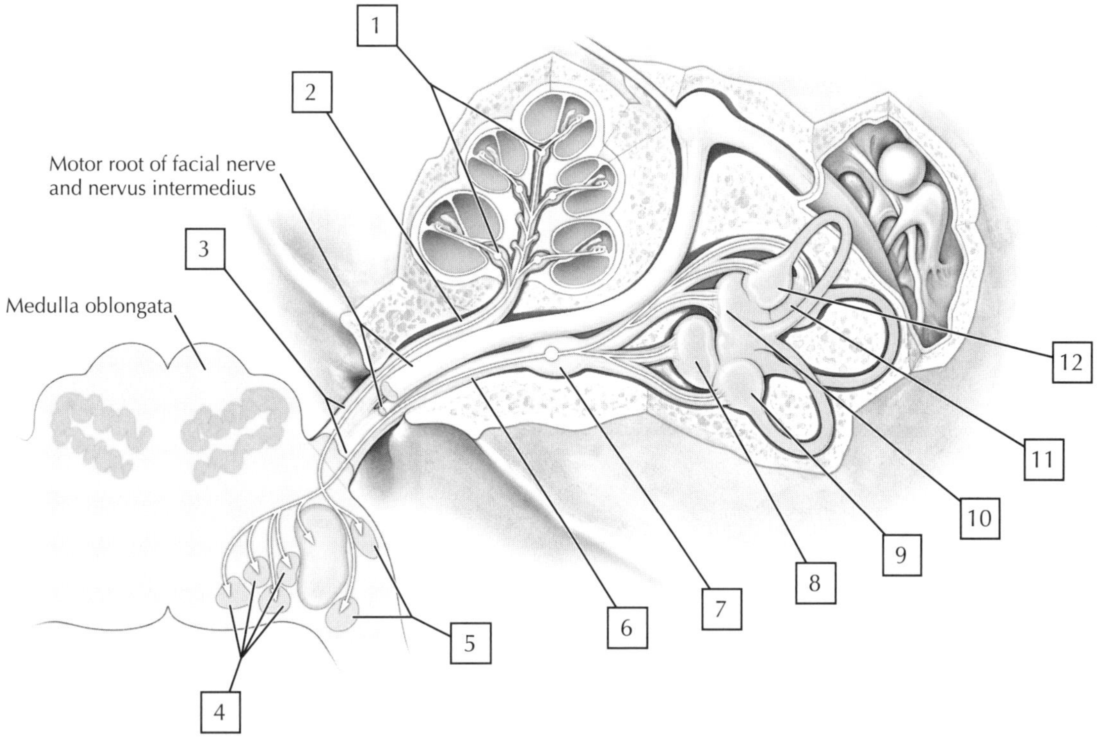
1
2
Motor root of facial nerve
and nervus intermedius
3
Medulla oblongata
4
5
6
7
8
9
10
11
12

Reticular Formation: General Pattern of Nuclei in the Brainstem

The reticular formation is the core of the brainstem, extending from the rostral spinal cord, through the interior of the medulla, pons, and midbrain, into portions of the diencephalon and septal nuclei. The neurons are called *isodendritic*, characterized by extensive dendritic arborizations and an axon that extends to many other neurons beyond the local territory of the cell body. These neurons are not interneurons. There are many components to the reticular formation, including a medial zone (mainly motor), a lateral zone (mainly sensory), and many individual nuclei. Some reticular formation groups include the raphe nuclei (serotonergic neurons with colocalized neuropeptides) and the brainstem noradrenergic and adrenergic chemically specific neurons. These serotonergic and noradrenergic neurons have axons with very extensive axonal arborizations that may provide varicose collaterals to the spinal cord, brainstem, cerebellum, diencephalon, basal ganglia, limbic forebrain, and widespread areas of the cerebral cortex, all from a single branching axon. These neurons are modulatory for the many regions to which they project, and help to regulate the excitability of many regions of the CNS (tuning the gain for excitability up or down for other excitatory and inhibitory inputs at the same time). Some neuroscientists also include the dopaminergic cell groups in the reticular formation. Other reticular formation regions include the paramedian reticular formation, the respiratory nuclei, cardiovascular regulatory regions of the brainstem, the periaqueductal gray, many hypothalamic regions, and the septal nuclei.

Clinical Note

The reticular formation is the core of the brainstem and is necessary for consciousness and for many functions required for life. The lateral reticular formation receives polymodal sensory input, especially powerful from nociceptive stimuli and provide the neural substrate for the Ascending Reticular Activating System (ARAS); these neurons are essential for sleep–wakefulness cycles and arousal and are necessary for stimulating and arousing the cerebral cortex. Consciousness requires one intact hemisphere and an intact reticular formation. The medial reticular formation provides upper motor neuronal regulation of basic tone and posture through the medullary reticulospinal tract (flexor bias) and the pontine reticulospinal tract (extensor bias). Many nuclei and areas of the paramedian reticular formation provide regulation of autonomic/visceral function (GI, cardiac, vascular, pulmonary, renal, others), and function as reticular formation autonomic centers, coordinated through the hypothalamic efferents. The serotonergic and noradrenergic nuclei regulate the set point of excitability for dozens of regions of the CNS and are involved in thermoregulation, feeding and drinking behavior, reproductive behavior, endocrine regulation, sympathetic and parasympathetic excitability, and many other essential functions. The serotonergic neurons of nucleus raphe magnus are particularly important for regulating the set point of sensitivity of the dorsal horn of the spinal cord to nociceptive inputs and permit endogenous opioid regulation of nociception. Major lesions of the reticular formation are lethal.

COLOR the following structures, using a separate color for each region.

- ☐ 1. **Dopaminergic cell groups**
- ☐ 2. **Paramedian reticular formation**
- ☐ 3. **Lateral reticular formation**
- ☐ 4. **Medial reticular formation**
- ☐ 5. **Respiratory nuclei**
- ☐ 6. **Caudal raphe nuclei**
- ☐ 7. **Noradrenergic and adrenergic cell groups (nuclei)**
- ☐ 8. **Rostral raphe nuclei**
- ☐ 9. **Periaqueductal gray**

Reticular Formation: General Pattern of Nuclei in the Brainstem

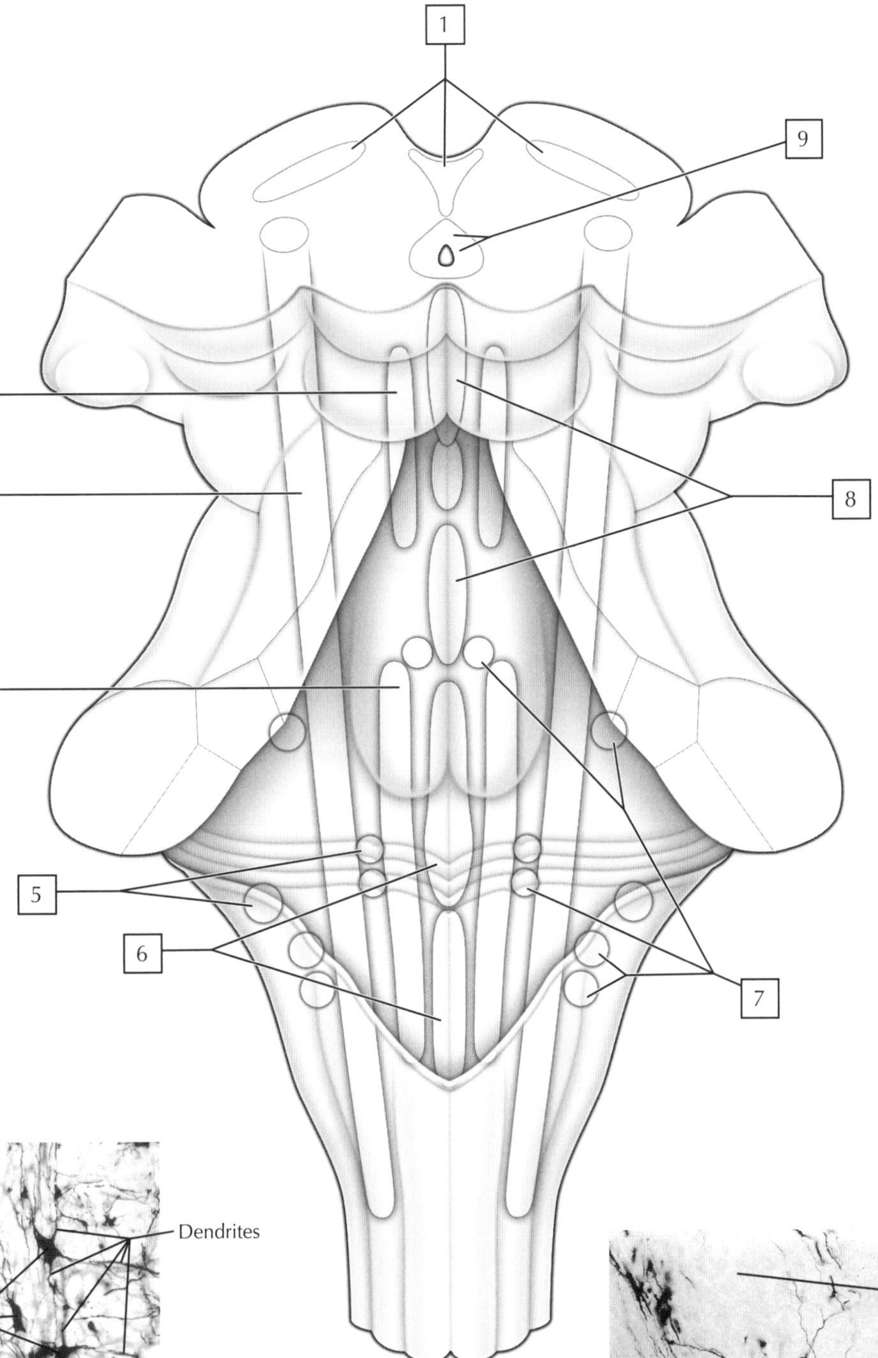

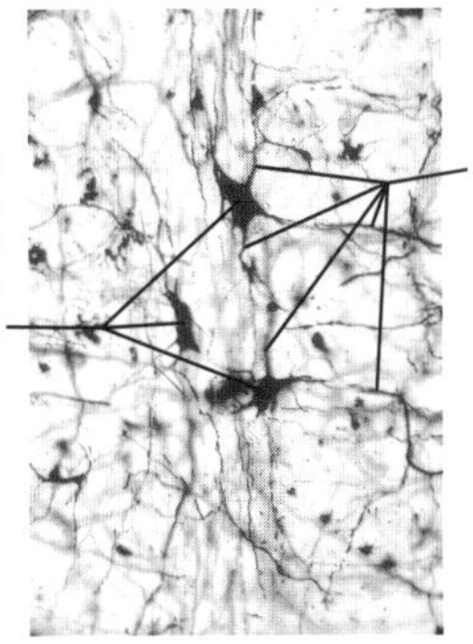

Nucleus raphe pallidus midline neurons with dendrites extending dorsally, ventrally, and laterally, and contributing to the formation of dendrite bundles, which help to coordinate firing of contributing neurons of this serotonergic reticular formation group. Golgi-Cox stain.

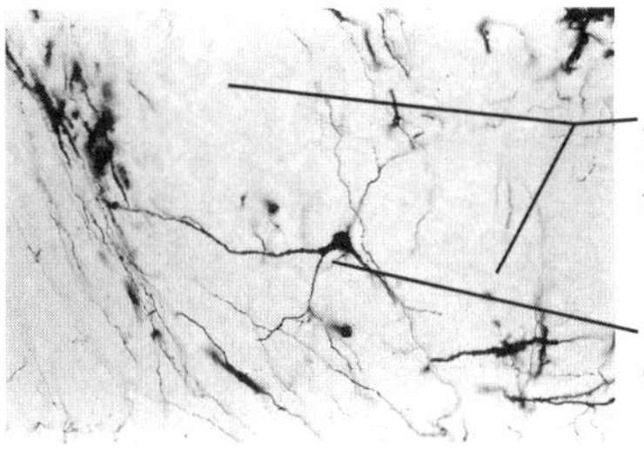

Nucleus raphe dorsalis neuron within the medial longitudinal fasciculus, with widespread dendrites branching into multiple regions. Golgi stain.

Dorsal view of the brainstem with the cerebellum removed

7 Cerebellar Organization: Lobes and Regions

The cerebellum has two systems of organization, anatomical organization and vertical (functional) organization. Anatomically, the cerebellum is subdivided into lobes, including the **anterior lobe,** the **posterior lobe,** and the **flocculonodular lobe** (consisting of the **nodulus** and the **flocculi**). The anterior and posterior lobes are demarcated by the **primary fissure.** The anterior lobe, consisting mainly of vermis and paravermis components, receives mainly unconscious proprioception from the spinal cord, associated with gait and coordination of leg movements. The posterior lobe (often called the *middle lobe*) makes up the bulk of the cerebellum and receives widespread information from the spinal cord, brainstem, and many sensory systems. It is associated with the coordination of limb and body movements, especially of the upper extremities. The flocculonodular lobe, consisting of the nodulus and flocculi, is associated mainly with the vestibular system, and maintenance of equilibrium.

Functionally, the vertical organization reflects the organization of the cerebellum into the vermis (midline region), paravermis (adjacent to the vermis), and the lateral hemispheres (the bulk of the cerebellum). These regions are associated with specific deep nuclei and their projections to specific upper motor neuronal cell groups.

VERTICAL REGION	DEEP CEREBELLAR NUCLEI	UPPER MOTOR NEURONAL SYSTEM
Vermis	Fastigial N., lateral vestibular N.	Vestibulospinal, reticulospinal tracts
Paravermis	Globose N, emboliform N.	Rubrospinal tract
Lateral hemisphere	Dentate N.	Corticospinal tract through the thalamus

COLOR the following structures, using a separate color for each structure (note, some of these structures overlap with each other).

- ☐ 1. **Lateral hemisphere**
- ☐ 2. **Paravermis**
- ☐ 3. **Vermis**
- ☐ 4. **Anterior lobe**
- ☐ 5. **Primary fissure**
- ☐ 6. **Posterior lobe**
- ☐ 7. **Flocculonodular lobe**
- ☐ 8. **Nodulus**
- ☐ 9. **Flocculi**

Clinical Note

Most lesions and damage to the cerebellum affect the lateral hemispheres. However, the anterior lobe can be damaged in early phases of chronic alcoholism, and the flocculonodular lobe can be damaged by a medulloblastoma tumor. The anterior lobe receives mainly unconscious proprioception from the spinal cord and consists mainly of vermis and paravermis components. Damage leads to a broad-based, staggering gait, sometimes with stiff legs and increased tone. Ataxia of leg movements is seen.

The flocculonodular lobe is associated mainly with vestibulocerebellar connections. It is needed for coordination of balance and equilibrium. A lesion in this lobe, such as a tumor, leads to the patient swaying, and sometimes falling, when standing. Upon attempted movement, there is a staggering gait, even though there is no tremor, and muscle tone is normal. There also is a loss of coordination of visual pursuit eye movements.

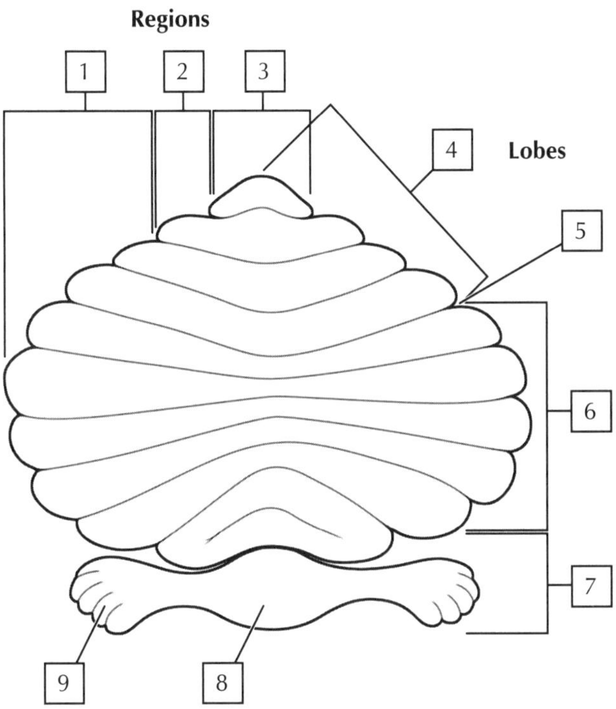

Dorsal view of the cerebellum, unfolded

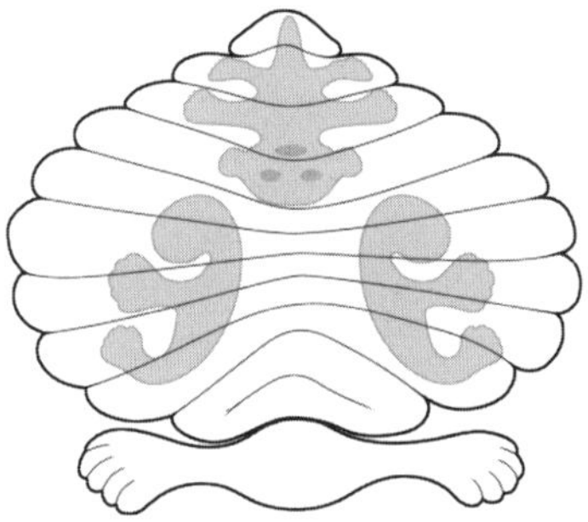

Unfolded schematic of cerebellum demonstrating body map areas

7 Cerebellar Anatomy

The cerebellum is a structure with extensive infolding, resulting in folia that permit a denser packing of gray matter than afforded by a smooth surface. The **cerebellar cortex** is found on the outside of the cerebellum; it is a three-layer structure (molecular layer [outer]; Purkinje cell layer; granule cell layer [inner]), beneath which is the white matter. The **deep cerebellar nuclei** (**dentate, globose and emboliform**, **fastigial**) are at the core of the cerebellum, located at the roof of the fourth ventricle. The three **cerebellar peduncles** (**superior, middle**, and **inferior**) interconnect the cerebellum with the rest of the brainstem and with the thalamus. The cerebellum sits above the **medulla** and **pons,** separated by the **fourth ventricle.** The cerebellar cortex is subdivided into 10 lobules, most of which are not of great individual clinical significance. The **vermis** is present in the midline, seen in the midsagittal section. The **tonsil of the cerebellum** is significant because it is a caudal portion of the cerebellum, which may herniate into the foramen magnum with a posterior fossa lesion or with an Arnold–Chiari malformation; this herniation can impinge on vital brainstem structures and quickly lead to death. There are a few anatomical landmarks of note for the cerebellum, including the **primary fissure** that separates the anterior and posterior lobes, and the **lateral recess of the fourth ventricle.**

COLOR the following structures, using a separate color for each structure.

- ☐ 1. **Cerebellar peduncles**
- ☐ 2. **Lateral recess of the fourth ventricle**
- ☐ 3. **Superior cerebellar peduncle**
- ☐ 4. **Primary fissure**
- ☐ 5. **Dentate nucleus**
- ☐ 6. **Cerebellar cortex**
- ☐ 7. **Vermis**
- ☐ 8. **Tonsil of the cerebellum**
- ☐ 9. **Medulla**
- ☐ 10. **Fourth ventricle**
- ☐ 11. **Pons**

Clinical Note

The greatest portion of the cerebellum is the lateral hemispheres, mainly the posterior (middle lobe. Damage to either the dentate nucleus and/or the superior cerebellar peduncle, or the lateral hemisphere results in a constellation of symptoms characterized as the classic lateral cerebellar syndrome. The deficits often are more severe with a dentate lesion or superior cerebellar peduncle lesion than with a cerebellar cortical lesion. The deep cerebellar nuclei provide the course adjustment for smoothing and coordinating motor activity, and the cerebellar cortex provides the fine adjustment.

The lateral cerebellar hemisphere damage results in an intention tremor (with movement, not at rest), decomposition of movement (loss of coordination of muscle movement across joints), dysdiadochokinesia (inability to perform rapid alternating movements), dysmetria with overshoot or undershoot when aiming to touch a stationary or moving target, hypotonus, pendular reflexes that do not readily dampen, breakdown of timing and rate called decomposition of movement, and disruption of the flow and coordination of speech. Note that these characteristics represent many results observed in a failed field sobriety test administered by police officers with suspected inebriated drivers. Acute alcohol consumption markedly affects cerebellar function and produces a chemically induced cerebellar syndrome.

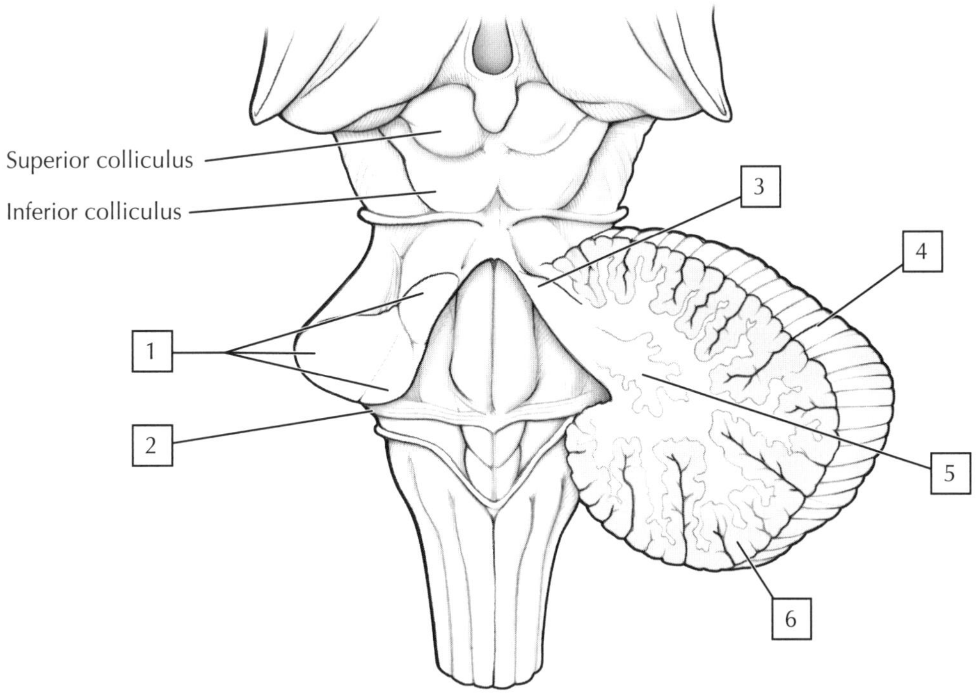

Dorsal view

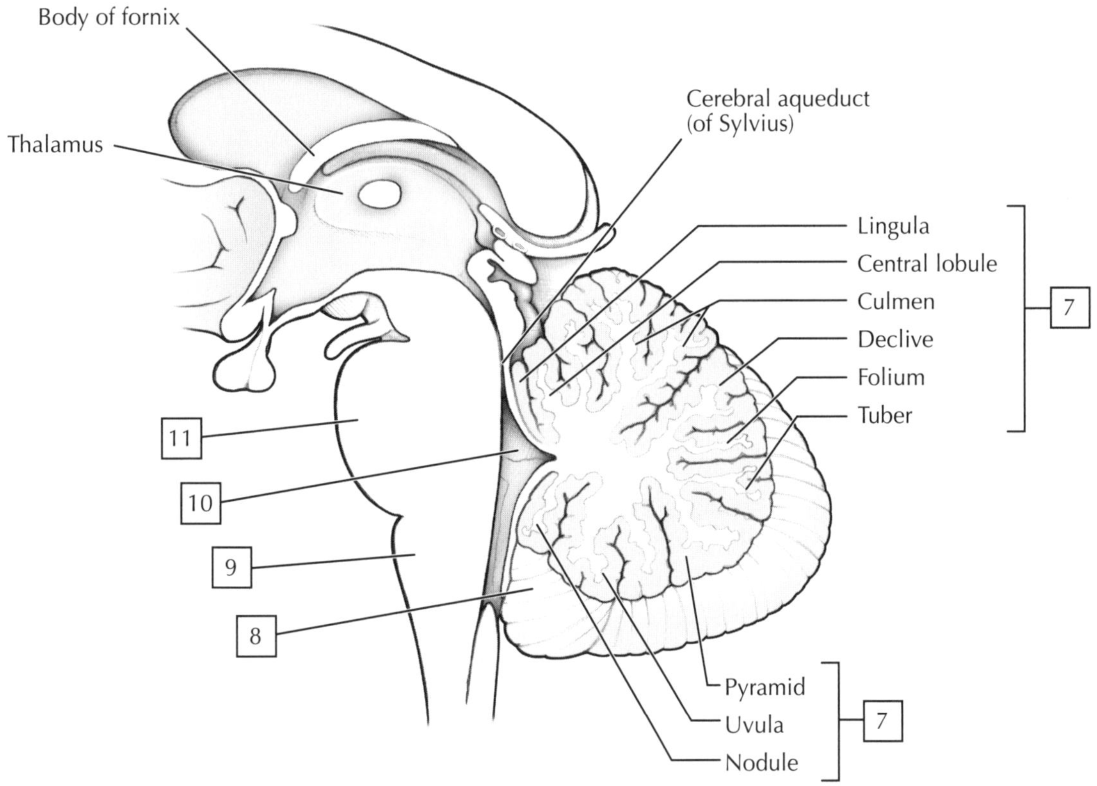

Midsagittal view

7 Deep Cerebellar Nuclei and Cerebellar Peduncles

The cerebellar peduncles interconnect the cerebellum with the brainstem and some thalamic structures. The **inferior cerebellar peduncle** carries spinocerebellar information and inputs from the brainstem reticular formation, trigeminal nuclei, caudal raphe nuclei, and the inferior olivary nucleus. Cerebellar efferents from primary and secondary vestibular sources exit through the inferior cerebellar peduncle. The **middle cerebellar peduncle** is exclusively a channel for the pontocerebellar connections from the more extensive corticopontocerebellar system providing information from the cerebral cortex to the cerebellum. The **superior cerebellar peduncle** provides input to the cerebellum from the ventral spinocerebellar tract, some trigeminal input, tectocerebellar input (superior and inferior colliculi), and input from the noradrenergic locus coeruleus. Efferent connections from the dentate nucleus to the red nucleus and ventral thalamus, and from the globose and emboliform nuclei mainly to the red nucleus, travel through the superior cerebellar peduncle.

The deep cerebellar nuclei are found lateral and dorsal to the **fourth ventricle;** they help to regulate upper motor neuronal systems. The **dentate nucleus** mainly regulates corticospinal tract activity through the ventral anterior and ventrolateral nuclei of the thalamus. The **globose and emboliform nuclei** regulate rubrospinal tract activity. The **fastigial nucleus** regulates vestibulospinal tract and reticulospinal tract activity. The cerebellar cortex also connects directly with the **lateral vestibular nucleus,** whose projections to lower motor neurons of the spinal cord provide powerful extensor (antigravity) drive. Therefore the lateral vestibular nucleus is often considered to be a fifth deep cerebellar nucleus.

COLOR the following structures, using a separate color for each structure.

- ☐ 1. **Emboliform nucleus**
- ☐ 2. **Dentate nucleus**
- ☐ 3. **Superior cerebellar peduncle**
- ☐ 4. **Inferior cerebellar peduncle**
- ☐ 5. **Lateral vestibular nucleus**
- ☐ 6. **Middle cerebellar peduncle**
- ☐ 7. **Fourth ventricle**
- ☐ 8. **Fastigial nucleus**
- ☐ 9. **Globose nucleus**

Clinical Note

The cerebellar peduncles, deep nuclei, and cerebellar cortex can be damaged by injuries, tumors, vascular infarcts, and other insults (e.g., toxic damage, herniation). A superior cerebellar artery vascular lesion can deprive the superior and middle cerebellar peduncles and the deep cerebellar nuclei on the ipsilateral side of blood, resulting in long-lasting cerebellar damage including ipsilateral limb ataxia, dysmetria, decomposition of movement, dysdiadochokinesia, intention (movement) tremor, hypotonus, and other characteristics of lateral cerebellar damage. The superior cerebellar artery also supplies some midbrain structures with blood; an infarct may result in eye movement problems and nystagmus.

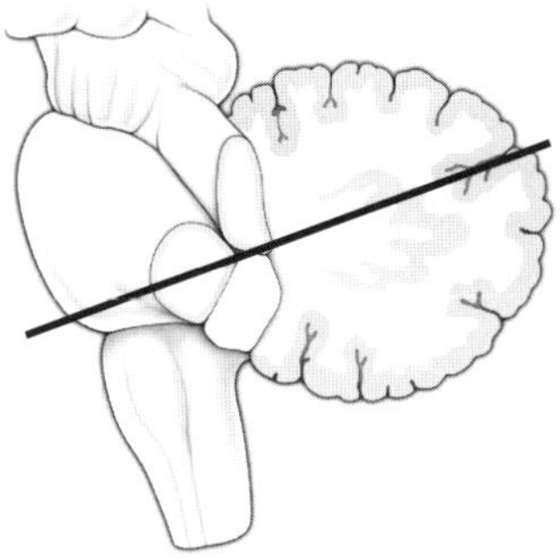

Level of section

Peduncle	Input (efferents)	Output (efferents)
Inferior (restiform body)	Spinocerebellar Dorsal Rostral Cuneocerebellar Olivocerebellar Reticulocerebellar Trigeminocerebellar Raphe–cerebellar	Fastigiobulbar, Uncinate fasciculus } To vestibular and reticular nuclei Direct cerebellovestibular (to lateral vestibular nucleus [LVN])
Juxtarestiform body	Vestibulospinal (primary, secondary)	
Middle (brachium pontis)	Pontocerebellar	
Superior (brachium conjunctivum)	Ventral spinocerebellar Trigeminocerebellar Tectocerebellar Superior colliculus Inferior colliculus Coeruleo-cerebellar	Dentatothalamic Dentatorubral Dentatoreticular Interpositus-rubral connections (globose, emboliform)

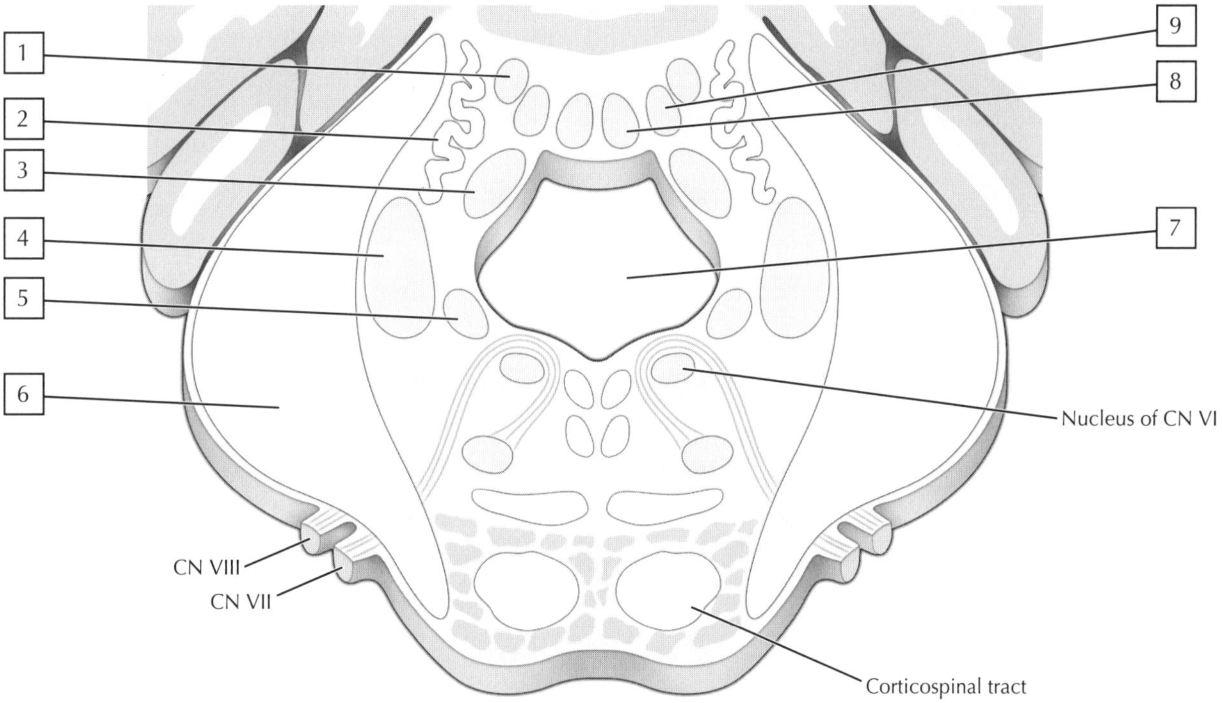

7 Brainstem Arterial Syndromes

The brainstem is supplied with blood by the **vertebrobasilar system**, called the **posterior circulation**. The vertebral arteries and the basilar artery give rise to alternating arterial branches, including **medial penetrating branches**, **short circumferential branches**, and **long circumferential branches**. The medial penetrating branches supply exiting CNs (e.g., CN XII), the corticospinal system, and sometimes sensory structures (e.g., medial lemniscus). Infarcts in the medial penetrating branches result in "**alternating hemiplegias**," which refers to ipsilateral CN damage and contralateral upper motor neuronal symptoms from damage to the corticospinal system. The circumferential branches (named branches), such as the **posterior inferior cerebellar artery (PICA)**, **anterior inferior cerebellar artery (AICA)**, and the **superior cerebellar artery**, provide blood to a zone of the medulla, pons, or midbrain. An infarct in one of these branches of the vertebrobasilar system results in a complex of sensory, motor, and autonomic symptoms that would appear inexplicable without a thorough knowledge of brainstem anatomy and the specific zones supplied by these arteries.

COLOR the following zones or territories, using a separate color for each zone or territory.

- ☐ 1. **Medial midbrain syndrome (Weber syndrome)**
- ☐ 2. **Paramedian midbrain syndrome (Benedikt syndrome)**
- ☐ 3. **Lateral pontine syndrome (AICA syndrome)**
- ☐ 4. **Medial pontine syndrome (Medial basilar infarct)**
- ☐ 5. **Lateral medullary syndrome (PICA syndrome, Wallenberg syndrome)**
- ☐ 6. **Medial medullary syndrome**

Clinical Note

For each of these six arterial syndromes, look closely at the structures in the territory of the affected region that is deprived of blood. List these structures and try to predict what symptoms would be expected, and on which side of the body. These syndromes are described in anatomical and functional (clinical) detail in *Netter's Atlas of Neuroscience*, fourth edition, 2022.

A. Midbrain

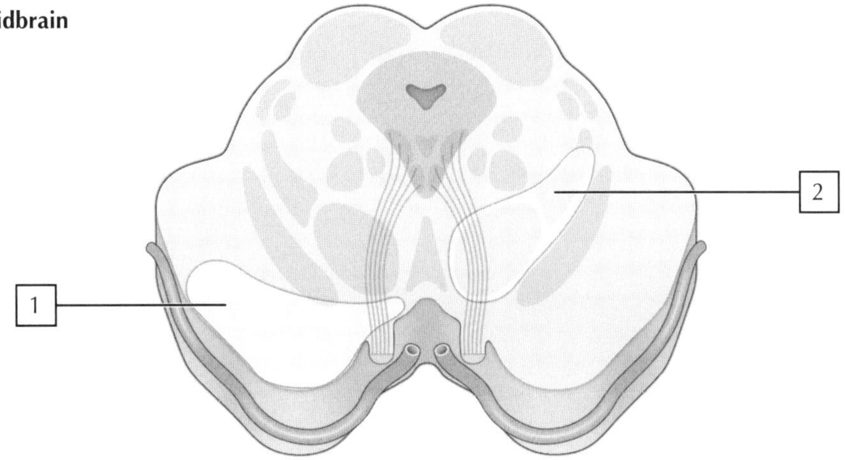

B. Pons

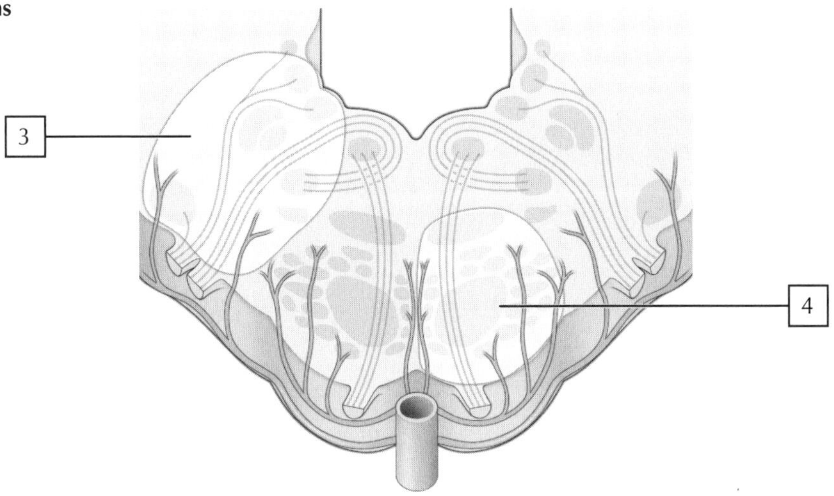

C. Medulla

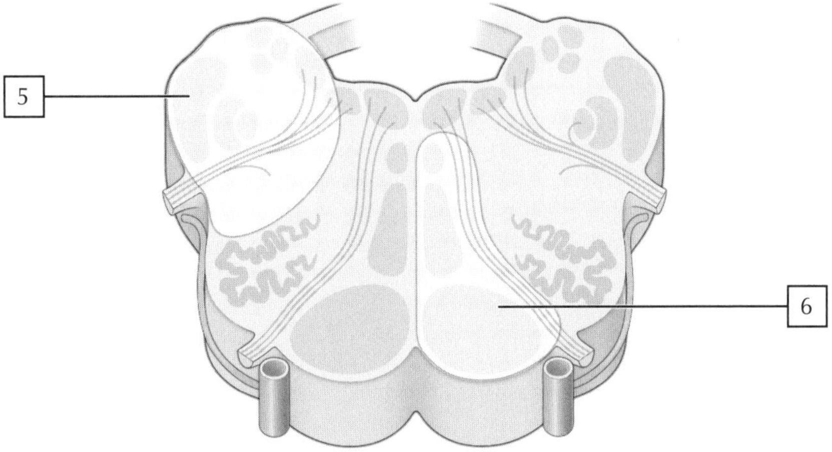

Chapter 8 Forebrain: Diencephalon and Telencephalon

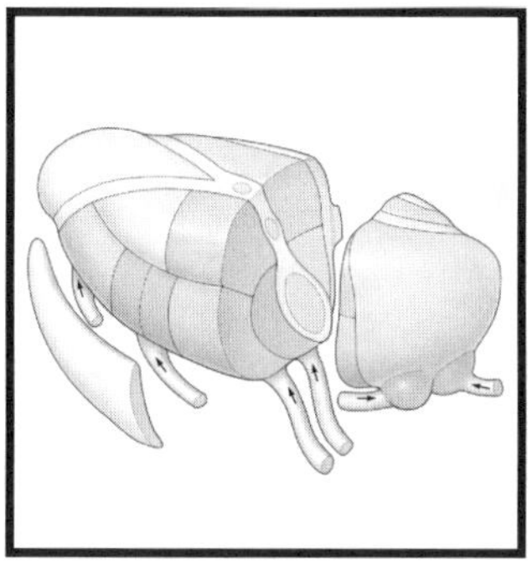

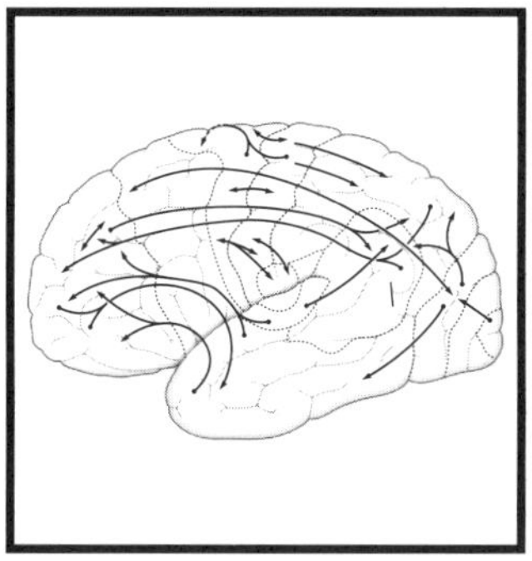

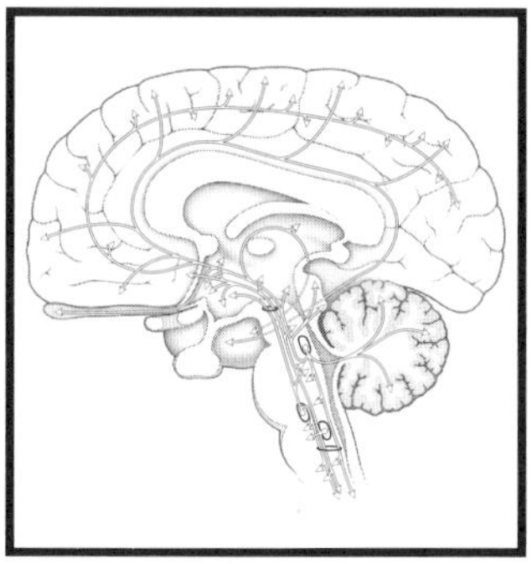

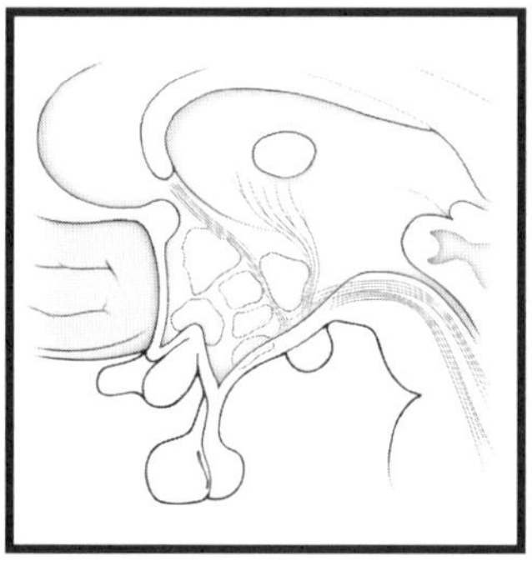

8 Thalamic Nuclei and Interconnections With the Cerebral Cortex

The thalamus is sometimes called *the gateway to the cerebral cortex*. Many thalamic nuclei convey extensive sensory, motor, and autonomic information to specific regions of the cortex and receive extensive reciprocal communication from cortical zones to which they project. All sensory systems except the olfactory system communicate with the cerebral cortex through the thalamus. The thalamus is not just a relay station; the projection nuclei contain networks of interneurons that modulate thalamic input via instructions from the cortex and help to pulse information to the cortex in appropriate "packages" to avoid bombarding it with unprocessed information. Specific thalamic nuclei project to circumscribed regions of the cortex. Nonspecific thalamic nuclei send diffuse projections to widespread regions of the cortex and to other thalamic nuclei. The reticular nucleus of the thalamus helps to modulate the excitability of other thalamic nuclei.

THALAMIC NUCLEUS	CORTICAL REGION TO WHICH IT PROJECTS
Specific Sensory Projection Nuclei	
Ventral posterolateral (VPL)	Postcentral gyrus (somatosensory)
Ventral posteromedial (VPM)	Lateral postcentral gyrus (trigeminal)
Lateral geniculate nucleus (LGN)	Occipital cortex (visual)
Medial geniculate nucleus (MGN)	Temporal lobe transverse gyrus of Heschl (auditory)
Pulvinar	Parietal cortex Occipital cortex (visual association cortex, 18 and 19)
Specific Motor-Related Nuclei	
Ventral lateral (VL)	Precentral gyrus (motor)
Ventral intermedial (VI)	Precentral gyrus (motor)—for dentate-rubro-thalamic-connections to the motor cortex, target of deep brain stimulation
Ventral anterior (VA)	Frontal cortex (premotor and supple-mental motor)
Specific Autonomic-Related Nuclei	
Anterior (Ant)	Anterior cingulate cortex
Lateral dorsal (LD)	Cingulate cortex, anterior parietal cortex
Medial dorsal (MD)	Frontal cortex
Nuclei Related to Association Areas	
Pulvinar	Parietal cortex
Lateral posterior (LP)	Parietal cortex
Nonspecific Thalamic Nuclei	
Intralaminar nuclei	
Centromedian	Widespread cortical regions: diffuse connections
Parafascicular	Widespread cortical regions: diffuse connections
Medial ventral anterior nucleus (VA)	Widespread cortical regions: diffuse connections
Reticular nucleus of the thalamus	Other thalamic nuclei

COLOR the following structures using a separate color for each structure.

- ☐ 1. **Ventral posterolateral nucleus (VPL)**
- ☐ 2. **Ventral posteromedial nucleus (VPM)**
- ☐ 3. **Lateral geniculate nucleus (body) (LGN)**
- ☐ 4. **Medial geniculate nucleus (body) (MGN)**
- ☐ 5. **Pulvinar**
- ☐ 6. **Centromedian (CM)**
- ☐ 7. **Medial dorsal nucleus (MD)**
- ☐ 8. **Lateral dorsal nucleus (LD)**
- ☐ 9. **Anterior nucleus (ANT)**
- ☐ 10. **Ventral anterior nucleus (VA)**
- ☐ 11. **Ventrolateral and ventral intermedial nuclei (VL and VI)**
- ☐ 12. **Reticular nucleus**

Clinical Note

The thalamus receives its blood supply from a host of small penetrating arteries. Individual thalamic nuclei are rarely damaged selectively due to vascular infarcts. When part of the thalamic blood supply is involved and ischemia ensues, the resultant symptoms can include changes in consciousness and alertness, affective disorders, memory dysfunction, motor disorders, altered somatic sensation, visual dysfunction, and altered perception and hallucinations. Some specific lesions in the thalamus can result in paroxysms of excruciating neuropathic pain, called "**thalamic syndrome**."

Thalamocortical radiations

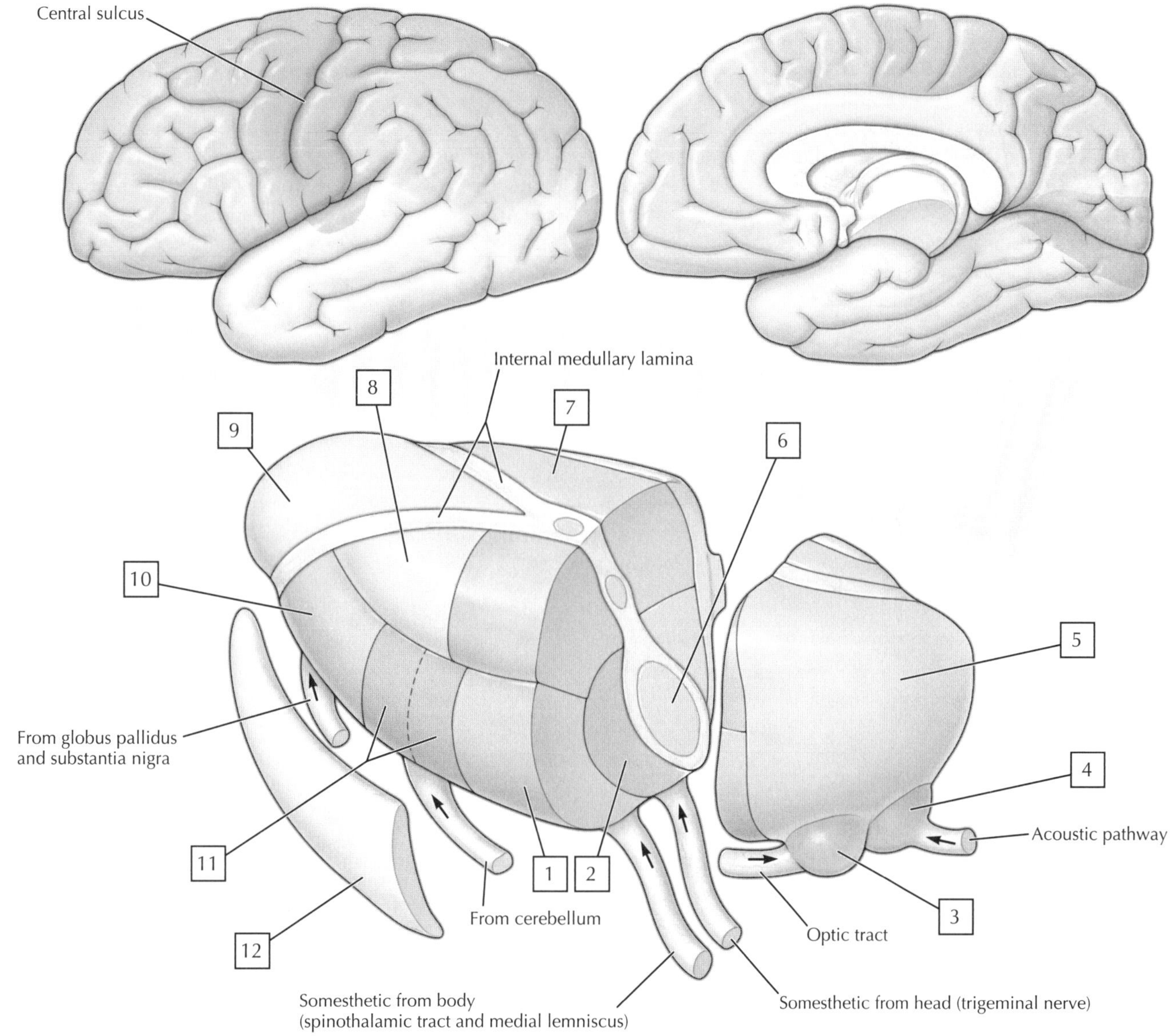

8 Hypothalamus and Pituitary Gland

The hypothalamus is a small region of the diencephalon that regulates **neuroendocrine functions** through the **pituitary gland (hypophysis)** and **visceral/autonomic functions** (e.g., temperature regulation, food and appetite regulation, thirst and water balance, reproduction and sexual behavior, parturition and lactation, respiratory and cardiovascular function, gastrointestinal function, stress responses, and reparative homeostatic states). There are many hypothalamic nuclei located in rostral-to-caudal zones (preoptic zone, anterior or supraoptic zone, tuberal zone, posterior or mammillary zone) and medial-to-lateral zones (periventricular zone, medial zone, lateral zone).

For neuroendocrine regulation, the **paraventricular and supraoptic nuclei** produce oxytocin and vasopressin and send projections through the **supraopticohypophyseal tract,** which channels through the **infundibulum (pituitary stalk)** to the **neurohypophysis (posterior lobe of the pituitary gland)**, at which site oxytocin and vasopressin are released into the general circulation. The arcuate nucleus and other nuclei that produce releasing factors and inhibitory factors for anterior pituitary hormones send projections to the contact zone of the **median eminence.** There the releasing factors are secreted into the hypophyseal-portal vascular system, which delivers very high concentrations of these factors directly to cells of the **anterior pituitary gland (the adenohypophysis)**.

The **mammillary nuclei (body)** constitute part of a limbic loop of interconnections previously proposed to be part of the Papez circuit for memory function. The mammillary nuclei receive inputs from the hippocampal formation via the **fornix**, and project to the anterior nucleus of the **thalamus** via the **mammillothalamic tract**.

COLOR the following structures, using a separate color for each structure.

- ☐ 1. **Fornix**
- ☐ 2. **Paraventricular nucleus**
- ☐ 3. **Supraoptic nucleus**
- ☐ 4. **Arcuate nucleus**
- ☐ 5. **Infundibulum (pituitary stalk)**
- ☐ 6. **Hypophysis (pituitary gland)**
- ☐ 7. **Adenohypophysis (anterior lobe of the pituitary gland)**
- ☐ 8. **Neurohypophysis (posterior lobe of the pituitary gland)**
- ☐ 9. **Mammillary nuclei (body)**
- ☐ 10. **Mammillothalamic tract**
- ☐ 11. **Supraopticohypophyseal tract**

Clinical Note

The posterior pituitary is an essential site for the release of **oxytocin and vasopressin (arginine vasopressin)**. Arginine vasopressin, also called **antidiuretic hormone**, is a key regulator of water balance. If this system is damaged, the patient will experience **diabetes insipidus**, with very high output of dilute urine and subsequent high fluid intake. Damage to the anterior pituitary or the **releasing and inhibitory factors** involved in regulation of anterior pituitary hormone secretion may result in a wide range of dysfunctions such as loss of corticosteroid secretion (adrenocorticotropic hormone), hypothyroidism (thyroid-stimulating hormone), sexual hormone dysregulation (follicle-stimulating hormone and luteinizing hormone), loss of growth hormone secretion, and others. This wide range of dysfunctions can occur with **pan-hypopituitarism**, or because of a **hypophysectomy** due to a tumor. In some situations, a hormone-secreting tumor (**pituitary adenoma**) may release large amounts of growth hormone into the circulation, resulting in **acromegaly** (excessive growth, dense bony growth, coarse features).

This necessitates removal of the tumor and replacement of whatever anterior pituitary hormones are lost following the surgery.

A. Visceral components

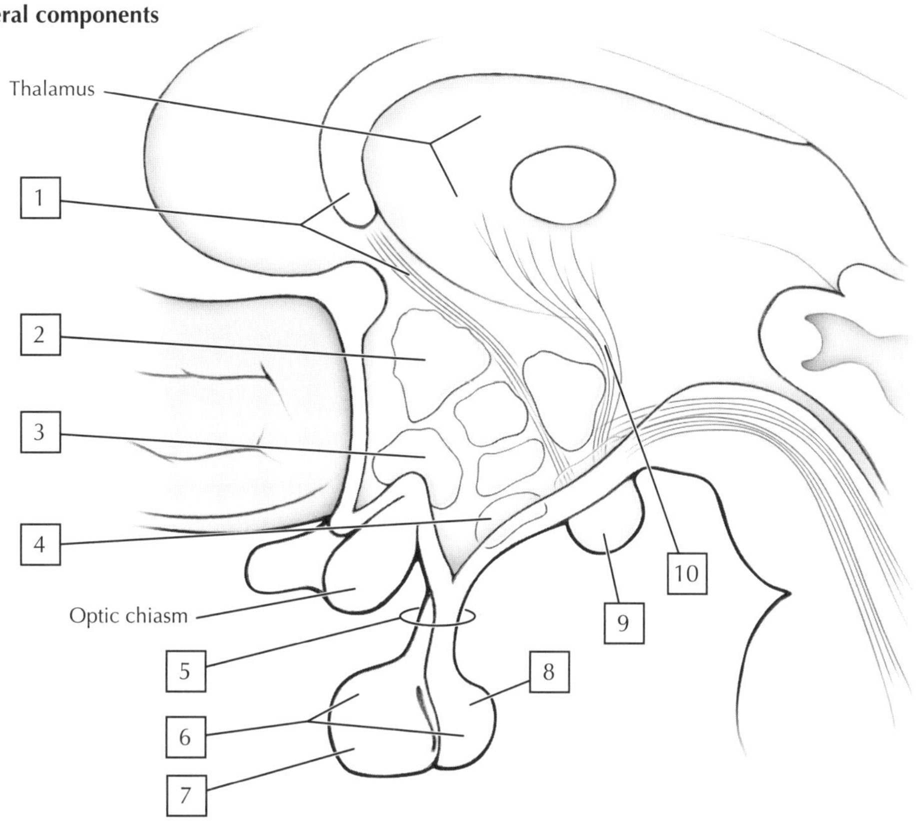

B. Neuroendocrine components

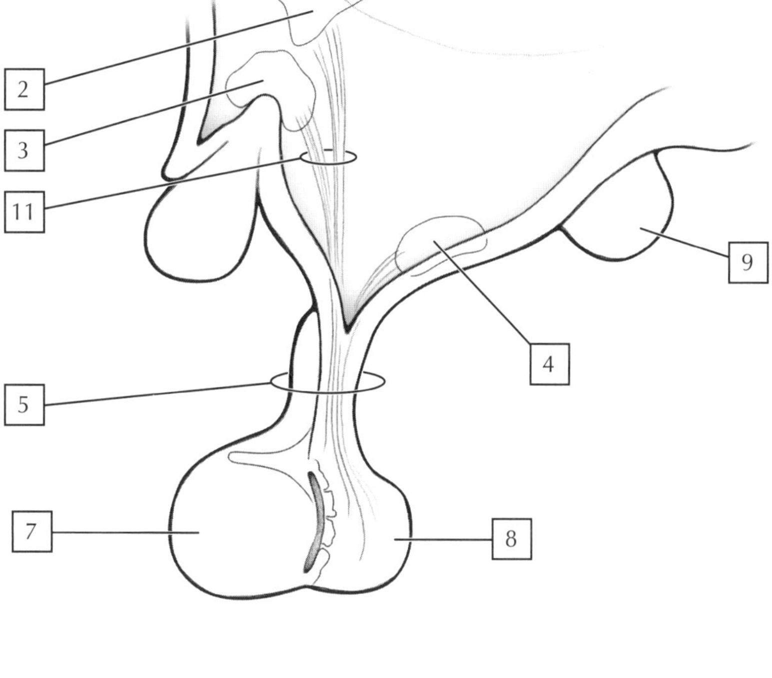

8 Schematic of Hypothalamic Nuclei

Hypothalamic nuclei possess unique afferent and efferent connections and are associated physiologically with specific visceral or neuroendocrine functions. **Hypothalamic areas** are larger collections of neurons involved in regulation of complex visceral/autonomic functions. The magnocellular neurons of the **supraoptic nucleus** mainly synthesize vasopressin; those of the **paraventricular nucleus** mainly synthesize oxytocin. Both nuclei release both of these hormones into the general circulation in the posterior pituitary. **Parvocellular neurons of the paraventricular nucleus** are key regulatory neurons in modulating both sympathetic and parasympathetic activity in the brainstem and spinal cord and also synthesize corticotropin-releasing factor (CRF) for release into the hypophyseal-portal vascular system at the median eminence. In addition, the **anterior hypothalamic area** helps to regulate the parasympathetic nervous system, and the **posterior hypothalamic area** helps to regulate the sympathetic nervous system. The **dorsomedial nucleus, ventromedial nucleus,** and **lateral hypothalamic area** regulate feeding, drinking, and reproductive behaviors. The **preoptic area (medial and lateral nuclei)** regulates cyclic neuroendocrine behavior and thermoregulation. The **suprachiasmatic nucleus** receives input regarding the light/dark cycle from the optic tract and regulates circadian rhythms and diurnal cycles. The **periventricular nucleus** and **arcuate nucleus** provide dopaminergic neuronal regulation in the median eminence over anterior pituitary hormone secretion. The **periarcuate region** is the principal source of beta-endorphin-producing neurons, and helps to regulate analgesic responses. Many hypothalamic nuclei (preoptic regions, suprachiasmatic nucleus), along with forebrain regions (nucleus basalis) and brainstem regions (reticular formation, nucleus solitarius, raphe nuclei, locus coeruleus), regulate the sleep–wake cycle. **Mammillary nuclei (complex)** may help to regulate memory function through limbic circuitry. Many regions of the hypothalamus are subject to influences from interleukins and are interposed into more complex circuitry for regulating autonomic functions, visceral functions, affective behavior, stress responses, and general illness behavior.

COLOR the following structures, using a separate color for each structure.

- ☐ 1. **Paraventricular nucleus**
- ☐ 2. **Lateral hypothalamic area**
- ☐ 3. **Dorsomedial nucleus**
- ☐ 4. **Lateral preoptic nucleus (area)**
- ☐ 5. **Anterior hypothalamic area**
- ☐ 6. **Medial preoptic nucleus (area)**
- ☐ 7. **Supraoptic nucleus**
- ☐ 8. **Suprachiasmatic nucleus**
- ☐ 9. **Ventromedial nucleus**
- ☐ 10. **Mammillary nuclei (complex)**
- ☐ 11. **Periventricular nucleus**
- ☐ 12. **Posterior hypothalamic area**

Clinical Note

The hypothalamus is the regulatory zone over neuroendocrine output (both anterior pituitary hormones and posterior pituitary hormones, oxytocin, and vasopressin) and visceral/autonomic functions. Some of the hypothalamic regulation is coordinated with motor and sensory processing, as in the case of feeding behavior, drinking behavior, and reproductive behavior. Some regulatory functions are achieved through direct connections and some through multiple and polysynaptic connections (e.g., regulation of nausea).

The hypothalamic circuitry undertaking such regulation is subject to influences from the limbic forebrain and the cerebral cortex. For example, if one sees something frightening or perceives a threat in the environment, many cortical and limbic structures (including the amygdaloid nuclei for providing the emotional context of the observed objects) interpret that threat and quickly recruit the appropriate hypothalamic and motor circuitry to achieve an appropriate behavior response, such as fleeing, freezing, or acting calmly. Similarly, it is possible through mental contemplation to recall events or situations that provoke feelings of rage, sorrow, joy, or other emotions. In such a situation, the cognitive activities may elevate blood pressure, produce feelings of anxiety, and change both autonomic activity (e.g., sympathetic activation) and neuroendocrine activity (e.g., activation of the hypothalamic–pituitary–adrenal axis using corticotropin-releasing factor, adrenocorticotropic hormone, and cortisol secretion). Thus the hypothalamus is at the crossroads of limbic–hypothalamic–autonomic and neuroendocrine regulation and is subject to the effects of cortical activity.

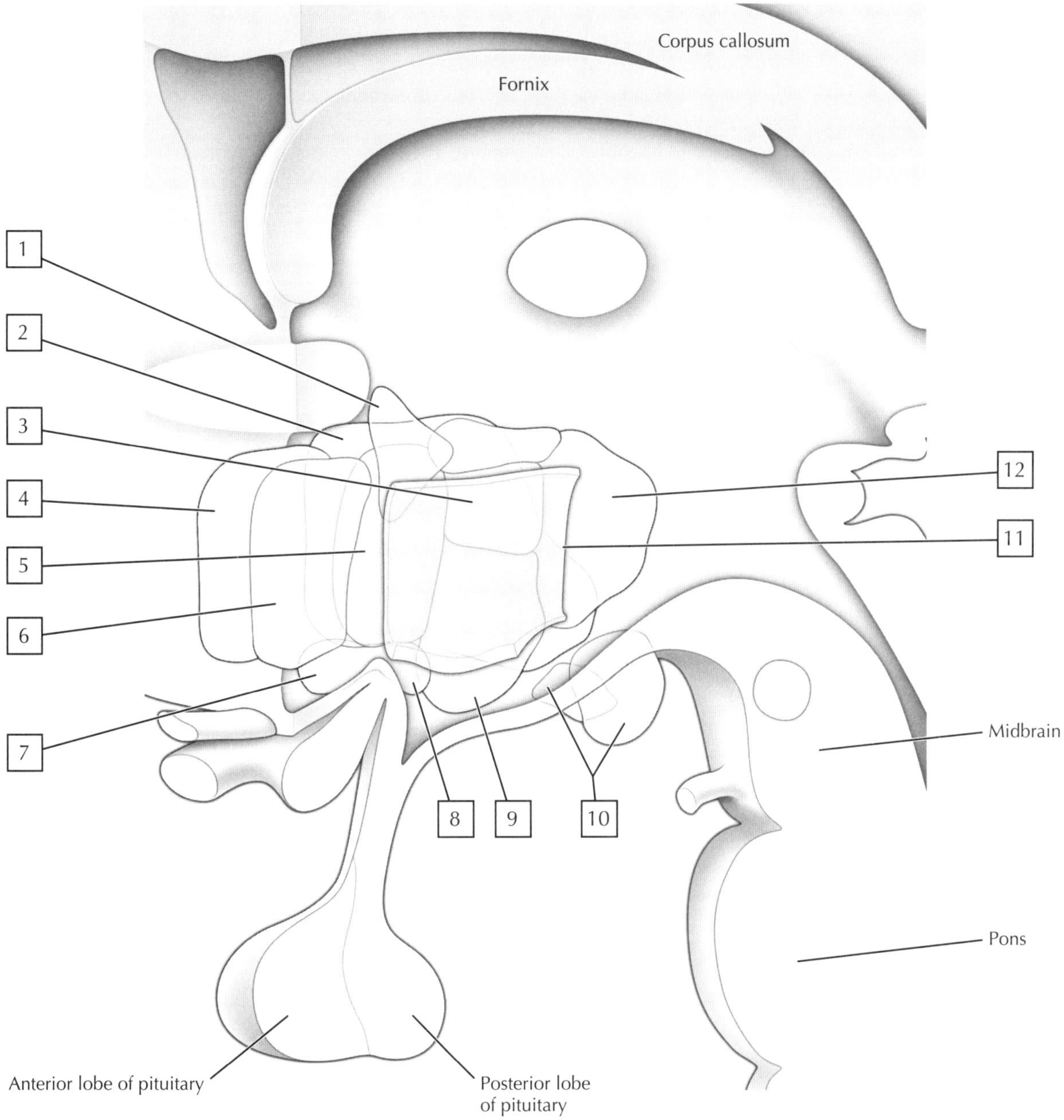
Corpus callosum
Fornix
1
2
3
4
5
6
7
8
9
10
11
12
Midbrain
Pons
Anterior lobe of pituitary
Posterior lobe of pituitary

8 Axial Section Through the Forebrain

An **axial section** through the forebrain is a true horizontal section with no tilt; early axial-type imaging sections were termed **horizontal** sections and were tilted 25 degrees from a true axial section. This axial section is taken at the level of the head of the caudate nucleus, the midthalamus, and the full representation of the internal capsule. These structures are key landmarks for interpreting axial brain imaging, providing a view of the important regions, the ventricles, and the symmetry of the two sides. The **anterior limb of the internal capsule** separates the **head of the caudate nucleus** medially from the **putamen** and **globus pallidus** laterally. The **genu (knee) of the internal capsule** is the innermost bend of the "V" shape, with the head of the caudate nucleus anteriorly and the **thalamus** posteriorly. The **posterior limb of the internal capsule** separates the thalamus medially from the putamen and globus pallidus laterally. The **lateral ventricles** are present in two places in this section, the **anterior horn** frontally and the **temporal pole** posteriorly. Lateral to the putamen are, successively, the **external capsule,** the **claustrum,** the **extreme capsule**, and the **insular cortex,** lying in the depths of the lateral fissure.

COLOR the following structures, using a separate color for each structure.

- ☐ 1. **Head of the caudate nucleus**
- ☐ 2. **Anterior limb of the internal capsule**
- ☐ 3. **Claustrum**
- ☐ 4. **External capsule**
- ☐ 5. **Putamen**
- ☐ 6. **Globus pallidus**
- ☐ 7. **Genu of the internal capsule**
- ☐ 8. **Insular cortex**
- ☐ 9. **Thalamus**
- ☐ 10. **Posterior limb of the internal capsule**
- ☐ 11. **Lateral ventricles—temporal pole**
- ☐ 12. **Lateral ventricles—anterior horn**

Clinical Note

This axial section is useful for observing potential pathology involved in many types of forebrain disorders. Diseases of the **basal ganglia** (caudate nucleus, putamen, globus pallidus) and **associated nuclei** (the subthalamus and the substantia nigra) may show degenerative changes, such as the flattening and shrinking of the head of the caudate nucleus in **Huntington disease**. Clinically, Huntington disease presents with choreiform (brisk, dance-like) movements, emotional problems, and cognitive decline. Small lacunar infarcts may be visible in the thalamus or the cortical white matter. Demyelinating plaques in **multiple sclerosis** may be seen in the cerebral white matter. An infarct in the **internal capsule** may indicate the occurrence of a stroke. The most frequently involved portions in an infarct in the internal capsule are the genu and posterior limb. Such an insult results in contralateral hemiplegia (soon resolving into spastic hemiplegia with hypertonus, hyperreflexia, and pathological reflexes), a contralateral drooping lower face, and contralateral loss of sensation on the body.

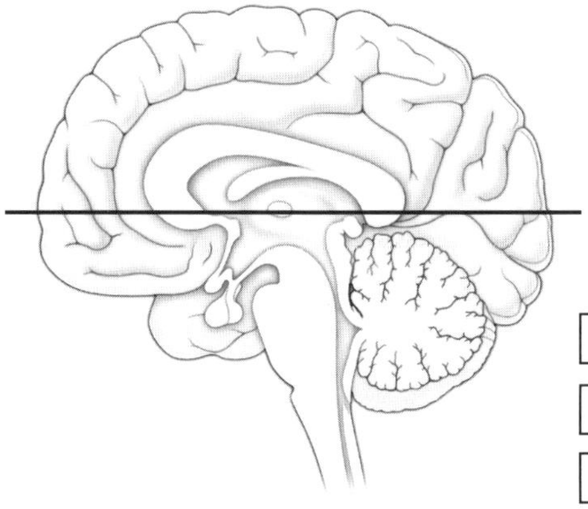

Level of section (head of caudate and midthalamus)

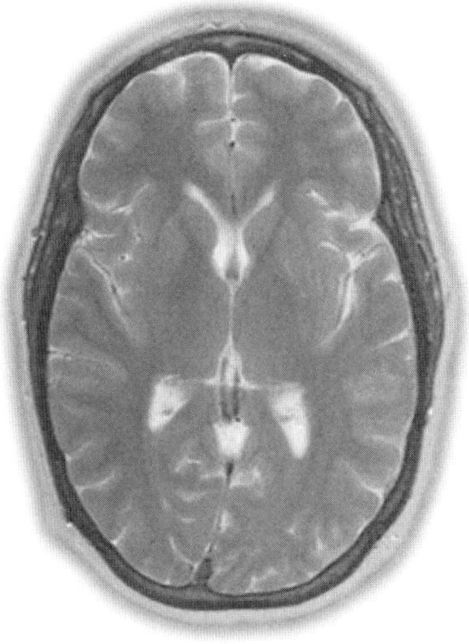

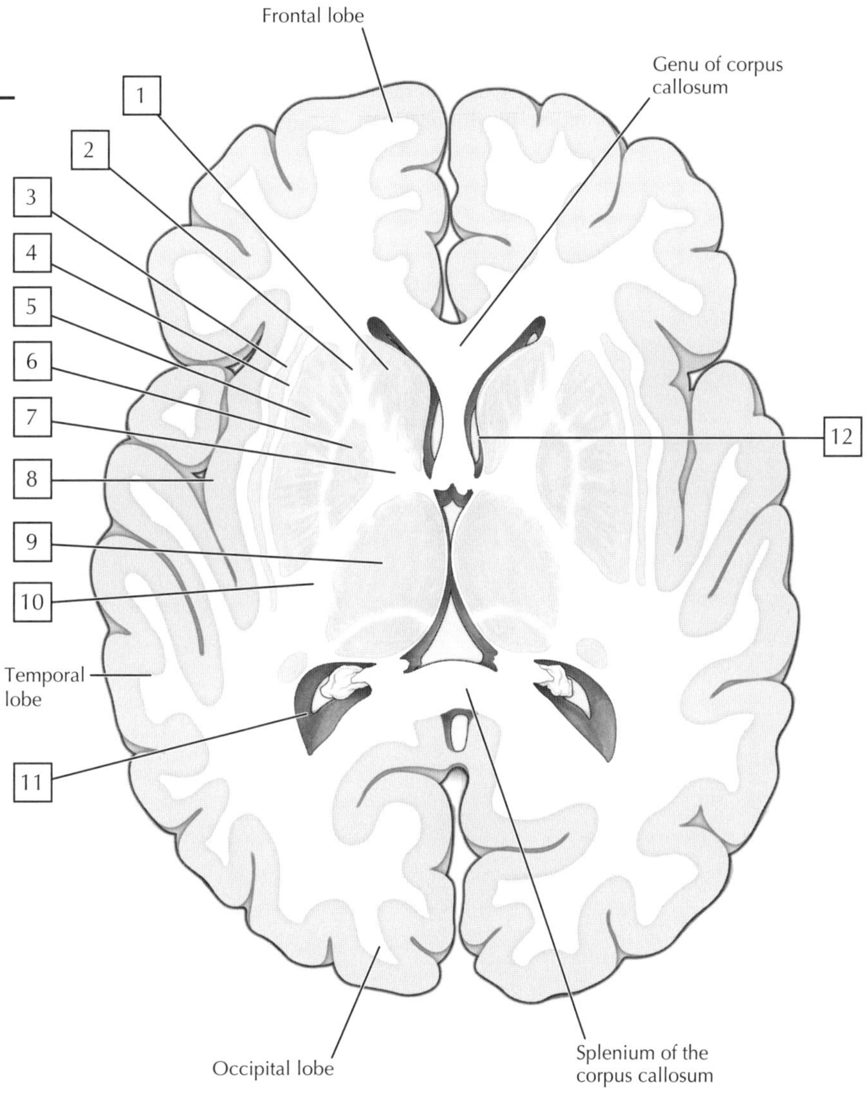

8 Coronal Section Through the Forebrain

This coronal section is a key section through the forebrain showing the anterior commissure, the columns of the fornix, many structures of the basal ganglia, and many limbic forebrain structures. The **anterior limb of the internal capsule** and the **anterior commissure** are major white matter zones in the interior of the forebrain. The anterior limb of the internal capsule separates the **head of the caudate nucleus** medially from the **putamen** and **globus pallidus** laterally. The anterior commissure interconnects corresponding regions of the temporal lobes. Both the **frontal pole of the lateral ventricles** and the **third ventricle** can be seen. In the medial pole of the anterior temporal lobe is the **amygdaloid complex** of nuclei. In the region just below the anterior commissure, termed the "substantia innominata," is the **nucleus basalis (of Meynert)**, an important region of forebrain cholinergic neurons. Along the midline of the frontal lobe is the **cingulate cortex**, with the **cingulum** (major forebrain tract carrying noradrenergic, serotonergic, dopaminergic, and cholinergic axons projecting to the cerebral cortex) just above the **body of the corpus callosum**. The **columns of the fornix** convey projections from the CA1 and CA3 regions of the hippocampus to the septal nuclei, nucleus accumbens, preoptic and anterior regions of the hypothalamus, and other limbic structures. The **insular cortex**, regulating some visceral activities, is located in the depths of the lateral fissure.

COLOR the following structures, using a separate color for each structure.

- ☐ 1. **Cingulate cortex**
- ☐ 2. **Columns of the fornix**
- ☐ 3. **Head of the caudate nucleus**
- ☐ 4. **Anterior limb of the internal capsule**
- ☐ 5. **Putamen**
- ☐ 6. **Insular cortex**
- ☐ 7. **Globus pallidus**
- ☐ 8. **Anterior commissure**
- ☐ 9. **Nucleus basalis (of Meynert)**
- ☐ 10. **Amygdala (amygdaloid complex)**
- ☐ 11. **Frontal pole of the lateral ventricle**
- ☐ 12. **Body of the corpus callosum**

Clinical Note

The nucleus basalis, found in the substantia innominata just beneath the region of the anterior commissure, contains a major collection of central cholinergic neurons whose axons send diffuse projections to many regions of the cerebral cortex and limbic forebrain. These neurons have been found to degenerate in the brains of some patients with Alzheimer disease and have been described as important for short-term memory function and cognitive function. Many pharmaceutical and nutritional efforts have been made to provide choline or supportive cholinergic-enhancing medications in the attempt to improve memory function. Despite some experimental success in animal models, these approaches have not been more than marginally successful in humans, probably because of the widespread neuronal damage that already has occurred by the time the patient is diagnosed with significant cognitive decline.

Nuclei in the amygdala are important in providing an emotional context for sensory stimuli, especially fear responses. The amygdala may be damaged bilaterally by **contrecoup injury** (damage opposite to the site of the direct trauma) following a blow to the head. The resultant "**Klüver–Bucy**" syndrome is accompanied by a loss of fear to dangerous objects, loss of short-term memory function, indiscriminate hyperactive sexual responses, and other altered behaviors. In circumstances where the amygdala is damaged more selectively bilaterally, the loss of fear responses is present and the patient cannot recognize fearful facial expressions in others.

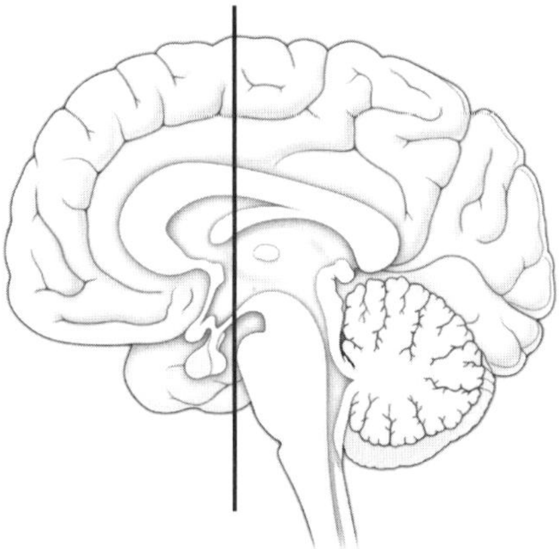

Level of section (anterior commissure/columns of fornix)

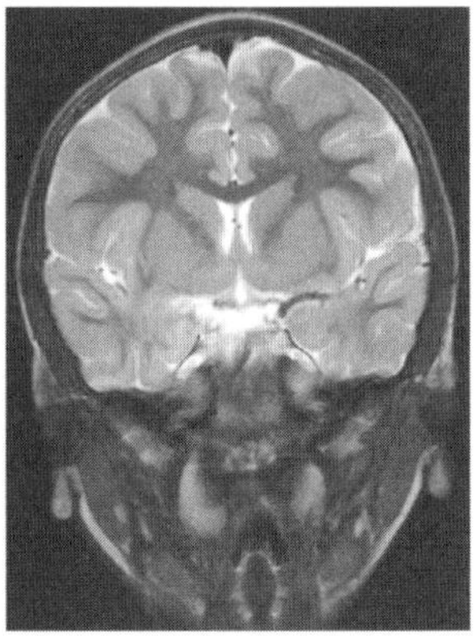

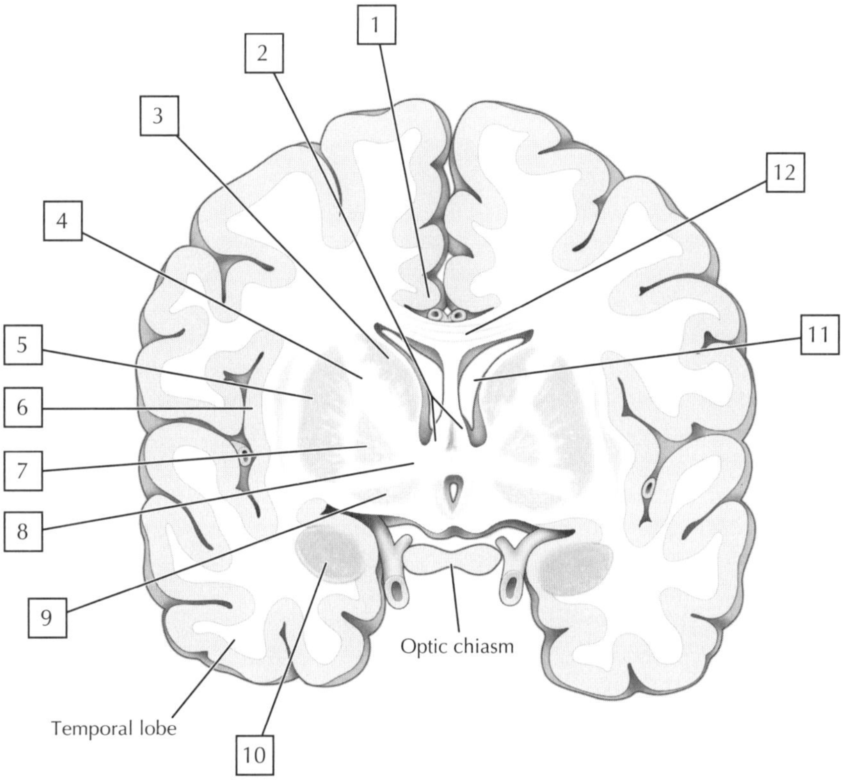

8 Layers of the Cerebral Cortex

The cerebral cortex is a six-layer neuronal structure, located on the exterior of the forebrain. It is sometimes called the neocortex, to distinguish it from phylogenetically older cortex with fewer layers (three-layer archicortex-hippocampus; and five-layer paleocortex–olfactory-related cortex). The major neuronal cell types proliferate in the ventricular zone during fetal development and migrate to the exterior of the central nervous system following radial glia. The cortex has two **pyramidal cell layers, layer V (large pyramidal layer)** and **layer III (small pyramidal cell layer)**. The pyramidal cells possess extensive basolateral dendritic arborizations and a branching apical dendrite running perpendicular to the surface. The pyramidal neurons serve as projection neurons, with axons that leave the cortex and may travel long distances to their targets.

There are two **granule cell layers, layer IV (the major granule cell layer)** and **layer II**. Granule cells are local circuit neurons with small cell bodies, local dendritic arborizations, and local axonal distribution. The granule cells receive **thalamic inputs (specific afferents)** and **other afferents and association fibers** and modulate the excitability of other cortical neurons.

Sensory cortex (e.g., postcentral gyrus) possesses a large granule cell layer IV, receiving abundant specific afferents from the thalamus. Pyramidal neurons in the sensory cortex are sparse but are functionally important components of the vertical columns. **Motor cortex** (e.g., precentral gyrus) possesses large pyramidal layers V and III and has sparse numbers of granule cells. The motor cortex gives rise to abundant efferents to subcortical regions of the brain as well as to other regions of the cerebral cortex. **Association cortex** has a balance of pyramidal cell layers and granule cell layers as it receives inputs from some specific afferents and other inputs and gives rise to extensive **efferent projections to other parts of the cortex.**

Noradrenergic axonal inputs from the locus coeruleus in the pons **and serotonergic raphe axonal inputs from the rostral brainstem nuclei** send very fine varicose axons into the cerebral cortex, with massive arborizations into all six layers. These noradrenergic and serotonergic axons modulate the excitability of other neurons and their synaptic responsiveness.

COLOR the following structures, using a separate color for each structure.

- ☐ 1. **Pyramidal cell layer V in motor cortex and association cortex**
- ☐ 2. **Pyramidal cell layer III in motor cortex**
- ☐ 3. **Motor axons from pyramidal cells in motor cortex**
- ☐ 4. **Granule cell layer IV in sensory cortex**
- ☐ 5. **Granule cell layer II in sensory cortex**
- ☐ 6. **Specific afferents (thalamic inputs) to sensory cortex**
- ☐ 7. **Other afferents and association fiber inputs to association cortex**
- ☐ 8. **Efferent projections to other parts of the cortex from association cortex**
- ☐ 9. **Noradrenergic axonal inputs from the locus coeruleus**
- ☐ 10. **Serotonergic axonal inputs from rostral raphe nuclei**

Clinical Note

Sensory cortex serves as the receiving zone for specific inputs in the major sensory systems. Motor cortex acts as the final major cortical output to lower motor neurons of the brainstem and spinal cord, and to other motor structures such as the upper motor neurons in the brainstem. In between sensory cortex and motor cortex are extensive networks of connectivity for processing stimuli and to provide past memory and emotional context to those stimuli. This connectivity is then processed back to the premotor and supplemental motor cortices and the motor cortex to elicit an appropriate behavioral response. The two hemispheres interact with each other through commissural connections of the corpus callosum and the anterior commissure.

Disruption of these major cortically related axonal systems may result in specific sensory and/or motor deficits, apraxias and agnosias, aphasias, and altered behavioral responses.

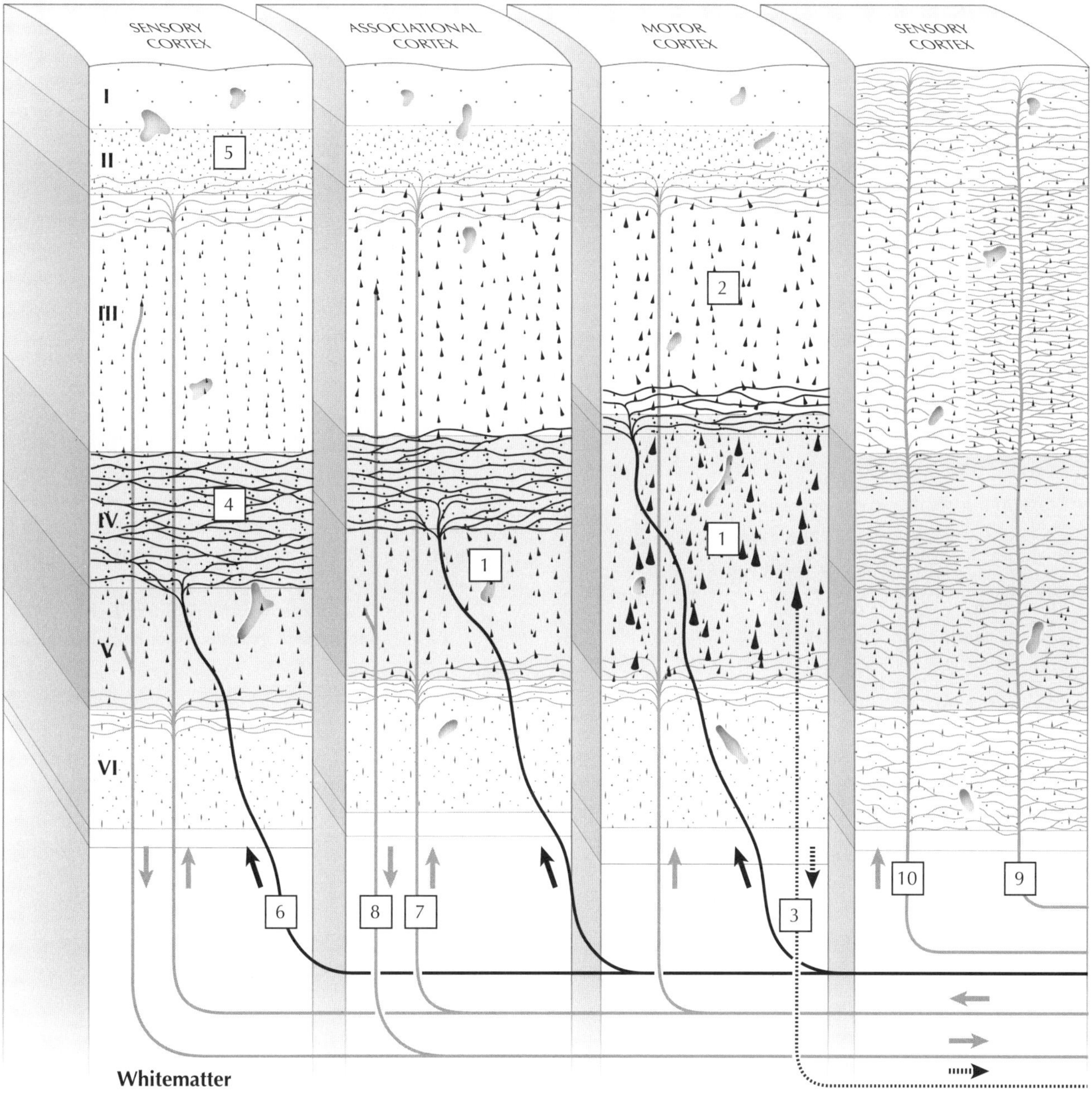

SENSORY CORTEX
ASSOCIATIONAL CORTEX
MOTOR CORTEX
SENSORY CORTEX
I
II
III
IV
V
VI
1
2
3
4
5
6
7
8
9
10
Whitematter

8 Vertical Columns: Functional Units of the Cerebral Cortex

Specific afferents conveying information to sensory cortices often bring very precise information about the stimulus that activated the lemniscal pathway to the thalamus, and hence the thalamic projections to the cortex. This information does not just get dumped into general banks of the cortex but terminates in precise **vertical columns** that cut through all six layers of the cerebral cortex. The vertical columns are 0.5 to 1.0 mm in diameter, based on the horizontal dendritic spread of the major pyramidal cell associated with the vertical column. These vertical columns project abundantly to each other, an important basis for the convergence of information for interpretation of the sensory world. The key neurons involved are the **small pyramidal cells,** the **granule cells,** and at least one **large pyramidal cell.** The key afferent fibers are **corticocortical afferents** and **thalamic afferents** (specific afferent projections). The key efferent fibers in the vertical column are the **cortical projections to subcortical structures,** and **corticocortical efferents to other nearby vertical columns.**

COLOR the following structures, using a separate color for each structure.

- ☐ 1. **Small pyramidal cell**
- ☐ 2. **Granule cell**
- ☐ 3. **Large pyramidal cell**
- ☐ 4. **Corticocortical afferent to the vertical column**
- ☐ 5. **Thalamic afferent (specific afferent) to the vertical column**
- ☐ 6. **Cortical projection from the vertical column to subcortical structures**
- ☐ 7. **Corticocortical efferents (projections) to nearby vertical columns**
- ☐ 8. **Outline the vertical column in this illustration**

Clinical Note

Vertical columns of neurons are critical for the orderly processing of sensory information from its raw form that arrives through the thalamus, through the sophisticated processing that allows us to make a detailed fine-grained analysis of the outside world. For example, a vertical column in the primary visual cortex (area 17) may receive an input corresponding to a point source of light that impinges on the retina in a precise position, perhaps activating just a few or even one cone initially. Then, several vertical columns, each responding to a contiguous set of points on the retina, may collectively project to nearby vertical columns whose optimal stimulus is these multiple point sources of light; this results in an optimal response to a bar of light. Several such vertical units may further project to another vertical unit that best responds to a curved arc of light on the retina. Continuing with this type of **convergence**, there may be a vertical column that responds optimally to a stimulus representing the image of your grandmother. This is actually called "**the grandmother cell theory**." What it points out is the incredible precision and connectivity, along with massive integration that is necessary for the brain to achieve what we take for granted thousands of times per day: an accurate picture of the objects and stimuli in our environment, even when they are moving or we are moving.

Damage to some of these projections and convergence circuits may result in agnosia, a failure to recognize some objects. Some of the agnosias are quite striking, showing the consequences of damage to the aforementioned sequential processing. Some agnosias result in the inability to recognize animate and inanimate objects from each other, the position of objects in the environment (right side up vs. upside down), or even the faces of familiar people whose voices are clearly recognizable.

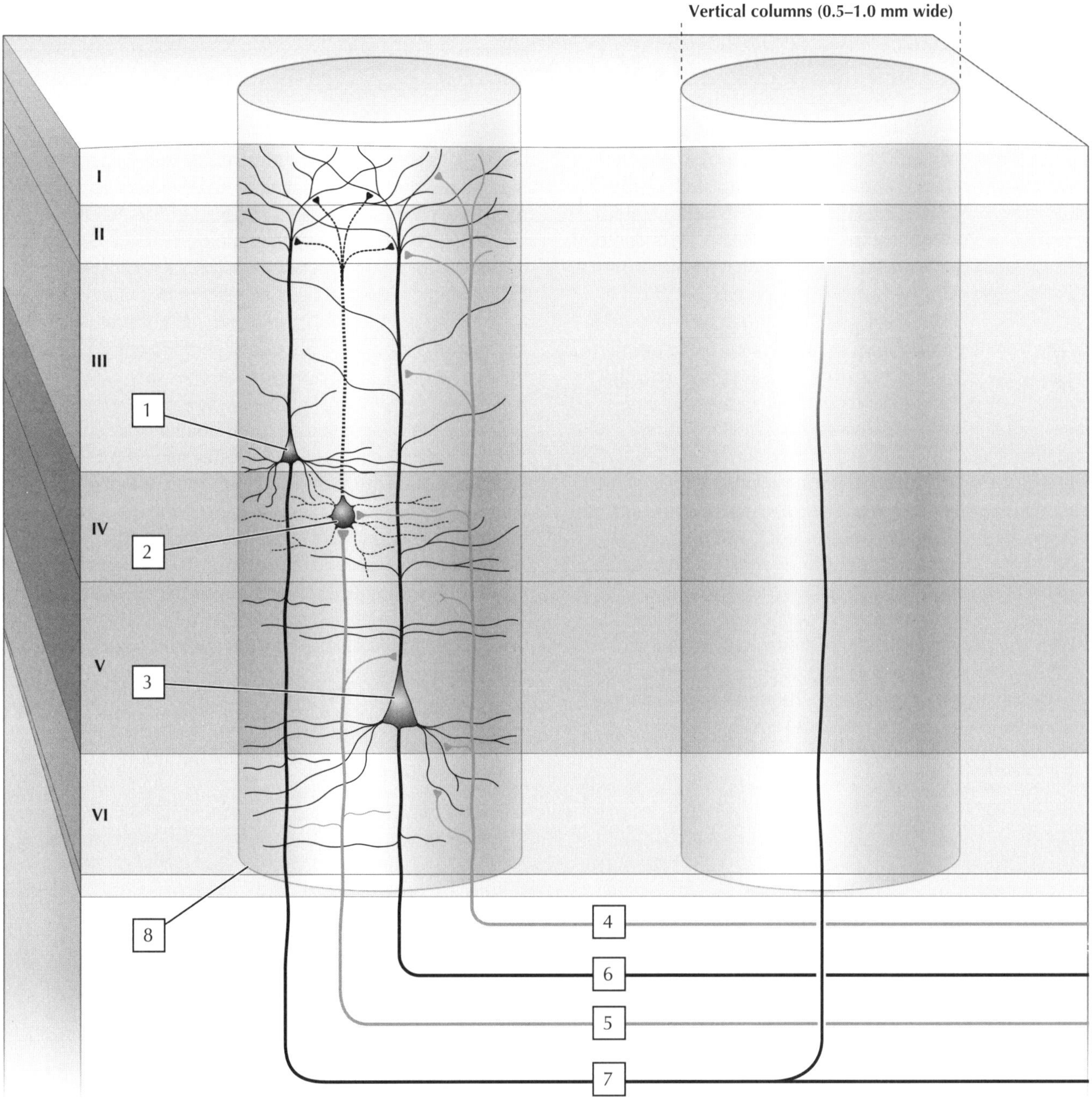
Vertical columns (0.5–1.0 mm wide)
I
II
III
IV
V
VI
1
2
3
4
5
6
7
8

8 Efferent Connections of the Cerebral Cortex

The cerebral cortex has hundreds of specific zones and regions, some of them consolidated into specific gyri or areas; some parts of association areas are not yet fully understood. One way to identify some of the functional roles of regions of the cerebral cortex is to examine the connectivity of those regions. At the most fundamental level, thousands of vertical units interconnect with other functional units, with permutations and combinations that are vast. As an added feature, connectivity can expand or contract, depending on functional demands. For example, if a digit is amputated, the cortical regions for processing that now-absent information will accept and accommodate information from adjacent areas.

Connectivity of the cerebral cortex on a nonmicro level that can be identified by tracing studies or recording studies falls into three categories: (1) **association fibers**, (2) **commissural fibers**, and (3) **projection fibers**. The association fibers can be categorized into short association fibers projecting to nearby regions of the ipsilateral hemisphere and long association fibers projecting to distant regions of the ipsilateral hemisphere. Projections from the primary visual cortex (area 17) to the association visual cortex (areas 18 and 19) are short association connections, whereas projections between expressive and receptive language regions of the left hemisphere (Broca's area and Wernicke's area) are long association areas. The commissural fibers interconnect similar regions of the left and right hemispheres through the corpus callosum and the anterior commissure (for parts of the temporal lobe). The projection fibers are vast in scope and number and represent connections with lower motor neuron groups, upper motor neurons in the brainstem, the pontine nuclei for connectivity with the cerebellum, the basal ganglia and related nuclei, secondary sensory nuclei and sensory structures such as the colliculi, reciprocally connected regions of the thalamus, hypothalamus and autonomic-related structures, some limbic forebrain structures, and other structures.

COLOR the following structures, using a separate color for each structure.

- ☐ 1. **Long association fibers**
- ☐ 2. **Short association fibers**
- ☐ 3. **Commissural fibers**
- ☐ 4. **Projection fibers**

Clinical Note

Damage to cortical efferent connections can occur with trauma, tumors, demyelinating diseases, forebrain infarcts, and many other pathological conditions. Damage to long association fibers can disconnect regions of the cortex that are necessary for integrative activity, such as language function, coordinated sensory integration, and many behaviors. Damage to commissural fibers, sometimes done deliberately to prevent the spread of seizures from one side to the other, can disconnect the two hemispheres from knowing what each one is doing and cause dysfunctional responses and behavior requiring simultaneous coordination of both sides of the cortex.

Damage to the projection fibers, especially with lesions in the internal capsule, can disconnect the cortex from lower motor neurons, upper motor neurons in the brainstem, the basal ganglia and the cerebellum, the hypothalamus and limbic forebrain structures, and the reciprocally connected thalamic nuclei. This may lead to an array of problems, especially on the contralateral side, such as contralateral hemiplegia and lower facial droop, contralateral hemianopia, and other motor, sensory, and behavioral deficits.

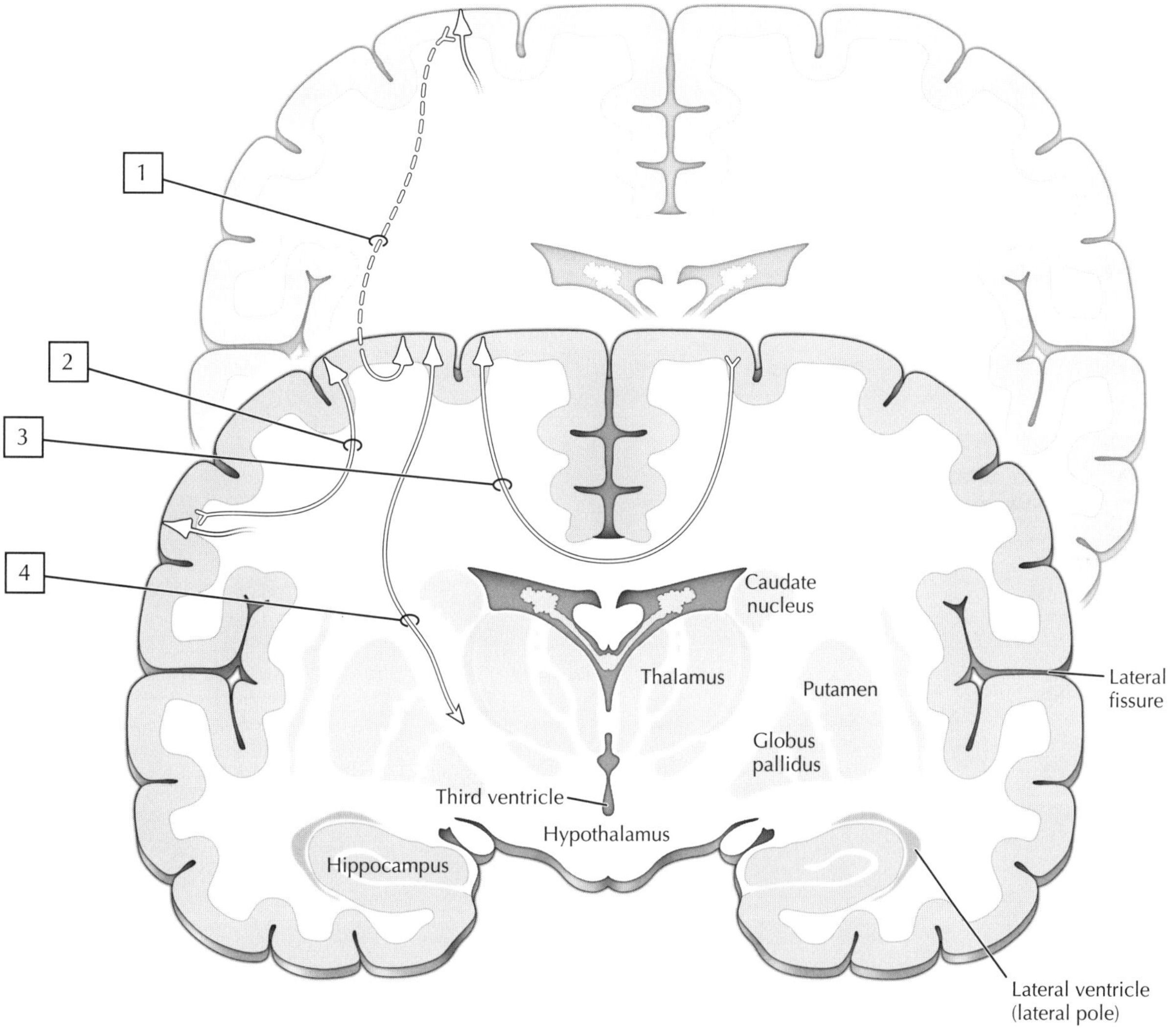
1
2
3
4
Caudate nucleus
Thalamus
Putamen
Lateral fissure
Globus pallidus
Third ventricle
Hypothalamus
Hippocampus
Lateral ventricle (lateral pole)

8 Cortical Association Fibers

Cortical association pathways provide essential communication between and among cortical areas necessary for coordinated activities and behaviors. These association fibers may connect a primary sensory area with the adjacent sensory association cortex, may connect multiple sensory cortical areas with the complex association cortex (integration of sensory perception), may interlink critical regions for language function, and may interlink regions important for cognitive function and emotional behavior and their analysis. These named association pathways include the **superior longitudinal fasciculus**, the **uncinate fasciculus**, the **frontocingulate pathway**, the **cingulum**, the **superior occipitofrontal fasciculus**, and the **inferior occipitofrontal fasciculus**. These large white matter bundles have numerous fiber systems entering, exiting, and traversing them.

COLOR the following structures, using a separate color for each structure.

- ☐ **1. Superior longitudinal fasciculus**
- ☐ **2. Uncinate fasciculus**
- ☐ **3. Frontocingulate pathway**
- ☐ **4. Cingulum**
- ☐ **5. Superior occipitofrontal fasciculus**
- ☐ **6. Inferior occipitofrontal fasciculus**

Clinical Note

Damage to interconnections on the left side between Broca's area (frontal cortex) and Wernicke's area (parietal–temporal cortex), with both of these areas left intact, will result in the patient's inability to repeat complex words or sentences, in the absence of classical expressive or receptive aphasia. This is known as **conductive aphasia**. Disconnection between major regions of the cortex through some of these large association bundles may result in dementia, inattention, emotional changes, and memory dysfunction; these problems usually occur without the presence of movement disorders or aphasias. The cingulum is the major route through which the noradrenergic, serotonergic, dopaminergic, and cholinergic projections travel to the cortex. This bundle can be damaged by **multiinfarct dementia** (not by demyelinating diseases, because these pathways consist of small, unmyelinated axons) removing these vital neurotransmitter actions in the cortex. This may result in depression, bipolar disorder, and attention deficits. Bilateral damage to frontal projection pathways may result in euphoria or inappropriate affect (pseudobulbar affect), and disconnection between the frontal lobe and limbic forebrain structures may result in psychotic behavior.

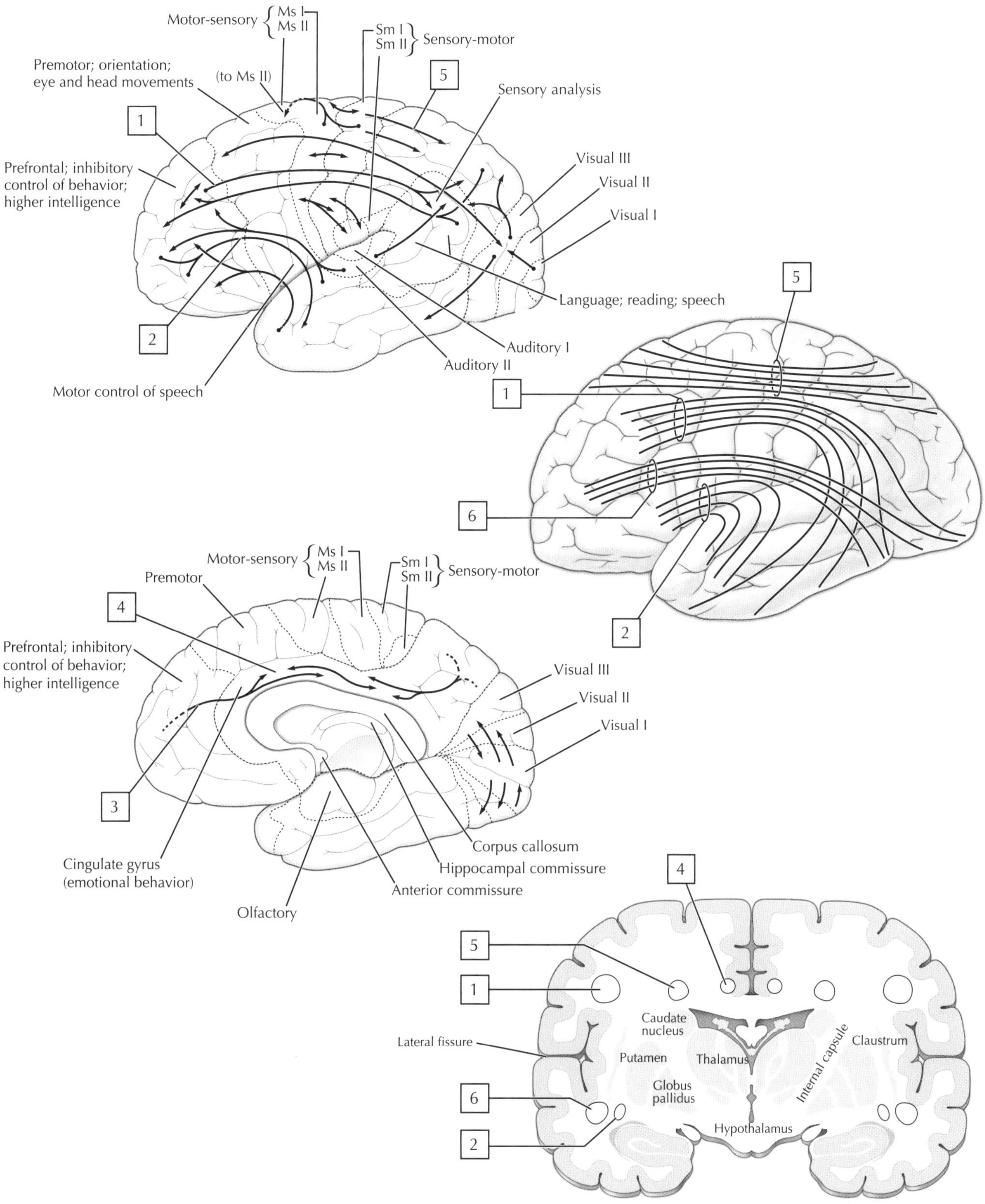
Motor-sensory
Ms I
Ms II
Sm I
Sm II
Sensory-motor
Premotor; orientation; eye and head movements
(to Ms II)
5
Sensory analysis
1
Prefrontal; inhibitory control of behavior; higher intelligence
Visual III
Visual II
Visual I
Language; reading; speech
2
Auditory I
Auditory II
Motor control of speech
5
1
6
2
Motor-sensory
Ms I
Ms II
Sm I
Sm II
Sensory-motor
Premotor
4
Prefrontal; inhibitory control of behavior; higher intelligence
Visual III
Visual II
Visual I
3
Corpus callosum
Hippocampal commissure
Anterior commissure
Cingulate gyrus (emotional behavior)
Olfactory
4
5
1
Caudate nucleus
Lateral fissure
Putamen
Thalamus
Internal capsule
Claustrum
Globus pallidus
6
2
Hypothalamus

Aphasias and Cortical Areas of Damage

The left hemisphere is the dominant hemisphere for language in all right-handed individuals, and in most left-handed individuals. Cerebral infarcts or damage from tumors and other lesions can produce cortical gray matter lesions in the inferior frontal cortex (Broca's area) or the parietotemporal cortex (Wernicke's area). Demyelination or other pathological conditions can produce damage to long association pathways interconnecting language areas. Major types of aphasia are (1) **Broca's aphasia** (also called expressive aphasia); (2) **Wernicke's aphasia** (also called receptive aphasia); and (3) **global aphasia.** These aphasias are disorders of language function, not just disorders of speech. With lesions in the brainstem, there may be dysphonia due to cranial nerve involvement, and with lesions in the cerebellum, there may be uncoordinated speech. However, in these brainstem or cerebellum disorders, expression or reception of language is intact.

COLOR the following structures, using a separate color for each structure.

- ☐ 1. **Cortical region affected in Broca's aphasia, on lateral view of the brain**
- ☐ 2. **Cortical region affected in Wernicke's aphasia, on lateral view of the brain**
- ☐ 3. **Cortical region affected in global aphasia, on lateral view of the brain**
- ☐ 4. **Forebrain region affected in Broca's aphasia, in coronal section**
- ☐ 5. **Forebrain region affected in Wernicke's aphasia, in coronal section**
- ☐ 6. **Forebrain region affected in global aphasia, in coronal section**

Clinical Note

Broca's aphasia involves difficulty expressing language. There is sparseness in word production, great difficulty finding proper words to use, with halting, slow, and effortful expression. This aphasia is sometimes called **nonfluent aphasia**. With left-sided damage to the Broca's area, there are often accompanying problems, including contralateral hemiplegia (motor/premotor cortex), contralateral loss of sensation on the body (somatosensory cortex), gaze palsy (frontal eye fields), and spatial neglect contralaterally (parietal cortex). **Frontotemporal dementia** is characterized by cognitive decline and expressive aphasia.

Wernicke's aphasia involves difficulty understanding language. There is excessive verbal expression, usually with use of incorrect words and expressions (called paraphasic errors), with fluent, mixed, nonunderstandable utterances. Sometimes the patient can only say a few specific words, and repeats them with meaningless repetition. This condition is sometimes called **fluent aphasia**. With left-sided damage in the parieto-temporal region, there are often accompanying problems, including contralateral hemianopia (optic radiations) or upper quadrantanopia (Meyer's loop in the temporal lobe). The rare right-sided lesion may be accompanied by constructional apraxia.

Global aphasia involves difficulty with all language function, hence the name of global aphasia. In a patient with severe left hemispheric damage, there is no ability to express or understand language. This is accompanied by severe right hemiplegia. Many other problems accompany global aphasia, including contralateral hemisensory loss, contralateral gaze palsy, contralateral spatial neglect, or contralateral hemianopia. The lesion is usually so extensive that there is edema and increased intracranial pressure, leading to decreased consciousness or even coma.

Primary progressive aphasia is a slow, progressive aphasia that occurs in the absence of an acute event.

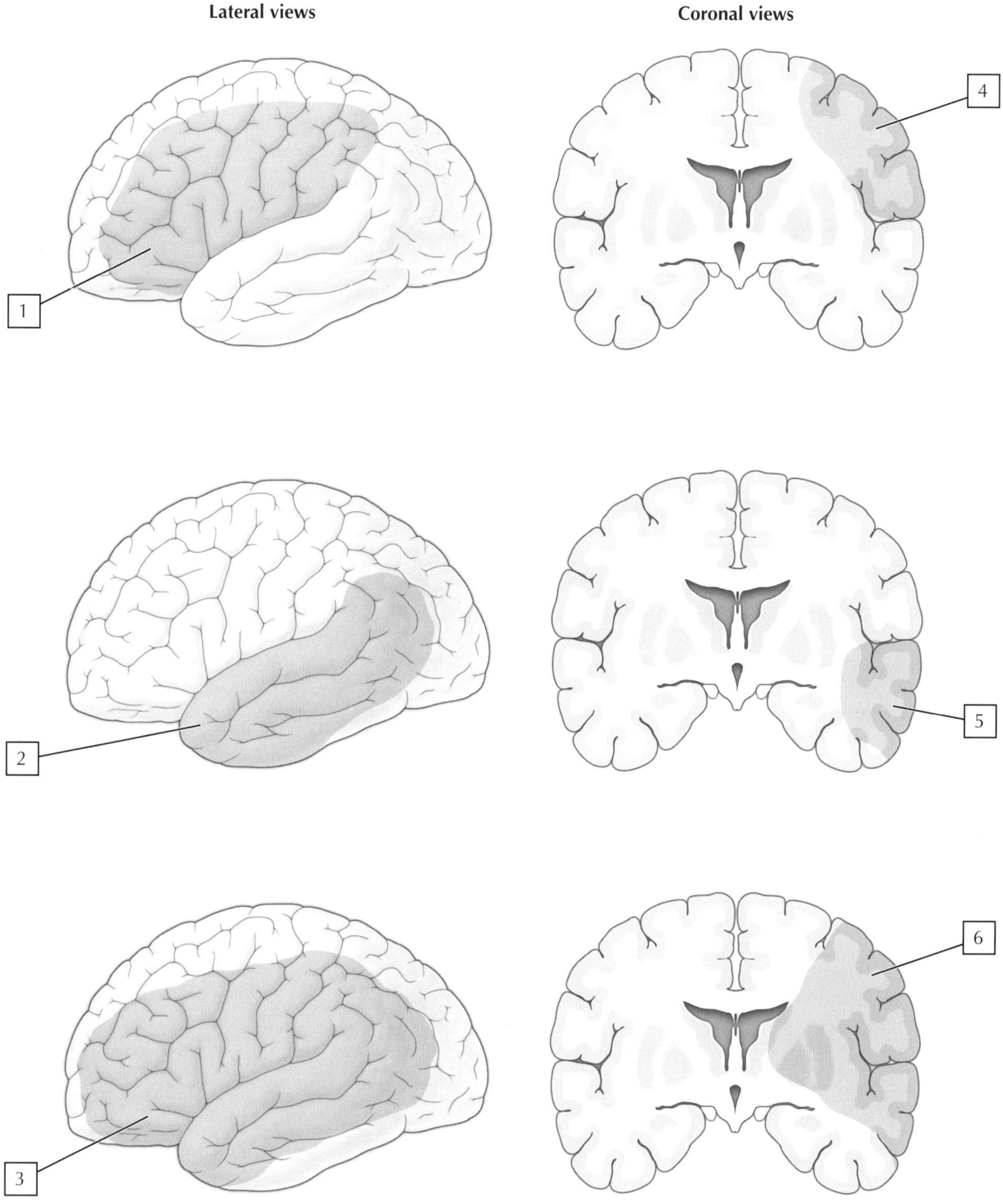
Lateral views
Coronal views
1
2
3
4
5
6

8 Noradrenergic Pathways

The use of fluorescence histochemistry for visualization of catecholamines (dopamine, norepinephrine) and indoleamines (serotonin, or 5-hydroxytryptamine) in the 1960s and 1970s led to the discovery of chemically specific neurons whose cell bodies are found in the brainstem and whose fine, unmyelinated axons send extensive, diffuse, varicose boutons to virtually every major region of the central nervous system. The anatomy of these newly discovered systems was confirmed by immunohistochemistry using antibodies that labeled the major enzymes in the catecholamine and serotonin synthetic pathways. The noradrenergic and serotonergic connections are mainly modulators of the excitability of other transmitter systems in the regions to which they project.

Noradrenergic cell bodies are found in the **locus coeruleus** in the pons (group A6) and in several cell groups in the reticular formation in the medulla (**A1** and **A2**) and pons (**A5** and **A7**). Axonal projections from single neurons in the locus coeruleus branch to the cerebral cortex, hippocampal formation and other limbic forebrain structures, hypothalamus, thalamus, cerebellum, brainstem nuclei, and the spinal cord. These neurons modulate the excitability of structures such as the cerebellum (both excitatory and inhibitory systems) and the spinal cord dorsal horn (regulating the set point for sensitivity to nociceptive inputs). The locus coeruleus projections travel in the **dorsal noradrenergic bundle** and the **descending noradrenergic bundle**. The cortical connections from the locus coeruleus continue from the dorsal noradrenergic bundle into the **cingulum** and into a more **dorsal noradrenergic forebrain pathway through the white matter**. Neurons of A5 and A7 send axons into many regions of the brainstem, the hypothalamus, and the spinal cord; these axons travel in the **ventral noradrenergic bundle** and the **descending noradrenergic bundle**. A1 and A2 neurons send axons into brainstem regions, the hypothalamus, and the spinal cord, traveling in the same bundles as A5 and A7 projections. Overlapping with these widespread connections are the serotonergic projections and terminations of the raphe nuclei.

Noradrenergic systems help to regulate attention and alertness, the sleep–wake cycle, responses to stressors such as pain, neuroendocrine control, visceral functions (thermoregulation, feeding and drinking behavior, reproductive behavior, and autonomic regulation), and emotional behavior, to name a few major regulatory roles.

COLOR the following structures, using a separate color for each structure.

- ☐ 1. **Cingulum**
- ☐ 2. **Dorsal noradrenergic forebrain pathway through the white matter to the cortex**
- ☐ 3. **Dorsal noradrenergic bundle**
- ☐ 4. **Ventral noradrenergic bundle**
- ☐ 5. **Locus coeruleus**
- ☐ 6. **Groups A5 and A7 in the pons**
- ☐ 7. **Groups A1 and A2 in the medulla**
- ☐ 8. **Descending noradrenergic bundle**

Clinical Note

Central noradrenergic projections from the locus coeruleus to limbic forebrain structures and to the cerebral cortex are an important substrate for the catecholamine hypothesis of affective disorders. More than 50 years ago, Bunney and Schildkraut hypothesized that this noradrenergic system was critical to the occurrence and treatment of depression, suggesting that diminished noradrenergic activity at these sites contributed to depression. In the same era, it was also recognized that serotonin was similarly involved, and that diminished serotonin also contributed to depression. Psychiatrists noted that all three major classes of drugs used for treating depression (monoamine oxidase inhibitors, tricyclic antidepressants, and psychomotor stimulants) enhanced noradrenergic neurotransmission. The major metabolite of central norepinephrine, 3-methoxy-4-hydroxyphenylglycol (MHPG), was noted to be diminished in many depressed individuals. Further observations suggested that altered central noradrenergic neurotransmission in the brain of depressed patients may also affect the modulation of the paraventricular nucleus of the hypothalamus (the parvocellular component), leading to enhanced peripheral stress hormone secretion of both cortisol and norepinephrine.

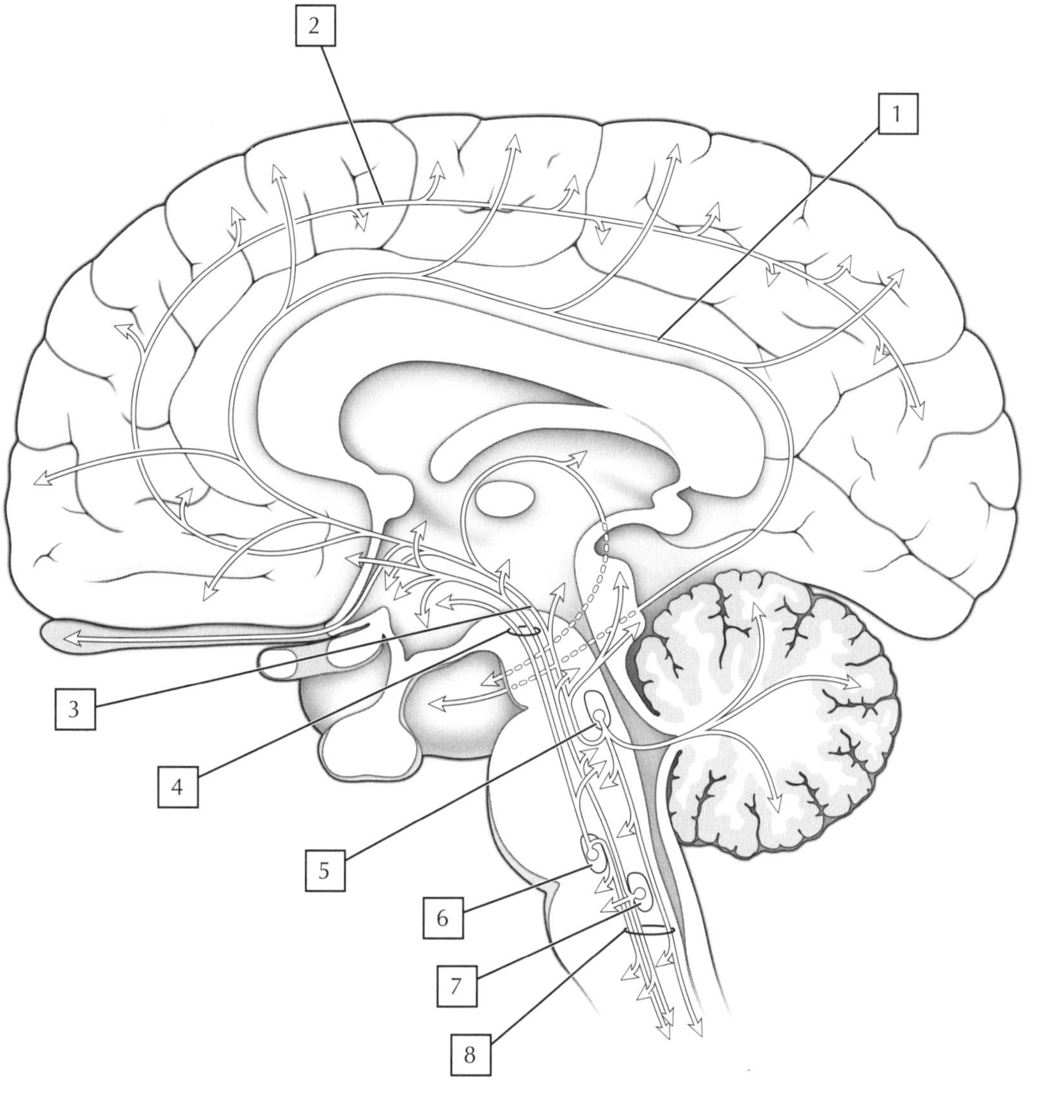
1
2
3
4
5
6
7
8

8 Serotonergic Pathways

Serotonergic (5-hydroxytryptamine) neurons are found in the raphe nuclei of the brainstem, and in lateral wings of neurons that extend from the raphe nuclei into the reticular formation. The serotonergic neurons project to every subdivision of the central nervous system. Serotonergic neurons in the rostral (midbrain) raphe nuclei, **nucleus raphe dorsalis** and **nucleus centralis superior**, send extensive varicose axons that innervate the cerebral cortex, many limbic forebrain structures (e.g., hippocampus, amygdala), the **basal ganglia**, many hypothalamic nuclei and areas, and some nuclei in **the thalamus**. These projections travel through the **ascending serotonergic pathway** with axons to the cortex traveling further through the **cingulum** and more dorsal forebrain white matter. Serotonergic neurons in the caudal raphe nuclei **(nucleus raphe pontis, nucleus raphe magnus**, **nucleus raphe pallidus**, and **nucleus raphe obscurus**) innervate many regions of the brainstem and spinal cord, and the cerebellum. These axonal projections travel through the **descending serotonergic pathway**. Of particular importance are the serotonergic connections from neurons in nucleus raphe magnus to the dorsal horn of the spinal cord, where opioid analgesia and modulation of pain reactivity occur, especially directed toward the enkephalin-producing neurons in the dorsal horn.

The ascending serotonergic systems influence emotional behavior, exert widespread modulation of neuroendocrine and visceral hypothalamic functions, influence sleep–wakefulness cycles, and modulate the processing of afferent inputs. The descending serotonergic systems modulate the excitability of autonomic preganglionic neurons and lower motor neurons (enhancing excitability).

COLOR the following structures, using a separate color for each structure.

- ☐ 1. **Cingulum**
- ☐ 2. **Ascending serotonergic pathway**
- ☐ 3. **Nucleus raphe dorsalis**
- ☐ 4. **Nucleus centralis superior**
- ☐ 5. **Nucleus raphe pontis**
- ☐ 6. **Nucleus raphe magnus**
- ☐ 7. **Nucleus raphe pallidus and nucleus raphe obscurus**
- ☐ 8. **Descending serotonergic pathway**
- ☐ 9. **Basal ganglia**
- ☐ 10. **Thalamus**

Clinical Note

Pharmacological agents that influence serotonin or serotonin receptors exert influences on depression, other cognitive and emotional states, pain modulation, some movement disorders, migraine headaches, and other conditions. With the discovery of serotonergic tricyclic antidepressant medications that block the reuptake of serotonin, more target medications were used for treatment of depression. Serotonin-specific reuptake inhibitors are used extensively for treatment of unipolar depression, but many side effects have been noted, such as weight gain and diminished libido, reflecting the wide range of activities modulated by serotonin. The choice of uptake inhibitors now includes noradrenergic-specific, serotonin-specific, and mixed uptake inhibitors. The extent of involvement of the serotonin systems in depression has recently been questioned.

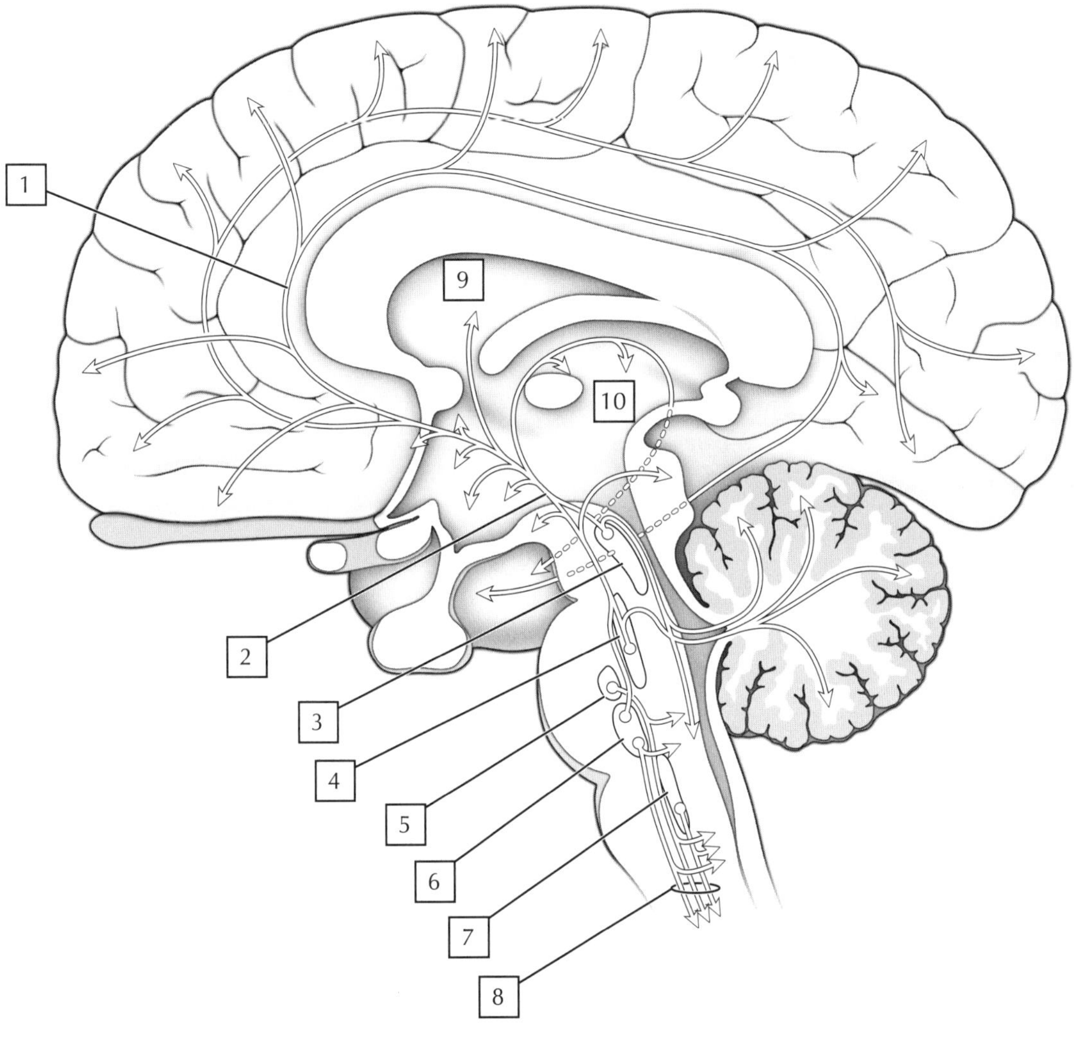
1
2
3
4
5
6
7
8
9
10

8 Dopaminergic Pathways

Dopamine (DA) neurons are found in the midbrain and the hypothalamus. Although the unmyelinated, varicose axons of DA neurons are highly branched, they have more circumscribed projections than the serotonergic and noradrenergic axons. The DA systems are relatively discrete. In the midbrain, DA neurons in the **substantia nigra**, **pars compacta**, send axons through the **nigrostriatal pathway** mainly to the **striatum** (caudate nucleus and putamen), and also to the globus pallidus and subthalamus, which are all components of the basal ganglia. In addition, in the midbrain, DA neurons in the **ventral tegmental area** and zones of the midbrain reticular formation send **mesolimbic projections (pathway)** to the **nucleus accumbens,** the amygdala, and the hippocampus, and **mesocortical projections (pathway)** to the frontal cortex and more sparsely to other cortical association areas such as the **entorhinal cortex**, through the **cingulum**. DA neurons in the **hypothalamus** are found in the arcuate nucleus and the periventricular nucleus. They give rise to small pathways, the **tuberoinfundibular dopamine pathway** from the arcuate nucleus to the contact zone of the median eminence, where DA acts as prolactin inhibitory factor, and the **intrahypothalamic dopamine pathway**, which influences other neuroendocrine and visceral hypothalamic functions.

COLOR the following structures, using a separate color for each structure.

- ☐ 1. **Cingulum**
- ☐ 2. **Nucleus accumbens**
- ☐ 3. **Mesolimbic and mesocortical dopamine pathways**
- ☐ 4. **Nigrostriatal pathway**
- ☐ 5. **Hypothalamus**
- ☐ 6. **Tuberoinfundibular dopamine pathway**
- ☐ 7. **Ventral tegmental area**
- ☐ 8. **Entorhinal cortex**
- ☐ 9. **Substantia nigra, pars compacta**
- ☐ 10. **Striatum**

Clinical Note

The DA nigrostriatal pathway is well known for its involvement in Parkinson disease, in which DA neurons in substantia nigra, pars compacta degenerate and DA nerve terminals in the striatum are extensively diminished. While the DA influences on the striatum include helping the basal ganglia in the planning and execution of cortical activities, the most conspicuous deficits in Parkinson disease are motor problems (hence, the term movement disorder), including bradykinesia (difficulty initiating or stopping movement), a resting tremor, muscle rigidity through all ranges of motion, and postural instability. The principal treatment is aimed at replacing the diminished DA with levodopa or a DA agonist. In addition, deep brain stimulation is also used to rebalance physiological interactions in the basal ganglia circuitry in an attempt to ameliorate some of the motor symptoms.

The mesolimbic projection from the ventral tegmental area to nucleus accumbens is important in motivation and reward, in biological drives, and in addictive behaviors, including substance abuse. The mesocortical projection to the frontal lobe helps to regulate frontal cortical function and attention mechanisms. Many neuroleptic and antipsychotic medications (D2 receptor antagonists) target these limbic and cortical DA systems and are used in treatment of schizophrenia, obsessive-compulsive disorder, attention deficit-hyperactivity disorder, Tourette syndrome, and other neuropsychiatric disorders. Some investigators have hypothesized that schizophrenia may be associated with increased activity in the mesolimbic DA system and decreased activity in the mesocortical DA system and its frontal cortical projections.

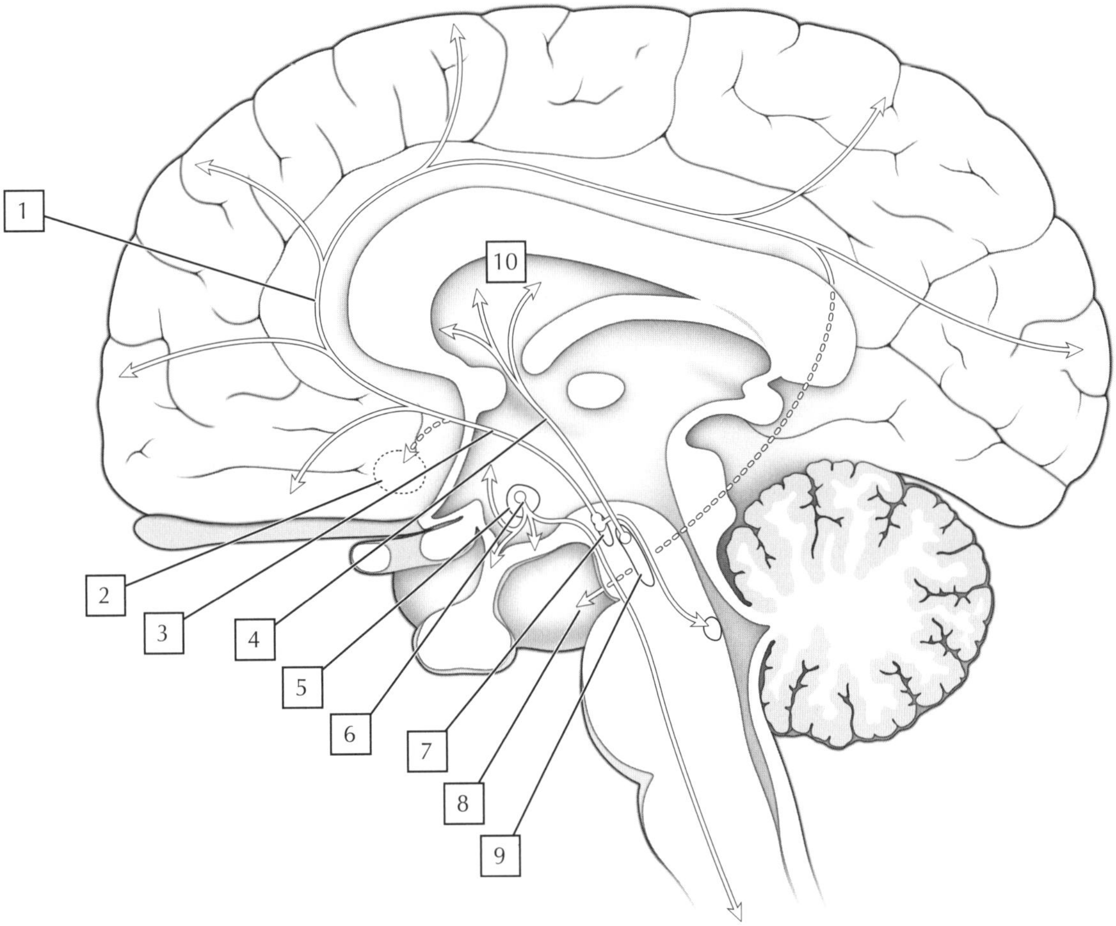
1
2
3
4
5
6
7
8
9
10

Central Cholinergic Pathways

Acetylcholine is used as the principal neurotransmitter in all lower motor neurons in the spinal cord and brainstem, in all autonomic preganglionic neurons and in postganglionic neurons of the parasympathetic system. These acetylcholine-using neurons are called **cholinergic**. Small cholinergic interneurons are found in the striatum, where they interact with other chemically specific systems such as dopamine and serotonin to regulate tone, posture, initiation or cessation of movement, or selection of movement patterns.

Important central cholinergic neuronal groups are found in the basal forebrain, in the **nucleus basalis (of Meynert)**, found in substantia innominata, and in the **nucleus of the diagonal band**. These cholinergic neurons provide the principal input to the cerebral cortex through the **ascending cholinergic pathway** and subsequent projections through the **cingulum.** Cholinergic neurons in the **medial septal nucleus** send axons to the **hippocampal formation** with a projection through **the fornix** and are involved in the consolidation of short-term memory. A **brainstem tegmental cholinergic group** of neurons provide cholinergic input to the brainstem, cerebellum, and the **thalamus**, using a **descending cholinergic pathway**, and some ascending projections. Cholinergic innervation of the thalamus modulates arousal and the sleep–wake cycle and is important in the initiation of rapid eye movement sleep.

COLOR the following structures, using a separate color for each structure.

- ☐ 1. **Cingulum**
- ☐ 2. **Ascending cholinergic pathway**
- ☐ 3. **Nucleus basalis (of Meynert)**
- ☐ 4. **Hippocampal formation**
- ☐ 5. **Brainstem tegmental cholinergic group of neurons**
- ☐ 6. **Descending cholinergic pathway**
- ☐ 7. **Medial septal nucleus**
- ☐ 8. **Thalamus**
- ☐ 9. **Fornix**

Clinical Note

In patients with **Alzheimer disease**, the loss of central forebrain cholinergic neurons correlates with cognitive impairment and loss of consolidation of short-term memory. In keeping with a cholinergic deficit, many patients with Alzheimer disease also have a loss of high-affinity choline uptake (needed for the synthesis of acetylcholine) and loss of central muscarinic and nicotinic cholinergic receptors. Some therapeutic agents target the cholinergic system, such as the cholinesterase inhibitor tetrahydroaminoacridine (attempt to prolong the presence of acetylcholine at cholinergic synapses). Attempts to provide dietary choline or lecithin to boost precursor availability for acetylcholine synthesis have not met with much success. However, these efforts target only one neurotransmitter system, in the face of extensive neuronal degeneration, alterations in other neurotransmitter systems (e.g., substance P, corticotropin-releasing factor, somatostatin, norepinephrine, neuropeptide Y), and altered receptor expression and distribution. By the time cognitive impairment is evident, and some short-term memory loss occurs, the disease has probably been present for at least a decade or more.

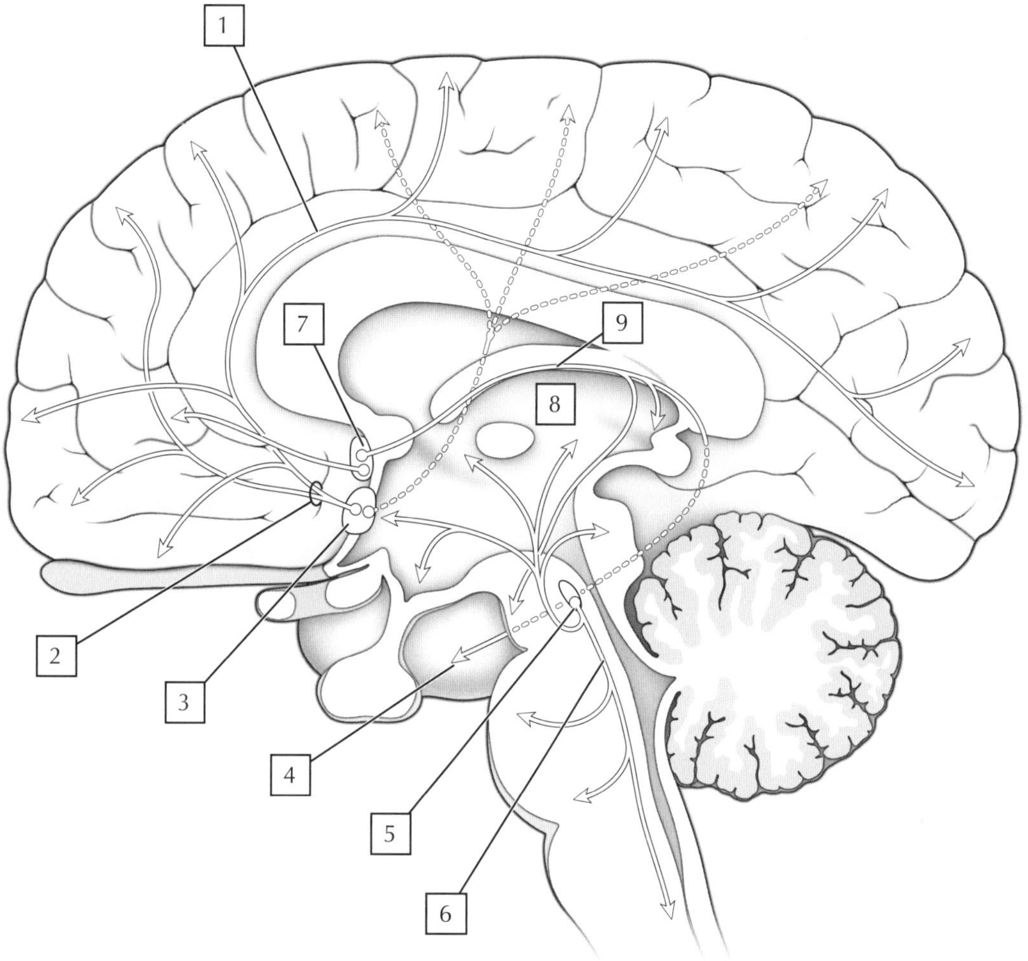
1
2
3
4
5
6
7
8
9

8 Endogenous Opioid Systems

The brain has three endogenous opioid peptide systems, **β-endorphin** (β-end), **dynorphins**, and **met-enkephalin**. They interact with three major opioid receptors: **mu**, **kappa**, and **delta** and are derived from larger peptides posttranslationally cleaved to the smaller opioid peptides in the neuronal cytoplasm, and transported to the nerve terminals via anterograde axonal transport.

β-endorphin, derived from **proopiomelanocortin** (**POMC**), is synthesized mainly in the **arcuate nucleus** (sometimes called **peri-arcuate region**) of the hypothalamus, and, to a lesser extent, in **nucleus solitarius**. These neurons project to some thalamic sites, many limbic structures, hypothalamic nuclei and regions, and brainstem sites (especially related to modulation of spinoreticular nociception [e.g., the periaqueductal gray, parabrachial nuclei, noradrenergic and serotonergic nuclei, reticular formation]). β-end neurons in nucleus solitarius innervate dorsal horn neurons in the spinal cord.

β-endorphin inhibits the activity of the stress axes (e.g., inhibition of corticotropin-releasing factor neurons in the hypothalamus); its release is stimulated by exercise, eating, sexual activity, and many relaxing activities. β-end is important in **analgesia** (brainstem circuits activate serotonergic neurons in nucleus raphe magnus to mediate analgesia through met-enkephalin neurons in the dorsal horn of spinal cord), amelioration of anxiety, appetitive behaviors, temperature regulation, and other visceral functions. β-end interacts with all three receptor types, but especially mu receptors for opioid analgesia. Overdose with mu agonists results in respiratory suppression and can cause death; the **mu antagonist naloxone** can block that response and rescue someone experiencing an overdose.

Dynorphins are synthesized from posttranslational processing of **prodynorphin**. Dynorphin neurons are found in the hippocampus, entorhinal cortex, amygdala, bed nucleus of the stria terminalis, nucleus accumbens, striatum, brainstem visceral/autonomic-related nuclei, and spinal cord. Dynorphins act via kappa receptors and inhibit many excitatory circuits.

Dynorphins modulate pain responses, stress responses, appetitive behaviors, temperature regulation, learning and memory, and emotional responsiveness. Dynorphin circuits are involved in neurological and neuropsychiatric disorders, such as seizures, depression, schizophrenia, and addictive behaviors.

Met-enkephalin is cleaved from **proenkephalin A**, and is found mainly in **small local-circuit neurons** in widespread areas of the CNS, including the cerebral cortex, basal ganglia, amygdala, hippocampus, bed nucleus of the stria terminalis, nucleus accumbens, thalamic and hypothalamic sites, many brainstem visceral/autonomic-related nuclei, and dorsal horn of the spinal cord. met-enkephalin acts on both delta and mu receptors and integrates sensory information related to pain perception and emotional context. It also modulates memory, visceral hypothalamic functions, and DA release in limbic and cortical systems involved in addictive behaviors, reward, motivation, and cortical functions.

COLOR the following structures:

- ☐ 1. **Thalamus**
- ☐ 2. **Amygdala**
- ☐ 3. **Arcuate nucleus (peri-arcuate region) of the hypothalamus**
- ☐ 4. **Caudate nucleus**
- ☐ 5. **Putamen**
- ☐ 6. **Hypothalamus**
- ☐ 7. **Dorsal horn of the spinal cord**
- ☐ 8. **Hippocampus**
- ☐ 9. **Dentate gyrus of the hippocampus**
- ☐ 10. **Globus pallidus**
- ☐ 11. **Nucleus accumbens**
- ☐ 12. **Nucleus raphe magnus**

Clinical Note

The U.S. is facing an opioid use crisis. Opiates, including morphine, heroin, fentanyl (synthetic opiate), and prescription opiates (e.g., oxycodone, hydrocodone), can produce analgesic responses and pain relief for severe acute pain, and sometimes for long-term pain (depending on the source, severity, and duration) that is unresponsive to other agents. Opiates also are used recreationally for pleasurable responses and euphoria, but can produce strong dependence, cravings, significant side effects, and addictive behaviors.

Fentanyl is a highly potent (50–100 times stronger than morphine) addictive synthetic opiate. It is responsible for over 75% of overdoses and deaths (100,000+ per year) in the U.S. Fentanyl produces a very rapid and powerful suppression of respiration, often occurring before naloxone can be given, or medical help can arrive. Fentanyl can be used clinically for acute, severe pain, but the main source of fentanyl is illicit manufacturing outside the U.S., and illegal transport across U.S. borders, with some fentanyl tablets looking like candy. The problem appears to be getting worse, and overdoses and deaths continue to increase. The medical and drug enforcement challenge is to keep opiates available for patients who need them, while stopping the flood of fentanyl and other illicit opiates from causing more deaths and damage.

Endogenous Opioids:
Beta Endorphin

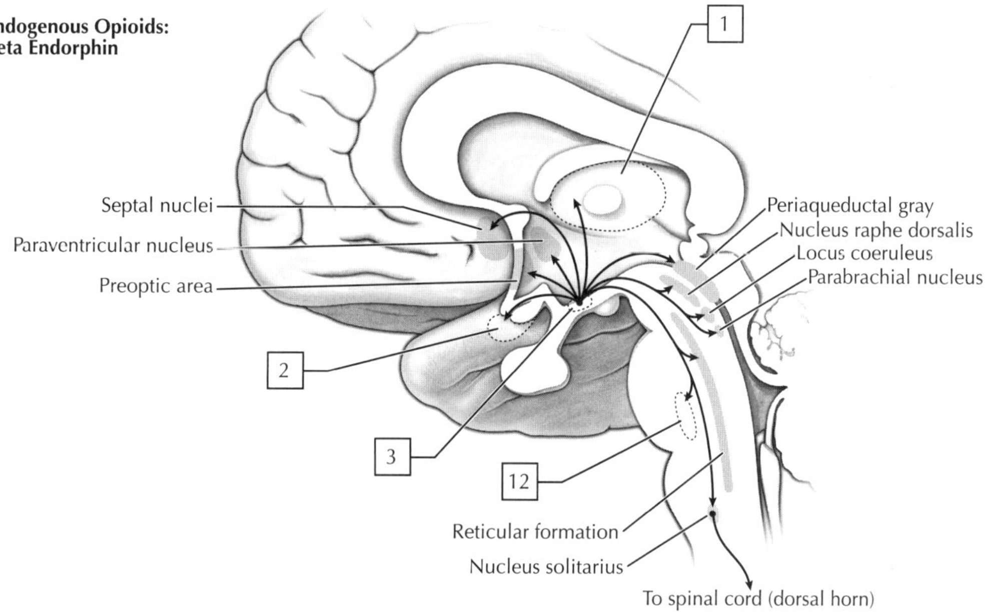

Endogenous Opioids:
met-Enkephalin

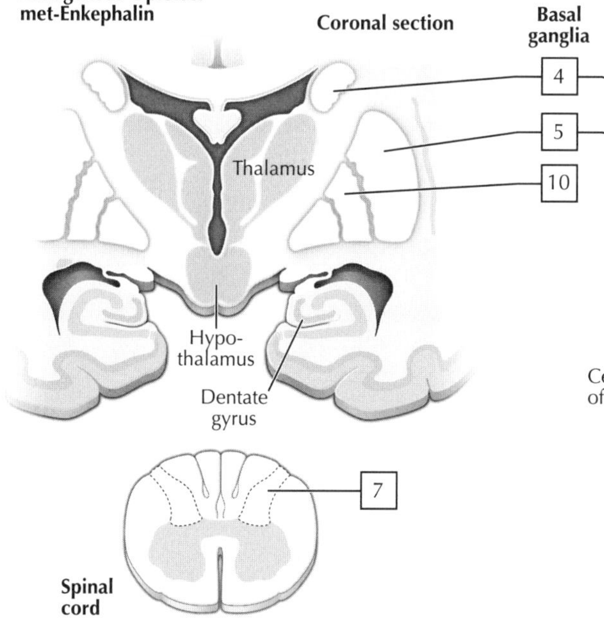

Endogenous Opioids:
Dynorphins

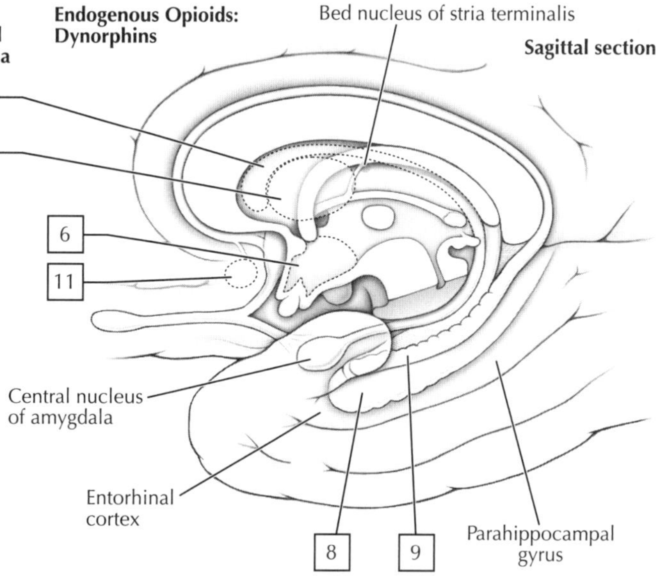

SECTION II REVIEW QUESTIONS

1. Match the following structures on the figure with information about their role or activities:

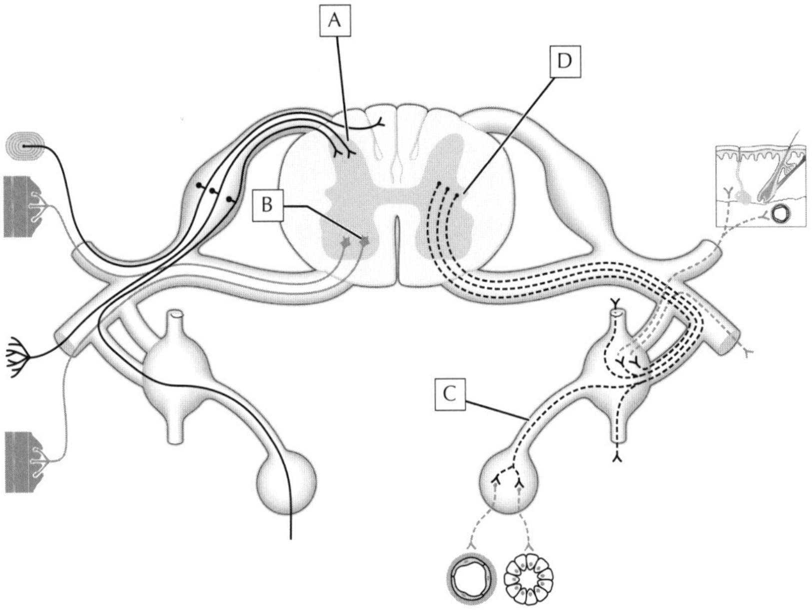

(1) ______________________

(2) ______________________

(3) ______________________

(4) ______________________

(1) Site of location of preganglionic sympathetic neurons
(2) Location of preganglionic sympathetic axons after they leave the sympathetic chain and head for synapsing in collateral ganglia
(3) Site of termination of nociceptive signals transduced by bare nerve endings
(4) Site of lower motor neurons that innervate skeletal muscle

2. Match the information provided with the sites of brainstem involvement in this illustration.

Midbrain

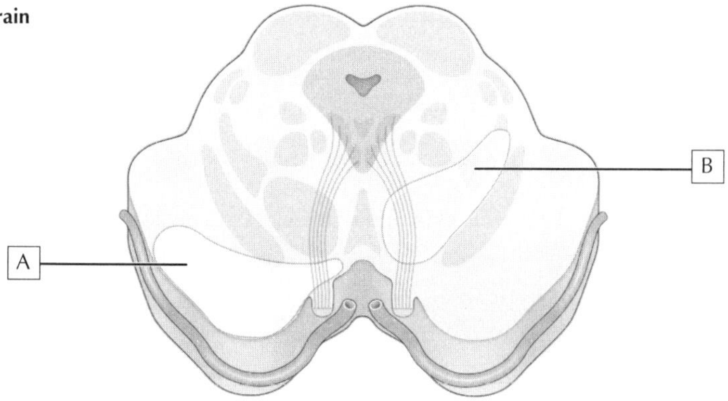

Pons

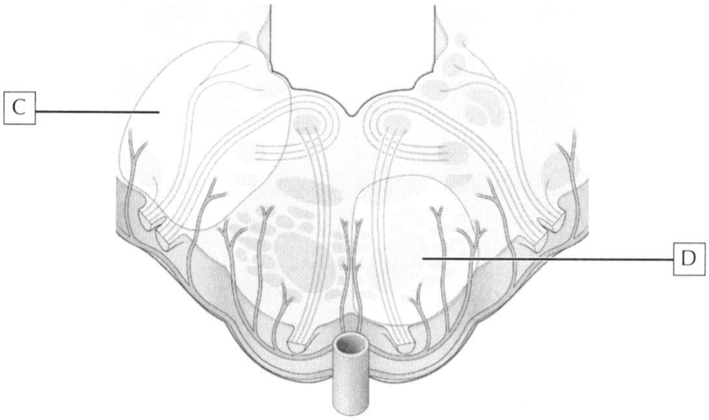

Medulla

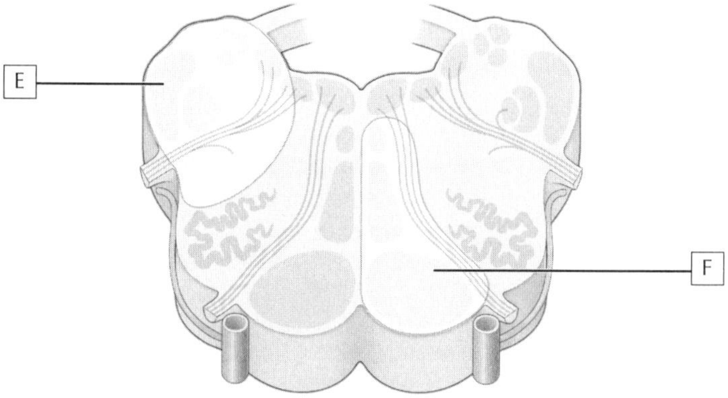

(1) ______________________

(2) ______________________

(3) ______________________

(4) ______________________

(5) ______________________

(6) ______________________

(1) Most likely to produce a tremor or movement disorder

(2) Most likely to result in both contralateral motor weakness and contralateral loss of fine, discriminative touch

(3) Most likely to result in loss of pain and temperature sensation on the ipsilateral side of the face and the contralateral side of the body

(4) Most likely to result in contralateral hemiparesis and ipsilateral paralysis of lateral eye movement

(5) Most likely to result in contralateral loss of all sensation from the body and ipsilateral paralysis of the muscles of mastication

(6) Most likely to result in contralateral hemiplegia and loss of ipsilateral pupillary constriction to light shined in either eye

3. A herniated disc impinges on a nerve root. What is the most likely consequence?
   A. Radiating pain in the distribution of the dermatome
   B. Anesthesia in the distribution of the dermatome
   C. Loss of pain sensation but not fine, discriminative touch in the distribution of the dermatome
   D. Reflex contraction of all muscles contacted by the afferents in the nerve root
   E. No consequence unless the nerve roots above and below are also impinged upon

4. In a hemisection injury of the spinal cord (a Brown–Séquard lesion) at a midthoracic level, which of the following findings is most likely to occur?
   A. Contralateral spastic paralysis below the level of the lesion
   B. Contralateral loss of fine, discriminative touch below the level of the lesion
   C. Contralateral loss of pain and temperature sensation below the level of the lesion
   D. Horner syndrome on the ipsilateral side
   E. Bowel and bladder paralysis

5. From where is the major control for the gamma motor neurons derived?
   A. Monosynaptic connections from Ia afferents
   B. Cascading nociceptive afferents through the dorsal horn neuronal system
   C. Descending upper motor neuronal projections
   D. Direct synaptic activation by projections from deep cerebellar nuclei
   E. Collaterals from spinocerebellar pathways

6. What cells respond best to angular acceleration (movement) of the head?
   A. Hair cells in the organ of Corti on the basilar membrane
   B. Hair cells in the macula of the utricle
   C. Hair cells in the ampullae of the semicircular ducts
   D. Hair cells in the macula of the saccule

7. The dopamine projections from the brainstem to the forebrain provide regulatory control over reward, motivation, biological drives, and addictive behaviors through which major structure?
   A. Hippocampal formation
   B. Amygdala
   C. Caudate nucleus and putamen
   D. Nucleus basalis
   E. Nucleus accumbens

8. What structure serves as a blood–nerve barrier, protecting peripheral axons from damaging circulating toxins?____________________

9. Which secondary sensory channel carries information for conscious interpretation by the cerebral cortex?____________________

10. To what stimulus does a Pacinian corpuscle best respond?____________________

11. How is the action of acetylcholine terminated in the neuromuscular junction?____________________

12. What kind of information is processed in the substantia gelatinosa of the spinal cord? ____________________

13. Where do vagal afferents mainly terminate?____________________

14. What part of the brainstem provides basic control of body tone and posture, processes long-lasting pain from the body, and is necessary for the maintenance of consciousness?____________________

15. Which thalamic nucleus is most likely to assist the cerebral cortex with long-term goal orientation?____________________

16. Which nuclei of the hypothalamus produce and transport oxytocin and vasopressin to the posterior pituitary gland?____________________

17. Which central nervous system structures contain cholinergic neurons that project to forebrain cortical and limbic areas, and may be diminished in their activity in patients with Alzheimer disease?____________________

18. Which chemically specific neuronal system plays a key role in regulating opiate analgesia in the dorsal horn of the spinal cord?____________________

19. What structure serves as a blood–nerve barrier, protecting peripheral axons from damaging circulating toxins?
   A. Epineurium
   B. Perineurium
   C. Endoneurium
   D. Schwann cell sheath
   E. Myelin sheath

20. Lemniscal channels, such as the dorsal column system, carry:
   A. Reflex afferents that connect with lower motor neurons and preganglionic autonomics
   B. Unconscious proprioceptive afferents that connect with spinocerebellar pathways
   C. Unconscious proprioceptive afferents that signal the basal ganglia
   D. Afferents that process information for conscious interpretation by the cortex
   E. Efferent connections going to targets of the autonomic nervous system

21. What stimulus does a pacinian corpuscle best respond to?
    A. Vibratory stimulus
    B. Light moving touch
    C. Steadily applied pressure
    D. Maximal stretch on a joint
    E. Nociceptive stimulus

22. What is the major route of inactivation of acetylcholine at the neuromuscular junction following release?
    A. Presynaptic reuptake
    B. Diffusion out of the synaptic cleft
    C. Chemical inactivation by choline acetyltransferase
    D. Rapid hydrolysis by acetylcholinesterase
    E. Postsynaptic uptake into the muscle

23. The substantia gelatinosa of the spinal cord gray is mainly focused on processing what information?
    A. Spinocerebellar unconscious proprioceptive information
    B. Fine, discriminative touch
    C. Fast signaling of pain and temperature sensation
    D. Muscle stretch reflex information
    E. Slow, excruciating nociceptive information

24. Where do vagal afferents mainly terminate?
    A. Dorsal horn of the spinal cord
    B. Dorsal motor (autonomic) nucleus of the vagus
    C. Nucleus ambiguus
    D. Nucleus solitarius (nucleus of the solitary tract)
    E. Hypothalamic nuclei

25. Which of the following activities is not part of reticular formation regulation?
    A. Neuroendocrine transduction at the median eminence
    B. Motor control of basic tone and posture
    C. Sleep and wakefulness
    D. Sensory processing of severe, long-lasting pain
    E. Maintenance of consciousness

26. The cerebellum compares the state of the structures associated with movement in the body (muscles, joints, tendons, ligaments, other afferents) with the plans and directions for movement coming from the cerebral cortex. These plans from the cortex are conveyed to the cerebellum via:
    A. Pontocerebellar projections
    B. Spinocerebellar pathways
    C. Brainstem reticular formation projections
    D. Thalamic pathways
    E. Basal ganglia pathways

27. Which thalamic nucleus is most likely to assist the cerebral cortex with long-term goal orientation and executive functions?
    A. Medial dorsal
    B. Intralaminar
    C. Ventrolateral and ventral anterior
    D. Medial geniculate nucleus
    E. Pulvinar

28. What system of axons plays the key role in release of oxytocin and vasopressin (antidiuretic hormone) into the systemic blood?
    A. Median forebrain bundle
    B. Dorsal longitudinal fasciculus
    C. Supraopticohypophyseal tract
    D. Tuberoinfundibular tract
    E. Fornix

29. What major structures contain cholinergic neurons that project to forebrain cortical and limbic areas, and may be diminished in their activity in Alzheimer disease?
    A. Nucleus basalis and medial septal nucleus
    B. Ventral tegmental area and nucleus accumbens
    C. Caudate nucleus and putamen
    D. Locus coeruleus and brainstem reticular formation
    E. Substantia nigra, pars compacta, and the arcuate nucleus of the hypothalamus

30. The cerebral cortex has regulatory input to all structures with direct connections, except to:
    A. Basal ganglia (caudate and putamen)
    B. Thalamus
    C. Brainstem cranial nerve motor nuclei
    D. Cerebellum
    E. Anterior horn cells in the C7 spinal cord

31. Which chemically specific system plays a key role in regulating opiate analgesia in the dorsal horn of the spinal cord?
    A. Cholinergic pathway from nucleus basalis
    B. Serotonergic pathway from nucleus raphe magnus
    C. Noradrenergic pathway from the locus coeruleus
    D. Dopaminergic pathway from the ventral tegmental area
    E. Glutamate pathway from the hippocampal formation

ANSWER KEY

1. (1) D, Lateral horn of the spinal cord
   (2) C, Splanchnic nerve
   (3) A, Dorsal horn of the spinal cord
   (4) B, Ventral horn of the spinal cord
2. (1) B, Paramedian midbrain syndrome (Benedikt syndrome)
   (2) F, Medial medullary syndrome
   (3) E, Lateral medullary syndrome (posterior inferior cerebellar artery syndrome or Wallenberg syndrome)
   (4) D, Medial pontine syndrome (medial basilar infarct)
   (5) C, Lateral pontine syndrome (anterior inferior cerebellar artery syndrome)
   (6) A, Medial midbrain syndrome (Weber syndrome)
3. A
4. C
5. C
6. C
7. E
8. Perineurium
9. Lemniscal
10. Vibratory sensation
11. Hydrolysis (cleavage) by acetylcholinesterase
12. Nociception—Severe, chronic pain
13. Nucleus solitaries
14. Reticular formation
15. Medial dorsal
16. Supraoptic and paraventricular nuclei
17. Nucleus basalis (of Meynert, nucleus of the diagonal band, and medial septal nucleus)
18. Serotonin from nucleus raphe magnus
19. B
20. D
21. A
22. D
23. E
24. D
25. A
26. A
27. A
28. C
29. A
30. D
31. B

Chapter 9 Sensory Systems

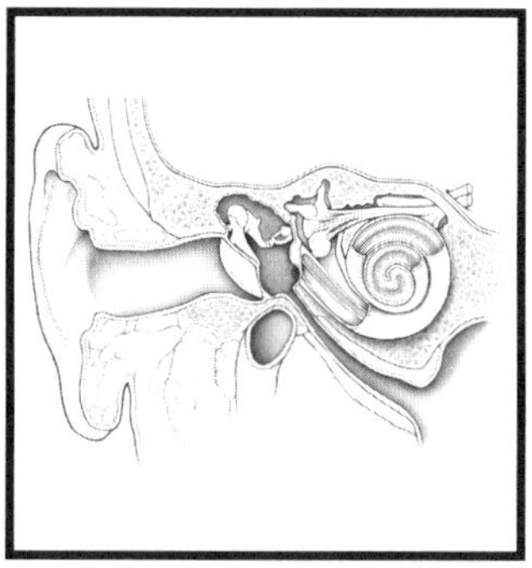

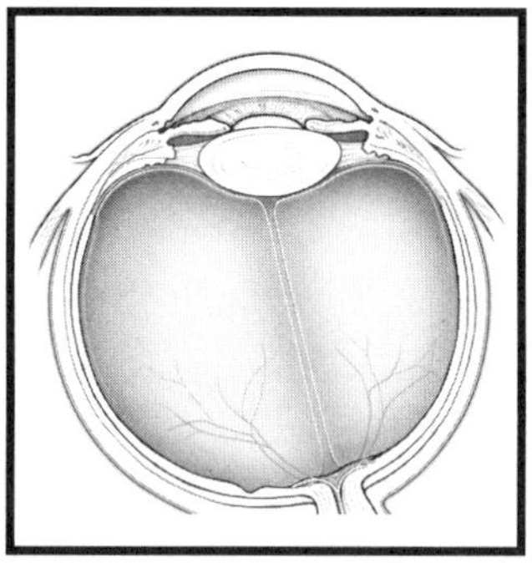

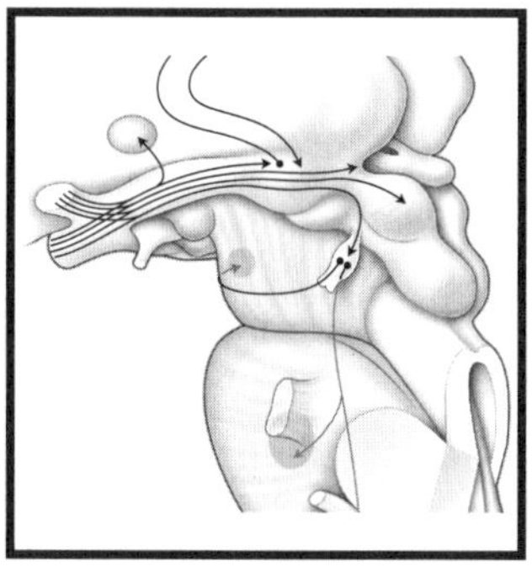

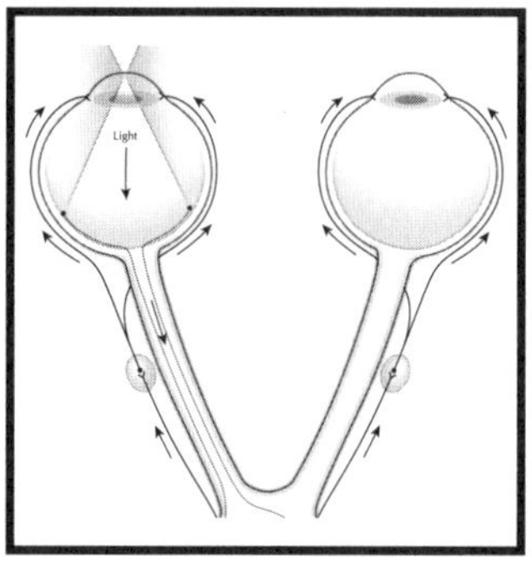

9 Somatosensory System: Spinocerebellar Pathways

Proprioceptive somatosensory information from the muscles, joints, tendons, ligaments, and adjacent tissues is conveyed to the **cerebellum** through a two-neuron chain as spinocerebellar pathways, terminating in both the deep nuclei and the cerebellar cortex as mossy fibers on the granule cells. Proprioceptive information from the joints, tendons, and ligaments (indicated in the plate as Ib-Golgi tendon organ axons) convey "whole muscle" information to the cerebellum through terminations on **dorsal horn neurons** for the upper body (above T6) and on **border cells in the dorsal horn** for the lower body (T6 and below). The neurons for the upper body convey secondary sensory projections to the cerebellum through the **rostral spinocerebellar tract,** and those for the lower body through the **ventral spinocerebellar tract**. The rostral spinocerebellar tract enters the cerebellum through the inferior cerebellar peduncle, terminating ipsilaterally. The ventral spinocerebellar tract crosses the midline through the **anterior white commissure** at the approximate level of entry of the primary sensory information, ascends contralaterally at the ventrolateral edge of the lateral funiculus, enters the cerebellum through the **superior cerebellar peduncle,** and mainly crosses again, terminating in the cerebellum ipsilateral to the origin of information.

Proprioceptive somatosensory information from the muscle spindles is indicated in this plate as Ia (primary muscle spindle afferents), conveying "individual muscle fiber" information to the cerebellum through the **lateral (accessory) cuneate nucleus** for the upper body and through the **nucleus dorsalis (of Clarke)** for the lower body. The tract for the upper body is the **cuneocerebellar tract** and for the lower body is the **dorsal spinocerebellar tract;** both of these tracts enter the cerebellum through the **inferior cerebellar peduncle.**

The cerebellum monitors the status of both individual muscle fiber information and whole muscle information on a moment-to-moment basis, providing continuous information to keep the brain informed about the status of proprioception in the periphery, and provides feedback regarding the results of both unconscious and volitional muscle activity.

COLOR the following structures, using a separate color for each structure.

- ☐ 1. **Cerebellum**
- ☐ 2. **Cuneocerebellar tract**
- ☐ 3. **Inferior cerebellar peduncle**
- ☐ 4. **Lateral (accessory) cuneate nucleus**
- ☐ 5. **Rostral spinocerebellar tract**
- ☐ 6. **Dorsal horn neurons for the upper body**
- ☐ 7. **Dorsal spinocerebellar tract**
- ☐ 8. **Border cells (Cooper-Sherrington) in the dorsal horn for the lower body**
- ☐ 9. **Nucleus dorsalis (of Clarke)**
- ☐ 10. **Anterior white commissure**
- ☐ 11. **Ventral spinocerebellar tract**
- ☐ 12. **Superior cerebellar peduncle**

Clinical Note

The spinocerebellar system with its four major tracts plays a critical role in permitting skilled and successful movement and activities. The spinocerebellar system informs the central nervous system (CNS) through the spinocerebellar tracts of the precise status of the muscle spindles, tendons, ligaments, joints, and other tissues on a moment-to-moment basis and allows the forebrain and brainstem to receive detailed feedback about the success of the upper motor neuronal systems in regulating motor behavior. If the brain does not receive this proprioceptive feedback, it is unable to assess the success of its initiation of motor activity and cannot make accurate adjustments. Therefore myelopathies of the lateral funiculus of the spinal cord (e.g., from a herniated disc) when they first impinge on and damage the spinocerebellar tracts result in loss of coordination and in ataxia. In the periphery, if the joint receptors and other proprioceptors are damaged and cannot send continuous information into the spinocerebellar system, the ability of skilled movements will be seriously impaired.

Thus the primary proprioceptive axons, the secondary sensory nuclei in the spinal cord, the spinocerebellar tracts, and the cerebellum must be fully functional and intact to permit skilled movement and sophisticated behavior.

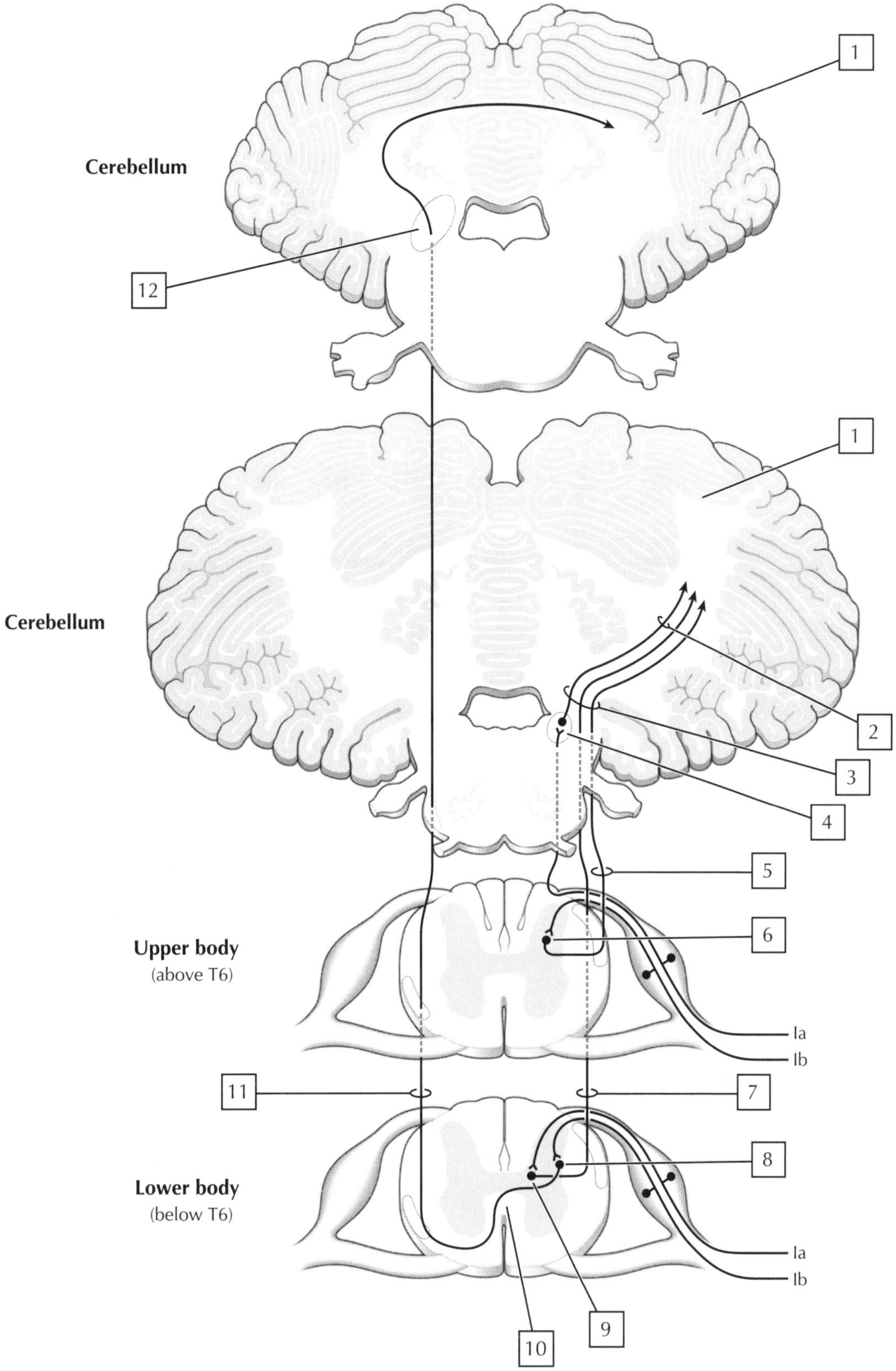

1
Cerebellum
12
1
Cerebellum
2
3
4
5
6
Upper body
(above T6)
Ia
Ib
11
7
8
Lower body
(below T6)
Ia
Ib
9
10

Somatosensory System: Dorsal Column System and Epicritic Modalities

The lemniscal somatosensory systems convey information from the periphery into the CNS, ultimately bringing this information for conscious interpretation in the cerebral cortex. A host of encapsulated sensory receptors translate fine discriminative touch, pressure, vibratory sensation, and joint position sense (epicritic modalities) into action potentials in myelinated primary sensory axons whose cell bodies are in the dorsal root ganglia. These myelinated axons enter the spinal cord through the dorsal roots, then turn rostrally to travel in the dorsal columns as **fasciculus gracilis** (below T6) and **fasciculus cuneatus** (T6 and above). These primary sensory axons terminate in nuclei gracilis and cuneatus, where further processing occurs. **Nuclei gracilis and cuneatus** give rise to crossing fibers in the medulla **(decussation of the medial lemniscus, or internal arcuate fibers)** and ascend in the medial medulla as the **medial lemniscus,** widely separated from the lateral spinothalamic/spinoreticular system. As the medial lemniscus ascends through the brainstem, the tract moves laterally, running adjacent to the spinothalamic/spinoreticular system. The medial lemniscus terminates in the **ventral posterolateral (VPL) nucleus of the thalamus,** where further processing occurs through cortical regulation of the interneurons in this nucleus. The VPL nucleus of the thalamus sends projections through the **posterior limb of the internal capsule** to end in the postcentral gyrus (primary sensory cortex, or S1) in the rostral portion of the parietal lobe contralateral to the source of the primary sensory input. This entire system is topographically organized, with the upper part of the body represented laterally on the **postcentral gyrus (Brodmann areas 3a, 3b, 1, 2)**, and the lower part represented medially into the midline portion of the postcentral gyrus, part of the paracentral lobule. Some areas have far greater representation on the postcentral gyrus than others. The digits and perioral area have huge representation, while the back and proximal limbs have far smaller representation.

The two regions of Area 3 receive most of the thalamic somatosensory input for initial processing. Area 3a receives proprioceptive input from thalamic nucleus VPL. Area 3b receives information about touch and somatosensory stimuli from thalamic nucleus VPL and regions of the pulvinar. Areas 3a and 3b project to areas 1 and 2 for further somatosensory analysis. Area 1 processes information about texture; area 2 processes information about size, shape, and proprioception. Damage results in astereognosis, agraphesthesia, hypesthesia, hemineglect if the right hemisphere is damaged, and reduced nociception, thermoreception, and crude touch. These latter protopathic modalities are conveyed for further interpretation to the insular cortex and cingulate cortex, especially for emotional context. Areas 3, 1, and 2 of the primary somatosensory cortex also project to the SII cortex (area 43), superior parietal cortex (areas 5 and 7), and the primary motor cortex (area 4).

The spinocervical system is a supplemental source of epicritic information processed through primary sensory axons traveling in the dorsolateral portion of the lateral funiculus in the **spinocervical tract,** to the ipsilateral **lateral cervical nucleus** in C1 and C2 of the spinal cord. The lateral cervical nucleus sends ipsilateral connections to nuclei gracilis and cuneatus, and some crossed projections into the medial lemniscus.

COLOR the following structures, using a separate color for each structure.

- ☐ **1. Postcentral gyrus**
- ☐ **2. Posterior limb of the internal capsule**
- ☐ **3. VPL nucleus of the thalamus**
- ☐ **4. Medial lemniscus**
- ☐ **5. Fasciculus gracilis**
- ☐ **6. Fasciculus cuneatus**
- ☐ **7. Spinocervical tract**
- ☐ **8. Lateral cervical nucleus (in C1 and C2)**
- ☐ **9. Decussation of the medial lemniscus**
- ☐ **10. Nucleus cuneatus**
- ☐ **11. Nucleus gracilis**

Clinical Note

The dorsal column/medial lemniscal system carries fine discriminative touch, pressure, vibratory sensation, and joint position sense, the primary epicritic somatosensory modalities. These primary modalities are necessary for additional cortical "modalities" such as stereognosis (the ability to determine the structure and nature of an object by touch alone, e.g., a coin in your pocket), two-point discrimination (the ability to determine that two simultaneously applied stimuli at varying distances are actually two separate stimuli), graphesthesia (the ability to interpret a letter or number traced on the palm), and others. These epicritic modalities are essential to allow exquisitely fine sensations necessary for skilled activities. Damage to the primary sensory myelinated axons in the periphery (e.g., demyelinating disease), dorsal columns (e.g., combined systems degeneration), dorsal column nuclei (e.g., brainstem vascular lesions), medial lemniscus (e.g., brainstem lesions), VPL nucleus of the thalamus (e.g., vascular lesions), posterior limb of the internal capsule (e.g., vascular lesions, strokes), or postcentral gyrus (e.g., tumor, stroke, trauma) all lead to loss of sensation of epicritic modalities.

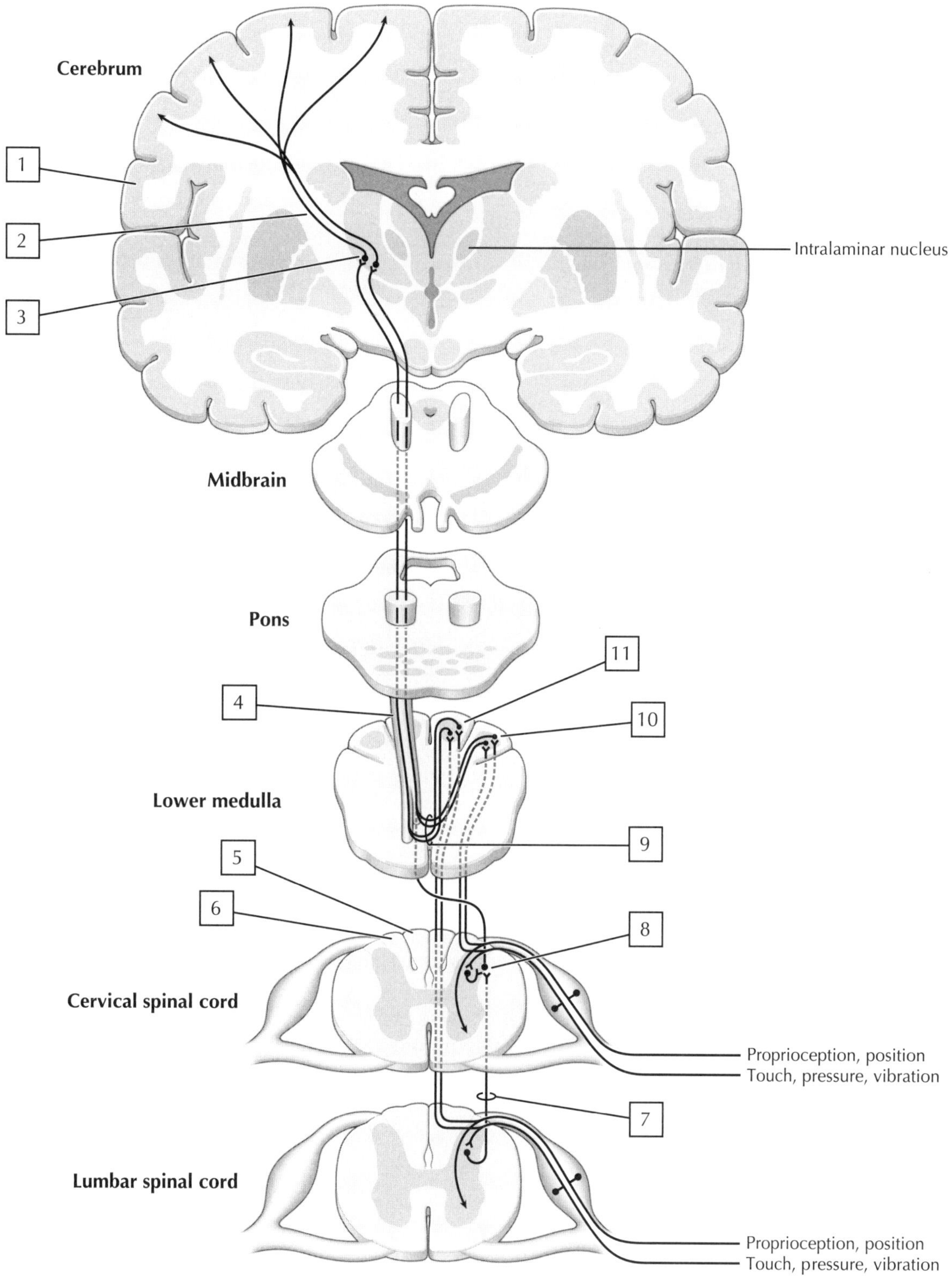
Cerebrum
1
2
3
Intralaminar nucleus
Midbrain
Pons
11
4
10
Lower medulla
9
5
6
8
Cervical spinal cord
Proprioception, position
Touch, pressure, vibration
7
Lumbar spinal cord
Proprioception, position
Touch, pressure, vibration

9 Somatosensory System: Spinothalamic and Spinoreticular Systems and Protopathic Modalities

Pain (nociception) and temperature sensation are considered protopathic modalities and are viewed as two interactive but parallel systems. "Fast pain" and general awareness of temperature sensation are considered acutely perceived lemniscal modalities that are interpreted by the cerebral cortex, but the perception does not outlast the duration of the stimulus; these modalities are tested neurologically using light pinprick sensation and perception of cool or warm water in small test tubes. Information is processed in the periphery by receptors associated with small myelinated axons (A-delta fibers) or unmyelinated C fibers. These axons enter the spinal cord through the dorsal roots and terminate on **dorsal horn neurons in Laminae I and V**. These dorsal horn neurons send axons across the midline in the **anterior white commissure**; these axons then ascend as the **spinothalamic tract** in the ventrolateral funiculus. These spinothalamic axons terminate on neurons in the **VPL nucleus of the thalamus**, separate from those contacted by axons of the medial lemniscus. VPL neurons send axons through the **posterior limb of the internal capsule** to both the **primary sensory cortex (SI) on the (postcentral gyrus)** and the **SII sensory cortex**, just posterior to the lateral portion of the postcentral gyrus.

The "slow pain" system derives from **bare nerve endings associated with C fibers**. This nociceptive input is interpreted by the brain as long-lasting, excruciating, burning, and agonizing pain, outlasting the period of nerve stimulation. These axons enter the dorsal roots and terminate on **neurons in the substantia gelatinosa,** followed by a **cascade of neuronal connections** through the dorsal horn and intermediate gray. Axons from this system (especially from lamina VII) cross into the anterolateral funiculus through the anterior white commissure. Some axons remain ipsilateral, with cascades of connections into the brainstem. The spinoreticular axons terminate in the **lateral reticular formation, parabrachial nuclei**, **deep layers of the superior colliculus and the periaqueductal gray**, and other brainstem sites. This **spinoreticular system** ultimately connects with the **nonspecific nuclei of the thalamus**, such as the **centromedian nucleus**. The information is then sent to widespread areas of the cortex, and to limbic structures that provide emotional context for the excruciating pain. The constant bombardment of the spinoreticular system with nociceptive input can result in centrally reinforced pain that can exist even in the absence of peripheral stimuli. The connections of the spinoreticular system are shown in the illustration only on the contralateral side.

COLOR the following structures, using a separate color for each structure.

- ☐ 1. **Cerebral cortex—postcentral gyrus**
- ☐ 2. **Posterior limb of the internal capsule**
- ☐ 3. **Ventral posterolateral (VPL) nucleus of the thalamus**
- ☐ 4. **Spinothalamic/spinoreticular ascending system in the ventrolateral funiculus**
- ☐ 5. **Anterior white commissure**
- ☐ 6. **Bare nerve ending C fibers contributing to the slow pain system**
- ☐ 7. **Pain and temperature axons contributing to the fast pain system**
- ☐ 8. **Dorsal horn neuronal cascade associated with the slow pain system**
- ☐ 9. **Dorsal horn laminae I and V**
- ☐ 10. **Lateral reticular formation**
- ☐ 11. **Parabrachial nuclei**
- ☐ 12. **Deep layers of the superior colliculus and the periaqueductal gray**
- ☐ 13. **Nonspecific thalamic nuclei (centromedian nucleus)**

Clinical Note

Pathological activation of the spinoreticular system, resulting in agonizing pain, occurs with conditions such as complex regional pain syndrome (CRPS), formally called *reflex sympathetic dystrophy,* phantom limb pain, causalgia, pain from terminal cancer, painful diabetic neuropathy, and other pain syndromes that bring about central activation and persistence of the slow pain system. Widespread areas of the limbic forebrain and cerebral cortex are activated via nonspecific thalamic nuclei, to the extent that little attention can be focused on other more specific sensory inputs.

Opioid analgesics can, in some cases, ameliorate agonizing pain for a brief period, but they are not a highly effective long-term solution, especially with issues of dependency, cognitive side effects, and often severe autonomic consequences. Some therapeutic approaches use membrane-stabilizing agents (e.g., antiseizure meds), low-dose antidepressants, dorsal column stimulation, and other approaches to attempt to dampen the highly activated slow pain system.

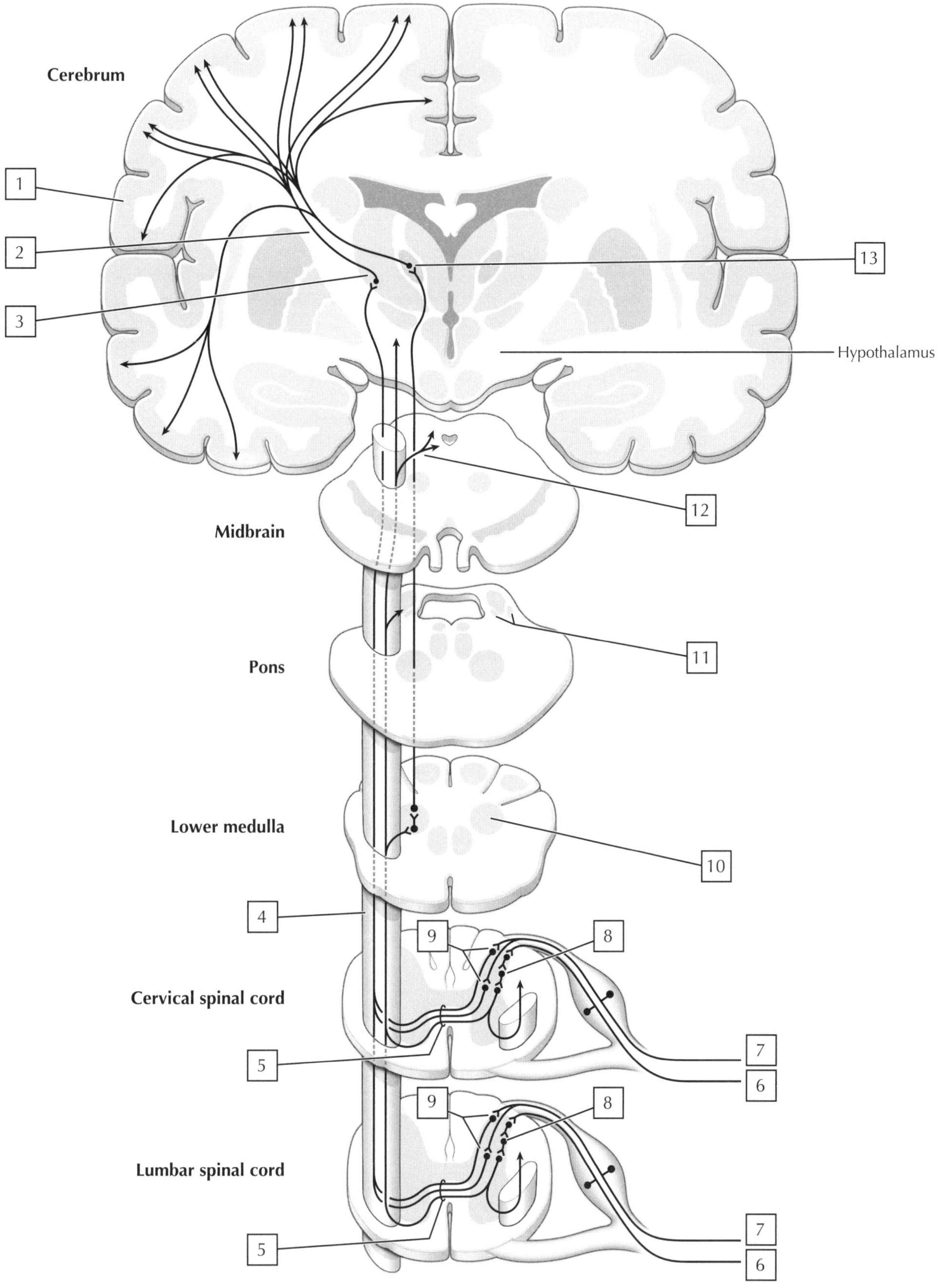
Cerebrum
1
2
3
13
Hypothalamus
12
Midbrain
11
Pons
Lower medulla
10
4
9
8
Cervical spinal cord
5
7
6
9
8
Lumbar spinal cord
7
5
6

9 Mechanisms of Neuropathic Pain and Sympathetically Maintained Pain

The cascading, self-reinforcing "slow pain" system can be activated by initial peripheral bombardment of the dorsal horn neuronal system by continuing input from C fibers associated with bare nerve endings, leading to activation of the **spinoreticular system** and its higher central connections. The neurons in **substantia gelatinosa** and the **cascading dorsal horn/intermediate neurons** recruit additional neuronal activation through a converging system. Ordinarily, with acute nociceptive input, stimulation of the large diameter mechanoreceptor-associated axons can dampen the pain system through **gating** (i.e., a stimulation of inhibitory interneurons that inhibits the transmission of nociception through the cascading system). This is the physiological basis for dorsal column stimulation by a TENS unit (transcutaneous electrical nerve stimulation) and the well-known phenomenon of lightly rubbing an area of skin just injured. In some cases of prolonged nociceptive input, these inhibitory neurons responsible for gating of pain are destroyed by **excitotoxic damage (apoptosis) due to excessive glutamate release** (called glutamate storm).

With prolonged nociceptive input, the cascading pain system can be self-driven and self-reinforcing, as may occur with the central phenomenon of CRPS. With such injury, dorsal horn neurons can express **alpha-adrenergic receptors on their bare nerve endings** and their **cell bodies,** providing a mechanism for sympathetically driven activation of these primary sensory neurons by norepinephrine and epinephrine (hence, the former name of reflex sympathetic dystrophy). Other mechanisms of neuropathic pain (the central activation of chronic severe pain that often occurs even in the absence of peripheral stimulation) are lowered threshold of C fibers to further activation, inadequate gating of pain, loss of inhibition of nociceptive dorsal horn activation through glutamate excitotoxicity, or inability of descending serotonin and noradrenergic central axons to modulate and dampen the dorsal horn cascade.

COLOR the following structures, using a separate color for each structure.

- ☐ 1. **Central serotonergic and noradrenergic pathways**
- ☐ 2. **Site of expression of alpha receptors on primary sensory cell bodies in the dorsal root ganglion**
- ☐ 3. **Site of lowered axonal threshold excitability**
- ☐ 4. **Site of expression of alpha receptors on bare nerve endings**
- ☐ 5. **Enkephalin neurons in the dorsal horn**
- ☐ 6. **Site where glutamate excitotoxicity may occur**
- ☐ 7. **C fibers contributing input to the dorsal horn neuronal cascade**
- ☐ 8. **Dorsal horn neuronal cascade**
- ☐ 9. **Zone in the dorsal horn of gating of pain**

Clinical Note

Complex regional pain syndrome (CRPS) is a neuropathic response to injury. In some cases of nerve damage or nerve compression, usually associated with direct trauma, a sprain, a crush injury, an injection directly into a nerve, a postsurgical state, or even minor trauma, a pathological reaction takes place that drives and activates the cascading dorsal horn neuronal system and establishes a self-reinforcing activation of the CNS "slow pain" system. This reaction affects the upper extremity more than the lower extremity. Patients describe the resulting nociception as stabbing, burning, or agonizing pain, sometimes spreading to the mirror image region on the contralateral limb. The patient experiences **allodynia** (extreme sensitivity to touch) and **hyperesthesia** (extreme sensitivity to painful stimuli). When these phenomena occur in the territory of one nerve (as was originally observed during the civil war), it is called **causalgia**.

In circumstances where alpha-adrenergic receptors proliferate on the bare nociceptive nerve endings and on the dorsal root ganglion cell bodies, norepinephrine may evoke severe **neuropathic pain**, and other sympathetically related phenomena may be noted, such as changes in skin appearance due to altered vascular flow (**vasomotor changes**), atrophic skin and nails (**trophic changes**), altered sweating and skin temperature (**sudomotor changes**), and altered bone density on a triphasic bone scan. Treatment of CRPS is difficult at best but must be initiated very quickly after diagnosis to optimize chances for success.

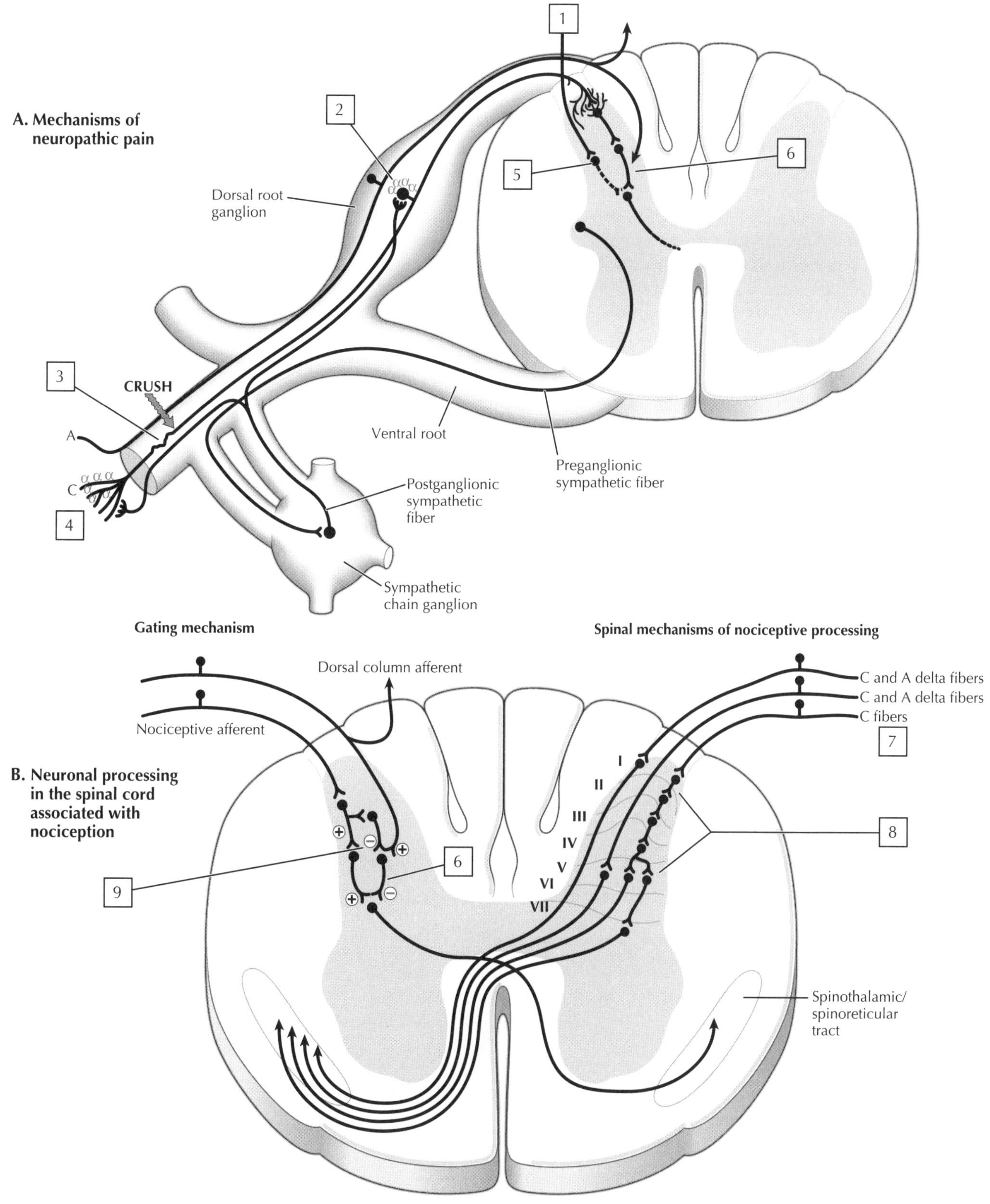
A. Mechanisms of neuropathic pain
1
2
Dorsal root ganglion
5
6
3
CRUSH
A
C
4
Ventral root
Preganglionic sympathetic fiber
Postganglionic sympathetic fiber
Sympathetic chain ganglion
Gating mechanism
Spinal mechanisms of nociceptive processing
Dorsal column afferent
Nociceptive afferent
C and A delta fibers
C and A delta fibers
C fibers
7
B. Neuronal processing in the spinal cord associated with nociception
I
II
III
IV
V
VI
VII
8
9
6
Spinothalamic/ spinoreticular tract

Descending Control of Ascending Somatosensory Systems

The **dorsal horn of the spinal cord** is a key site at which the cascading nociceptive "slow pain" system can be modified by other central structures. These central regions include the sensory **cortex (SI)** (through **corticonuclear fibers**) and **limbic forebrain structures,** the **β-endorphin neurons in the hypothalamus,** through the **periaqueductal gray of the midbrain** (containing **enkephalin neurons**), and through the **raphe nuclei** (and **descending serotonergic pathways**) and **locus coeruleus** (and **descending noradrenergic pathways**). **Enkephalin-containing neurons in the dorsal horn** are a target of the descending serotonergic and noradrenergic pathways, which themselves are driven by the β-endorphin neurons of the **periarcuate region of the hypothalamus**. The cerebral cortex is usually quite able to influence the ascending sensory information it receives from the various sensory systems for fine-grained analysis of the outside world. However, the bombardment of the cortex from nonspecific thalamic nuclei, driven by the cascade of the spinoreticular "slow pain" system, can overwhelm cortical focus on other specific stimuli and divert attention inward toward the excruciating pain, thus incapacitating the individual.

COLOR the following structures, using a separate color for each structure.

- ☐ 1. **Axons from β-endorphin neurons in the hypothalamus**
- ☐ 2. **Cortical and limbic regions influencing dorsal horn pain processing**
- ☐ 3. **Locus coeruleus**
- ☐ 4. **Descending noradrenergic pathway**
- ☐ 5. **Descending serotonergic pathway**
- ☐ 6. **Enkephalin neuron in the dorsal horn of the spinal cord**
- ☐ 7. **Dorsal horn of the spinal cord**
- ☐ 8. **Corticonuclear fibers**
- ☐ 9. **Raphe nuclei (raphe magnus)**
- ☐ 10. **Periaqueductal gray of the midbrain with enkephalin neurons**

Clinical Note

The nociceptive, or protopathic, system usually quickly draws the attention of the cerebral cortex as a protective reaction to permit the initiation of movement or behavior to help remove the part of the body involved, or the entire individual, from the source of nociception. The limbic system can assess the potential emotional connotation of the stimulus and initiate appropriate responses through connections with the periarcuate region of the hypothalamus, the major source of β-endorphin neurons in the brain. These neurons can initiate central serotonergic and noradrenergic responses that influence enkephalin neurons in the dorsal horn of the spinal cord, the initial central zone processing incoming nociceptive information. The cortex and limbic system, working in concert, can determine the focus and the response to the potentially offending nociceptive stimuli. If the individual is vigorously involved in a contact sport, with total focus and sympathetic drive directed to the activity at hand, then a potentially major nociceptive injury may simply be ignored, even with significant damage. This mechanism of response is a survival adaptation to help an organism respond to a potentially life-threatening insult or injury. By contrast, if one is resting quietly in a chair, then nociceptive stimuli such as toothache, or an injury sustained in an athletic event, may become a major focus of attention and may be perceived as far more painful than was the case during the athletic event.

Psychological factors can contribute to the perception and severity of pain, but a default position of "it's all in your head" is frequently wrong and demeans the person experiencing very real pain. The **placebo effect**, involving cortical and limbic circuitry, can exert neuronal influence over the cascading circuitry involved in the spinoreticular system.

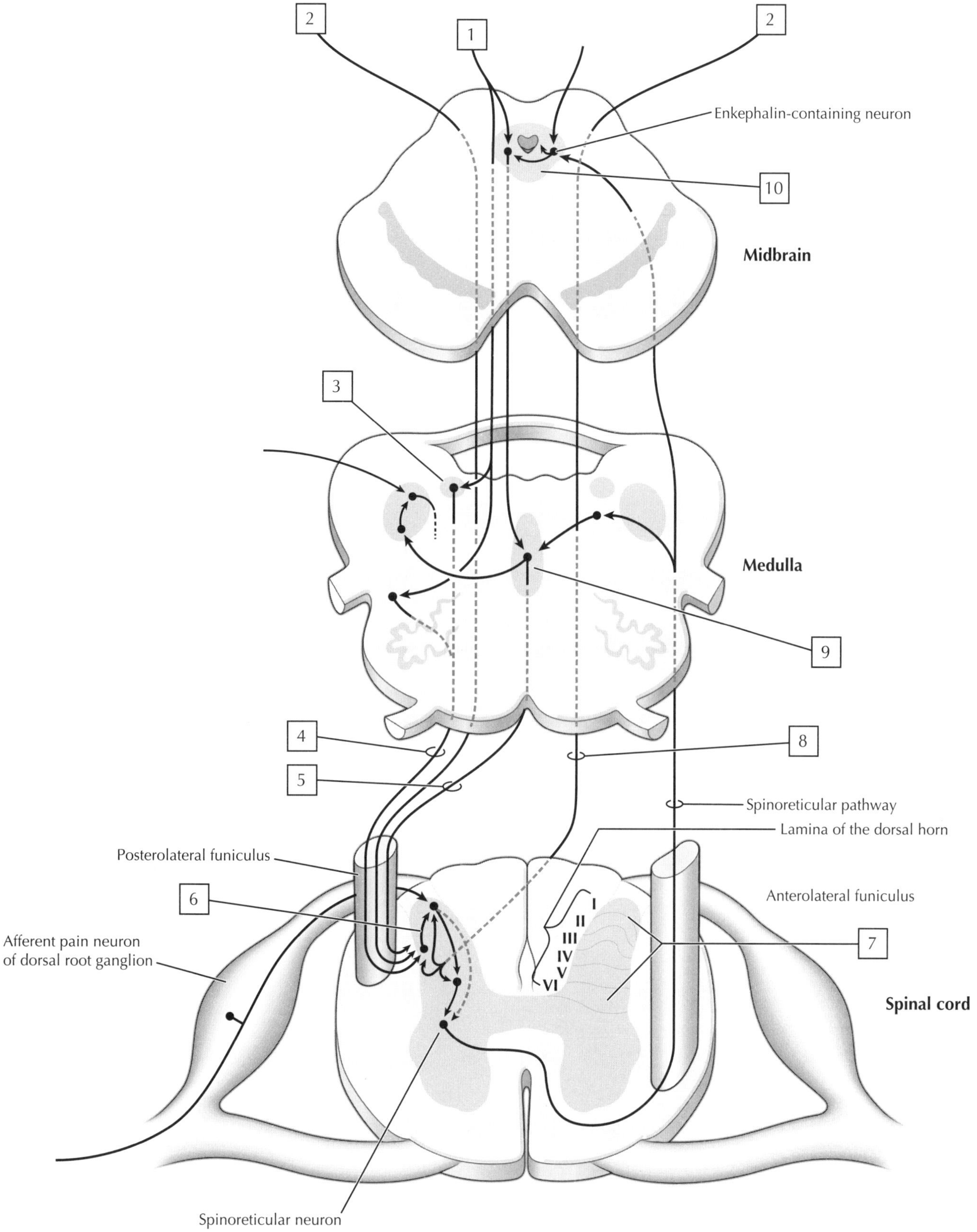

2
1
2
Enkephalin-containing neuron
10
Midbrain
3
Medulla
9
4
8
5
Spinoreticular pathway
Lamina of the dorsal horn
Posterolateral funiculus
Anterolateral funiculus
6
I
II
III
IV
V
VI
7
Afferent pain neuron of dorsal root ganglion
Spinal cord
Spinoreticular neuron

9 Trigeminal Sensory and Associated Systems

Axons of neurons in the **trigeminal (semilunar) ganglion (V)** supply the face, the anterior oral cavity, teeth, and gums with sensation. Axons from neurons in the geniculate ganglion (VII) and jugular ganglion (X) supply small zones of the external ear. Axons of neurons in the petrosal ganglion (IX) supply general sensation to the posterior oral cavity and pharynx, and project centrally into the trigeminal system. Primary sensory axons for the trigeminal and related systems (similar to the spinal cord dorsal column system) convey fine discriminative modalities and terminate in the rostral portion of the **descending (spinal) nucleus of V** and the **main (chief, principal) sensory nucleus of V**. These nuclei contribute axons to the **ventral trigeminothalamic tract**, also called the **ventral trigeminal lemniscus**, which terminates in the **ventral posteromedial (VPM) nucleus of the thalamus**, contralateral to the initial side of the sensory input. A portion of the main sensory nucleus also projects ipsilaterally to the VPM nucleus via the **dorsal trigeminothalamic tract**, also called the **dorsal trigeminal lemniscus**. This smaller sensory projection system, along with the taste system, travels ipsilaterally to the sensory cortex, perhaps for processing information regarding food.

Primary sensory axons for general sensation in the trigeminal and related systems terminate in the lower two-thirds of the descending nucleus of V (traveling through the primary sensory **descending [spinal] tract of V**); this nucleus sends crossed axons via the ventral trigeminothalamic tract to the VPM nucleus of the thalamus. Nucleus VPM sends its contralateral trigeminal sensory information through the **posterior limb of the internal capsule** to the **lateralmost portion of the primary sensory (SI) cortex on the postcentral gyrus**, consistent with its topographical organization.

Protopathic axons from the trigeminal and related systems terminate in the caudal portion of the descending nucleus of V, which in turn projects to a portion of the VPM nucleus of the thalamus. This is the equivalent of the "fast pain" system for the somatosensory system; caudally, this nucleus is contiguous with **substantia gelatinosa of the spinal cord.** C fibers conveying severe, long-lasting pain (e.g., chronic dental pain) terminate in the caudal portion of the descending nucleus of V, which sends projections bilateral to the lateral reticular formation, parabrachial nucleus, and **intralaminar nuclei** (e.g., **centromedian nucleus**) of the thalamus, the equivalent of the "slow pain" system for the somatosensory system.

The **mesencephalic nucleus of V** is a primary sensory nucleus, the only one within the CNS. Its axons supply muscle spindles in the masticatory muscles and the extraocular muscles, and mediate muscle stretch reflexes.

COLOR each of the following structures, using a separate color for each structure.

- ☐ 1. **Posterior limb of the internal capsule**
- ☐ 2. **Dorsal trigeminothalamic tract**
- ☐ 3. **Ventral trigeminothalamic tract**
- ☐ 4. **Descending (spinal) tract of V**
- ☐ 5. **Descending (spinal) nucleus of V**
- ☐ 6. **Substantia gelatinosa of the spinal cord**
- ☐ 7. **Trigeminal (semilunar) ganglion**
- ☐ 8. **Main (chief, principal) sensory nucleus of V**
- ☐ 9. **Mesencephalic nucleus of V**
- ☐ 10. **Ventral posteromedial (VPM) nucleus of the thalamus**
- ☐ 11. **Intralaminar (nonspecific) nuclei (e.g., centromedian) of the thalamus**
- ☐ 12. **Lateral portion of the primary sensory cortex on the postcentral gyrus**

Clinical Note

The descending nucleus and tract of V and the spinothalamic/spinoreticular system are found in the ventrolateral quadrant of the medulla in the territory of the posterior inferior cerebellar artery as well as the vertebral artery. A vascular occlusion in either of these arteries will result in loss of pain and temperature sensation on the ipsilateral face and the contralateral body, while sparing the motor system. The protopathic trigeminal system extending from the caudal descending nucleus of V is also involved in processing paroxysms of excruciating pain from the face in a disorder called **trigeminal neuralgia**, where even minor stimuli (touch, chewing) on a trigger point results in bursts of pain. This condition is mainly treated with antiseizure medications.

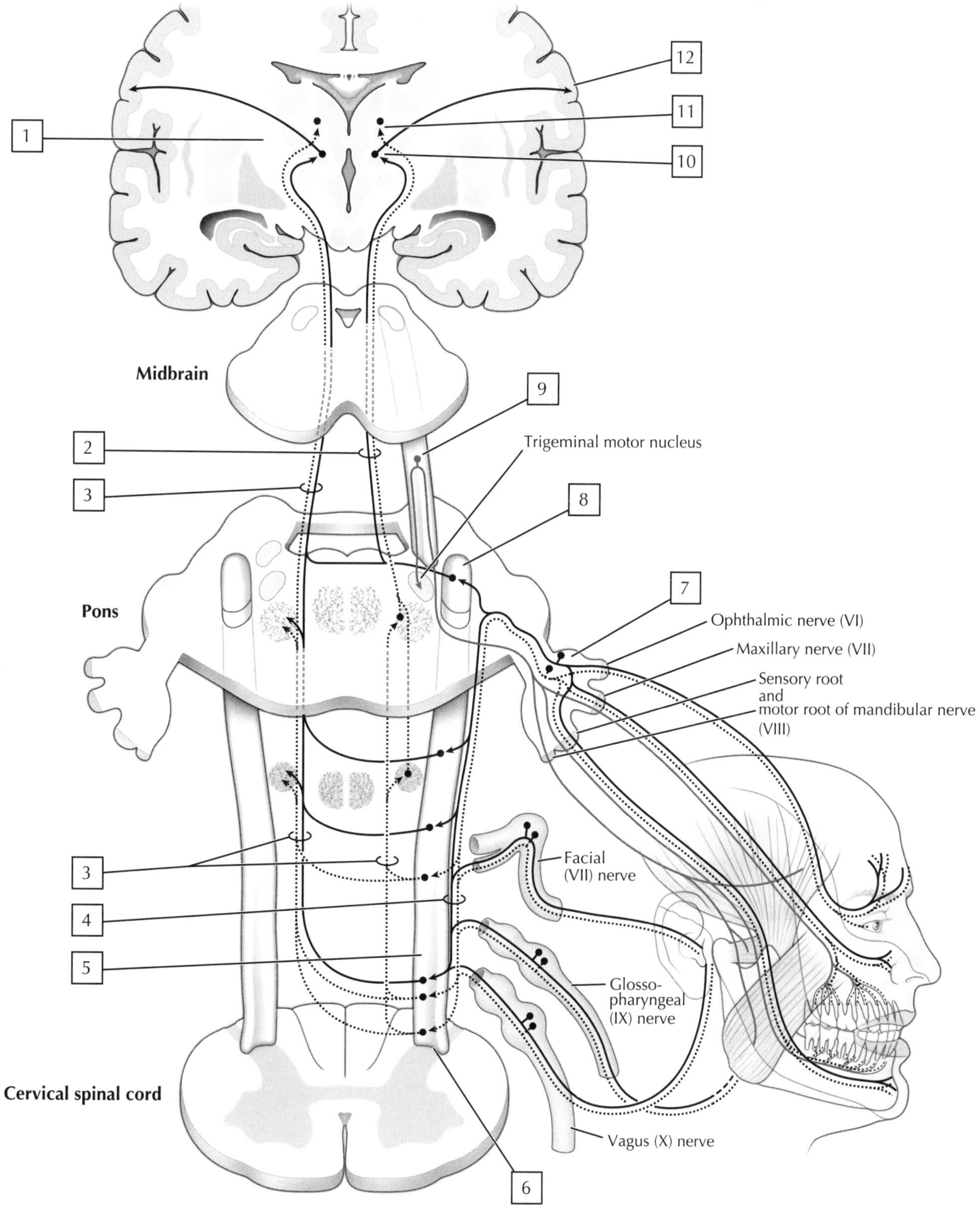
12
11
1
10
Midbrain
9
Trigeminal motor nucleus
2
3
8
Pons
7
Ophthalmic nerve (VI)
Maxillary nerve (VII)
Sensory root
and
motor root of mandibular nerve
(VIII)
Facial
(VII) nerve
3
4
5
Glosso-
pharyngeal
(IX) nerve
Cervical spinal cord
Vagus (X) nerve
6

9 Pain-Sensitive Structures of the Head and Pain Referral

Many types of primary headaches, including migraine headaches, tension headaches, and neuralgias, can arise from stimulation of pain structures in the head and neck. Pain-sensitive structures of the neck region include **afferent nerves of the occipital region**, the **dura of the posterior fossa**, and **the vertebrobasilar arteries**; this nociceptive information is conveyed to the **dorsal horn cascading neuronal system of the spinal cord** via the **dorsal root ganglia of C1–C3**. The **ophthalmic nerve (V1)** conveys nociceptive information from the head and scalp and retrobulbar sites to the descending nucleus of V. Additional nociceptive information from the **dural sinuses, middle meningeal artery**, **temporal artery**, **proximal cerebral arteries**, **internal and external carotid arteries**, and **tentorium cerebelli** is also conveyed via the ophthalmic nerve into the descending nucleus of V. This information ascends to the VPM nucleus, mainly contralaterally, and then activates lateral cortical regions of the postcentral gyrus.

COLOR each of the following structures, using a separate color for each structure.

- ☐ 1. **Cerebral dural sinuses (e.g., superior sagittal sinus)**
- ☐ 2. **Middle meningeal artery**
- ☐ 3. **Temporal artery**
- ☐ 4. **Proximal cerebral artery**
- ☐ 5. **Tentorium cerebelli**
- ☐ 6. **Internal and external cerebral arteries**
- ☐ 7. **Ophthalmic nerve (V1)**
- ☐ 8. **Dorsal root ganglia of C1–C3**
- ☐ 9. **Dorsal horn cascading neuronal system of the spinal cord**
- ☐ 10. **Afferent nerves of the occipital region**
- ☐ 11. **Dura of the posterior fossa**
- ☐ 12. **The vertebrobasilar arteries**

Clinical Note

Dural structures, arteries, and muscles are pain-sensitive structures in the head and neck. Some headaches result from arterial constriction, such as temporal arteritis and migraine headaches. Tension headaches can result from contracted muscles. Irritative lesions of the trigeminal or glossopharyngeal nerves can produce painful neuralgias, the equivalent of the nucleus pulposus of a herniated disc impinging on a dorsal root. There are secondary causes of headache. Tumors, abscesses, or hematomas may impinge on dural structures or arteries. A ruptured Berry aneurysm may lead to bleeding into the subarachnoid space (subarachnoid hemorrhage), producing “the worst headache of my life.” Infectious processes, such as meningitis or meningeal irritation, can result in an excruciatingly painful headache, with nuchal rigidity and muscle guarding.

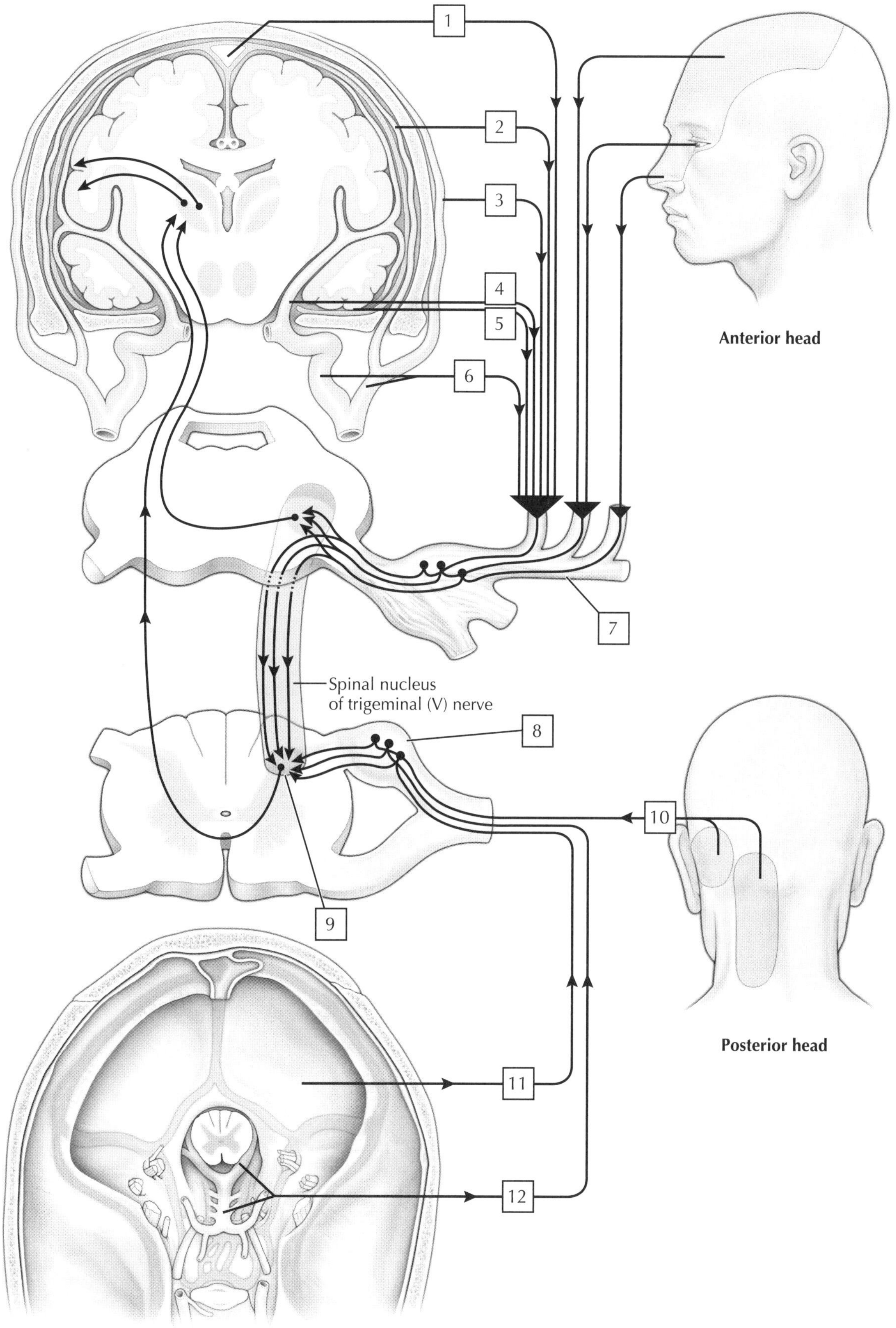
1
2
3
4
5
6
7
Spinal nucleus
of trigeminal (V) nerve
8
9
10
11
12
Anterior head
Posterior head

9 Taste Pathways

Taste is detected by **taste buds** on **papillae**. There are an estimated 3000–10,000 taste buds on a human tongue, each approximately 0.03 mm wide and 0.06 mm deep. Chemical transduction occurs by neurotransmitter release (acetylcholine, ATP, glutamate, norepinephrine, serotonin, GABA) from taste buds, activating receptors on peripheral nerve endings of the geniculate (CN VII), petrosal (CN IX), and nodose (CN X) ganglia that supply the taste buds in the fungiform, foliate, and vallate papillae. A scheme of distribution of specific tastes was developed over 100 years ago and has been commonly cited. In this scheme, sweet sensation occurs on the tip of the tongue, stimulated by sugar. Sour sensation occurs on the sides of the tongue, stimulated by acids. Salt sensation occurs on the tip and anterior tongue, stimulated by inorganic salts, and bitter sensation occurs on the back of the tongue, stimulated by organic agents and some salts such as calcium and magnesium. More careful investigation demonstrates that these tastes can be detected on almost all parts of the tongue, as well as the soft and hard palates. The "standard" scheme may indicate the most sensitive regions of the tongue for some of these tastes. A fifth taste has been described by investigators, reflecting a unique taste sensation called "umami." This taste is the result of glutamate sensation, sometimes called "savory." Some investigators have proposed a sixth taste related to detection of starch.

Primary sensory axons for taste derive from the **geniculate ganglion (VII)** for the anterior two-thirds of the tongue, from the **petrosal (inferior) ganglion (IX)** for the posterior one-third of the tongue and from the **nodose (inferior) ganglion (X)** for the epiglottis and palate (especially present in children). Central axons from these ganglia terminate in the **rostral nucleus of the solitary tract (nucleus solitarius)** in the **medulla**. This gustatory portion of rostral nucleus solitarius supplies axons to the **preganglionic parasympathetic nuclei** supplying the salivary glands, and to the **dorsal motor (autonomic) nucleus of X**, providing regulation of salivary secretion and gastric secretion in preparation for the consumption of food. In humans, rostral nucleus solitarius projects ipsilaterally to the **ventral posteromedial (VPM) nucleus in the thalamus** via the **solitariothalamic tract** and to the **parabrachial nucleus** in the pons. Projections from the parabrachial nucleus associated with taste go to the ipsilateral VPM nucleus (which projects to portions of the **lateral sensory cortex**), to the **hypothalamus** (lateral hypothalamic area, paraventricular nucleus), to some **amygdaloid nuclei**, and to the **insular cortex**, particularly the anterior portion. The insular cortex is considered to be the major region of gustatory perception. These limbic/hypothalamic projections likely account for the emotional, motivational, and behavioral aspects of a gustatory experience. Information from the trigeminal system and the olfactory system also integrate into the experience of enjoying a meal.

COLOR the following structures, using a separate color for each structure.

- ☐ 1. **Ventral posteromedial (VPM) nucleus of the thalamus**
- ☐ 2. **Lateral sensory cortex**
- ☐ 3. **Hypothalamus**
- ☐ 4. **Amygdala (amygdaloid nuclei)**
- ☐ 5. **Parabrachial nucleus of the pons**
- ☐ 6. **Geniculate ganglion (CN VII)**
- ☐ 7. **Rostral nucleus of the solitary tract (nucleus solitarius)**
- ☐ 8. **Medulla**
- ☐ 9. **Petrosal (inferior) ganglion (CN IX)**
- ☐ 10. **Nodose (inferior) ganglion (CN X)**
- ☐ 11. **Papillae on the tongue**
- ☐ 12. **Taste buds**

Clinical Note

For taste to have full expression in appreciation of a gustatory experience, the pathways noted above, the trigeminal system, and olfaction must be fully functional and physiologically responsive. Even a cold or nasal congestion, blocking sensitive olfaction, can result in food "tasting" bland. Exposure to many chemicals, including those related to smoking, alters taste. These chemicals include some medications and chemotherapeutic agents. Liver failure, exposure to radiation treatments, and some vitamin deficiencies can lead to altered taste sensation, lingering unpleasant tastes, or loss of appetite.

In the elderly, the onset of taste dysfunction may be an early marker for neurodegenerative disease. Loss of taste perception and olfaction can accompany a COVID-19 infection; these losses can persist as part of long-COVID.

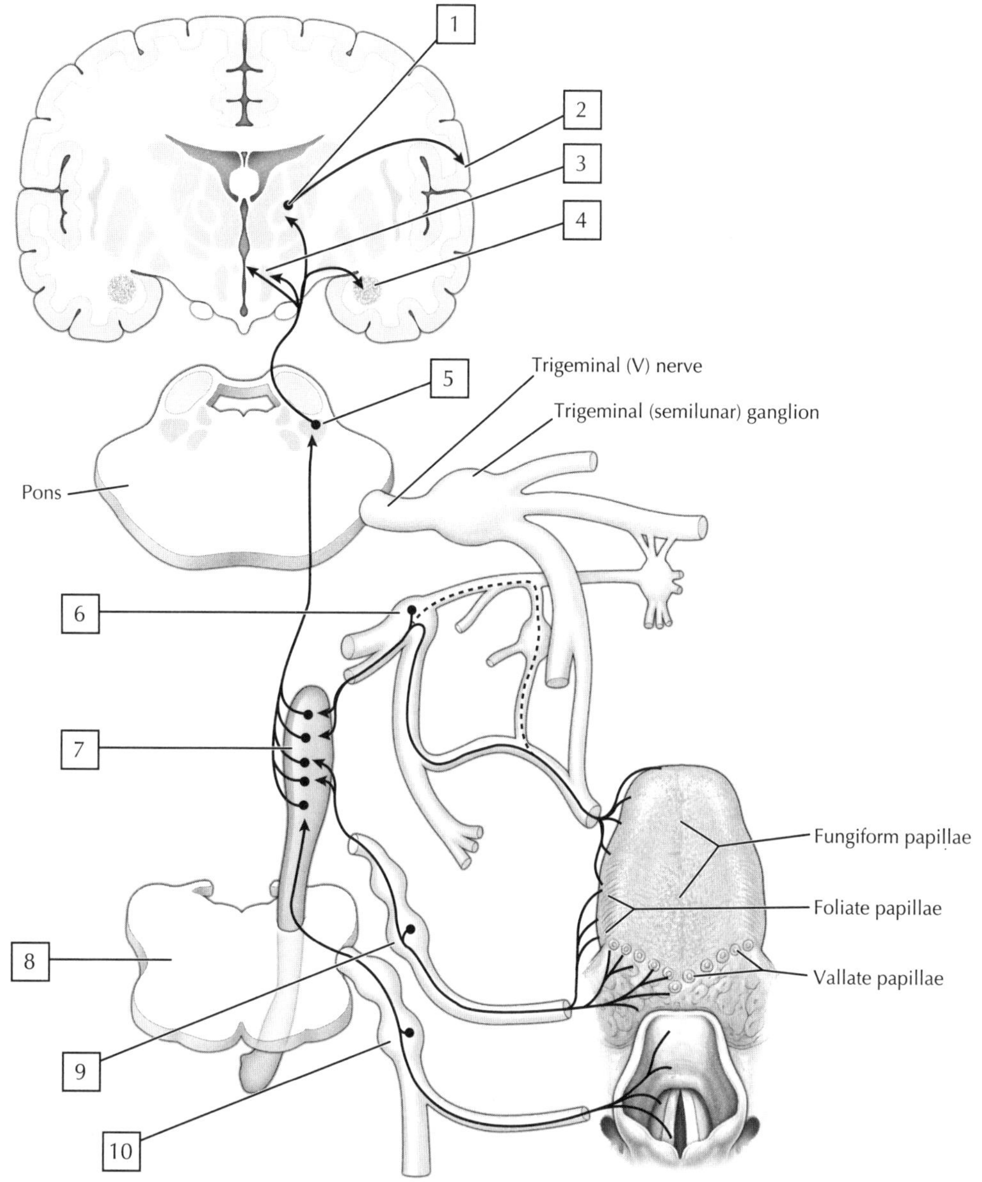

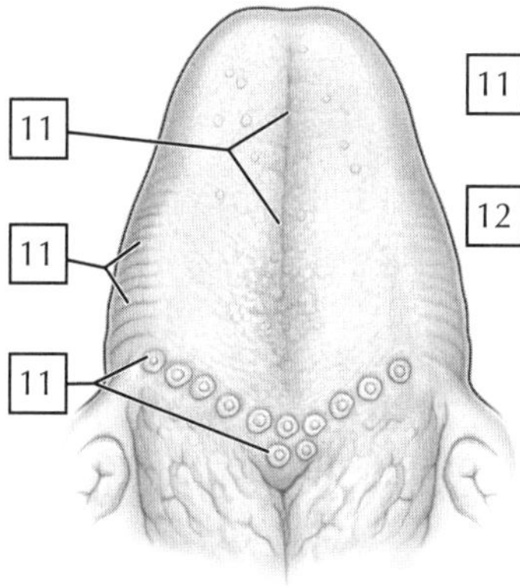

A. Tongue

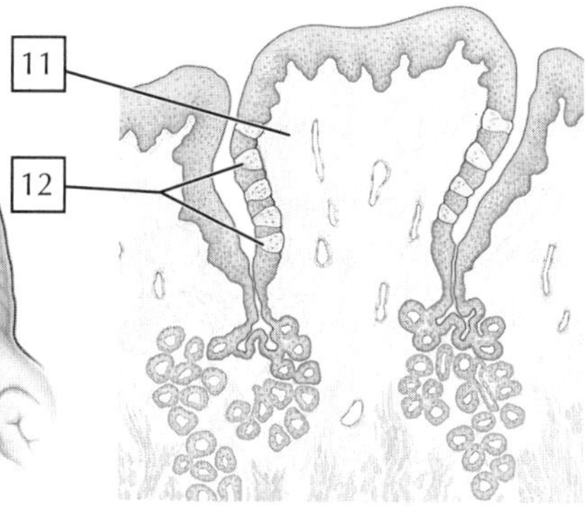

B. Section through vallate papilla

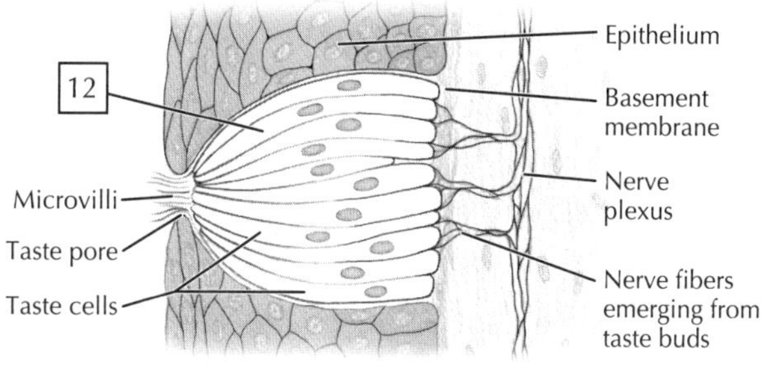

C. Taste bud

9 Peripheral Pathways for Sound Reception and the Bony and Membranous Labyrinths

Hearing involves a complex set of mechanisms for transducing sound waves through the external ear to produce fluid movements in the **cochlea** that stimulate hair cells, activating afferent nerve endings of the auditory nerve. Sound waves proceed through the **external auditory meatus**, causing distortion of the **tympanic membrane**. This movement of the tympanic membrane is leveraged by the ossicles **(malleus, incus, stapes)** to the **oval window**, at which movement of the perilymph initiates a fluid wave through the **scala vestibuli** and then the **scala tympani**, resulting in fluid movement in the **cochlear duct.** Fluid movement of the **endolymph** in the cochlear duct produces a differential force between the movement of the **hair cells** on the **basilar membrane** of the **organ of Corti** and the overlying **tectorial membrane**. Hair cell stimulation activates the primary afferent nerve endings, which send action potentials into central auditory structures. Low-frequency tones optimally stimulate the hair cells at the **apex of the cochlea (helicotrema)**, and high-frequency tones optimally stimulate hair cells at the **base of the cochlea**.

The **ampullae of the semicircular canals** of the vestibular system (responding to **angular acceleration, or movement**) and the **utricle** and **saccule** (responding to **linear acceleration or gravity** and also low-frequency vibration for the saccule) are closely associated with the cochlear components of the auditory system. These two components, auditory and vestibular, constitute the apparatus of **CN VIII (vestibulocochlear)**.

Clinical Note

Disruption of many portions of the auditory system may produce partial or total hearing loss. Damage to CN VIII, which can be a consequence of trauma, a tumor such as an acoustic Schwannoma, or other pathology, prevents the access of any messages in the periphery from reaching the CNS. Partial hearing loss can involve any frequencies, but the most significant are the frequencies of human communication (30–3000 Hz) of 40 or more decibels. The two principal types of hearing loss are sensorineural and conductive.

Conductive hearing loss involves damage in the outer and middle ear. Sound cannot be transduced to the inner ear to stimulate hair cells to activate primary sensory auditory axons. Sensorineural hearing loss involves damage to the hair cells in the organ of Corti, the cochlear nerve, or the central auditory pathways. Clinical testing can distinguish between the two forms of hearing loss. With conductive hearing loss, air conduction is impaired (damaged transduction) but bone conduction is intact. With sensorineural hearing loss, both air conduction and bone conduction are diminished. Bedside testing uses a 512-Hz tuning fork. The Weber test places the vibrating tuning fork on the center of the forehead; with a normal response, the patient hears the tuning fork equally in both ears. With a conduction deficit, the sound is heard best in the affected ear. With a sensorineural loss, the sound is heard best in the unaffected ear.

COLOR the following structures, using a separate color for each structure.

- ☐ 1. **Oval window**
- ☐ 2. **Stapes**
- ☐ 3. **Malleus**
- ☐ 4. **Incus**
- ☐ 5. **External auditory meatus**
- ☐ 6. **Tympanic membrane**
- ☐ 7. **Scala tympani**
- ☐ 8. **Cochlear duct**
- ☐ 9. **Scala vestibuli**
- ☐ 10. **Cochlea**
- ☐ 11. **Helicotrema of the cochlea**
- ☐ 12. **Vestibulocochlear nerve (CN VIII)**
- ☐ 13. **Ampullae of the semicircular canals**
- ☐ 14. **Utricle and saccule**

Peripheral Pathways for Sound Reception and the Bony and Membranous Labyrinths

A. Peripheral pathways for sound reception

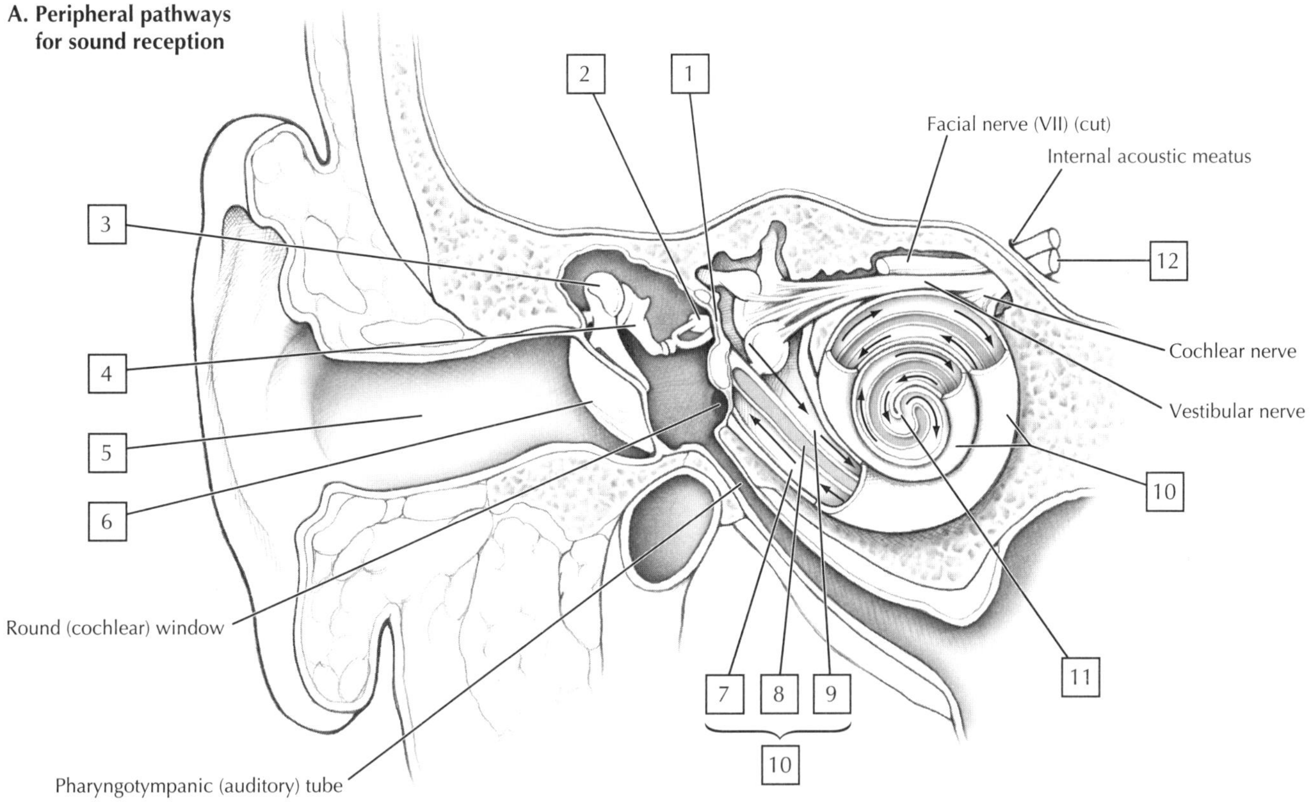

B. Bony and membranous labyrinths

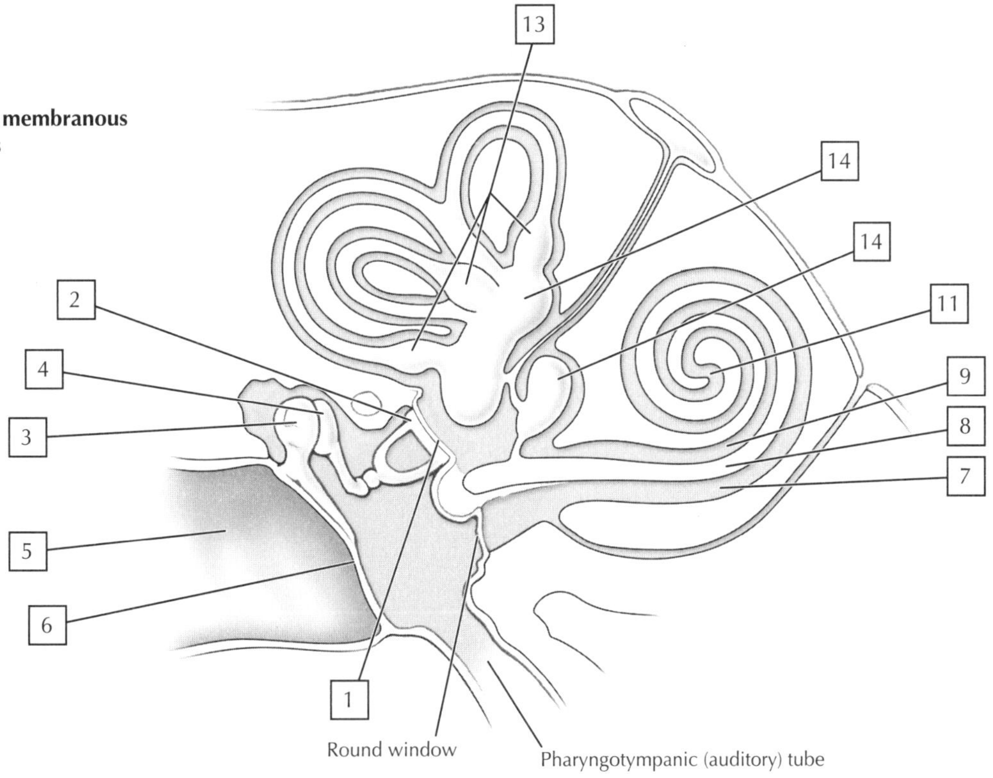

9 CN VIII Innervation of Hair Cells in the Organ of Corti

Inner and outer hair cells sit on the **basilar membrane** of the **organ of Corti**. **Hairs** protrude from the hair cell apical surface; they can be displaced laterally by movement of the overlying **tectorial membrane**. A fluid wave set up by the movement of the **stapes** at the **oval window** travels through the **scala vestibuli** and around the helicotrema through the **scala tympani**. This fluid wave is transmitted across the **cochlear duct** through the endolymph, a charged fluid at +80 mV, which causes a differential movement of the tectorial membrane (shearing forces) on the apical hairs on the hair cells. The potential difference of the endolymph contributes to the excitability of the hair cells. This causes the hair cells to release their neurotransmitter(s). The hair cells are innervated by the **peripheral process (axons) of the bipolar ganglion cells** of the **auditory (spiral) ganglion**. The central process of the ganglion cells (continuation of the axon) travels with the **auditory portion of CN VIII** and terminates in the cochlear nuclei of the brainstem.

COLOR the following structures, using a separate color for each structure.

- ☐ 1. **Inner and outer hair cells**
- ☐ 2. **Basilar membrane of the organ of Corti**
- ☐ 3. **Organ of Corti**
- ☐ 4. **Tectorial membrane**
- ☐ 5. **Cochlear duct**
- ☐ 6. **Scala vestibuli**
- ☐ 7. **Peripheral process of the bipolar ganglion cells**
- ☐ 8. **Auditory (spiral) ganglion**
- ☐ 9. **Scala tympani**
- ☐ 10. **Auditory portion of CN VIII**
- ☐ 11. **Oval window**
- ☐ 12. **Stapes**

Clinical Note

Specific sets of hair cells on specific portions of the spiral-shaped cochlea are optimally excited by movement in the cochlear duct precipitated by specific frequencies. The lowest frequencies maximally stimulate hair cells at the apex of the cochlea (helicotrema), and the highest frequencies maximally stimulate hair cells at the base of the cochlea. The hair cells can be damaged by many insults. Sustained loud noises above 85 dB (e.g., loud rock music) can damage hair cells responsive to the offending frequencies; hair cells in the basilar coils of the cochlea are especially susceptible to sustained high frequencies, such as the noise of jet engines, high-pitched machinery, gunshot noise, and loud industrial or environmental noise. Repeated exposure to these noises can cause permanent damage; ear protection is now required for construction sites, factory noises, airport personnel, and other potentially hazardous sites.

Some viral infections (e.g., mumps) and some medications such as quinine and antibiotics can damage hair cells. The outer hair cell membranes express a protein, prestin, which amplifies the deflection of their apical cilia in response to low volume sounds, enhancing auditory sensitivity. However, these hair cells are easily damaged by continuing loud sounds, resulting in diminished hearing, especially involving high-frequency sounds and contributing to presbycusis, diminished hearing with aging, a multifactorial process.

A. CN VIII nerve innervation of hair cells

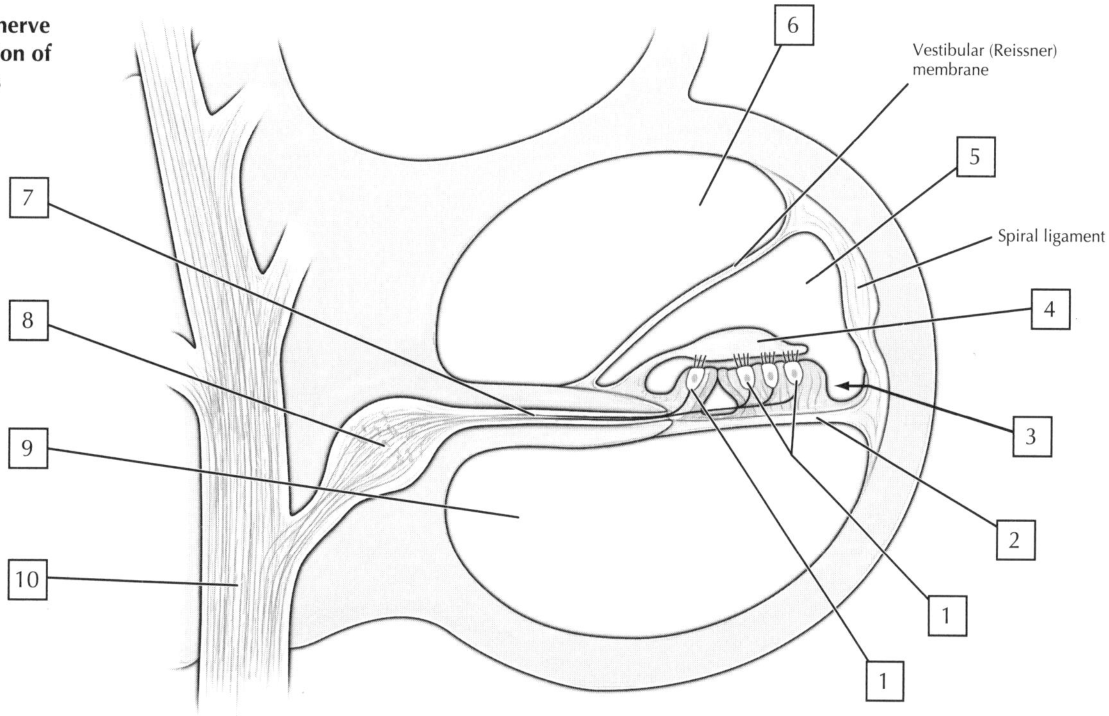

B. Mechanisms of sound transduction

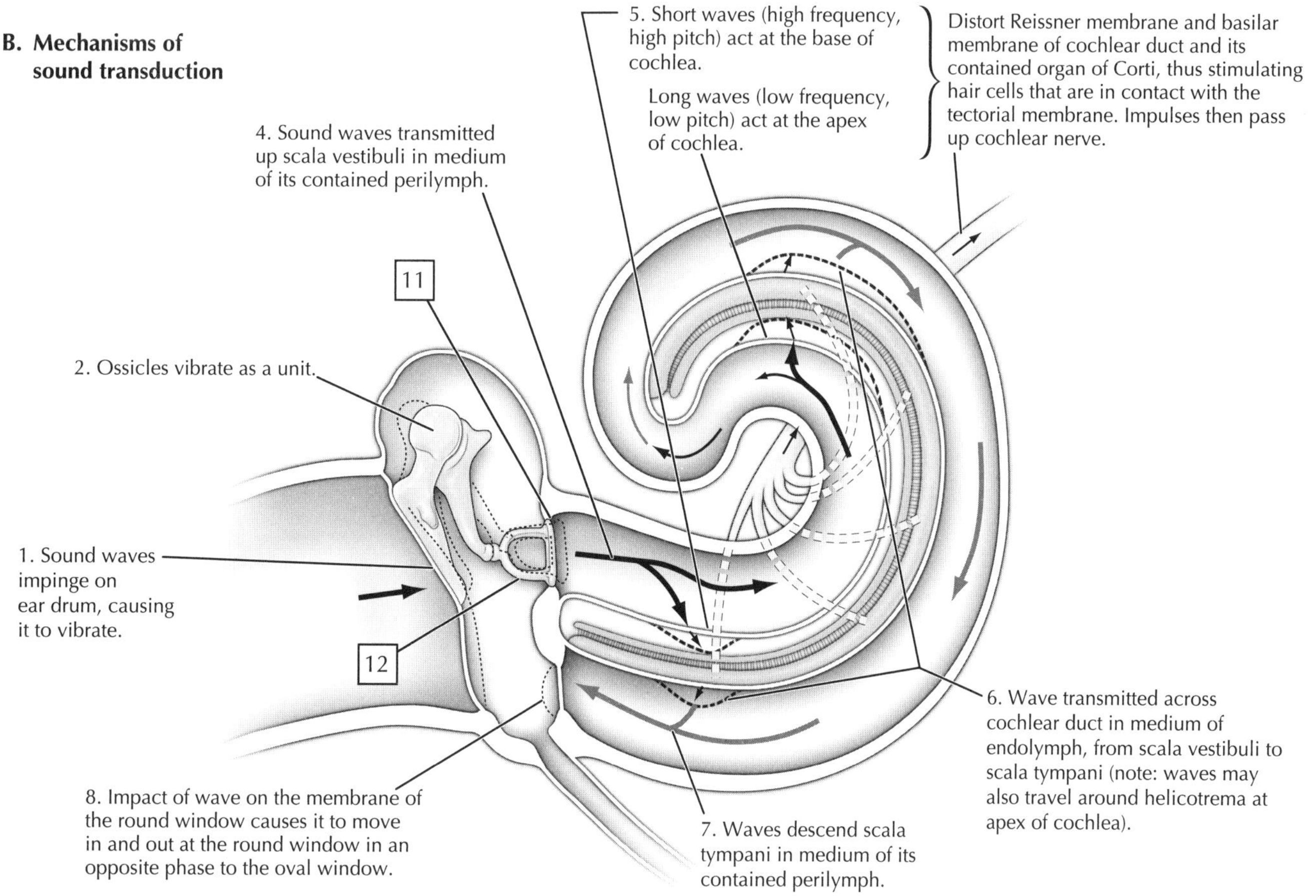

9 Central Auditory Pathways

Primary sensory neurons of the **spiral (auditory) ganglion**, when stimulated by neurotransmitters from specific **hair cells in the organ of Corti**, send their tonotopic (frequency-specific) information into the caudal pons of the brainstem, where the axons terminate in the **dorsal and ventral cochlear nuclei**. There are at least three tonotopic maps of the auditory world represented in the cochlear nuclei. The cochlear nuclei send axons into the **lateral lemniscus**, both ipsilateral and contralateral, through the **acoustic stria** (dorsal, intermediate, and ventral stria, **trapezoid body**). These axons of the cochlear nuclei terminate in the **nucleus of the inferior colliculus**, which in turn projects axons via the **brachium of the inferior colliculus** to the **medial geniculate nucleus (body) of the thalamus**. The medial geniculate nucleus sends tonotopic maps of the auditory world through the auditory radiations to the **transverse gyrus of Heschl** on the edge of the temporal lobe at the lateral fissure. Primary auditory cortex sends projections to association auditory cortex, and then via dorsal and ventral pathways that connect with the prefrontal cortex. The dorsal pathway travels through the inferior parietal lobule and conveys information about sound localization and movement. The ventral pathway travels through the temporal lobe and conveys information about identification and meaning of sound.

The lateral lemniscus also sends axons bilaterally to a host of brainstem nuclei, including the **superior olivary complex (nuclei)**, the nuclei of the lateral lemniscus, and the nuclei of the trapezoid body for additional processing of features of audition. The superior olivary complex helps to localize sound in space, which respond to the timing of a stimulus on hair cells on each side.

Sound is represented bilaterally at all levels through the central auditory afferent pathway. A unilateral lesion of the lateral lemniscus, medial geniculate nucleus, auditory radiations, and the auditory cortex will not produce contralateral deafness but diminished hearing with contralateral neglect to simultaneous auditory stimuli presented bilaterally.

The auditory system also has centrifugal connections, by which auditory structures can modulate the processing at more caudal levels. A specialized part of the centrifugal pathways is the olivocochlear bundle, projections from the superior olivary nuclear complex to the cochlea. This structure can modulate the auditory flow through the hair cells, thus focusing on specific frequencies of sound. This is an advantage when trying to localize and evaluate sound from a specific site or direction. It is sometimes called the "cocktail party" phenomenon, whereby one can focus on comments being made by a single individual among a crowd of conversing people.

COLOR the following structures, using a separate color for each structure.

- ☐ **1. Medial geniculate nucleus (body) of the thalamus**
- ☐ **2. Brachium of the inferior colliculus**
- ☐ **3. Nucleus of the inferior colliculus**
- ☐ **4. Lateral lemniscus**
- ☐ **5. Superior olivary complex (nuclei)**
- ☐ **6. Acoustic stria**
- ☐ **7. Trapezoid body**
- ☐ **8. Ventral cochlear nucleus**
- ☐ **9. Dorsal cochlear nucleus**
- ☐ **10. Transverse gyrus of Heschl in the temporal lobe**
- ☐ **11. Spiral (auditory) ganglion**
- ☐ **12. Hair cells in the organ of Corti**

Clinical Note

The auditory nerve is susceptible to damage from trauma (e.g., to the petrous portion of the temporal bone), tumors (e.g., an acoustic Schwannoma), infections, and other causes. The hair cells and auditory nerve also can be damaged by irritative lesions (endolymph pressure on hair cells in Meniere disease), which can produce tinnitus (a sense of ringing, buzzing, clicking, or annoying noises in the ear). With progressive damage, the irritative process can lead to a destructive lesion of hair cells, producing deafness as the tinnitus diminishes. An acoustic Schwannoma, often starting on the vestibular portion of CN VIII, can initially irritate the auditory apparatus, producing tinnitus, accompanying the vestibular symptoms of vertigo, dizziness, nystagmus, and balance problems. As the tumor further encroaches on the auditory nerve, continuing loss of hearing occurs. Often, these encapsulated, noncancerous tumors can be removed surgically, with restoration of some or all of the VIII nerve damage.

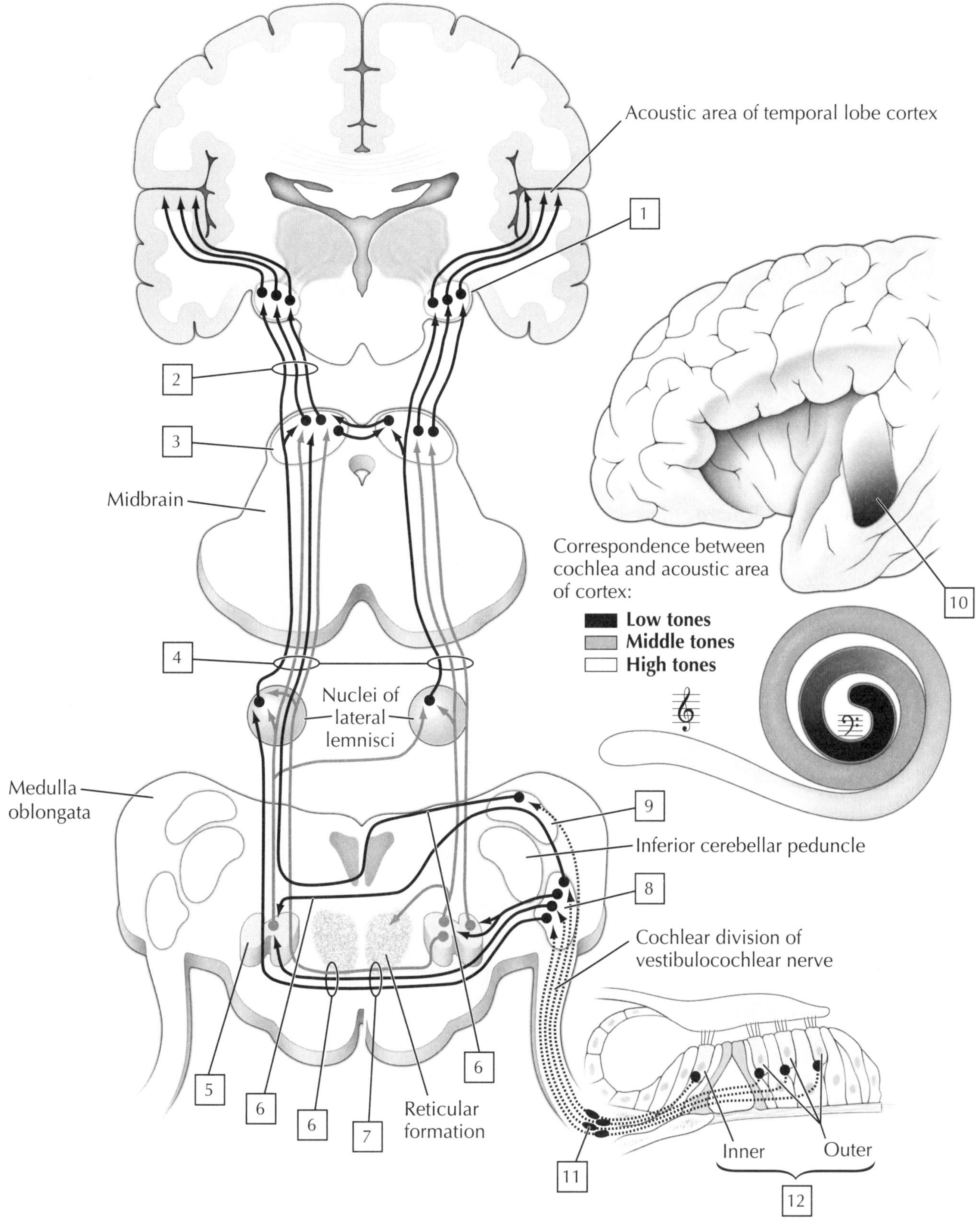
Acoustic area of temporal lobe cortex
1
2
3
Midbrain
4
Nuclei of lateral lemnisci
Medulla oblongata
9
Inferior cerebellar peduncle
8
Cochlear division of vestibulocochlear nerve
5
6
6
6
7
6
Reticular formation
Correspondence between cochlea and acoustic area of cortex:
Low tones
Middle tones
High tones
10
Inner
Outer
11
12

9 Vestibular Receptors

The vestibular receptors are hair cells, located in the **cristae within the ampullae of the semicircular canals** (angular acceleration or movement), the **utricle** (linear acceleration or gravity), and the **saccule** (linear acceleration and low-frequency vibration). Hair cells of the utricle and saccule have very **slowly adapting or nonadapting** responses; they are continuously active. The utricle is the site of response during **lateral tilt** of the head, and the saccule is the site of response during **head flexion and extension**. The three semicircular canals **(superior, horizontal, posterior)** are oriented orthogonally to each other. The **hair cells (type I and type II)** in the cristae within the ampullae sit on a basement membrane, with **hairs protruding from the apical surface**, consisting of one single **kinocilium** and several stereocilia. The hairs are embedded in a **gelatinous cupula**, which moves with fluid movement in the semicircular canal. Bending of the kinocilium results in depolarization of the hair cell, releasing neurotransmitter(s) from the cell, which stimulates the **primary sensory nerve endings of the vestibular primary sensory bipolar axons of the vestibular ganglion (Scarpa ganglion)**. The hair cells in the macula of the utricle and saccule are embedded in a gelatinous cupula, on top of which is an otolithic membrane. Small calcium carbonate crystals, called **otoconia**, sit on the membrane. They register the direction of gravity through pressure on the kinocilium of the hair cells.

COLOR the following structures, using a separate color for each structure.

- ☐ 1. **Saccule**
- ☐ 2. **Utricle**
- ☐ 3. **Superior semicircular canal**
- ☐ 4. **Horizontal semicircular canal**
- ☐ 5. **Posterior semicircular canal**
- ☐ 6. **Cristae within the ampullae of the semicircular canal**
- ☐ 7. **Gelatinous cupula**
- ☐ 8. **Otoconia**
- ☐ 9. **Hair cells type I and II**
- ☐ 10. **Kinocilium**
- ☐ 11. **Hairs protruding from the apical surface of hair cells**
- ☐ 12. **Primary sensory bipolar axons of the vestibular ganglion (Scarpa ganglion)**

Clinical Note

The vestibular and auditory systems can be damaged by increased endolymphatic pressure that gradually destroys hair cells in both systems. This process is called **Meniere's disease.** It presents clinically as abrupt episodes of severe vertigo that can last for many hours and are incapacitating. Nausea and vomiting occur during these attacks. Accompanying the vestibular symptoms are the auditory symptoms of tinnitus and progressive sensorineural deafness (hair cell destruction). This process is usually unilateral but can become bilateral. This process can proceed to total deafness and severe ongoing vertigo and vestibular dysfunction. In some cases, remission may occur.

A. Membranous labyrinth

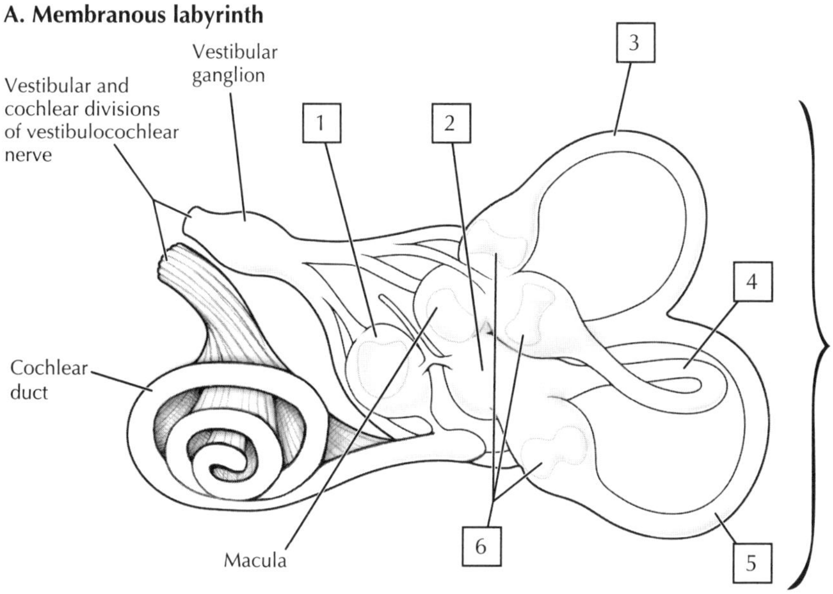

B. Position within base of skull

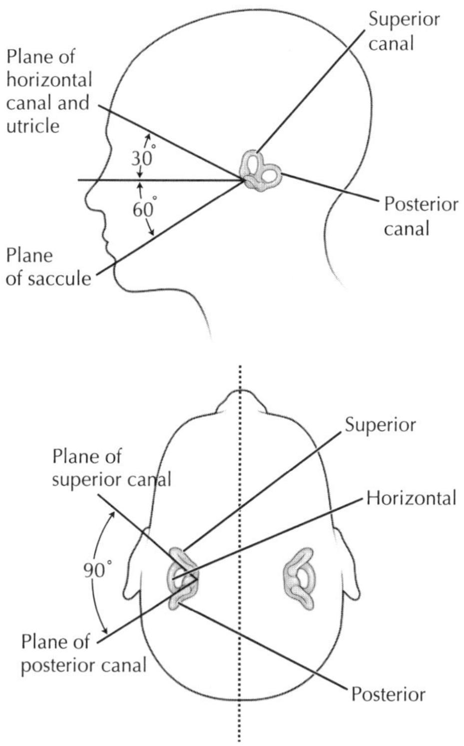

C. Section of crista

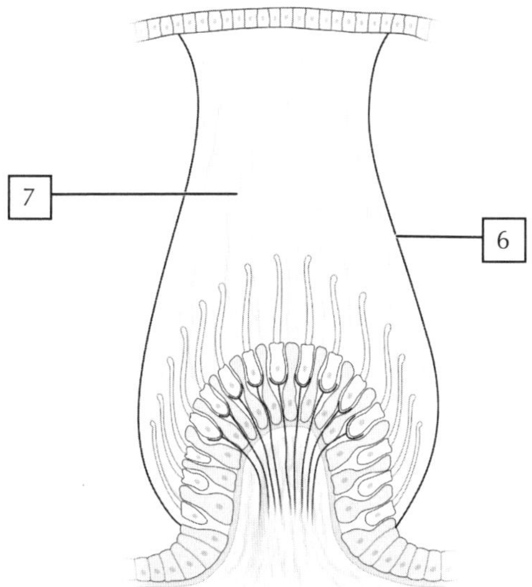

D. Section of macula

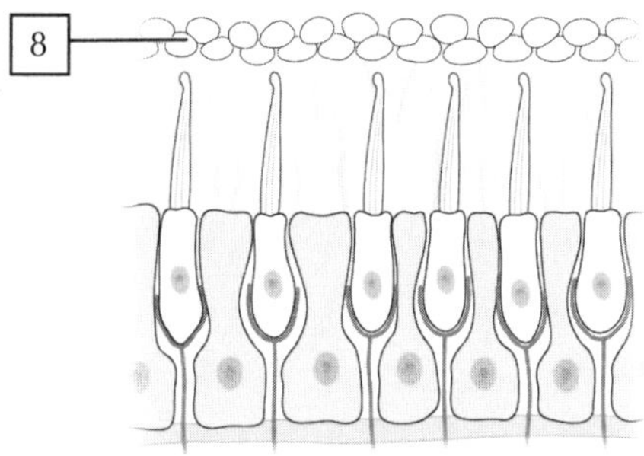

E. Structure and innervation of hair cells

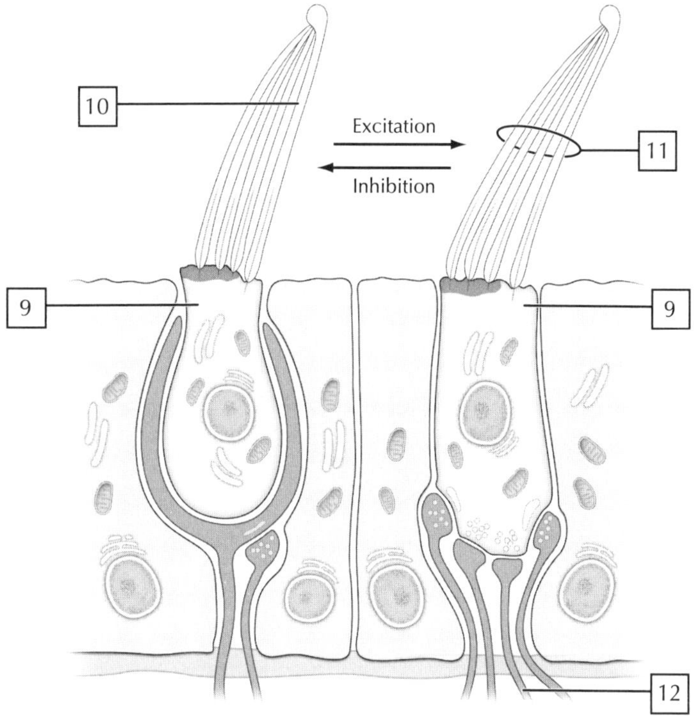

9 Central Vestibular Pathways

Hair cell stimulation in the **cristae of the ampullae of the semicircular canals**, and the **maculae of the utricle and saccule**, results in neurotransmitter release and activation of vestibular axons of the primary sensory **bipolar neurons of the vestibular ganglion**. Axons of vestibular primary sensory neurons enter the CNS and terminate in the four **vestibular nuclei (superior, medial, lateral, and inferior)** and the **cerebellum** (deep nuclei and cerebellar cortex of the vermis and flocculonodular lobe, called the vestibulocerebellum). The vestibular nuclei send projections to the lower motor neurons (LMNs) of the spinal cord, via the lateral and medial vestibulospinal tracts, to the extraocular nuclei, via the **medial longitudinal fasciculus (MLF)**, to the cerebellum, and to the reticular formation.

The **lateral vestibulospinal tract** (derived from the lateral vestibular nucleus) projects to all levels of the spinal cord and provides powerful antigravity activation of extensor LMNs, mainly through their associated interneurons. The **medial vestibulospinal tract** (derived from the medial vestibular nucleus) projects to cervical LMNs (mainly through associated interneurons) and regulates head and neck movements in response to vestibular changes. Multiple vestibular nuclei project to the vestibulocerebellum and modulate coordination of basic tone and posture, especially involving trunk musculature. Multiple vestibular nuclei project to the extraocular nuclei through the MLF and help to coordinate eye movement with head and neck movements. Thus the vestibular system provides interactive coordination of head and neck movements, eye movements, and body tone and posture in response to gravity and movement. Some projections from the vestibular nuclei may reach neurons in the thalamus near the posterior nuclei and the VPM nucleus. Some vestibular-related projections from the thalamus may reach area 2 of the lateral postcentral gyrus (for regulation of motion perception and spatial orientation), the insular cortex, and the parieto-temporal cortex.

COLOR the following structures, using a separate color for each structure.

- ☐ 1. **Medial longitudinal fasciculus (MLF)**
- ☐ 2. **Superior vestibular nucleus**
- ☐ 3. **Medial vestibular nucleus**
- ☐ 4. **Lateral vestibular nucleus**
- ☐ 5. **Inferior vestibular nucleus**
- ☐ 6. **Primary sensory vestibular projections to the vestibulocerebellum**
- ☐ 7. **Bipolar neurons of the vestibular ganglion**
- ☐ 8. **Cristae of the ampullae of the semicircular canals**
- ☐ 9. **Maculae of the utricle and saccule**
- ☐ 10. **Lateral vestibulospinal tract**
- ☐ 11. **Medial vestibulospinal tract**

Clinical Note

The vestibular system is a powerful driving force for antigravity muscle activity to permit the extensor musculature to strongly support the body and to allow basic tone and posture that are necessary for behavioral activity and survival. If one wants to achieve fine, skilled movements, which are mainly flexor movements driven by volitional corticospinal activity, it is necessary to provide temporary inhibition of some of the extensor drive. If the cerebral cortex (corticospinal system) and red nucleus (rubrospinal system) are removed from influencing the vestibular nuclei (as occurs with progressive increased intracranial pressure that damages the forebrain and midbrain), then the vestibular nuclei operate without inhibition. As a consequence, the lateral vestibulospinal system powerfully drives extension of all four limbs (called decerebrate rigidity, more properly spasticity) and neck extension (called opisthotonus). Selective damage in the MLF, a common occurrence in the demyelinating disease of multiple sclerosis, results in internuclear ophthalmoplegia, a disorder of conjugate lateral gaze. Adduction is impaired on the side of the MLF lesion, and attempted lateral gaze produces diplopia.

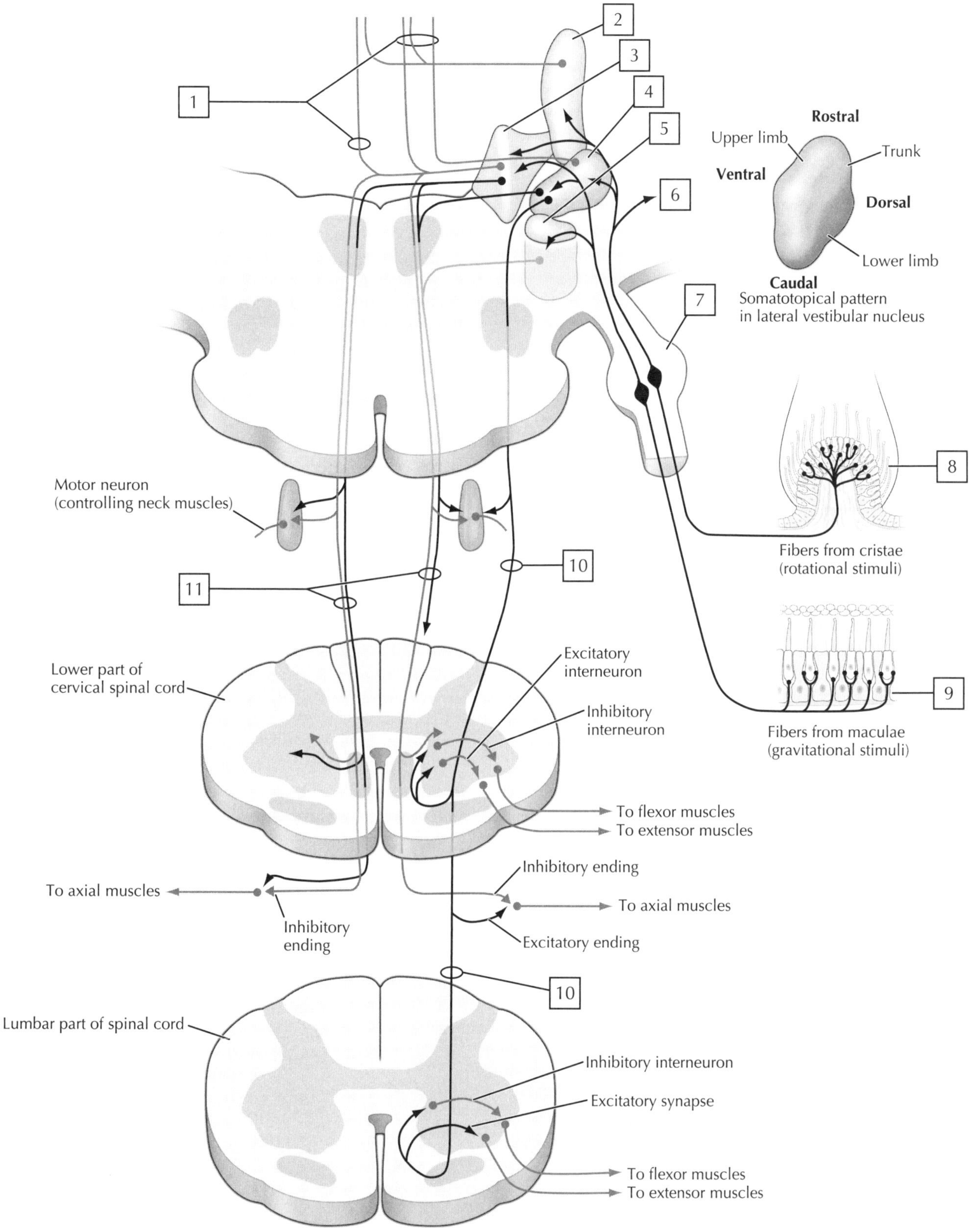

1
2
3
4
5
6
Rostral
Upper limb
Trunk
Ventral
Dorsal
Lower limb
Caudal
Somatotopical pattern in lateral vestibular nucleus
7
8
Fibers from cristae (rotational stimuli)
9
Fibers from maculae (gravitational stimuli)
Motor neuron (controlling neck muscles)
10
11
Lower part of cervical spinal cord
Excitatory interneuron
Inhibitory interneuron
To flexor muscles
To extensor muscles
Inhibitory ending
To axial muscles
To axial muscles
Inhibitory ending
Excitatory ending
10
Lumbar part of spinal cord
Inhibitory interneuron
Excitatory synapse
To flexor muscles
To extensor muscles

9 Anatomy of the Eye

The eye consists of three layers, sometimes called tunics. The outer layer is a tough, fibrous protective layer. The largest portion is the opaque **sclera,** continuous posteriorly with the outer sheath of the optic nerve. The smaller anterior portion is the transparent **cornea,** which provides a majority (90%) of the refraction of light.

The middle vascular layer, sometimes called the uveal tract, consists of the **choroid**, the **ciliary body** from which the **lens** is suspended, and the **iris**. The choroid is the vascular component of the posterior portion of the eye. The ciliary body consists of meridional and circular ciliary muscle fibers, and the ciliary process from which the transparent lens is suspended by the **zonular fibers**. The iris is the contractile anterior portion of the vascular layer and contains the **pupillary dilator muscle** and the **pupillary constrictor muscle**.

The inner layer is made up of the **neuroretina**, the nonpigmented epithelium of the ciliary body, and the pigmented epithelium of the iris. The neuroretina contains photoreceptors (rods and cones) that permit the transduction of light into neural signals, and several neuronal cell types that process the information for transmission into other central structures for further visual processing. The neuroretina is a CNS structure, and its vasculature is CNS vasculature.

Aqueous humor is secreted from the vasculature of the iris into the **posterior chamber** and flows through the aperture of the pupil into the **anterior chamber**. The aqueous humor is absorbed through the **canals of Schlemm** at the **iridocorneal angle** into the venous drainage of the eye. The gelatinous **vitreous humor**, secreted by nonpigmented epithelial cells of the ciliary body, fills the interior of the eyeball, providing support for the spherical structure of the eye.

Ideally, refraction of light coming into the eye will focus directly on the retina. Refractive errors can result in the light focusing either in front of the retina (in the interior of the eye), or behind the retina. **Myopia** (**nearsightedness**) occurs when light is focused in front of the retina; this may occur when the eye is elongated from front to back. Near vision is clear and far vision is blurry. Myopia is present in approximately 42% of the U.S. population. Correction of myopia can be accomplished through the use of concave lenses. **Hyperopia** (**farsightedness**) is when light is focused behind the retina; this may occur when the eye is shortened from front to back. Far vision is clear and near vision is blurry, or sometimes all vision is blurry. Hyperopia is present in 5% to 10% of the population, and often is diagnosed in childhood. Correction of hyperopia can be accomplished through the use of convex lenses. **Astigmatism** is an imperfection in the eye's curvature, with uneven contours; it can be treated with corrective lenses or with **LASIK** treatment. LASIK is a laser-based reshaping of the cornea, used for correction of myopia, hyperopia, and astigmatism. It can have side effect, such as glare, halos, and overshoot and undershoot, with continuing refraction errors.

COLOR the following structures, using a separate color for each structure.

- ☐ **1. Sclera**
- ☐ **2. Choroid**
- ☐ **3. Neuroretina**
- ☐ **4. Ciliary body**
- ☐ **5. Zonular fibers**
- ☐ **6. Canals of Schlemm at the iridocorneal angle**
- ☐ **7. Iris**
- ☐ **8. Lens**
- ☐ **9. Cornea**
- ☐ **10. Anterior chamber**
- ☐ **11. Posterior chamber**
- ☐ **12. Vitreous humor**

Clinical Note

As light enters the eye, it is refracted to permit the visual images to focus on the retina. The cornea provides a majority of the refraction of the incoming light, but it is a fixed structure that cannot be neurally regulated. The lens, suspended by the zonular fibers from the ciliary process, also provides a smaller portion (10%) of light refraction, but can be regulated by the tension on the lens capsule by ciliary muscle fibers, innervated by the parasympathetic portion of CN III (oculomotor nerve). Accommodation for near vision is accomplished by the activity of the nucleus of Edinger–Westphal (EW) via CN III to the ciliary ganglion, whose axons travel in the short ciliary nerves and supply myelinated axons to both the ciliary muscle and the pupillary constrictor muscle. When the ciliary muscle contracts, it lifts the ciliary body upward and inward, releasing tension on the zonular capsular fibers, resulting in the bunching of the lens for greater refraction of light. Accommodation for near vision diminishes with age, called **presbyopia**, due to a loss of elasticity of the lens for accommodation for near vision, and may require refractive lenses to aid in properly focusing light on the retina. Both the cornea and the lens can become opacified, clouding or blocking the visual image impinging on the retina.

A **cataract** is a blurring or clouding of the lens, interfering with clear vision. Cataracts that interfere with vision usually can be surgically corrected. A lens with cataracts can be replaced with a high-tech toric lens that allows clear near and far vision, eliminating the need for glasses with corrective lens or for contact lenses.

Horizontal section

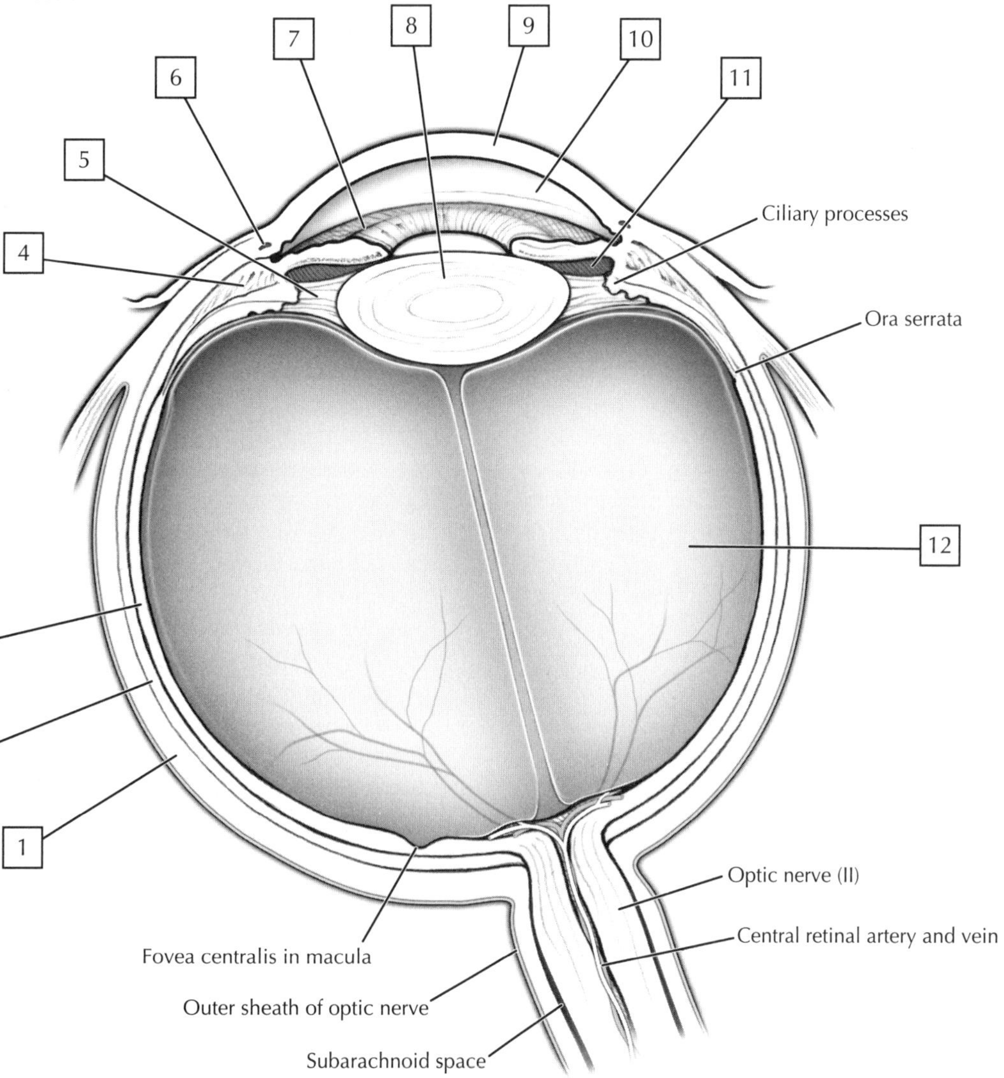

Anterior and Posterior Chambers of the Eye

The CNS can regulate both the refraction of light through the **lens** and the size of the pupillary aperture through the parasympathetic control from CN III (oculomotor) via the nucleus of EW, and its preganglionic axonal connections with the **ciliary ganglion** whose myelinated axons subsequently bring about contraction of the ciliary muscle. When the **ciliary muscle** contracts, both **meridional fibers** and **circular fibers** pull the **ciliary body** and its **ciliary process** up and in. Consequently, tension on the **zonular fibers** is reduced, and the lens becomes more convex or "fattens," permitting greater refraction of light. The ciliary ganglion also provides control over the aperture of the pupil, along with the sympathetic **superior cervical ganglion**. The ciliary ganglion activates the **pupillary constrictor muscle**, constricting the pupil. The superior cervical ganglion activates the **pupillary dilator muscle**, dilating the pupil. In a condition known as closed-angle glaucoma, the dilation of the pupil can be accompanied by blockage of absorption of the aqueous humor into the **canals of Schlemm (a venous sinus)** by physical obstruction from the **folds of the iris**. The aqueous humor is secreted from the vasculature of the iris into the **posterior chamber**, flows through the pupillary aperture into the **anterior chamber**, and is absorbed into the venous sinus (canals of Schlemm). This process of aqueous humor production and absorption is similar to the process of cerebrospinal fluid secretion and absorption; the production and absorption must be precisely balanced to keep the pressure appropriate and constant. Blockage of absorption of aqueous humor causes increased intraocular pressure in the eye, and blockage of absorption of cerebrospinal fluid causes increased intracranial pressure in the brain. The vitreous humor is secreted by the nonpigmented epithelial cells of the ciliary body into the posterior portion of the eye.

COLOR the following structures, using a separate color for each structure.

- ☐ **1. Canals of Schlemm (a venous sinus)**
- ☐ **2. Anterior chamber**
- ☐ **3. Folds of the iris**
- ☐ **4. Lens**
- ☐ **5. Pupillary constrictor muscle**
- ☐ **6. Pupillary dilator muscle**
- ☐ **7. Posterior chamber**
- ☐ **8. Zonular fibers**
- ☐ **9. Ciliary process**
- ☐ **10. Ciliary muscle circular fibers**
- ☐ **11. Ciliary muscle meridional fibers**
- ☐ **12. Ciliary body**

Clinical Note

The production and absorption of aqueous humor through the posterior chamber, anterior chamber, and the canals of Schlemm must be precisely matched. If absorption of aqueous humor is blocked, increased intraocular pressure occurs. Increased intraocular pressure can result in increased pressure on the optic nerve head, with atrophy and damaged vision; this damage can progressively increase to total blindness. Glaucoma is the most prevalent cause of optic nerve damage, especially with age; it is clinically detectable through ophthalmoscopy and tonometry. In wide-angle glaucoma (most common), the canals of Schlemm undergo a sclerotic process, obstructing absorption of aqueous humor. In narrow-angle glaucoma (acute or closed-angle), dilation of the pupil can cause obstruction of aqueous humor absorption by the bunched folds of the iris, precipitating a painful, swollen, red eye. This is an emergency situation that requires pharmacologically induced pupillary constriction.

A. Anterior and posterior chambers

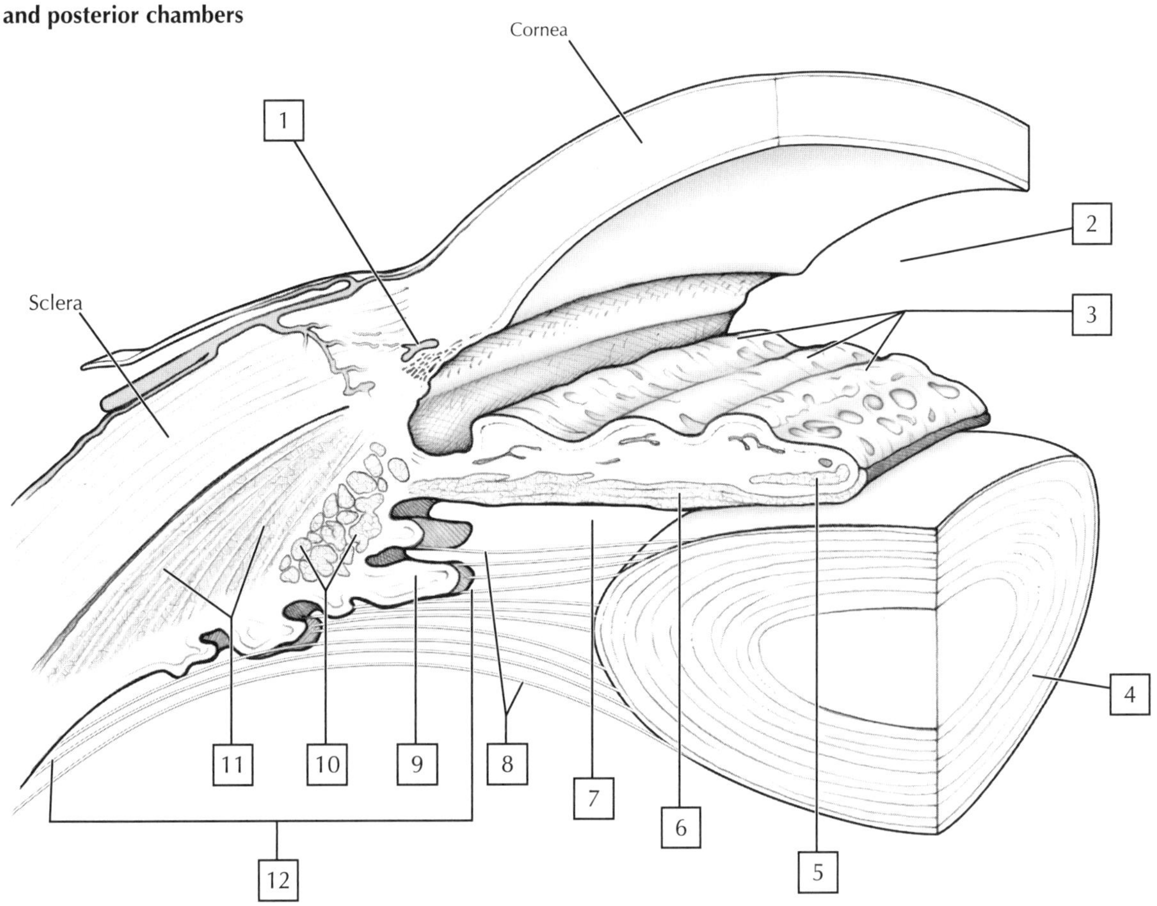

B. Lens and supporting structures

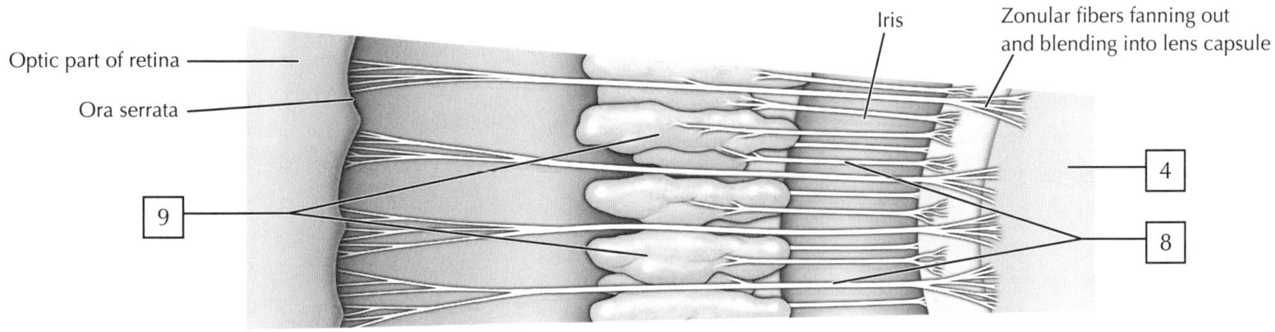

9 Retina: Retinal Layers

The retina is a thin layer of CNS tissue at the inner surface of the posterior eyeball, supplied with blood from the central retinal artery and arteries of the choroid. The retina contains the **photoreceptors (**120 million **rods** and 6–7 million **cones)** and other neuronal cell types. The cones transduce light for color vision and are concentrated in the central region for focused vision, the fovea centralis (0.4 mm) in the macula (3 mm). The rods transduce light for black-and-white vision and are present throughout the nonfoveal retina. When the photoreceptors transduce light into electrical messages, the information flows through the **bipolar cells** to the **ganglion cells.** The ganglion cells give rise to **axons, which travel in the optic nerve** and enter deeper portions of the CNS. **Horizontal cells** and **amacrine cells** assist in the horizontal flow of retinal information, and **Muller cells** provide glial support for the neurons. In the fovea centralis, for color vision (a region of only cones), there is close to a one-to-one association of cones with bipolar cells and then ganglion cells. In the periphery, there is enormous convergence of rods onto bipolar cells, which then converge onto a single ganglion cell. Therefore acuity is achieved through the fovea and macular region. In the periphery, the rods are highly sensitive to impinging light in the dark.

The rods transduce light into an electrical signal through use of a photopigment, **rhodopsin.** When light strikes the rod, it converts **all-*cis*-retinal** to **all-*trans*-retinal**. This process results in calcium influx into the rod, with a decrease in sodium conductance, resulting in hyperpolarization of the rod in the light. Retinal signal transduction involves extensive interaction of neuronal hyperpolarization and depolarization. Cones use **opsin photopigments** for blue, green, red, and all-***cis***-retinal. Photopigments are members of a large family of G-protein coupled receptors (a chain of 340–370 amino acids, embedded in a lipid membrane) that recognize specific wavelengths of light and transduce them into electrical signals to permit visual stimulation of the retinal photoreceptors.

There are three categories of cones: (1) S cones, which absorb blue light (short wavelength, hi-frequency); (2) L cones, which absorb red light (long wavelength, low-frequency); and (3) M cones, which absorb green light (intermediate wavelength and frequency, between blue and red). Bipolar neurons and ganglion cells in the retina are ON or OFF in their responsiveness to light, with horizontal cells acting to achieve lateral inhibition. There are two types of ganglion cells: (1) P cells—smaller cells responsible for reporting fine features and color for high visual acuity, ending on parvocellular neurons in the lateral geniculate nucleus (LGN); and (2) M cells—larger cells responsible for reporting movement and contrast of illumination, ending on magnocellular neurons in the LGN. Both types of ganglion cells are smaller close to the macula, compared with farther from the macula.

COLOR the following structures, using a separate color for each structure.

- ☐ 1. **Ganglion cell axons traveling in the optic nerve layer**
- ☐ 2. **Ganglion cells**
- ☐ 3. **Muller cells**
- ☐ 4. **Amacrine cells**
- ☐ 5. **Bipolar cells**
- ☐ 6. **Horizontal cells**
- ☐ 7. **Photoreceptors (rods)**
- ☐ 8. **Photoreceptors (cones)**
- ☐ 9. **Rhodopsin**
- ☐ 10. **All-*cis*-retinal**
- ☐ 11. **All-*trans*-retinal**

Clinical Note

The visual pathway from the macular region is essential for high-acuity (**photopic**) color vision. In old age, a common visual problem is **macular degeneration**, which results in gradual deterioration of high-acuity (central) vision, inability to read, and inability to interact with the environment. **Dry macular degeneration** (80%) is a degeneration or thinning of the retina, accompanied by "**drusen,**" visible with ophthalmoscopy as clumps of protein. **Wet macular degeneration** (20%) involves growth of abnormal blood vessels under the retina. These vessels cause leakage and scarring of the retina, with rapid loss of vision. The peripheral visual pathway, using high-convergence rods, is active in night vision (**scotopic**).

The retina is attached to the choroid at the **ora serrata**, in the zone adjacent to the nonpigmented epithelium of the ciliary body. If the retina separates from the choroid at the ora serrata, a **detached retina** may occur. This can result in distorted or impaired vision, as the tissue-paper-thin retina separates from part of its blood supply from the choroid. Retinal reattachment often is achieved through a laser procedure.

A. Retinal layers and connectivity

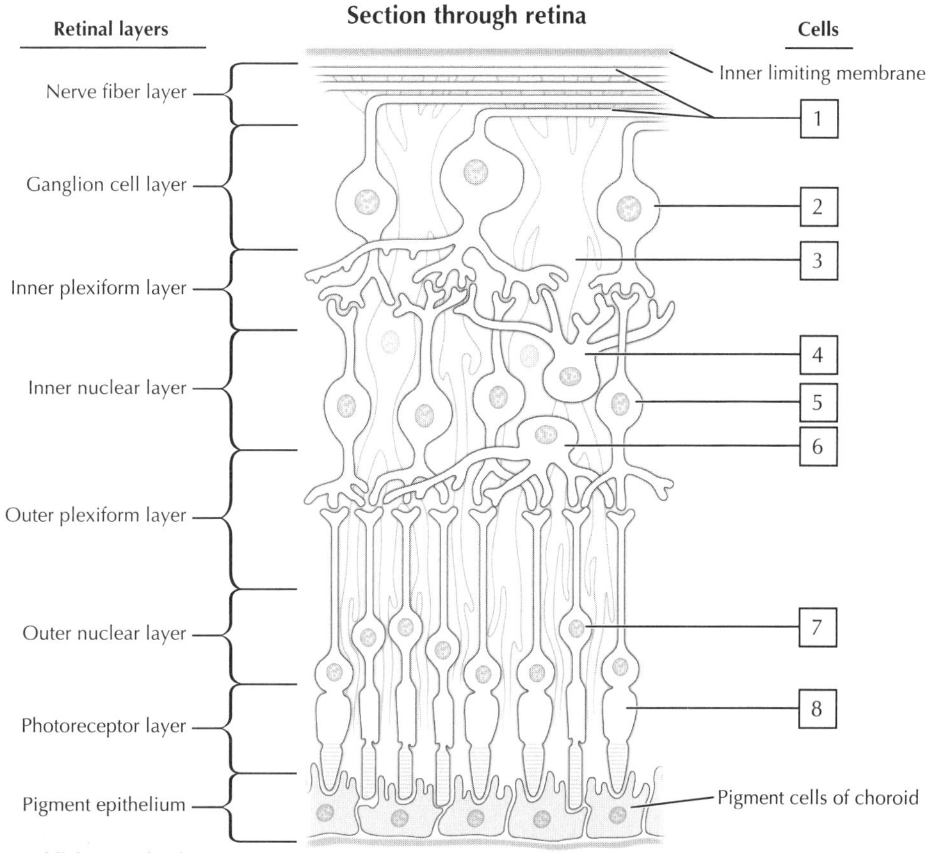

B. Rod and cone structures and light transduction

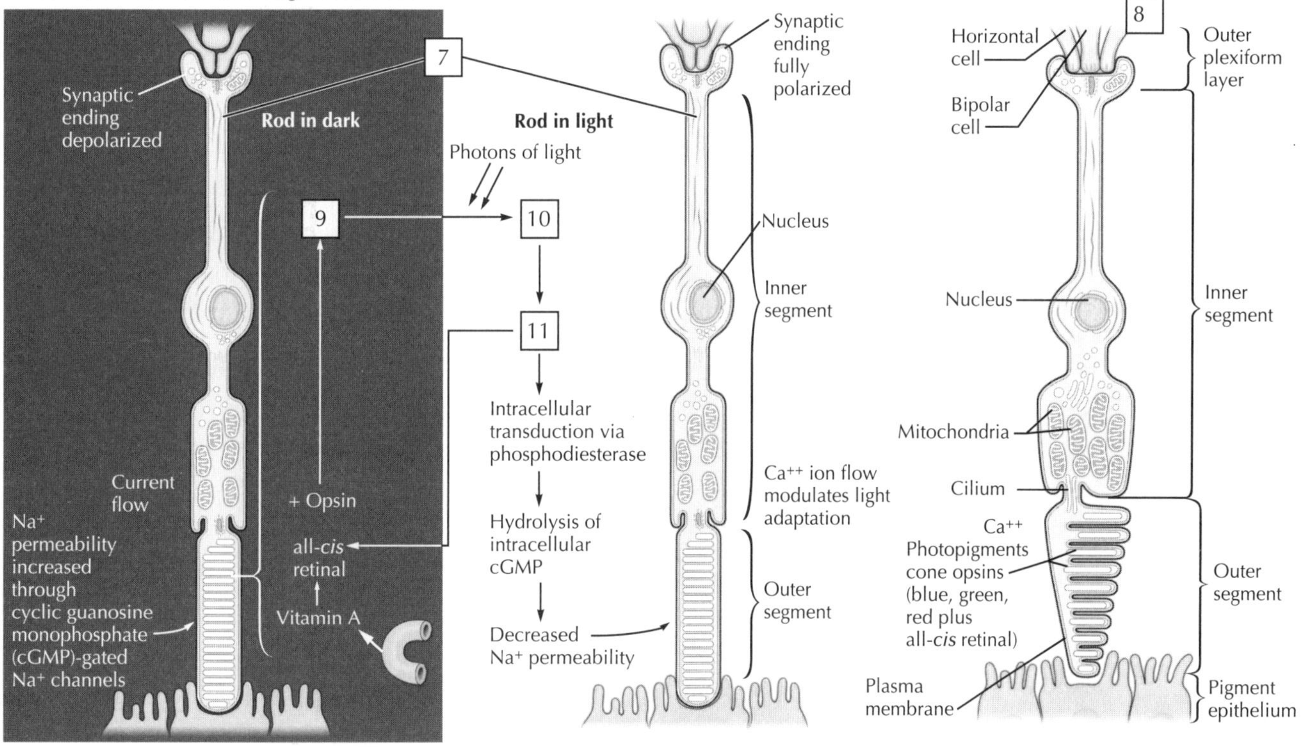

9 Anatomy and Relationships of the Optic Chiasm

The retinal ganglion cells of each retina send their axons into the ipsilateral **optic nerve**. The optic nerves come together at the **optic chiasm**, where the ganglion cell axons resort themselves. The axons carrying information from the **temporal (lateral) hemiretinas** continue ipsilaterally into the **optic tract**. The axons carrying information from the **nasal (medial) hemiretinas cross at the optic chiasm** and travel in the contralateral **optic tract**. Thus axons from the nasal hemiretina of one eye and the temporal hemiretina of the other eye travel together (congruently) in each optic tract, carrying visual images from the contralateral visual field (visual world). In the optic chiasm, the **inferior nasal ganglion cell axons cross in the anterior portion**, and the **superior nasal ganglion cell axons cross in the posterior portion**.

The ganglion cell axons terminate in many structures in the brain, but for the main interpretation of visual images, they synapse on thalamic specific projection neurons in **the lateral geniculate nucleus (body)** (LGN). The LGN neurons send axons into the **optic radiations**, which course posteriorly through temporal and occipital white matter, terminating in the **primary visual cortex** on the banks of the **calcarine fissure** in the occipital lobe.

COLOR the following structures, using a separate color for each structure.

- ☐ 1. **Temporal hemiretinas**
- ☐ 2. **Nasal hemiretinas**
- ☐ 3. **Optic nerve**
- ☐ 4. **Optic chiasm**
- ☐ 5. **Optic tract**
- ☐ 6. **Lateral geniculate nucleus (body)**
- ☐ 7. **Optic radiations**
- ☐ 8. **Primary visual cortex**
- ☐ 9. **Inferior nasal ganglion cell axons (crossing in the anterior portion of the optic chiasm)**
- ☐ 10. **Superior nasal ganglion cell axons (crossing in the posterior portion of the optic chiasm)**

Clinical Note

The ganglion cell axons traverse the optic nerve, the optic chiasm, and the optic tract. If the optic nerve is damaged (e.g., from a demyelinating lesion in multiple sclerosis called optic neuritis), all ganglion cell axons from the ipsilateral retina can be affected, resulting in **ipsilateral blindness**. If the optic chiasm is damaged (e.g., from a pituitary adenoma), the tumor encroaches on crossing fibers starting with damage to the crossing inferior nasal fibers, resulting in an **upper bitemporal quadrantanopia**. If the encroachment continues, it can damage all of the crossing fibers of the optic chiasm, resulting in a total **bitemporal hemianopia**. If the optic tract is damaged, the axons from the ipsilateral temporal hemiretina and from the contralateral nasal hemiretina are affected, resulting in a **contralateral hemianopia**.

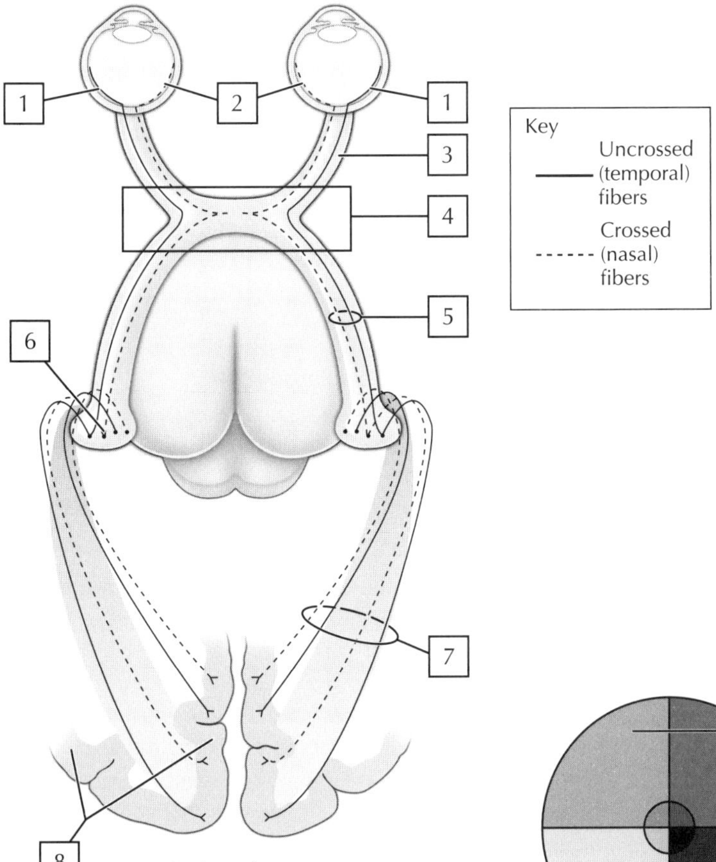

Optic pathway (superior view)

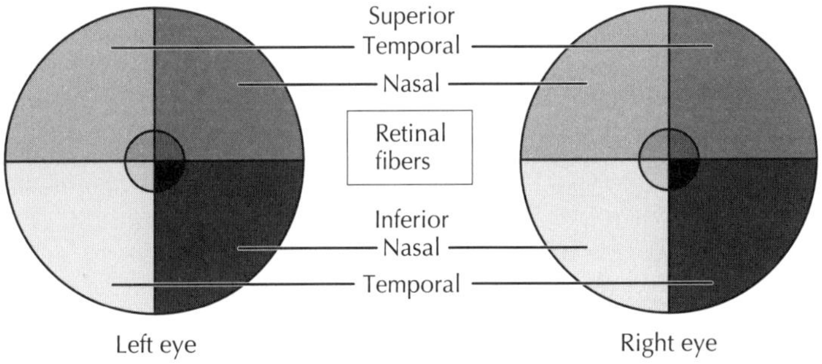

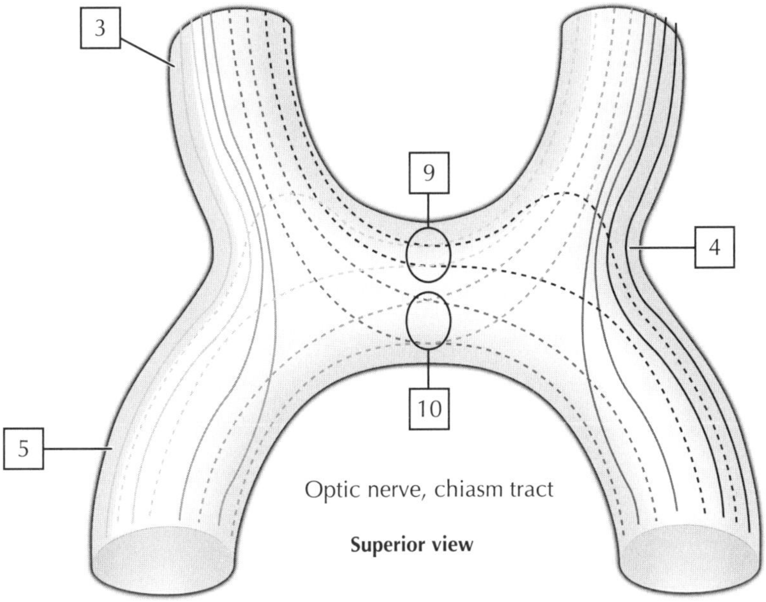

Optic nerve, chiasm tract

Superior view

9 Visual Pathways to the Thalamus, Hypothalamus, and Brainstem

Ganglion cell axons in each **optic tract** carry information about the contralateral visual field. These axons terminate in many CNS sites. The main visual pathway terminates in the **lateral geniculate nucleus (LGN)**, which is the thalamic portion of the **retino-geniculo-calcarine pathway** for the interpretation of the visual world. This pathway involves the LGN projections into the **optic radiations** to the **primary visual cortex (area 17)** on the banks of the calcarine fissure, also called the V1 cortex.

The ganglion cell axons also terminate in the upper layers of the **superior colliculus**, which projects to the **pulvinar** of the thalamus, whose neurons, in turn, sends axons to the **secondary (association) visual cortex, areas 18 and 19** also known as the V2 and V3 visual cortex. Some optic tract axons terminate directly in the pulvinar. This is a second visual pathway and is involved in localization of objects in space as well as tracking responses, helping to move the eyes to novel or moving stimuli. The superior colliculus also gives rise to the **tectospinal tract,** which provides visual input to LMNs in the cervical region for head and neck movements in response to moving visual stimuli. The superior colliculus receives substantial ipsilateral input from the primary visual cortex. The superior colliculus also sends projections into the **brainstem reticular formation.**

Retinal ganglion cell axons terminate in the hypothalamus in the **suprachiasmatic nucleus** and provide daylight information to the hypothalamus related to control of circadian rhythms and diurnal cycles; the suprachiasmatic nucleus connects with parvocellular neurons of the paraventricular nucleus of the hypothalamus, which projects to the sympathetic preganglionic neurons of the T1–T2 spinal cord for sympathetic control of melatonin synthesis and release in the pineal gland. Loss of this input disrupts these cycles and rhythms. Retinal ganglion cell axons also terminate in the **pretectum,** providing visual information used for initiating the pupillary light reflex. The ganglion cell axons also terminate in the **nucleus of the inferior accessory optic tract** and may assist in brainstem responses for visual tracking and connect with the preganglionic sympathetic neurons in T1 and T2 of the intermediolateral cell column for regulation of the superior cervical ganglion and its influences on the production of melatonin by the pineal gland supplied by sympathetic fibers. Some parvocellular neurons of the paraventricular nucleus of the hypothalamus also project directly to T1 and T2 via the median forebrain bundle and the lateral brainstem tegmentum.

COLOR the following structures, using a separate color for each structure.

- ☐ 1. **Optic radiations**
- ☐ 2. **Optic tract**
- ☐ 3. **Suprachiasmatic nucleus of the hypothalamus**
- ☐ 4. **Lateral geniculate nucleus (LGN)**
- ☐ 5. **Nucleus of the inferior accessory optic tract**
- ☐ 6. **Superior colliculus**
- ☐ 7. **Pretectum**
- ☐ 8. **Pulvinar**
- ☐ 9. **Brainstem reticular formation**
- ☐ 10. **Tectospinal tract**

Clinical Note

The influx of light to the brain is an important contributor to appropriate regulation of circadian rhythms and diurnal cycles. It was previously thought that rhythms such as cyclic production of cortisol during the 24-hour day were innate rhythms built into the architecture of the hypothalamus. However, human experiments in which individuals lived for months in caves, with no outside or ambient daylight, demonstrated that some of these rhythms had cycles other than 24 hours. It appears that light impinging on the organism, through projections to the suprachiasmatic nucleus of the hypothalamus, entrains these rhythms to 24-hour cycles. Melatonin produced by the pineal gland is a hormone related to sleep, also entrained by light exposure. Air travel through multiple time zones produces "jet lag," which may require many days in the new site to normalize the disrupted rhythms and cycles. Some travelers take melatonin supplements in an attempt to alleviate the effects of jet lag.

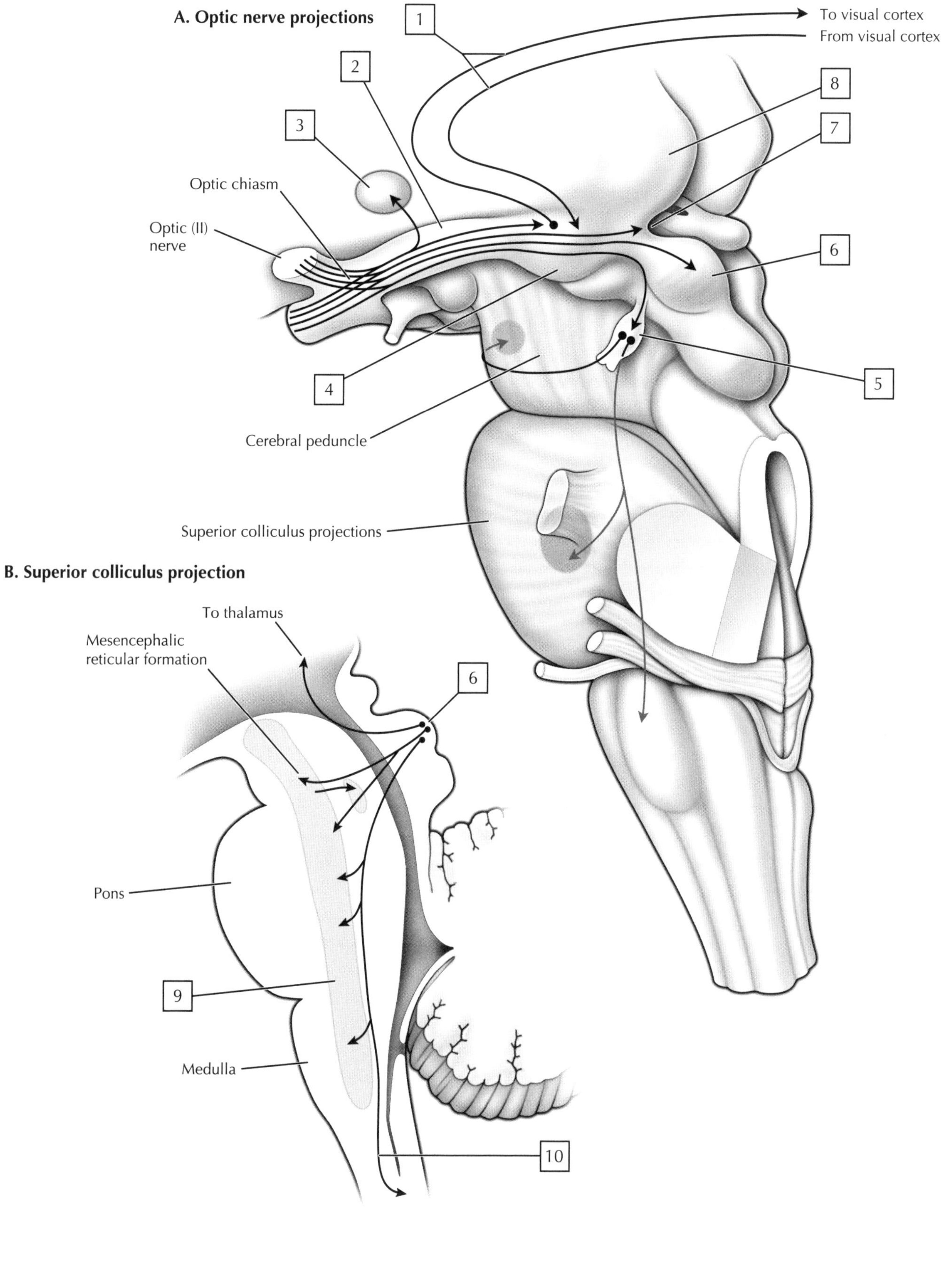
A. Optic nerve projections
1
To visual cortex
From visual cortex
2
8
3
7
Optic chiasm
Optic (II) nerve
6
5
4
Cerebral peduncle
Superior colliculus projections
B. Superior colliculus projection
To thalamus
Mesencephalic reticular formation
6
Pons
9
Medulla
10

9 Pupillary Light Reflex

The pupillary light reflex is a visual system reflex that produces bilateral pupillary constriction when light is shown in either eye. This reflex requires CN II (optic), CN III (oculomotor), and brainstem structures. The afferent limb of the reflex is the **retinal ganglion cell axonal projections in the optic nerve**, **chiasm**, and **tract**. These axons terminate in the **pretectum** on both sides (located rostral to the superior colliculus, in the rostral midbrain). The pretectum projects bilaterally to the parasympathetic component of CN III, the **nucleus of Edinger-Westphal (EW)** in the midbrain. Light shone in either eye activates the nucleus of EW on both sides. The efferent limb of the pupillary light reflex is the projections from neurons in the nucleus of EW via **CN III** to the **ciliary ganglion,** which sends its myelinated postganglionic parasympathetic axons via **short ciliary nerves** to the **pupillary sphincter (constrictor) muscle** to constrict both pupils. The postganglionic sympathetic fibers from the superior cervical ganglion innervate the pupillary dilator muscle, which can potentially counteract pupillary constriction in dark conditions when a large pupillary aperture is needed.

COLOR the following structures, using a separate color for each structure.

- ☐ 1. **Optic nerve**
- ☐ 2. **Optic chiasm**
- ☐ 3. **Optic tract**
- ☐ 4. **Nucleus of Edinger–Westphal (EW)**
- ☐ 5. **Pretectum**
- ☐ 6. **CN III (Oculomotor nerve)**
- ☐ 7. **Ciliary ganglion**
- ☐ 8. **Short ciliary nerves**
- ☐ 9. **Pupillary sphincter (constrictor) muscle**

Clinical Note

The pupillary light reflex is a very important reflex in neurology, showing the status of CN II and CN III, and indicating potential pathology in the CNS such as increased intracranial pressure. If the optic nerve is damaged on one side (e.g., demyelinating lesion in multiple sclerosis), then light shone in the affected eye will elicit no response (no constriction) in either eye (afferent pathway is damaged). If the light is shone in the unaffected eye, both pupils will constrict, including the pupil on the side with CN II damage. Damage to CN III (e.g., pressure on the oculomotor nerve as it exits the midbrain due to increased intracranial pressure that presses CN III against the free edge of the tentorium cerebelli) will result in a fixed, dilated pupil on the affected side that will not respond to light shone in either eye (efferent pathway is damaged). The pupil is fixed and dilated due to the unopposed actions of the sympathetics on the pupillary dilator muscle. The pupil on the unaffected side will constrict with light shone in either eye. Following a head injury, pupillary light reflexes are tested frequently to check for the potential of increased intracranial pressure from bleeding or swelling (edema), which can precipitate rapid brain herniation and deterioration of brain function.

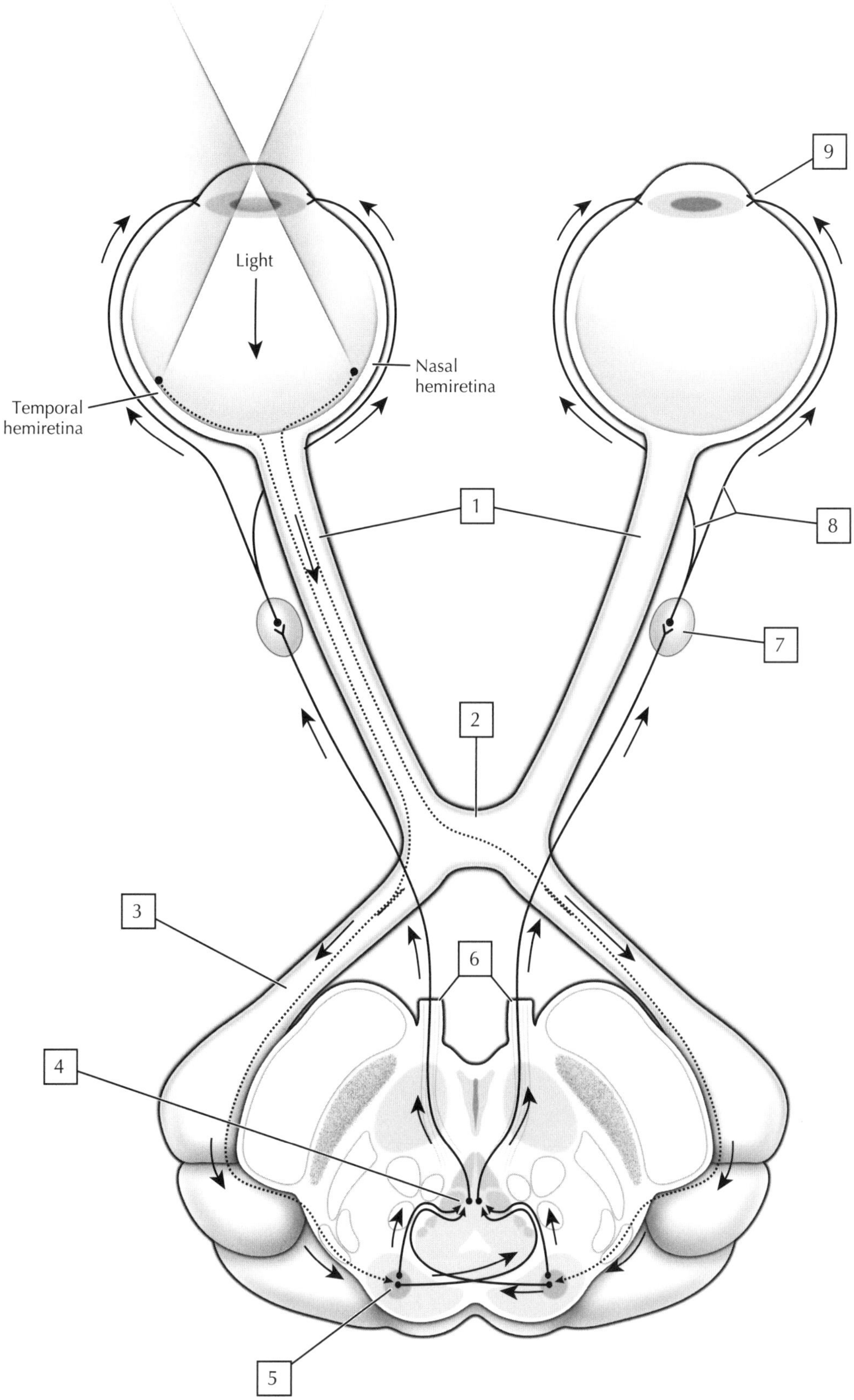
Light
Nasal hemiretina
Temporal hemiretina
1
2
3
4
5
6
7
8
9

9 Visual Pathway: The Retino-Geniculo-Calcarine Pathway

The ganglion cell axons from the retina distribute through the **optic nerve**, **optic chiasm**, and **optic tract**. The ganglion cell axons from the **temporal hemiretinas** continue ipsilaterally through the optic nerve and chiasm into the optic tract. The ganglion cell axons from the **nasal hemiretinas** cross in the optic chiasm and travel in the contralateral optic tract. As a consequence, projections from the nasal hemiretina of one side and the temporal hemiretina of the other side travel together in the optic tract; each optic tract carries information from congruent regions of the contralateral visual field. These axons terminate in the **lateral geniculate nucleus (LGN)**. Projections from the LGN neurons course through the white matter of the temporal lobe and occipital lobe as **optic radiations** and terminate in the **primary visual cortex** on the banks of the calcarine fissure in the occipital lobe. The portion of the optic radiations that course deepest into the temporal lobe is called **Meyer's loop** and represents information from the contralateral upper visual quadrant. Bilateral convergence (from congruent portions of both retinas) does not occur until the level of the primary visual cortex.

COLOR the following structures, using a separate color for each structure.

- ☐ 1. **Nasal hemiretinas**
- ☐ 2. **Optic nerve**
- ☐ 3. **Optic chiasm**
- ☐ 4. **Temporal hemiretinas**
- ☐ 5. **Optic tract**
- ☐ 6. **Lateral geniculate nucleus (LGN)**
- ☐ 7. **Meyer's loop in the temporal lobe**
- ☐ 8. **Optic radiations**
- ☐ 9. **Primary visual cortex**

Clinical Note

Damage to structures in the retino-geniculo-calcarine pathway, used for visual interpretation of the outside world produces classic pathology, reflecting the topographical organization of this entire pathway (called retinotopic organization). Damage to the optic nerve produces ipsilateral blindness. Damage to the optic chiasm results in bitemporal hemianopia, starting in the upper visual field and proceeding downward (likened to pulling down a shade on either side). Damage to the optic tract or the LGN produces contralateral hemianopia. Damage to Meyer's loop in the temporal lobe (mainly occurring because of a temporal lobe tumor or abscess) produces an upper contralateral quadrantanopia. Damage to the primary visual cortex on one side produces contralateral hemianopia, sometimes with macular sparing. Damage to the visual cortex on both sides (from a contrecoup injury due to head trauma) produces cortical blindness.

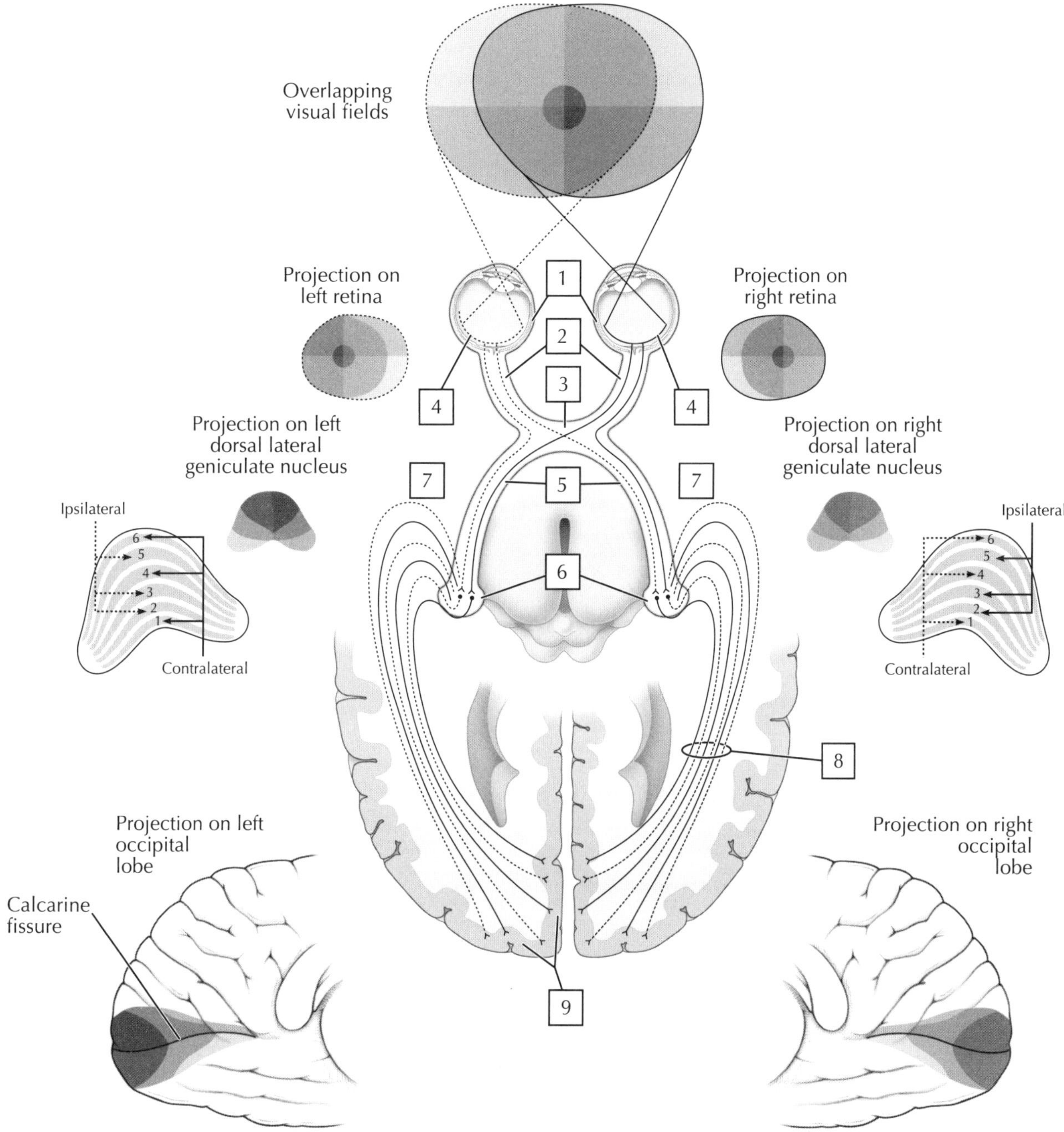

Overlapping visual fields
Projection on left retina
Projection on right retina
1
2
3
4
4
Projection on left dorsal lateral geniculate nucleus
Projection on right dorsal lateral geniculate nucleus
7
5
7
Ipsilateral
6
5
4
3
2
1
Contralateral
Ipsilateral
6
5
4
3
2
1
Contralateral
6
8
Projection on left occipital lobe
Projection on right occipital lobe
Calcarine fissure
9

Visual Pathways in the Parietal and Temporal Lobes

The projections of the retino-geniculo-calcarine pathway to the primary visual cortex are only the first step in conscious awareness and interpretation of objects in the visual world. The **primary visual cortex (area 17, or V1)** receives the visual information from the retina, begins the process of bilateral convergence of visual information, and initiates the first steps in evaluation of point sources of light and derived shapes, through simple, complex, and hypercomplex cortical cells, from which optimal convergent stimuli aid in the interpretation of points, lines, arcs, and more complex shapes. V1 projects information to the **association visual cortex (areas 18 and 19, V2 and V3)**, where further integration of information takes place. From the association visual cortex, further projections are sent to the **middle temporal area (MTA)**, whose neurons are direction selective and motion responsive. The MTA neurons send information to the **parietal lobe**, where spatial visual processing occurs related to motion and to the positional relationships among objects in the visual world. The association visual cortex also sends information to a region called **V4**, in the temporal lobe, where analysis of shape and color perception occurs. From V4, visual information continues into the **temporal lobe** as an **"object recognition pathway."** This region carries out high-resolution object recognition of faces, animate and inanimate objects, the orientation of objects, and classification of objects.

COLOR the following structures, using a separate color for each structure.

- ☐ 1. **Parietal lobe visual processing area**
- ☐ 2. **Middle temporal area (MTA)**
- ☐ 3. **Association visual cortex (areas 18 and 19, V2 and V3)**
- ☐ 4. **Primary visual cortex (area 17, V1)**
- ☐ 5. **Visual area V4**
- ☐ 6. **Temporal lobe region related to the object recognition pathway**

Clinical Note

Clinical observations of patients with discrete lesions in the temporal and parietal lobes have demonstrated visual deficits that go beyond hemianopias and quadrantanopias. Visual agnosias are a lack of recognition of objects in the visual field in the presence of intact visual acuity. Lesions in the occipitotemporal object recognition pathway for high resolution and form, especially in the mesial portion of the dominant hemisphere, can result in visual agnosias. Cortical color agnosias can occur with damage to V4 and subsequent occipital–temporal lobe regions. Discrete lesions in this occipital–temporal visual region (especially bilaterally) can result in facial agnosias, the inability to recognize a known individual's face (prosopagnosia), even though there is clear recognition of his/her voice. Some specific lesions in this occipital–temporal visual region may produce an inability to distinguish animate from inanimate objects, or distinguish whether an object is properly oriented.

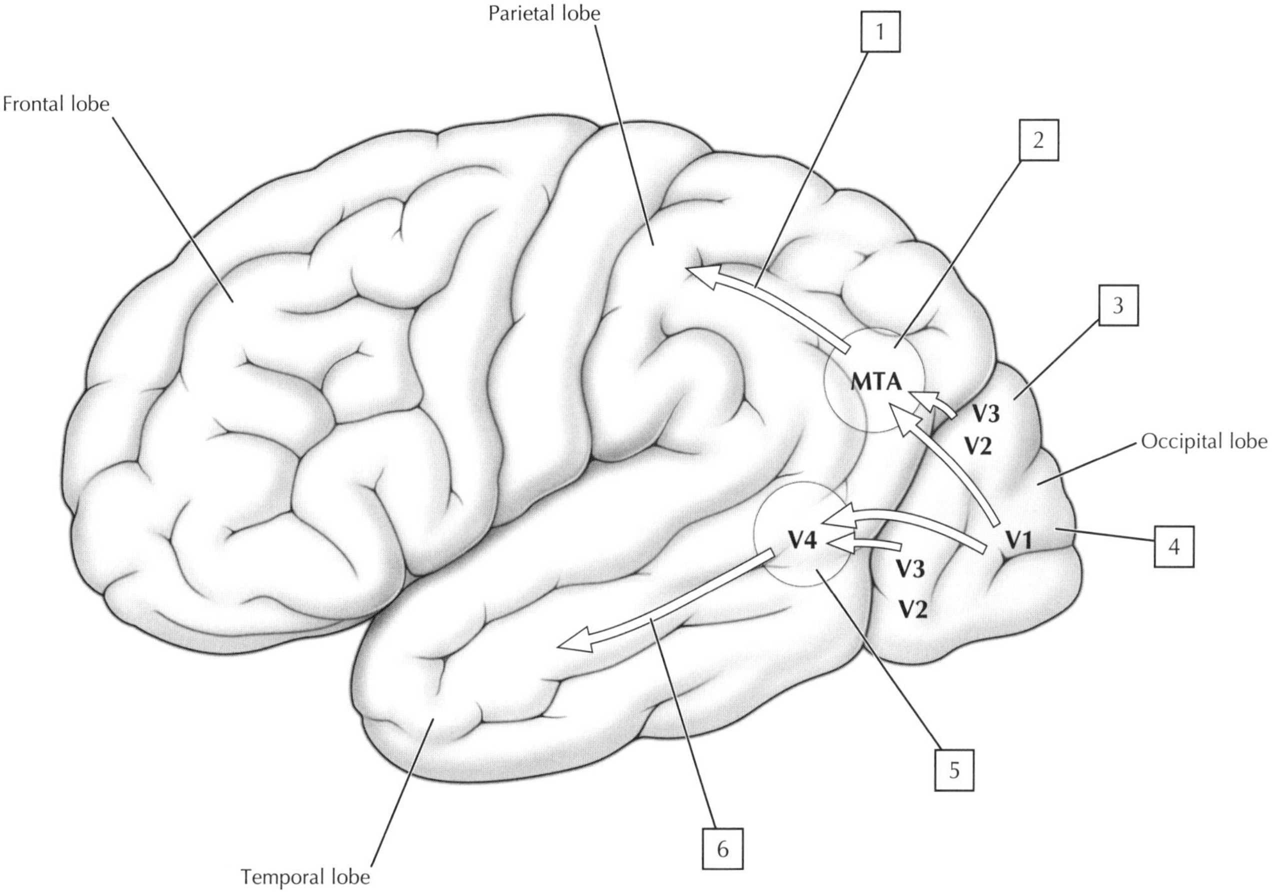
Parietal lobe
1
Frontal lobe
2
3
MTA
V3
V2
Occipital lobe
V4
V1
4
V3
V2
5
6
Temporal lobe

9 Visual System Lesions

This illustration provides a summary of the principle visual lesions in the retino-geniculo-calcarine pathway. It provides the reader with an exercise that tests understanding of the retinotopic organization in the key regions of the pathway.

COLOR the following structures and their lesions, using a separate color to indicate the site of the lesion.

- ☐ 1. **Optic nerve**
- ☐ 2. **Optic chiasm**
- ☐ 3. **Optic tract**
- ☐ 4. **Meyer's loop**
- ☐ 5. **Optic radiations (partial, medial portion)**
- ☐ 6. **Optic radiations (complete)**
- ☐ 7. **Occipital lobe lesion of the visual cortex**

Clinical Note

Homonymous hemianopia is the name given to a lesion from one half of the visual field that involves congruous portions of the visual field from the temporal hemiretina of one eye and the nasal hemiretina of the other eye. **Heteronymous hemianopia** is the name given to visual field lesions from noncongruent portions of the retina, such as optic chiasm lesions from a pituitary adenoma.

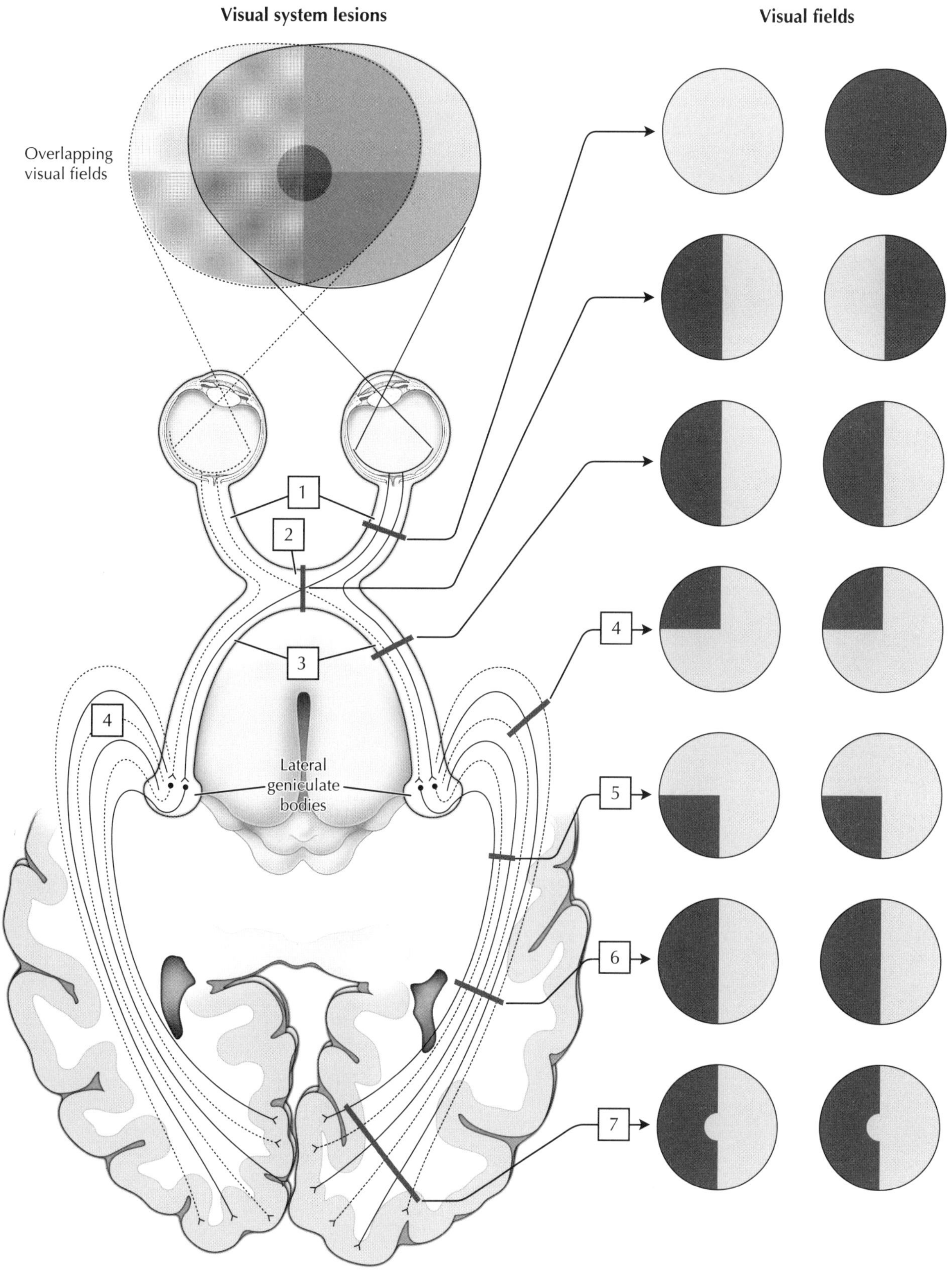
Visual system lesions
Visual fields
Overlapping visual fields
1
2
3
4
Lateral geniculate bodies
4
5
6
7

Chapter 10 Motor Systems

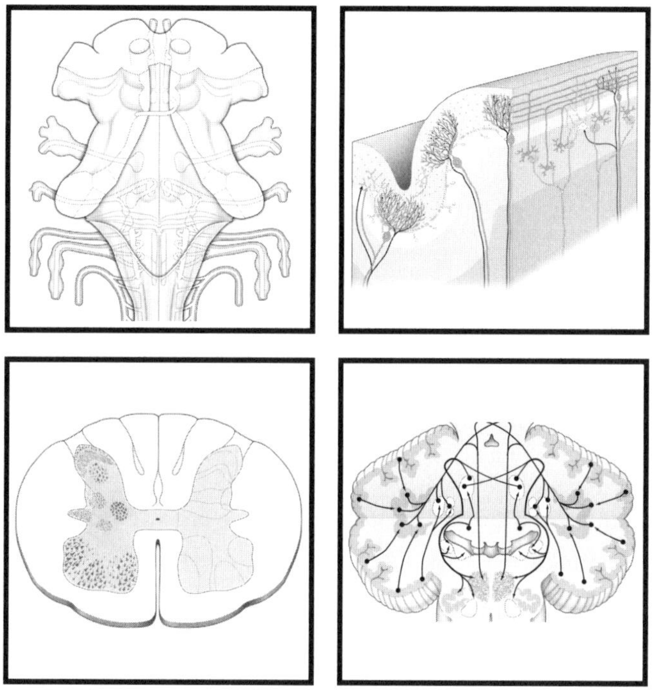

10 Alpha and Gamma Lower Motor Neurons

The starting point for all motor movement, behavior, and interactions with the environment is the **alpha lower motor neuron** (αLMN) and the group of skeletal muscle fibers (**extrafusal muscle fibers**) it supplies. This is called the motor unit. The αLMN uses acetylcholine (ACh) as its neurotransmitter at the motor end plate, **the neuromuscular junction**. Where fine motor control is needed (finger muscles, extraocular muscles), the motor units are small. Where strength is needed (quadriceps, gluteal muscles), the motor units are large. The αLMNs are found in the **anterior (ventral) horn of the spinal cord**. Embedded in the skeletal muscles and attached in parallel are the complex sensory/motor structures called **muscle spindles**. The muscle spindles possess central **nuclear bag fibers** and peripheral **nuclear chain fibers**, each possessing contractile components at the polar ends (**intrafusal muscle fibers**). These contractile elements are innervated by the **gamma LMNs (γLMN)**, which are also found in the anterior horn of the spinal cord, in proximity to the alpha LMNs. The γLMN ending on the bag fibers is a **plate ending**, and on the chain fibers is a **trail ending**. When the γLMNs fire action potentials, the muscle spindle contracts, putting tension on the nuclear bag and chain fibers.

Sensory fibers innervate the bag and chain fibers. The **Ia afferent fibers**, derived from cell bodies in the **dorsal root ganglia**, enwrap the equatorial region of the nuclear bag fibers with **annulospiral endings**; when activated, the Ia afferents report information on length and velocity (change in length with respect to time) into the central nervous system (CNS). This information is associated with reflex, cerebellar, and lemniscal channels. The reflex response occurs with Ia afferents entering through the dorsal root, traversing the **dorsal horn**, and **synapsing directly on the αLMNs** for the muscle fibers from which the muscle spindle was derived. This Ia activation results in contraction of the skeletal muscle fibers, restoring equilibrium. This response is known as the muscle stretch reflex, a hallmark of the neurological examination. The group II afferents form flower spray endings along the chain fibers, and report length information to the CNS, through cerebellar and lemniscal channels.

When brainstem and cortical upper motor neurons (UMNs) regulate αLMN activation, these UMN systems also simultaneously activate the γLMNs, a process known as α–γ coactivation. This ensures that the muscle spindle will always remain in its active state of sensory responsiveness through the Ia and group II afferents. Without this α-γ coactivation, the CNS would have no feedback on the state of motor activity.

COLOR the following structures, using a separate color for each structure.

- ☐ 1. **Dorsal horn**
- ☐ 2. **Ia afferent synapse on an alpha LMN**
- ☐ 3. **Dorsal root ganglion**
- ☐ 4. **Gamma lower motor neuron**
- ☐ 5. **Alpha lower motor neuron**
- ☐ 6. **Anterior horn of the spinal cord**
- ☐ 7. **Neuromuscular junction**
- ☐ 8. **Plate and trail endings**
- ☐ 9. **Nuclear bag fiber**
- ☐ 10. **Nuclear chain fiber**
- ☐ 11. **Annulospiral endings**
- ☐ 12. **Ia afferent fiber**

Clinical Note

The α and γ LMNs must have coordinated regulation from the UMNs to achieve optimal movement. Damage to or loss of αLMNs results in flaccid paralysis with loss of tone and reflexes. If remaining αLMNs sprout to reinnervate denuded skeletal muscle fibers, there will be abnormally large motor units, which occur frequently as a consequence of polio (postpolio syndrome). Damage to UMN systems will deprive the α and γ LMNs of their regulatory control, resulting in an abnormally strong and aberrant influence of sensory reflex connections and consequent spastic paresis, with hypertonus and hyperreflexia.

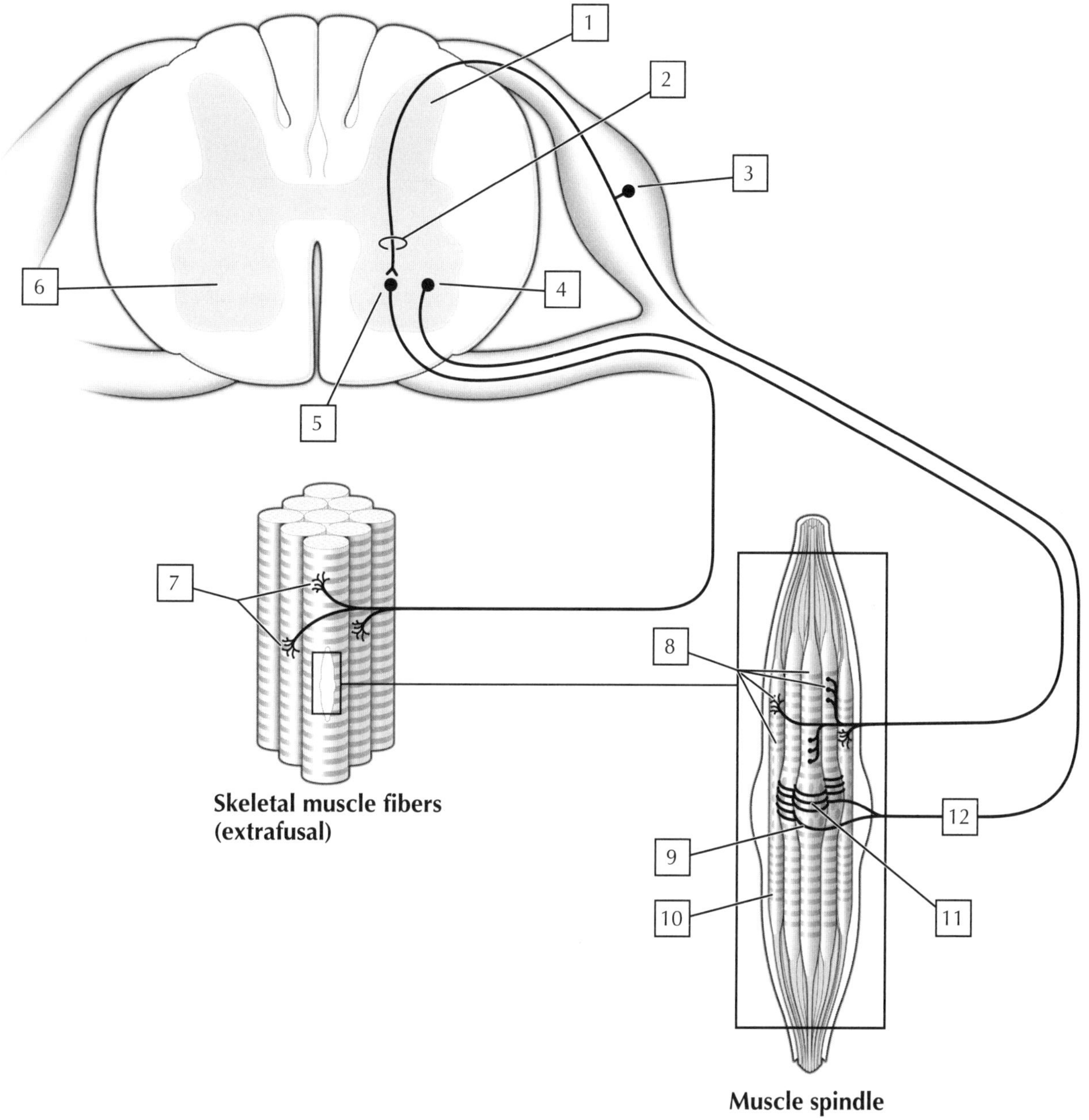
1
2
3
4
5
6
7
8
9
10
11
12
Skeletal muscle fibers (extrafusal)
Muscle spindle

10 Distribution of Lower Motor Neurons in the Spinal Cord

LMNs, both α and γ, are distributed in the **anterior (ventral) horn** of the spinal cord. The LMNs are topographically organized according to the spinal level associated with the skeletal muscle fibers innervated by the αLMNs, and also are distributed from medial to lateral for each spinal level: (1) distal limb muscles are supplied by **LMNs in the lateral part of the anterior horn**; (2) proximal limb muscles are supplied by **LMNs in the central part of the anterior horn**; and (3) trunk and neck muscles are supplied by **LMNs in the medial part of the anterior horn**. As an additional sorting of LMN location, **flexor LMNs** are found dorsally, and **extensor LMNs** are found ventrally, especially in the more lateral regions of the anterior horn. This organization is anatomically consistent with the location of the descending UMN systems. The lateral corticospinal tract and the rubrospinal tract descend in the **dorsolateral funiculus** and terminate in the more lateral portions of the anterior horn, where LMNs for distal musculature are found. The anterior corticospinal tract, the lateral vestibulospinal tract, and the reticulospinal tracts descend in the **anterior funiculus** and terminate in the more medial and central portions of the anterior horn, where LMNs for trunk and proximal muscles are found.

COLOR the following structures, using a separate color for each structure.

- ☐ **1. Dorsolateral funiculus**
- ☐ **2. Anterior horn of the spinal cord**
- ☐ **3. Anterior funiculus**
- ☐ **4. LMNs in the medial part of the anterior horn**
- ☐ **5. LMNs in the central part of the anterior horn**
- ☐ **6. LMNs in the lateral part of the anterior horn**
- ☐ **7. Site of extensor LMNs**
- ☐ **8. Site of flexor LMNs**

Clinical Note

The association of the αLMN with its associated skeletal muscle fibers must be robust and fully functional to achieve the desired behavior. If insufficient ACh is available to activate the muscle fibers at the neuromuscular junction, then the muscle may fail to contract because the muscle membrane response fails to reach threshold and fire the muscle action potential. This happens in myasthenia gravis, where autoantibodies block the nicotinic cholinergic receptors, leading to easy muscle fatiguability.

If released ACh is not rapidly hydrolyzed by acetylcholinesterase, ACh will continue to flood the neuromuscular junction, producing spasm and then a paralyzing block.

The LMN may demonstrate deterioration, either acutely because of a viral infection such as **polio** or other LMN disease, or gradually, as seen in **amyotrophic lateral sclerosis**, a disease characterized by combined LMN–UMN degenerative disease. With LMN deterioration, the LMN discharges may become aberrant and cause paroxysmal bursts of muscle fiber contraction, or twitching, seen visibly as **fasciculations**. These are called agonal bursts, as they signal a potential "death spiral" for the LMN. If the LMN actually dies, the associated muscle fibers will be denervated, will show denervation **atrophy**, will respond with small nonvisible membrane responses called **fibrillation** (detected electrophysiologically), and will ultimately demonstrate no power, no movement, no reflex responsiveness, and no tone.

A. Cytoarchitecture of the spinal cord gray matter

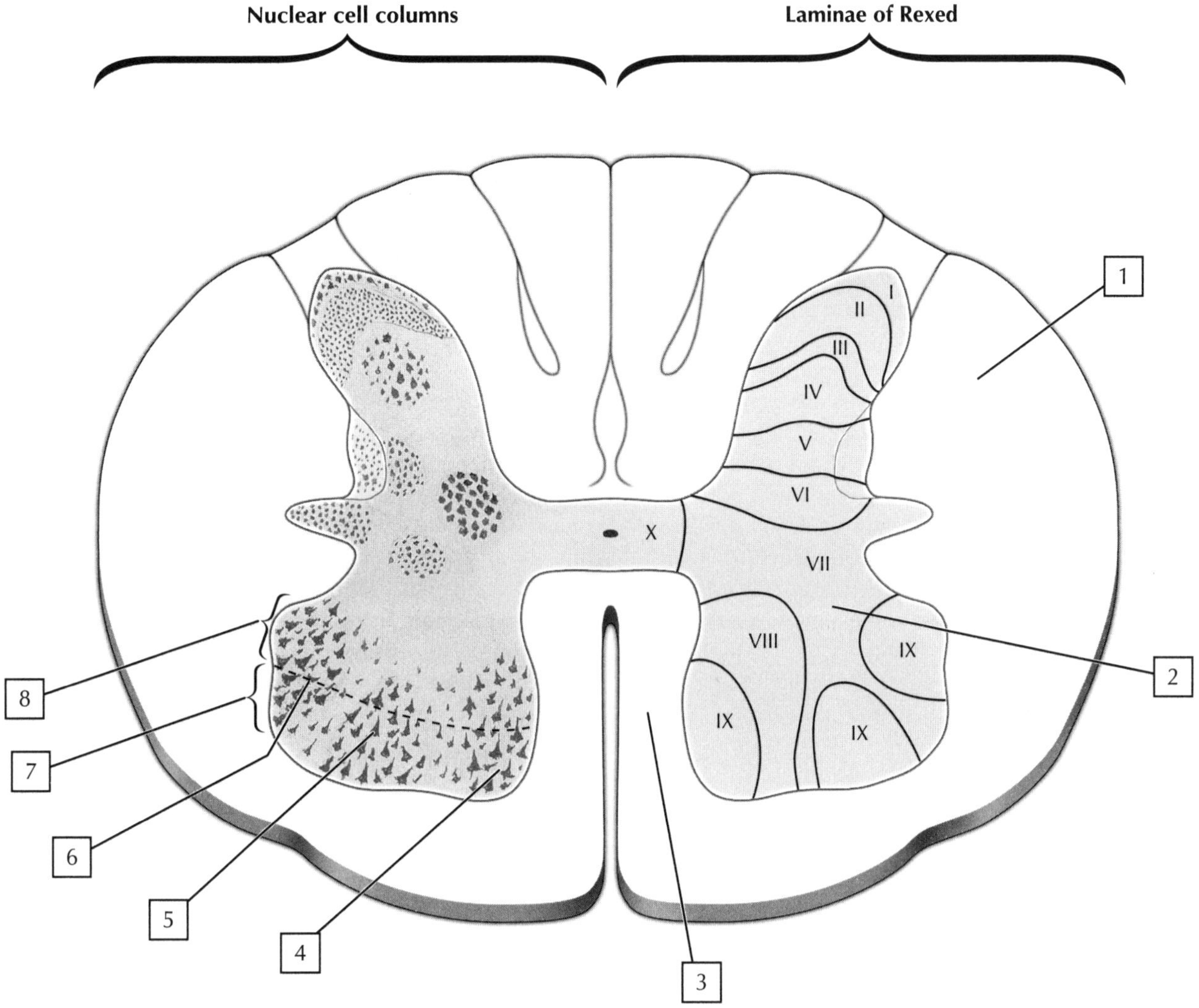

B. Representation of motor neurons

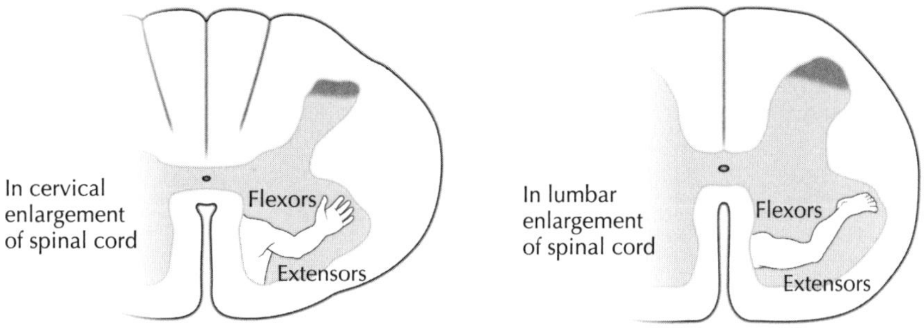

Distribution of Lower Motor Neurons in the Brainstem

The LMNs of the brainstem, normally described as the motor components of the cranial nerves (CNs), are found in the upper part of the cervical spinal cord, the medulla, the pons, and the midbrain. The LMNs are found in two longitudinal columns, both anatomically and embryologically. The medial column derives from the general somatic efferent system and includes the extraocular LMNs **(oculomotor, trochlear and abducens nuclei)** and the **hypoglossal nucleus.** The lateral column derives from the special visceral efferent system and includes the **trigeminal motor nucleus,** the **facial motor nucleus, nucleus ambiguus**, and the **spinal accessory nucleus**. These CN motor nuclei send their axons through CNS tissue, into the appropriate CN, and distribute to the associated skeletal muscle fibers in the head and neck. Not all of the CN motor nuclei receive inputs from muscle spindles, or have a γLMN counterpart. The trigeminal system has a primary Ia afferent "ganglion cell" system located within the CNS, the mesencephalic nucleus of V. This is the only primary sensory cell group found within the CNS. The Ia afferents are found mainly associated with the muscles of mastication (hence the existence of a testable jaw jerk reflex) and possibly with the extraocular muscles.

These LMN cell groups are under UMN regulation, similar to their spinal cord LMN counterparts. The brainstem LMN nuclei are particularly under the regulation of the corticobulbar tract, deriving from the lateralmost portion of the motor cortex and premotor cortex.

COLOR the following structures, using a separate color for each structure.

- ☐ **1. Oculomotor nucleus**
- ☐ **2. Trochlear nucleus**
- ☐ **3. Trigeminal motor nucleus**
- ☐ **4. Abducens nucleus**
- ☐ **5. Facial motor nucleus**
- ☐ **6. Nucleus ambiguus**
- ☐ **7. Hypoglossal nucleus**
- ☐ **8. Spinal accessory nucleus**

Clinical Note

The brainstem LMN cell groups are essential for survival. CNN III, IV, and VI are necessary for precise coordination of eye movements to allow a fine-grained analysis of the outside world through the visual system. A loss of binocular coordination can result in diplopia, vertigo, dizziness, and loss of coordinated activity. The trigeminal motor nucleus is necessary for mastication and food consumption (along with CNN XII and nucleus ambiguus). The facial nucleus regulates facial expression, an essential part of communication among individuals. Nucleus ambiguus is necessary for speaking and swallowing, and the hypoglossal nucleus aids in both processes. Because of their role in many important behavioral activities, they are closely regulated by the motor and premotor cortex on the lateral portion of the precentral gyrus.

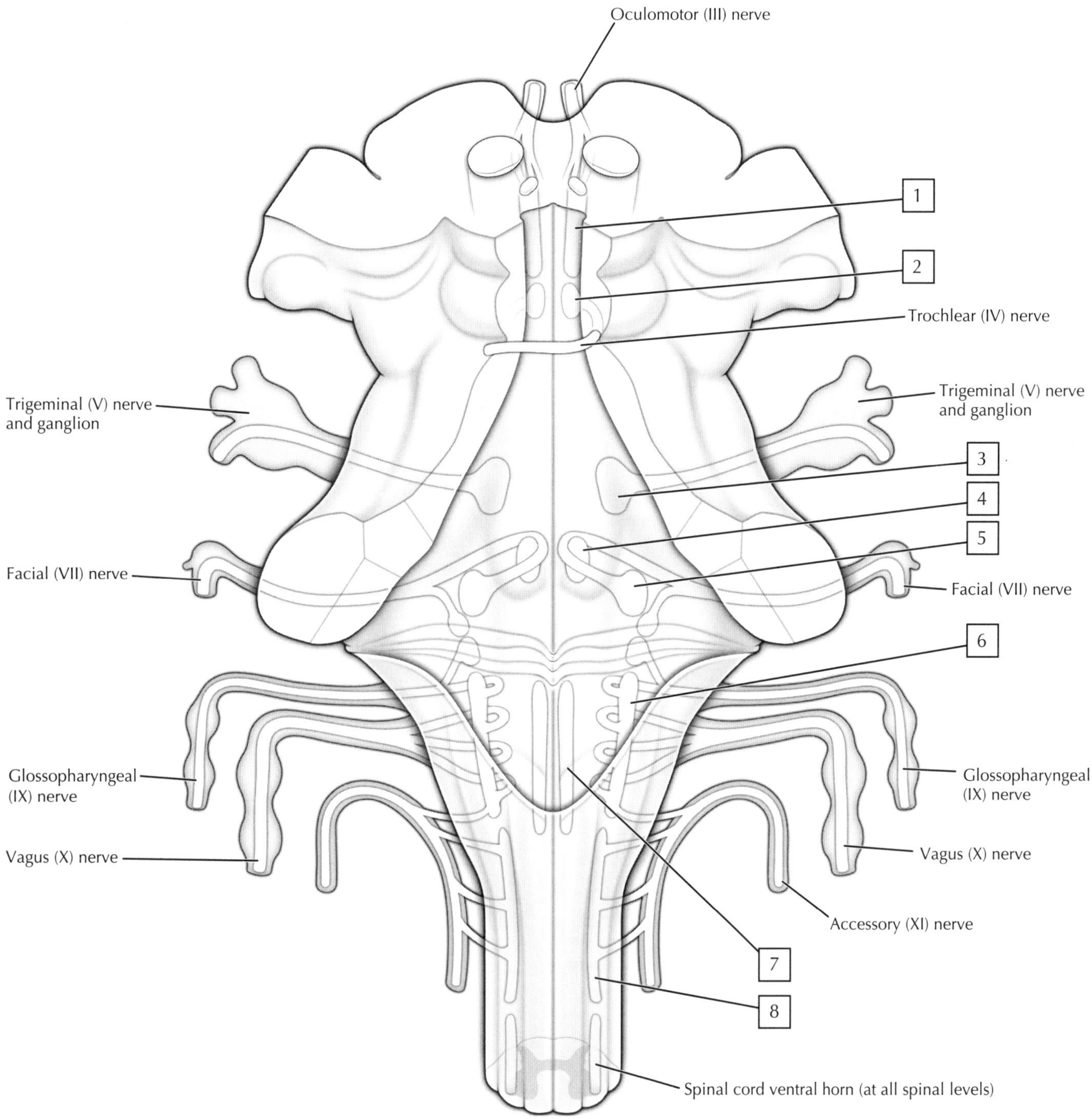
Oculomotor (III) nerve
1
2
Trochlear (IV) nerve
Trigeminal (V) nerve and ganglion
Trigeminal (V) nerve and ganglion
3
4
5
Facial (VII) nerve
Facial (VII) nerve
6
Glossopharyngeal (IX) nerve
Glossopharyngeal (IX) nerve
Vagus (X) nerve
Vagus (X) nerve
Accessory (XI) nerve
7
8
Spinal cord ventral horn (at all spinal levels)

Corticobulbar Tract

The corticobulbar tract (CBT) arises from the lateral portion of the primary motor cortex (area 4) and the premotor cortex (area 6). These regions of **motor**, **premotor cortex**, and **supplemental motor cortex** have a disproportionate representation of the head and neck region compared with most other regions of the body (except for hands). These cortical areas get inputs from many other forebrain regions, including limbic structures (e.g., amygdala), language centers, sensory cortical areas, and others. The **corticobulbar axons** descend through the **genu of the internal capsule**, continue through the **cerebral peduncle**, then through **fascicles of axons in the basis pontis** and the **medullary pyramid**. Axons leave these fiber systems and synapse in the motor cranial nerve nuclei (CNN) from the midbrain (extraocular) down to the spinal accessory nucleus (upper cervical spinal cord). The corticobulbar system distributes bilaterally to all cranial nerve motor nuclei **(CNN III, IV, VI, XII, V, VII for the upper face, nucleus ambiguus, and XI)** except the **facial motor nucleus** for the lower face, which receives exclusively contralateral connections.

COLOR the following structures, using a separate color for each structure.

- ☐ 1. **Motor and premotor cortex on precentral gyrus**
- ☐ 2. **Corticobulbar axons**
- ☐ 3. **Genu of the internal capsule**
- ☐ 4. **Bilateral corticobulbar distribution to CNN III and IV**
- ☐ 5. **Cerebral peduncle**
- ☐ 6. **Bilateral corticobulbar distribution to CNN VI**
- ☐ 7. **Fascicles in the basis pontis**
- ☐ 8. **Bilateral corticobulbar distribution to nucleus ambiguus, CNN XI, CNN XII, and spinal accessory nucleus**
- ☐ 9. **Medullary pyramid**
- ☐ 10. **Bilateral corticobulbar distribution to CNN VII for the upper face**
- ☐ 11. **Contralateral distribution to CNN VII for the lower face**

Clinical Note

The CBT distributes connections and functional control to both sides of the brainstem for all of the motor CNN except for the portion of CNN VII that distributes axons to lower facial muscles. This lower facial muscle system is controlled exclusively by contralateral CBT axons. If the genu of the internal capsule is damaged by a vascular (or other) lesion along with the posterior limb of the internal capsule, the result will be contralateral hemiplegia and contralateral drooping lower face (but not paralyzed upper face). This central facial palsy is distinguished from peripheral palsy, as seen in Bell palsy, which results in a total paralysis on the affected side, including inability to wrinkle the forehead or move any of the facial muscles. Clinical neurological testing has noted that some individuals demonstrate mainly contralateral corticobulbar connections to CNN XII, and mainly ipsilateral corticobulbar connections to the spinal accessory nucleus. These two unusual patterns of distribution may lead to some acute symptoms following a corticobulbar lesion, such as a stroke, but are unlikely to have long-term consequences.

Bulbar Palsy refers to consequences of LMN damage in the brainstem. In the era of the 1950s polio epidemic, bulbar palsy referred to damage of motor nuclei associated with CN IX, X, XI, and XII; in current understanding, bulbar palsy refers to LMN damage throughout the brainstem. The LMN damage is accompanied by loss of tone, loss of reflexes, atrophy of previously innervated muscles, and fasciculations (e.g., tongue muscles) during the death of the LMNs. **Pseudobulbar Palsy** is associated with bilateral damage to the CBT, leaving the brainstem LMNs intact but devoid of cortical (voluntary control). These lesions are accompanied by muscle hypertonus, hyperreflexia (e.g., brisk jaw jerk reflex and gag reflex), normal muscle bulk, and loss of voluntary motor movement of the innervated muscles. However, some limbic reactions (e.g., laughter at a joke) can provoke contraction of some of the muscles; such movement derives from descending regulation through pathways other than the CBT. Pseudobulbar palsy is often accompanied by excessive or exaggerated emotion or affect.

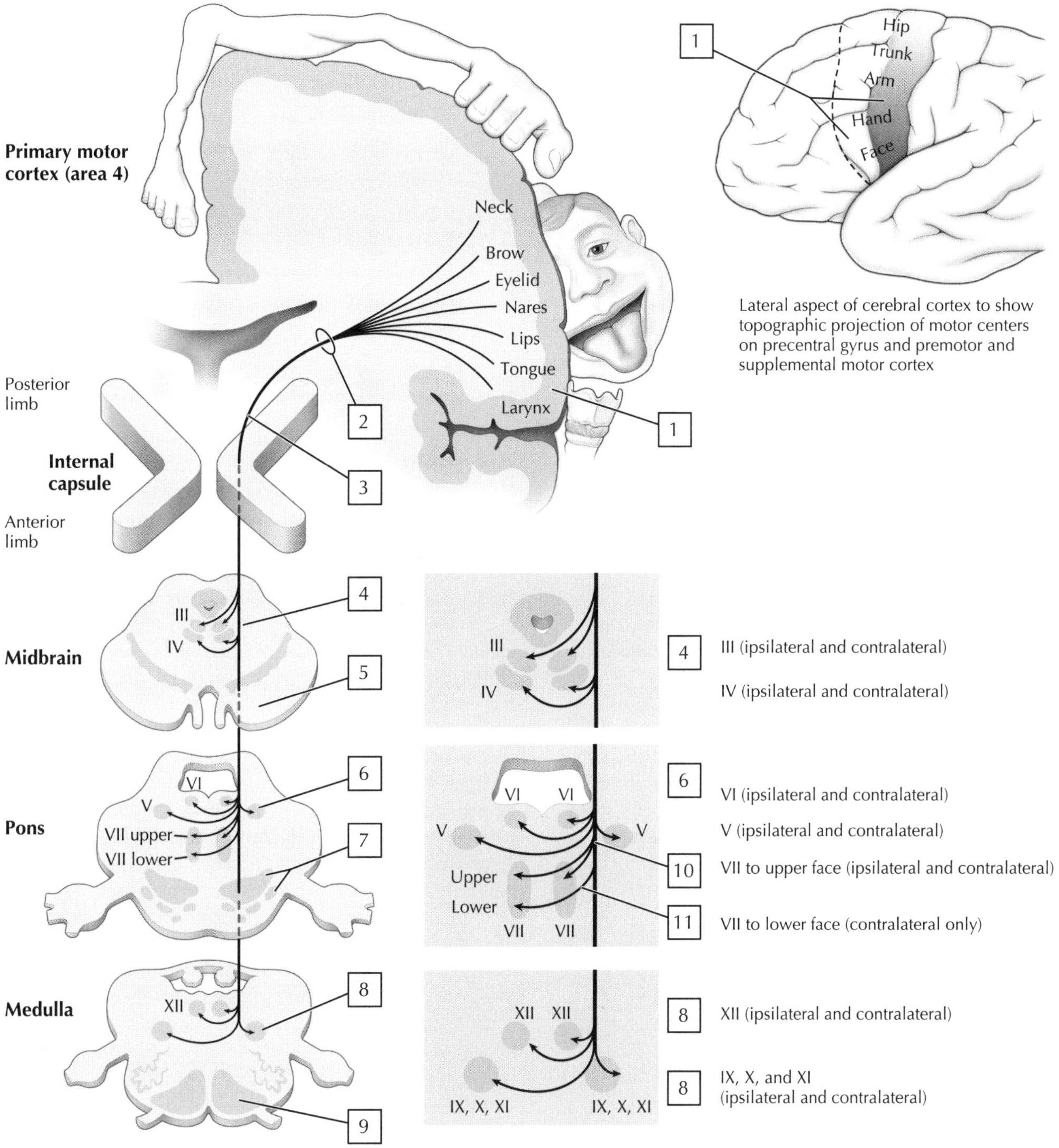

Lateral aspect of cerebral cortex to show topographic projection of motor centers on precentral gyrus and premotor and supplemental motor cortex

10 Corticospinal Tract

The **corticospinal tract (CST)** is the major UMN forebrain system that controls skilled voluntary movement and helps to regulate the broad array of spinal cord LMNs necessary for complex behavior, as opposed to basic tone and posture. The corticospinal tract arises from the main convexity of the **motor cortex** and the **premotor and supplemental motor cortex** (areas 4 and 6). **The primary motor cortex** (area 4) initiates the LMN activities to carry out the plans and programs of movement assembled by the premotor cortex and supplemental motor cortex. The **premotor cortex** (part of area 6) helps to select programs of motor activity, especially those based on visual inputs, sensory guidance, and mental images. The **supplemental motor cortex** (part of area 6) aids in the selection of motor activities based on complex sequences and programs of movement, and helps to guide movements involving the hands. **Prefrontal cortex, superior parietal cortex** (especially areas 5 and 7), and **regions of temporal cortex** help to guide movements through connections with the premotor and supplemental motor cortical areas.

Some authors report that the corticospinal tract also has an additional contribution from the postcentral gyrus, the primary sensory cortex (areas 3, 1, and 2). Although this sensory area sends axons that hitchhike with the corticospinal tract, they are not part of the UMN system that controls spinal cord LMNs; they are a system of **corticonuclear fibers** that terminate in secondary sensory nuclei (nucleus gracilis, cuneatus, dorsal horn of the spinal cord) and contribute to the regulation of lemniscal sensory input.

Corticospinal tract axons travel through the ipsilateral **posterior limb of the internal capsule**, **cerebral peduncle**, **fascicles in the basis pontis**, and the **medullary pyramids**. In the caudal region of the medulla, approximately 80% of the axons cross the midline in the **pyramidal decussation** (the demarcation between the medulla and the cervical spinal cord) and descend in the **lateral corticospinal tract** in the **dorsolateral funiculus**. These axons terminate in the lateral and central portion of the anterior horn of the spinal cord, especially the cervical cord (55% of axonal terminations), and help to control fine, skilled movements. These axons may directly synapse on LMNs (10%+ in humans) but mainly communicate with LMNs through associated premotor interneurons. The remaining 20% of the corticospinal axons continue to descend as the **anterior corticospinal tract** in the **anterior funiculus,** and then cross the midline through the **anterior white commissure**, ending mainly on LMNs and interneurons associated with trunk muscles and proximal muscles. Only a few corticospinal axons stay ipsilateral and end on ipsilateral LMNs or interneurons. The corticospinal axons end on and regulate both α and γ LMNs, and initiate α–γ coactivation.

COLOR the following structures, using a separate color for each structure.

- ☐ 1. **Corticospinal tract**
- ☐ 2. **Primary motor cortex on the precentral gyrus (area 4)**
- ☐ 3. **Premotor and supplemental motor cortex (area 6)**
- ☐ 4. **Posterior limb of the internal capsule**
- ☐ 5. **Cerebral peduncle**
- ☐ 6. **Fascicles in the basis pontis**
- ☐ 7. **Medullary pyramids**
- ☐ 8. **Decussation of the pyramids (pyramidal decussation)**
- ☐ 9. **Dorsolateral funiculus of the spinal cord**
- ☐ 10. **Lateral corticospinal tract**
- ☐ 11. **Anterior corticospinal tract**
- ☐ 12. **Anterior funiculus of the spinal cord**

Clinical Note

Corticospinal tract axons are rarely injured or damaged in isolation. In the posterior limb of the internal capsule, corticospinal tract axons are accompanied by **corticorubral** axons and other cortical outflow to other UMN systems. In the dorsolateral funiculus of the spinal cord, corticospinal tract axons are virtually always injured along with **rubrospinal tract** axons. The combination of disruption of the corticospinal and corticorubrospinal system results in classic UMN syndrome: (1) hemiparesis/hemiplegia (weakness) with pronator drift (arms outstretched with palms supinated, eyes closed, weak arm drifts down and pronates); (2) hypertonus (increased resistance to passive stretch, spasticity with clasp-knife response); (3) hyperreflexia, sometimes with clonus (alternating hyperresponsive muscle stretch reflexes); (4) plantar extensor response (sometimes called "Babinski reflex); and (5) pathological reflexes (e.g., brisk abdominal reflex, cremasteric reflex, withdrawal response, brisk autonomic responses).

In the only site where corticospinal tract axons travel in isolation, the medullary pyramids, disruption by infarct in a median arterial branch of the vertebrobasilar system results in clumsy finger and hand movements, mild hypotonus, and no spasticity. This not only provides evidence for the role of corticospinal tract axons in skilled hand movements but also reveals that an attempt to equate UMN system lesions in the posterior limb of the internal capsule or the dorsolateral funiculus of the spinal cord with "pyramidal tract syndrome" or lesions is incorrect.

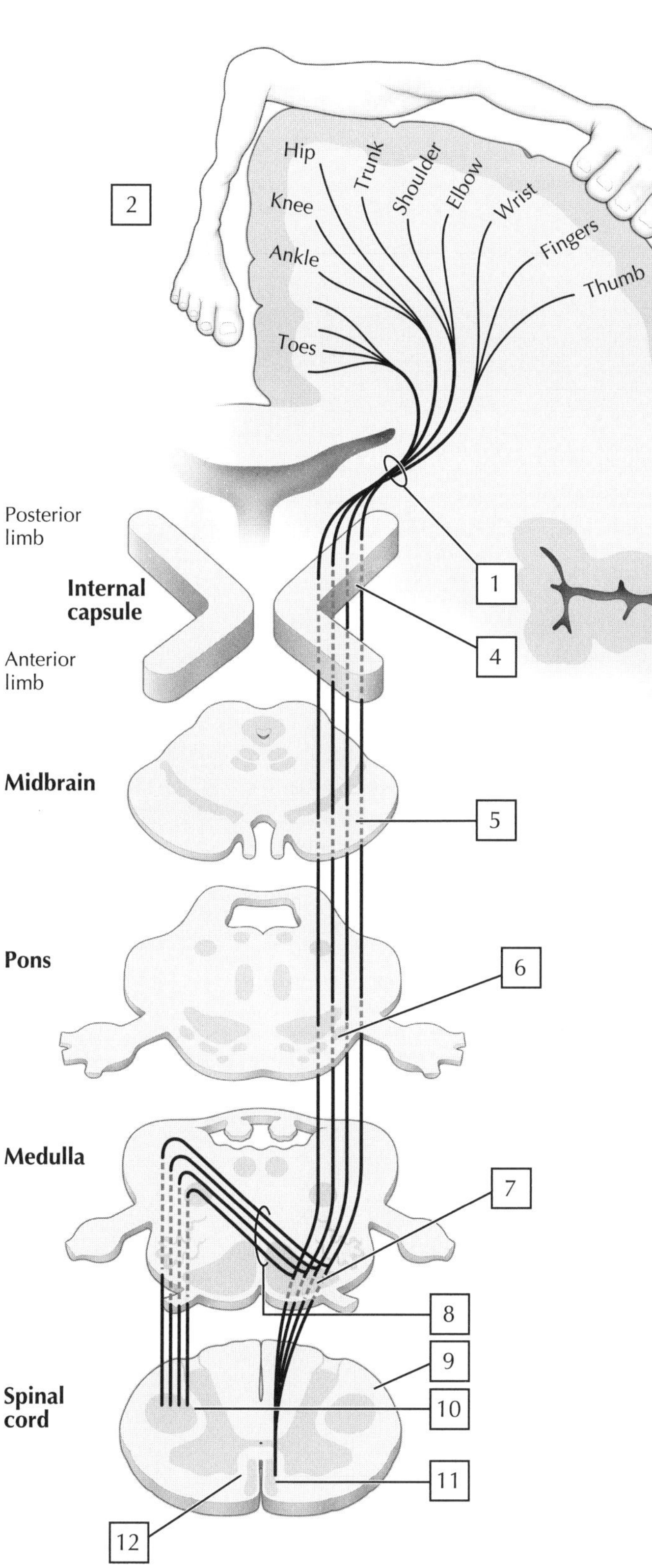

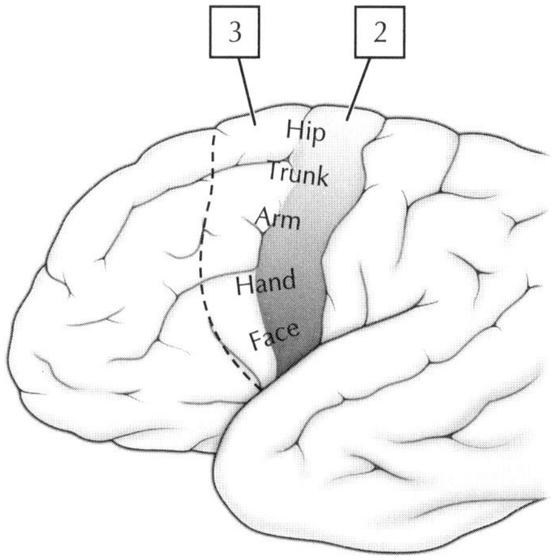

Lateral aspect of cerebral cortex showing topographic localization of motor centers on precentral gyrus and premotor and supplemental motor cortex

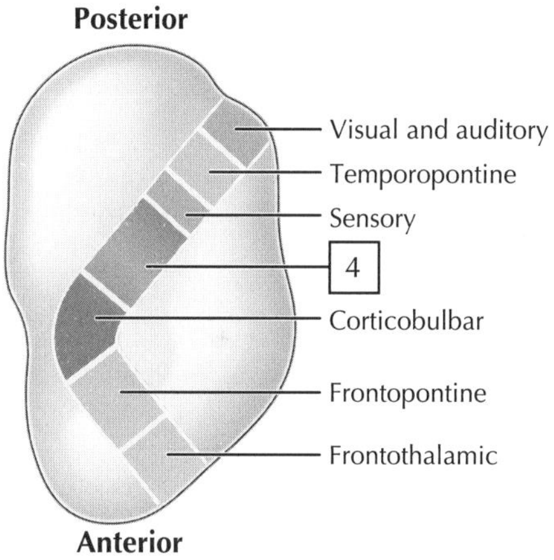

Horizontal section through internal capsule showing location of principal pathways

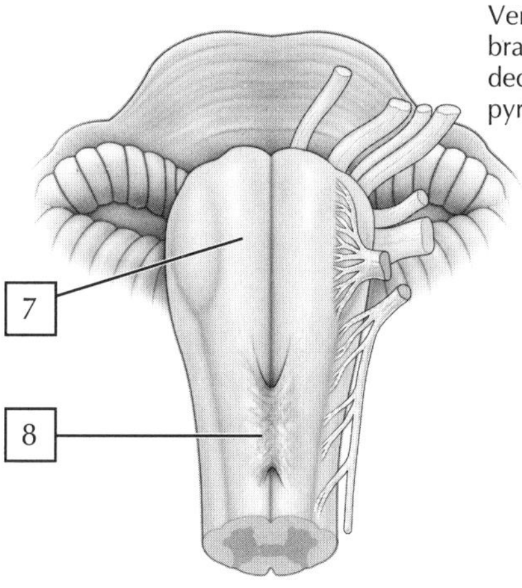

Ventral aspect of brain stem showing decussation of pyramids

Rubrospinal Tract

The **corticorubrospinal system** has sometimes been described as an indirect corticospinal system for proximal muscle control; the corticospinal tract is directed toward fine, skilled movements of the distal extremities. This system was dismissed by some as unimportant in humans because of how few magnocellular neurons are present in the human red nucleus, but functional considerations indicate that the corticorubrospinal system is significant in humans. The **red nucleus** is a large nucleus in the midbrain. It receives topographical input from the ipsilateral **primary motor cortex (area 4)**. Axons from cells in the red nucleus decussate in the midbrain in the **ventral tegmental decussation**, descend in the **lateral brainstem**, and continue into the **dorsolateral funiculus of the spinal cord**. The crossed **rubrospinal tract** travels alongside the crossed **lateral corticospinal tract**, with some intermixing of axons. Rubrospinal axons terminate mainly on pools of interneurons in the anterior horn, associated with both α and γ LMNs, in particular those associated with proximal musculature, especially **flexor LMNs** for the upper extremities.

The rubrospinal tract has a different functional bias in humans than in quadrupeds. In humans, rubrospinal axons drive flexion in the upper extremities and hold flexor movements in check in the lower extremities. Some axons from neurons in the red nucleus provide ipsilateral input to nuclei in the reticular formation, including the **medial reticular formation** associated with motor control of flexor tone and posture. The **cerebellum (globose and emboliform nuclei)** provides feedback information to the red nucleus.

COLOR the following structures, using a separate color for each structure.

- ☐ 1. **Primary motor cortex (area 4)**
- ☐ 2. **Input from the cerebellum (globose and emboliform nuclei) to the red nucleus**
- ☐ 3. **Red nucleus**
- ☐ 4. **Ventral tegmental decussation**
- ☐ 5. **Rubrospinal tract in the lateral brainstem**
- ☐ 6. **Lateral corticospinal tract**
- ☐ 7. **Rubrospinal tract influence on flexor LMNs**
- ☐ 8. **Rubrospinal tract in the dorsolateral funiculus of the spinal cord**
- ☐ 9. **Medial reticular formation**

Clinical Note

The red nucleus and rubrospinal tract are rarely damaged in isolation. The most common sites of damage are the posterior limb of the internal capsule (corticospinal axons and corticorubral axons) or the dorsolateral funiculus of the spinal cord (lateral corticospinal tract and rubrospinal tract). Damage in the dorsolateral funiculus leads to classic UMN syndrome **ipsilateral** to the lesion (the axons have already crossed) with spasticity, hypertonus, hyperreflexia, and pathological reflexes. Damage in the internal capsule leads to a similar clinical picture, **contralateral** to the lesion (the corticospinal and rubrospinal axons have not yet crossed). With damage to the cerebral cortex (and corticorubral axons), the red nucleus is disinhibited and the upper extremity is driven into a flexor posture with pronation (due to action of the disinhibited red nucleus), and the lower extremity is driven into extension (due to a combination of actions of several brainstem UMN groups), a condition called decortication. If the forebrain lesion extends more caudally, also removing the influence of the red nucleus, then the red nucleus flexor influence on the upper extremities is removed, and the limb musculature is driven mainly by the lateral vestibulospinal tract and the reticulospinal tracts. Both the lateral vestibulospinal tract and the pontine reticulospinal tract exert a powerful extensor influence on all four extremities (called decerebrate posture) and the neck musculature (opisthotonus). The switch from decortication to decerebration with removal of the influence of the red nucleus indicates the important functional role of this system. Decerebrate posture was sometimes called decerebrate rigidity, but the muscle tone is not reflective of rigidity (as is tone in Parkinson's disease), but spasticity.

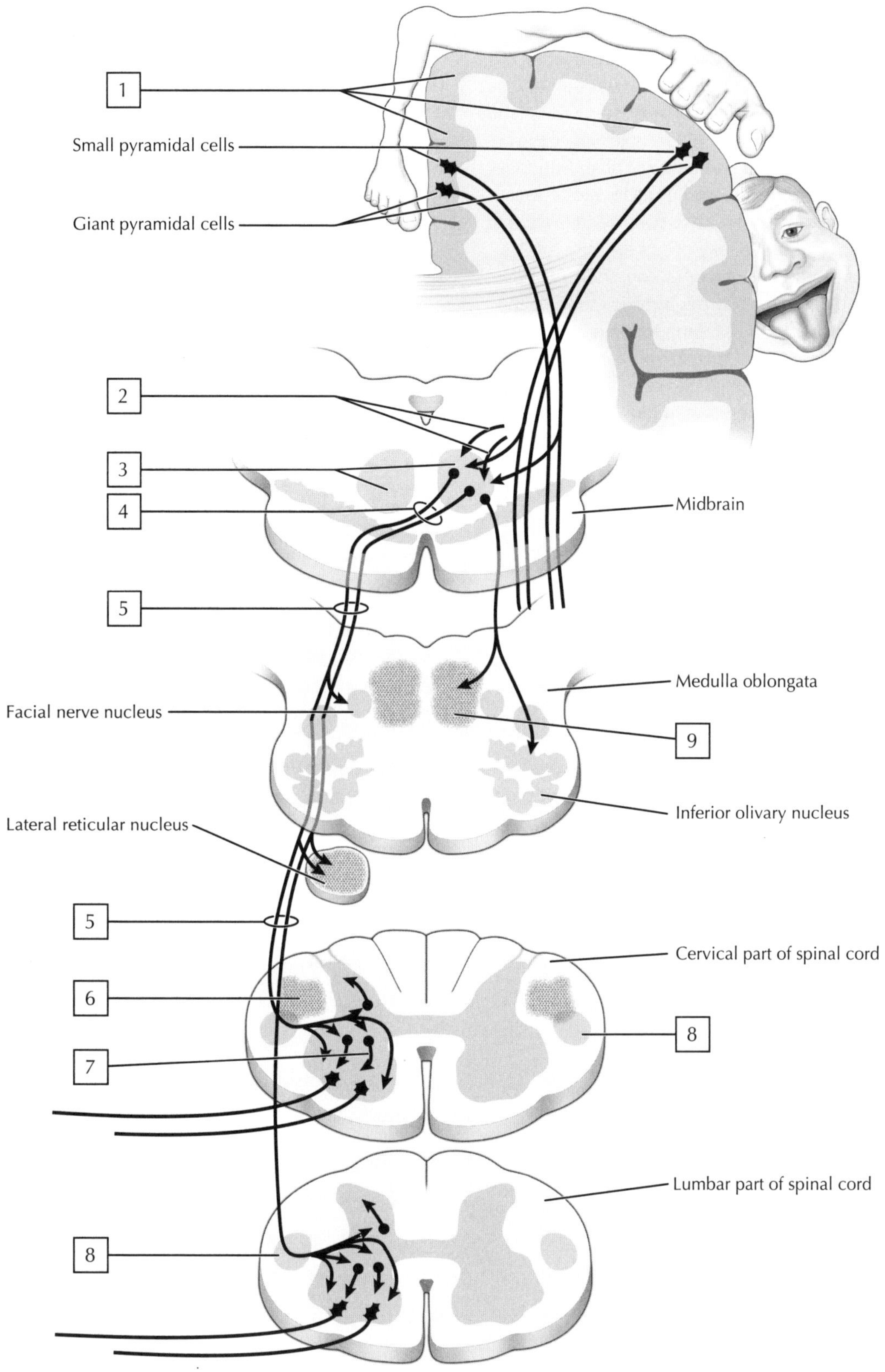
1
Small pyramidal cells
Giant pyramidal cells
2
3
4
Midbrain
5
Facial nerve nucleus
Medulla oblongata
9
Inferior olivary nucleus
Lateral reticular nucleus
5
Cervical part of spinal cord
6
8
7
Lumbar part of spinal cord
8

Vestibulospinal Tracts

The primary vestibular axonal projections carrying the information derived from the **macula of the utricle** and **saccule**, and the **cristae within the ampullae of the semicircular canals** (cell bodies in the **spiral ganglion**) terminate in the **vestibular nuclei in the brainstem** and in the **vestibulocerebellum** (vermis, flocculonodular lobe). The **lateral vestibulospinal tract** arises from neurons in the **lateral vestibular nucleus**, descends ipsilaterally, and travels through the anterior funiculus of the spinal cord to terminate mainly on interneurons associated with both **α and γ LMNs in the anterior horn at all levels of the spinal cord** directed particularly on LMNs controlling trunk and proximal muscles. This tract powerfully drives extensor LMNs (mainly through influences on adjacent interneurons). The lateral vestibular nucleus is held in check by the **anterior lobe of the cerebellum** and the **red nucleus**. Damage to the anterior lobe of the cerebellum (e.g., alcoholism) may initially produce a stiff-legged staggering gate. With forebrain damage, removal of the influence of the corticospinal system and the red nucleus results in disinhibition of the lateral vestibulospinal system, switching decortication (with upper extremity flexion) to decerebration (powerful extension of all four extremities).

The **medial vestibulospinal tract** arises from the **medial vestibular nucleus**. Its axons travel ipsilaterally in the brainstem near the midline and in the anterior funiculus of the spinal cord; they terminate in the **cervical spinal cord**, mainly on interneurons associated with α and γ LMNs that control neck movements.

These two UMN tracts help to provide vestibular influences on muscle tone (antigravity) and on neck muscle tone and movement. The **medial longitudinal fasciculus (MLF)**, with axons from all vestibular nuclei and other regions (parapontine reticular formation) to the **extraocular CNN**, helps to coordinate eye movements with neck movements and body tone and posture.

COLOR the following structures, using a separate color for each structure.

- ☐ 1. **Medial vestibular nucleus**
- ☐ 2. **Lateral vestibular nucleus**
- ☐ 3. **Vestibular nuclei in the brainstem**
- ☐ 4. **Vestibular axons projecting to the vestibulocerebellum**
- ☐ 5. **Spiral ganglion**
- ☐ 6. **Lateral vestibulospinal tract**
- ☐ 7. **Medial vestibulospinal axons terminating in the anterior horn of the cervical spinal cord**
- ☐ 8. **Medial vestibulospinal tract**
- ☐ 9. **Lateral vestibulospinal axons terminating in the anterior horn of the spinal cord, driving extensor LMNs**
- ☐ 10. **Macula of the utricle**
- ☐ 11. **Cristae within the ampullae of the semicircular canals**

Clinical Note

The lateral vestibulospinal system is the major driver of antigravity posture that permits one to actively engage in behaviors in one's surroundings. The antigravity posture is essential to maintain strength and mobility. By contrast, most skilled, dexterous movements are mainly flexor movements; to carry them out in skilled fashion, it is necessary to temporarily suppress the powerful antigravity tone for the superimposed voluntary flexor movements. This particularly occurs through cortical influences, red nucleus influences, and cerebellar influences, as well as Renshaw cell bias in the spinal cord. Impairment of the supraspinal inhibition of the antigravity responses results in altered tone and posture, damaged superimposed flexor responses, and serious neurological pathology.

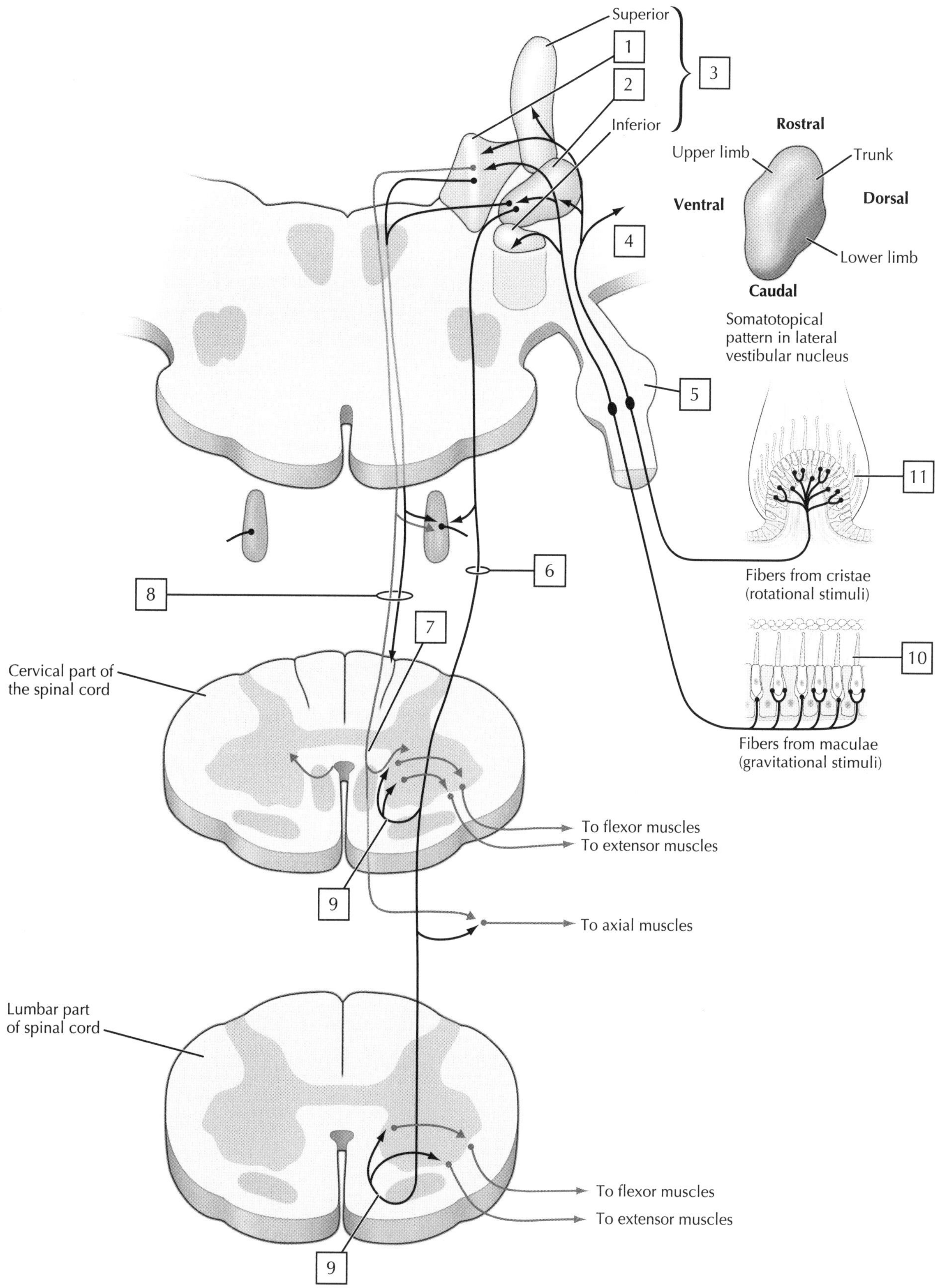

Superior
1
2
3
Inferior
Rostral
Upper limb
Trunk
Ventral
Dorsal
Lower limb
Caudal
Somatotopical pattern in lateral vestibular nucleus
4
5
11
Fibers from cristae (rotational stimuli)
6
8
7
10
Cervical part of the spinal cord
Fibers from maculae (gravitational stimuli)
To flexor muscles
To extensor muscles
9
To axial muscles
Lumbar part of spinal cord
To flexor muscles
To extensor muscles
9

10 Reticulospinal and Corticoreticulospinal Pathways

The reticulospinal tracts derive from the reticular formation, the isodendritic core of the brainstem, the site where the first basic UMN influences on LMNs are seen. They provide basic tone and postural responses and help to coordinate the LMNs for antigravity and movement responses. The pontine portion of this system derives from the **medial pontine reticular formation (nuclei pontis caudalis and oralis)**. The axons descend ipsilaterally as the **pontine (medial) reticulospinal tract** and terminate mainly on **interneurons associated with both α and γ LMNs** at all levels of the spinal cord. This tract has an **extensor bias**, especially on LMNs directed toward axial musculature, and helps to reinforce extensor responses from the lateral vestibulospinal system. This system does not depend on cortical input or drive, but responds strongly to nociceptive **inputs from the somatosensory and trigeminal systems**.

The medullary portion of this system derives from the **medial reticular formation in the medulla (nucleus gigantocellularis)**. Its axons descend bilaterally as the **medullary (lateral) reticulospinal tract** and exert a **flexor bias through interneurons associated with α and γ LMNs at all levels** of the spinal cord. These tracts are the core reticular system upon which the flexor-bias corticospinal and rubrospinal systems are superimposed. The **cortex helps to drive the medial reticulospinal system,** especially motor-related regions such as the primary motor cortex, premotor cortex, and supplemental motor cortex. In contrast to most of the other UMN descending systems, the reticulospinal tracts appear to not be somatotopically organized.

COLOR the following structures, using a separate color for each structure.

- ☐ 1. **Main regions of the cerebral cortex providing inputs and strong influence on medullary reticular formation**
- ☐ 2. **Medial pontine reticular formation (nuclei pontis, caudalis, and oralis)**
- ☐ 3. **Site of inputs to pontine reticular formation from somatosensory and trigeminal systems**
- ☐ 4. **Medial pontine reticular formation in the medulla (nucleus gigantocellularis)**
- ☐ 5. **Medullary (lateral) reticulospinal tract**
- ☐ 6. **Terminations of medullary reticulospinal tract on flexor-bias interneurons and LMNs**
- ☐ 7. **Terminations of pontine reticulospinal tract on extensor-bias interneurons and LMNs**
- ☐ 8. **Pontine (medial) reticulospinal tract**

Clinical Note

The **reticular formation** is the core of the brainstem, representing the first supraspinal or suprasegmental neuronal systems contributing to basic coordination of sensory, motor, and autonomic processes. The reticular formation neurons are called isodendritic and are not interneurons. They have large dendritic fields and have axons extending well beyond their local surrounds. The medial reticular formation is the motor component of region. It provides basic extensor and flexor tone through coordination of the LMN networks. It is not a sophisticated topographically organized system, as is the corticospinal system. The corticospinal system both bypasses the reticulospinal pathways with direct LMN connections and also provides some control over part of the reticulospinal system, the medullary portion, with a flexor bias. Any brainstem lesion or pathology that seriously threatens damage to these reticulospinal systems is likely to be incompatible with life.

Reticulospinal and Corticoreticulospinal Pathways

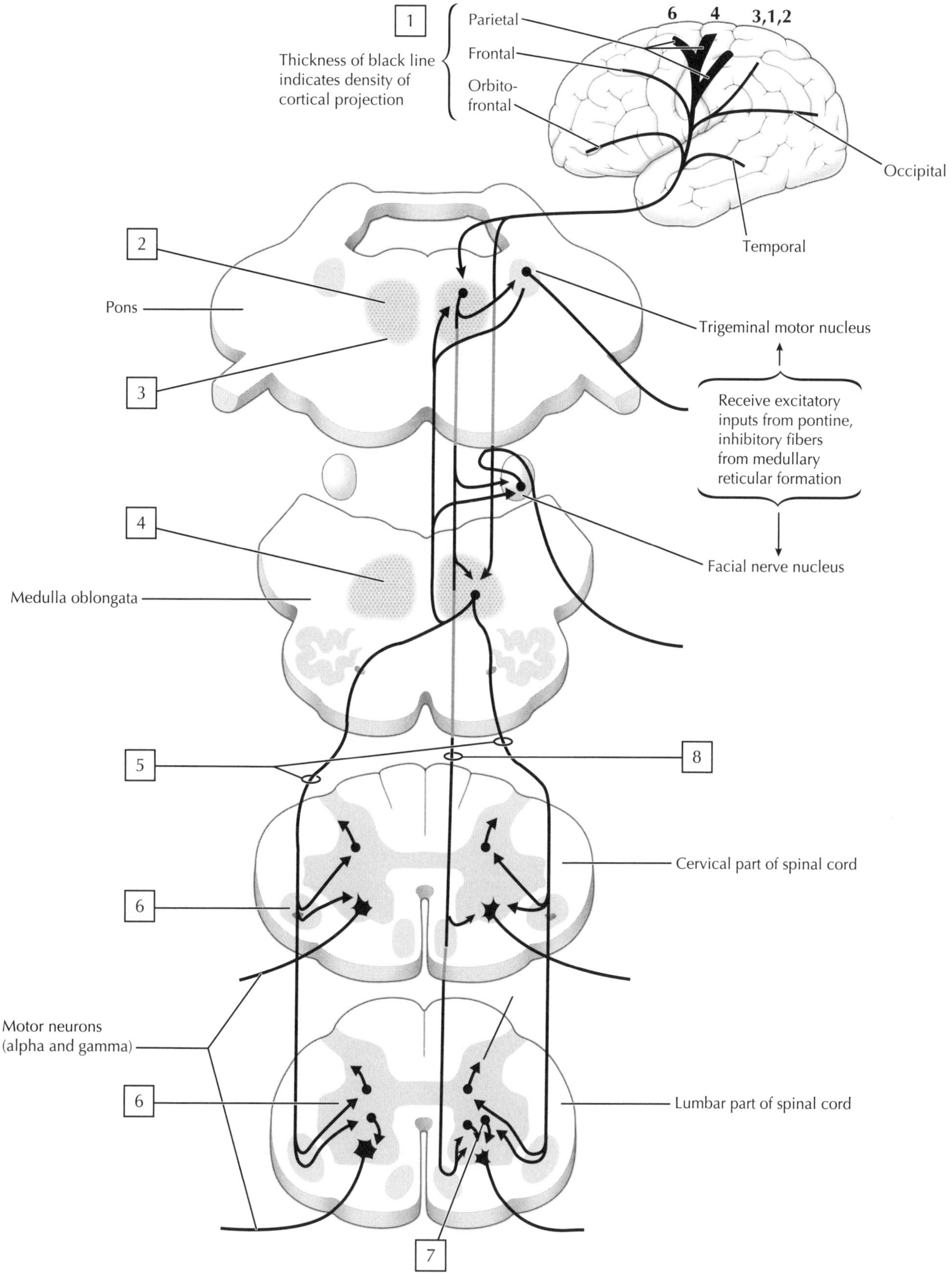

Tectospinal Tract and Interstitiospinal Tract

The **tectospinal tract** and **interstitiospinal tract** are UMN systems that provide visual (and auditory) regulatory control over neck movements and axial body movements, permitting proper reaction and orientation to stimuli that require coordination of body movement, head and neck movement, and proper orientation of the visual axis. The tectospinal tract originates from neurons in the deep layers of the **superior colliculus**. Its axons immediately decussate in the **dorsal tegmental decussation** and descend as the tectospinal tract, traveling with the **medial longitudinal fasciculus (MLF)**. These axons terminate, mainly through associated interneurons, on both **α and γ LMNs in the cervical spinal cord**, providing control over neck (and head) movements. With input from the retina, the visual cortex, visual cortical association areas, and the frontal eye fields, the tectospinal tract provides the means to respond to reflex movements and visual tracking through control of neck movements. The superior colliculus provides ascending connectivity through the **pulvinar** to the **visual association cortex** to assist in tracking responses. The inferior colliculus participates in reflex responses and startle responses through projections to the superior colliculus and the tectospinal tract.

The interstitiospinal tract arises from the **interstitial nucleus of Cajal** in the midbrain. It receives vestibular input through the ascending MLF and cortical input from the frontal eye fields. It helps to coordinate vertical and oblique eye movements and gaze centers related to the visual system. The interstitiospinal tract sends ipsilateral projections, traveling with the descending MLF, to **LMNs in the cervical spinal cord**, for controlling neck movements, and to **LMNs associated with axial trunk musculature** for controlling rotational movements of the body. This aids in keeping an appropriate fix on the visual horizon in response to reflex or tracking movements.

COLOR the following structures, using a separate color for each structure.

- ☐ **1. Tectospinal tract**
- ☐ **2. Superior colliculus**
- ☐ **3. Interstitial nucleus of Cajal**
- ☐ **4. Dorsal tegmental decussation**
- ☐ **5. Interstitiospinal tract**
- ☐ **6. Medial longitudinal fasciculus (MLF)**
- ☐ **7. Interstitiospinal tract terminations associated with LMNs in the cervical spinal cord**
- ☐ **8. Tectospinal tract terminations associated with LMNs in the cervical spinal cord**
- ☐ **9. Interstitiospinal tract terminations associated with axial truck musculature**

Clinical Note

The tectospinal tract and interstitiospinal tract, similar to the other brainstem UMN systems, are unconscious regulatory systems for specific pools of LMNs, mainly accessed through associated groups of interneurons. The tectospinal tract allows reflex responsiveness to visual stimuli, permitting rapid movement of the head and neck for continuing visual orientation. This is a critical component of visual tracking. This system also receives connectivity from the inferior colliculus to the superior colliculus to assist in rapid movement of the head and neck in response to sound. The interstitiospinal tract contributes to coordination of eye movements through gaze centers and the extraocular LMNs, and also regulates head and neck movements as well as axial rotational muscles to help coordinate body and head and neck movements for maintaining a clear fix on the visual horizon.

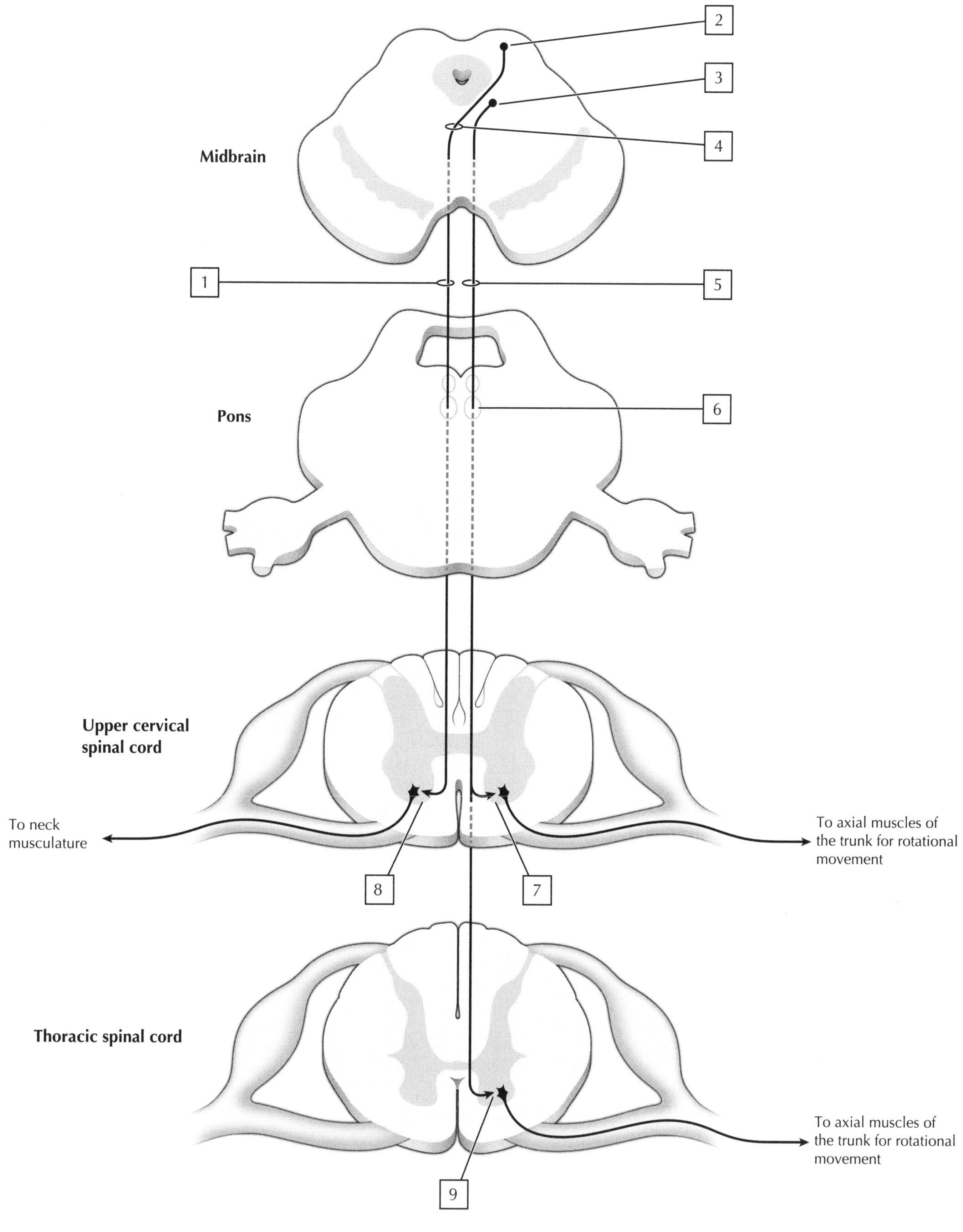
2
3
4
Midbrain
1
5
Pons
6
Upper cervical spinal cord
To neck musculature
To axial muscles of the trunk for rotational movement
8
7
Thoracic spinal cord
To axial muscles of the trunk for rotational movement
9

10 Central Control of Eye Movements

Central control of eye movements involves a complex regulation and coordination of **CNN III (oculomotor)**, **IV (trochlear)**, and **VI (abducens)**. A key coordinating center for this process is the **parapontine reticular formation (PPRF)**, also called the horizontal gaze center. The PPRF directly drives horizontal eye movements through connections to ipsilateral LMNs of the abducens nucleus, regulating the lateral rectus muscle. It also drives coordinated movement of the contralateral medial rectus muscle through **interneurons in the abducens nucleus** that ascend in the contralateral **medial longitudinal fasciculus (MLF)** to LMNs in the oculomotor nucleus. This permits the smooth coordination of the lateral rectus muscle on one side with the medial rectus muscle on the other side.

The PPRF receives input from several regulatory control systems: (1) the **vestibular nuclei**, permitting the coordination of horizontal eye movements; (2) the deep layers of the **superior colliculus** (neurons of origin for the tectospinal tract), which receive input from the **visual cortex (areas 17, 18, 19)**; (3) the **frontal eye fields (area 8)**, which coordinate cortically driven eye movements; and (4) the **interstitial nucleus of Cajal**, which receives inputs from the vestibular nuclei and the frontal eye fields. The interstitial nucleus of Cajal also acts as a coordinating (gaze) center for vertical and oblique eye movements, through connections with the oculomotor nucleus and the trochlear nucleus. The oculomotor nucleus and trochlear nucleus also receive inputs from the vestibular nuclei through ascending projections in the MLF.

COLOR each of the following structures, using a separate color for each structure.

- ☐ 1. **Visual cortex (areas 17, 18, 19)**
- ☐ 2. **Frontal eye fields (area 8)**
- ☐ 3. **Interstitial nucleus of Cajal**
- ☐ 4. **Superior colliculus and its projections to the PPRF**
- ☐ 5. **Oculomotor nucleus (CNN III)**
- ☐ 6. **Trochlear nucleus (CNN IV)**
- ☐ 7. **Medial longitudinal fasciculus (MLF)**
- ☐ 8. **Abducens nucleus (CNN VI)**
- ☐ 9. **Parapontine reticular formation (PPRF)**
- ☐ 10. **Vestibular nuclei**
- ☐ 11. **Interneurons in the abducens nucleus and their proximal axons entering the MLF**

Clinical Note

The MLF is a small axon bundle traversing the brainstem near the midline. This tract contains axons from the vestibular nuclei to the extraocular nuclei, axons from the interneurons in the abducens nucleus, axons from the PPRF, axons from the interstitial nucleus of Cajal (both the interstitiospinal tract and projections to the PPRF), and axons from the deep layers of the superior colliculus (tectospinal tract and projections to the PPRF). This small tract is frequently demyelinated in multiple sclerosis, despite its very small size. When this occurs, the coordinated activity for eye movements is disrupted. The most conspicuous clinical observation is **internuclear ophthalmoplegia**. When the MLF on one side is demyelinated (or damaged through another pathological process), the ipsilateral eye does not adduct. The contralateral eye abducts properly with attempted lateral gaze. This results in horizontal **diplopia** (double vision). The contralateral eye tries to move back to resolve the diplopia but is driven by the attempted lateral gaze, resulting in **nystagmus**.

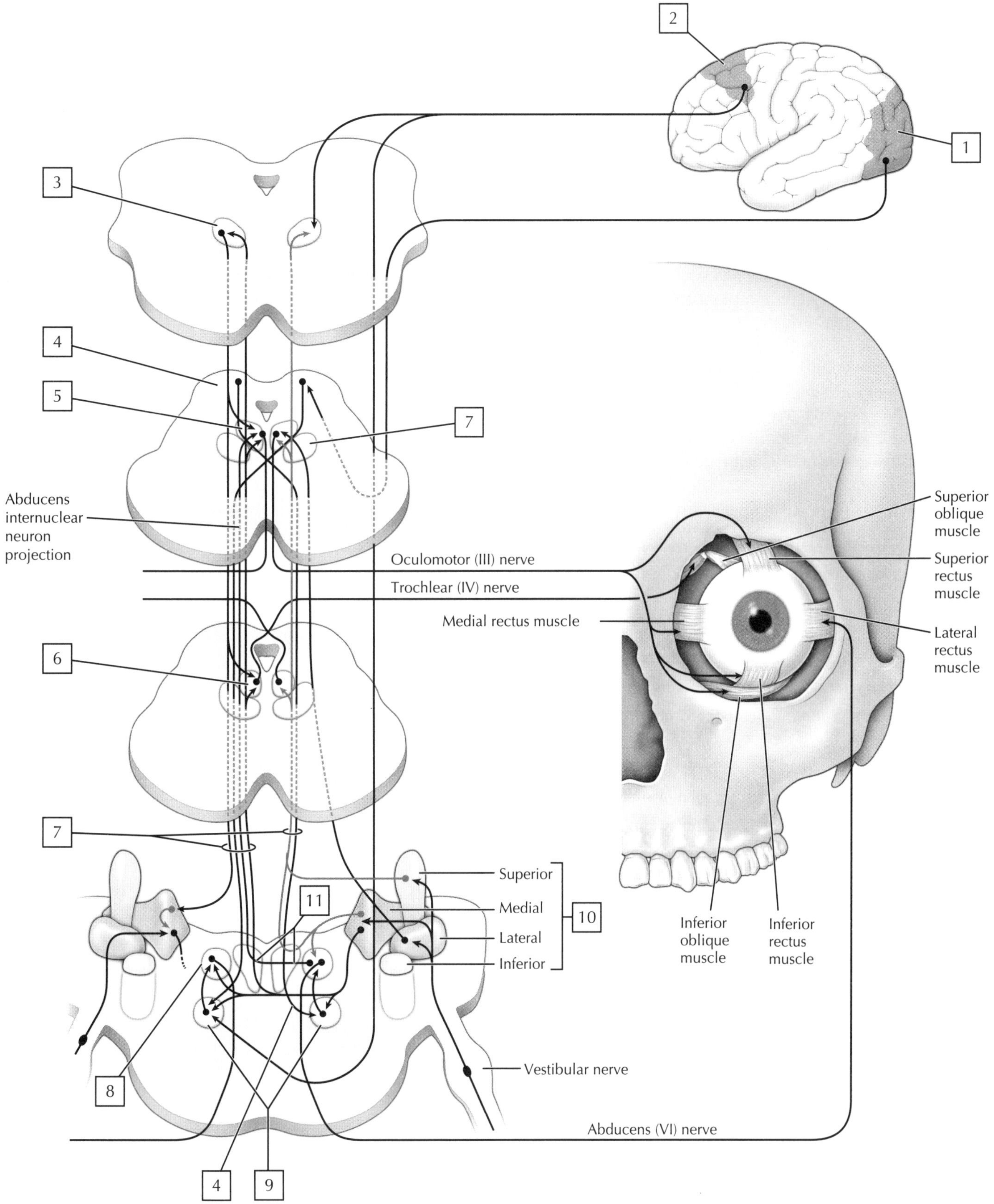

2
1
3
4
5
7
Abducens internuclear neuron projection
Oculomotor (III) nerve
Trochlear (IV) nerve
Medial rectus muscle
6
Superior oblique muscle
Superior rectus muscle
Lateral rectus muscle
7
Superior
Medial
Lateral
Inferior
10
11
Inferior oblique muscle
Inferior rectus muscle
Vestibular nerve
8
Abducens (VI) nerve
4
9

10 Central Control of Respiration

Inspiration and expiration are regulated by nuclei of the reticular formation in the brainstem. The **dorsal respiratory nucleus (ventrolateral nucleus solitarius)** sends contralateral projections to **LMNs of the phrenic nucleus** (diaphragm movements) and **thoracic LMNs for accessory respiratory muscles** (intercostal and other accessory muscles), regulating inspiration. The **ventral respiratory nucleus (nucleus retroambiguus)** sends contralateral projections to thoracic LMNs for accessory muscles regulating expiration. The dorsal and ventral respiratory nuclei mutually inhibit each other. The **medial parabrachial nucleus** functions as a **pacemaker**, with control over both the dorsal and ventral respiratory nuclei. Both **cortical** and **limbic (amygdala)** regions send input to the parabrachial pacemaker and can provide both voluntary and emotionally derived regulation of respiration.

Additional inputs may influence respiration. The dorsal respiratory nucleus receives inputs from the **carotid body** via **CN IX**; the carotid body detects carbon dioxide in a hypoxic state, and low blood pH, resulting in increased respiration. Chemosensors from the **aortic body** also send projections via **CN X** to the dorsal respiratory nucleus. **Central chemoreceptive zones in the lateral medulla** also project to the dorsal respiratory nucleus.

Clinical Note

The neural systems for control of respiration include the brainstem respiratory nuclei, the medial parabrachial nuclei, inputs from the cortex and limbic forebrain, and projections from the respiratory nuclei to LMNs in the phrenic nucleus and thoracic spinal cord. It is not surprising that disrupting this system at any point in the hierarchical neuronal control may produce disrupted respiration. If the forebrain is damaged (telencephalon and diencephalon), the patient will demonstrate **Cheyne–Stokes breathing** (crescendo-decrescendo breathing), with periods of hyperpnea followed by a period of apnea. If the damage extends into the midbrain and upper pons, as may occur during increased intracranial pressure and herniation, respiration is shallow with **hyperpnea**, accompanied by hypoxia. If the damage extends through the lower pons, the patient demonstrates **apneustic breathing**, with long inspiratory pauses prior to expiration. If the damage extends into the medulla, breathing is irregular with inspiratory gasps and periods of apnea (**ataxic breathing**). This pattern is likely to end with respiratory failure and death. In addition, excess presence of opioid peptides, particularly fentanyl, can suppress breathing and produce death, the major mechanism for death from opioid overdose.

COLOR the following structures, using a separate color for each structure.

- ☐ 1. **Cortical input to medial parabrachial nucleus**
- ☐ 2. **Amygdala input to medial parabrachial nucleus**
- ☐ 3. **Medial parabrachial nucleus (pacemaker)**
- ☐ 4. **Dorsal respiratory nucleus (ventrolateral nucleus solitarius)**
- ☐ 5. **CN X**
- ☐ 6. **Central chemoreceptive zones in the lateral medulla**
- ☐ 7. **Ventral respiratory nucleus (nucleus retroambiguus)**
- ☐ 8. **Aortic body**
- ☐ 9. **CN IX (glossopharyngeal)**
- ☐ 10. **Carotid body**
- ☐ 11. **LMNs of the phrenic nucleus**
- ☐ 12. **Thoracic LMNs for accessory respiratory muscles**

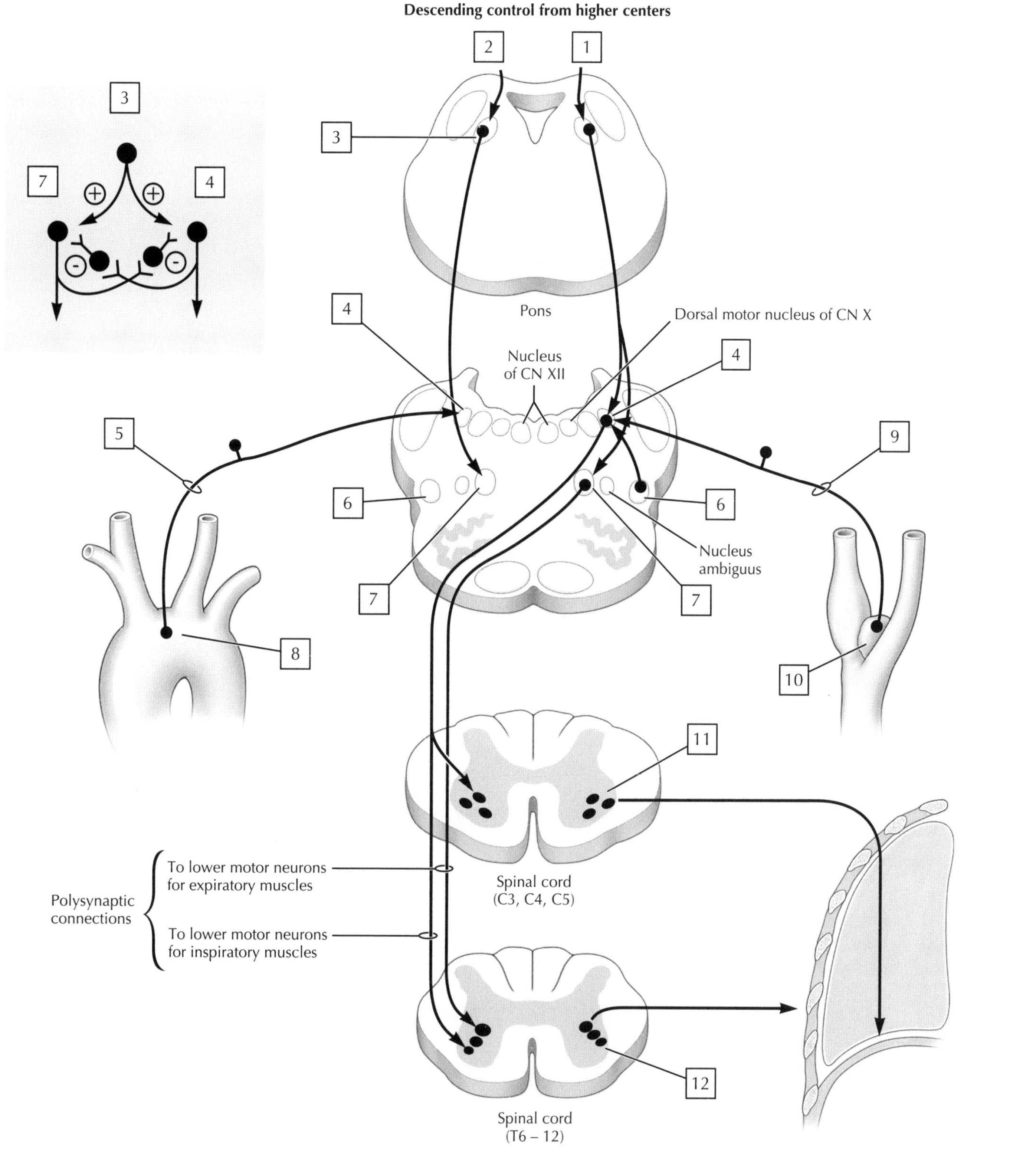

Descending control from higher centers
2
1
3
3
7
4
4
Pons
Dorsal motor nucleus of CN X
Nucleus
of CN XII
4
5
9
6
6
Nucleus
ambiguus
7
7
8
10
11
To lower motor neurons
for expiratory muscles
Polysynaptic
connections
To lower motor neurons
for inspiratory muscles
Spinal cord
(C3, C4, C5)
12
Spinal cord
(T6 – 12)

Cerebellar Organization and Neuronal Circuitry

The **cerebellum** is anatomically part of the brainstem (derived from the pons), receiving input from sensory, motor, and autonomic structures, and is particularly important for smoothing and coordinating motor activities, including voluntary movement, tone and posture, balance and coordination, and speech. It is also involved in autonomic control, learning and memory tasks, emotional reactivity, and cognitive tasks. The cerebellum receives input from all sensory systems except the olfactory system, and also receives massive input from the cerebral cortex, including the motor, premotor, and supplemental cortical areas, and many regions of association cortex, via the **cortico-ponto-cerebellar projections**.

The cerebellum is organized with **deep nuclei** at the core, and an outer **cerebellar cortex** interconnected with the deep nuclei through Purkinje cell axonal projections. The deep nuclei act as the "coarse adjustment" mechanism for cerebellar modification of motor activity, and the cerebellar cortex acts as the "fine adjustment" mechanism. Anatomically, from outer to inner, the cerebellum consists of the three-layered cerebellar cortex (an **outer molecular layer**, **Purkinje cell layer,** and deeper **granule cell layer**), white matter for inputs and outputs of the cerebellar cortex, the deep nuclei, and the cerebellar peduncles that provide inputs to, and outputs from, the cerebellum, deep nuclei included.

Purkinje cells are the major neurons in the cerebellar cortex, with orderly **dendritic trees** organized in parallel within the folds (folia). They receive inputs from the **climbing fibers** (from the **inferior olivary nuclei**) and **mossy fibers** (from all other nuclei) via the granule cell axons. The granule cell axons ascend into the outer molecular layer and run as **parallel fibers**, intersecting the planar dendritic trees of the Purkinje cells (up to 600 or more). Cerebellar **cortical interneurons (basket cells, outer stellate cells, Golgi cells)** regulate the excitability of Purkinje cell responses. **Noradrenergic axons** from locus coeruleus neurons distribute to all zones of the cerebellar cortex, and control the gain (excitability) of all neuronal types, including glutamate excitability and GABA inhibition in the same target neurons at the same time. The Purkinje cells send their axons to the deep nuclei, and provide fine-tuning of their regulation of the **upper motor neuronal systems.**

COLOR each of the following structures, using a separate color for each structure.

- ☐ 1. **Cerebellar cortex**
- ☐ 2. **Cerebellar deep nuclei**
- ☐ 3. **Upper motor neuronal systems**
- ☐ 4. **Parallel fibers intersecting Purkinje cell dendritic trees**
- ☐ 5. **Outer molecular layer**
- ☐ 6. **Granule cell layer**
- ☐ 7. **Mossy fibers to granule cells**
- ☐ 8. **Climbing fibers**
- ☐ 9. **Purkinje cells and layer**
- ☐ 10. **Purkinje cell dendritic trees**
- ☐ 11. **Cerebellar cortical interneurons (outer stellate cells, basket cells, Golgi cells)**
- ☐ 12. **Noradrenergic axons from locus coeruleus neurons**

Clinical Note

The cerebellar deep nuclei are considered the coarse adjustment mechanism for cerebellar smoothing and coordinating of motor activities, and the cerebellar cortex is considered the fine adjustment mechanism, acting through modifications of deep nuclei excitability. Classic cerebellar lesions of the lateral cerebellar hemisphere (middle or posterior lobe) result in ipsilateral alterations, including: (1) loss of coordination of movement, (2) ataxia, (3) gait disturbance, (4) mild hypotonia, (5) past-pointing, (6) decomposition of movement, (7) inability to perform rapid alternating movements (dysdiadochokinesia), (8) dysarthria, and other symptoms. If the deep nuclei and/or the cerebellar peduncles are damaged, the cerebellar dysfunction is severe and long lasting. If the cerebellar cortex is damaged without deep nuclei or peduncles involved, the initial symptoms are conspicuous, but may dissipate with time and rehabilitation.

A. General scheme

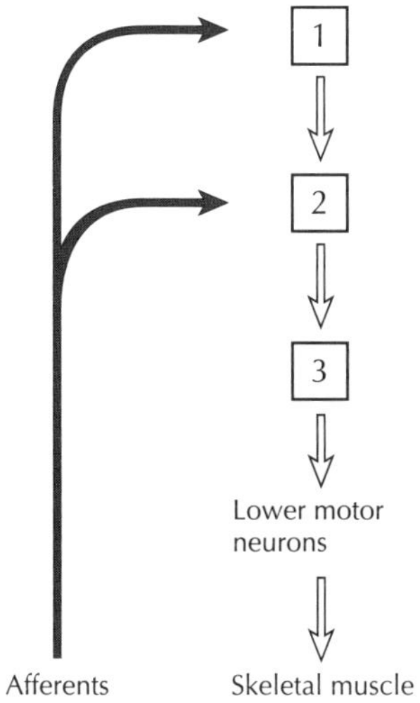

B. Deep nuclei relationship with afferents

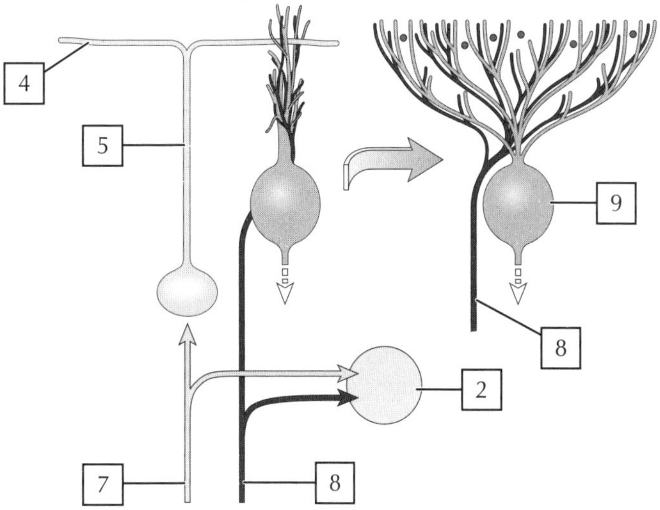

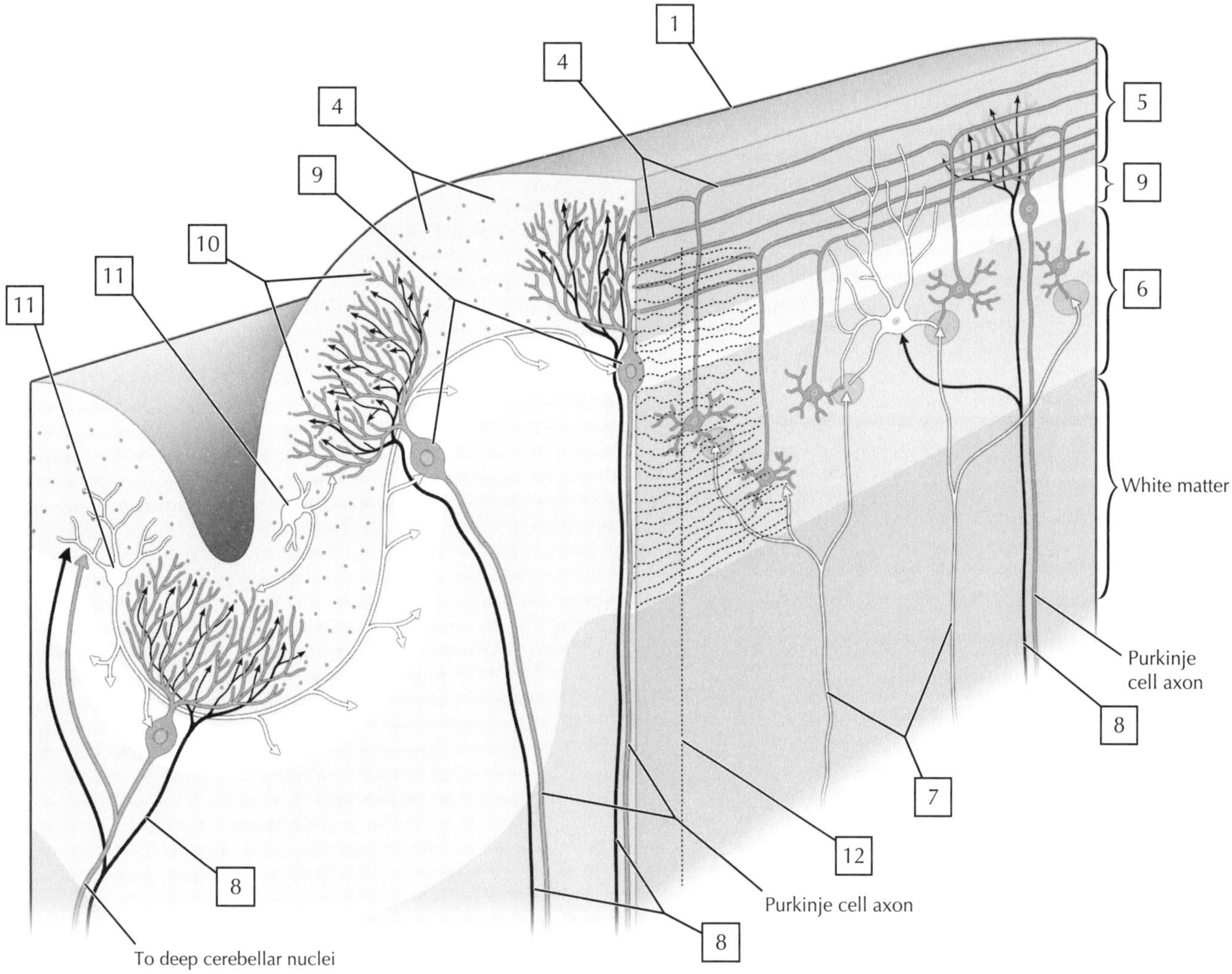

Cerebellar Afferents

Afferents (inputs) to the cerebellum enter through the **cerebellar peduncles** and project to both the **deep nuclei** (coarse adjustment) and the **cerebellar cortex** (fine adjustment). Somatosensory projections terminate in at least three topographical body representations in the cerebellar cortex. Somatosensory information from whole muscle activity projects to the cerebellum through the **ventral spinocerebellar tract** (lower body, below T6; crosses twice, once through the **anterior white commissure**, and then through the **superior cerebellar peduncle [SCP]**) and the **rostral spinocerebellar tract** (upper body, T6 and above, ipsilaterally through the **inferior cerebellar peduncle [ICP]**). Individual muscle fiber information projects to the cerebellum through the **dorsal spinocerebellar tract** (lower body, below T6) and the **cuneocerebellar tract** (upper body, T6 and above); both project ipsilaterally through the ICP.

The ICP also conveys information to the cerebellum from the **inferior olivary nuclei,** the brainstem **reticular formation, vestibular ganglion and nuclei,** and some **trigeminal nuclei**. The **middle cerebellar peduncle** conveys contralateral inputs from the **pontine nuclei,** as part of the **cortico-ponto-cerebellar system**. The SCP also conveys visual and auditory **tectocerebellar** input, some **trigeminal input**, and **noradrenergic projections** from the locus coeruleus.

This collective set of inputs allows the cerebellum to receive detailed, timely information on the status of muscles, joints, tendons, ligaments, comprehensive information from other sensory systems, and ongoing cortical activity. The cerebellum then processes the information as a comparator function to smooth and coordinate motor activity and other responses to sensory activity. The cerebral cortical input provides the cortical plan to compare with the state of the periphery. When correction and smoothing motor actions are taken, they are conveyed through UMN systems, not LMN systems.

COLOR the following structures, using a separate color for each structure.

- ☐ 1. **Reticular formation**
- ☐ 2. **Pontine nuclei**
- ☐ 3. **Inferior olivary nucleus**
- ☐ 4. **Vestibular ganglion and nuclei**
- ☐ 5. **Rostral spinocerebellar tract**
- ☐ 6. **Ventral spinocerebellar tract**
- ☐ 7. **Dorsal spinocerebellar tract**
- ☐ 8. **Cuneocerebellar tract**
- ☐ 9. **Inferior cerebellar peduncle (ICP)**
- ☐ 10. **Middle cerebellar peduncle**
- ☐ 11. **Superior cerebellar peduncle (SCP)**

Clinical Note

Damage to cerebellar inputs can produce a classic picture of cerebellar dysfunction, discussed in detail in the clinical note for Plate 10.12. Impingement of a herniated disc (nucleus pulposus) may produce both a radiculopathy and a myelopathy. As the disc impinges on the spinal cord, it first compresses the spinocerebellar tracts (especially the dorsal and ventral spinocerebellar tracts) at the lateral edge of the spinal cord, starting as clumsiness, ataxia, gait disturbance, and loss of coordination of movements. If deeper compression occurs to the descending lateral corticospinal tract and rubrospinal tract, ipsilateral UMN symptoms may predominate and mask some of the spinocerebellar damage.

Some forms of progressive neuronal degeneration may affect the cerebellar neurons and connections. **Friedreich ataxia** is a progressive autosomal recessive disorder that involves spinocerebellar tracts as well as other structures, and often is first seen with symptoms of ataxia, gait disturbance, dysmetria, decomposition of movements, and dysarthria. **Olivopontocerebellar atrophy** is a progressive, mainly autosomal dominant neurodegenerative disease that usually begins in middle age. It may start with gait disturbance and progress to limb ataxia and dysarthria. In addition, symptoms from basal ganglia damage also are seen, including dystonia, rigidity, and chorea.

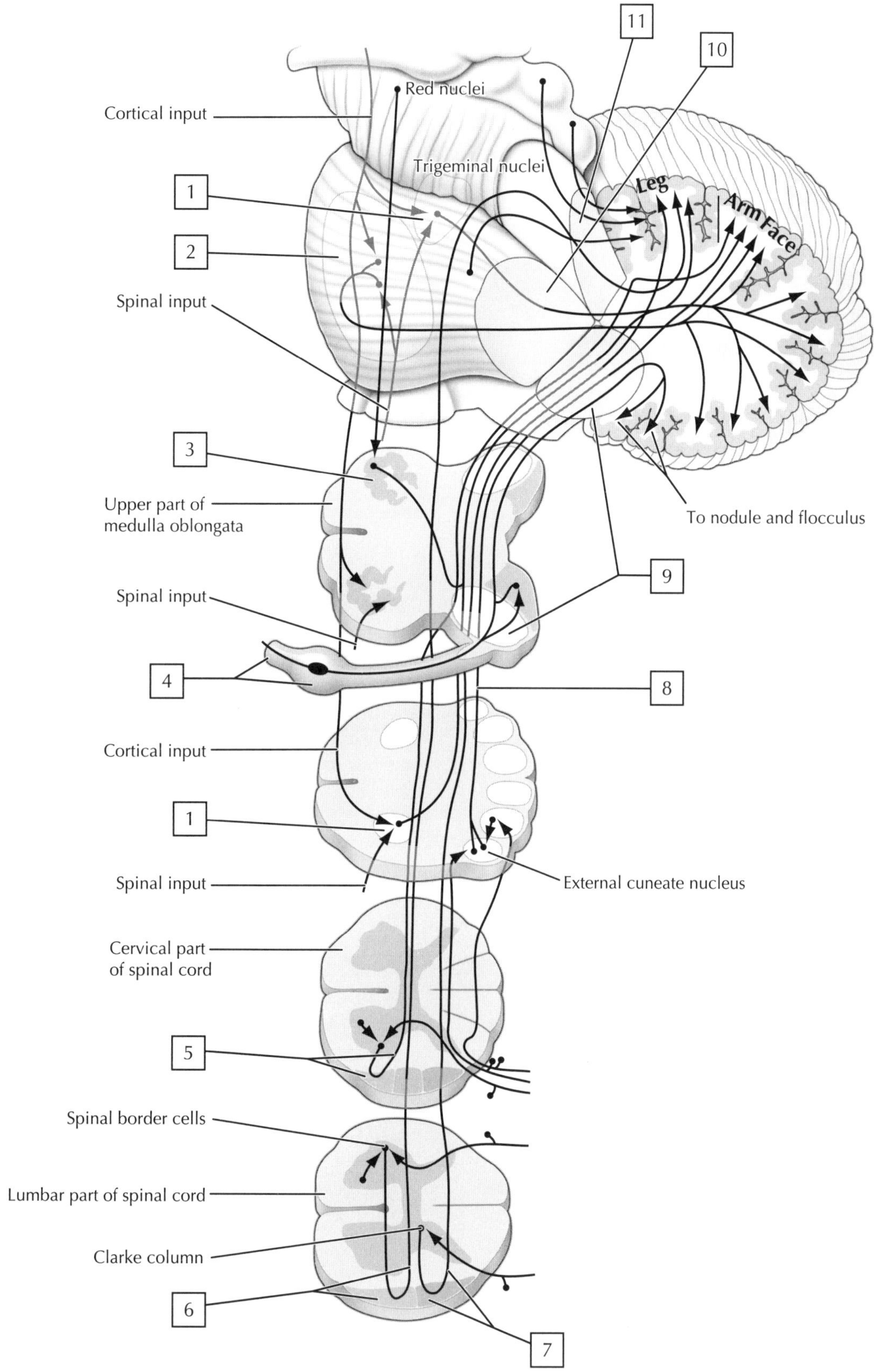
Red nuclei
Cortical input
Trigeminal nuclei
1
2
Spinal input
11
10
Leg
Arm
Face
3
Upper part of medulla oblongata
Spinal input
4
To nodule and flocculus
9
8
Cortical input
1
Spinal input
External cuneate nucleus
Cervical part of spinal cord
5
Spinal border cells
Lumbar part of spinal cord
Clarke column
6
7

Cerebellar Efferent Pathways

Cerebellar efferent pathways are organized according to the scheme of cerebellar cortex Purkinje cell axons to deep nuclei to **upper motor neurons (UMNs)**. The deep nuclei are the final output from the cerebellum to the UMNs. The **fastigial nucleus** receives input from the vermis (including anterior lobe) and flocculonodular lobe, and projects via the **ICP** to the vestibular and reticular nuclei, including the **lateral vestibular nucleus** (origin of the lateral vestibulospinal tract) and the **medial pontine and medullary reticular formation** (origin of the pontine and medullary reticulospinal tracts). Some Purkinje cell axons from the vermis and flocculonodular lobe project directly to the **lateral vestibular nucleus** through the ICP; this has led some neuroscientists to consider the lateral vestibular nucleus to be a **fifth deep cerebellar nucleus** (in addition to its role as a secondary sensory nucleus and a UMN cell group). The **globose and emboliform nuclei** receive input from the paravermis and project mainly to the **red nucleus** via crossed projections **(decussation) of the superior cerebellar peduncle (SCP)**; the red nucleus is the origin of the rubrospinal tract. A small portion of axons from the globose and emboliform nuclei project to the **ventral anterior (VA)** and **ventrolateral (VL) nuclei of the thalamus**. The **dentate nucleus** receives input from the lateral cerebellar hemispheres, and sends crossed projections through the decussation of the SCP to nuclei VA and VL of the thalamus, which in turn project axons through the **posterior limb of the internal capsule** to the **motor cortex, the premotor cortex, and the supplemental motor cortex**, the cortical regions of origin for the corticospinal tract. Thus the output of the cerebellum, especially the motor output, is directed systematically to the UMN systems to achieve smoothing and coordination of movements.

COLOR the following structures, using a separate color for each structure.

- ☐ 1. **Motor, premotor, and supplemental cortex (areas 4 and 6)**
- ☐ 2. **Posterior limb of the internal capsule**
- ☐ 3. **Ventrolateral nucleus of the thalamus**
- ☐ 4. **Ventral anterior nucleus of the thalamus**
- ☐ 5. **Decussation of the superior cerebellar peduncle (SCP)**
- ☐ 6. **Red nucleus**
- ☐ 7. **Fastigial nucleus**
- ☐ 8. **Globose nucleus**
- ☐ 9. **Emboliform nucleus**
- ☐ 10. **Inferior cerebellar peduncle (ICP)**
- ☐ 11. **Medial pontine and medullary reticular formation**
- ☐ 12. **Lateral vestibular nucleus**

Clinical Note

The cerebellum is a significant target for the toxic effects of pharmaceutical agents and environmental toxins. Some drugs, given in therapeutic dose ranges for a prolonged period, or taken in a toxic dose, can produce cerebellar symptoms, usually appearing as impairment of gait, and then limb ataxia. Potential damaging drugs include some antiseizure meds (phenytoin, carbamazepine, barbiturates, valproate), some cancer chemotherapeutic agents, and some psychoactive agents (especially neuroleptics). Toxic agents damaging to the cerebellum include organophosphates, some organic solvents, and some heavy metals (methylmercury, lead, thallium).

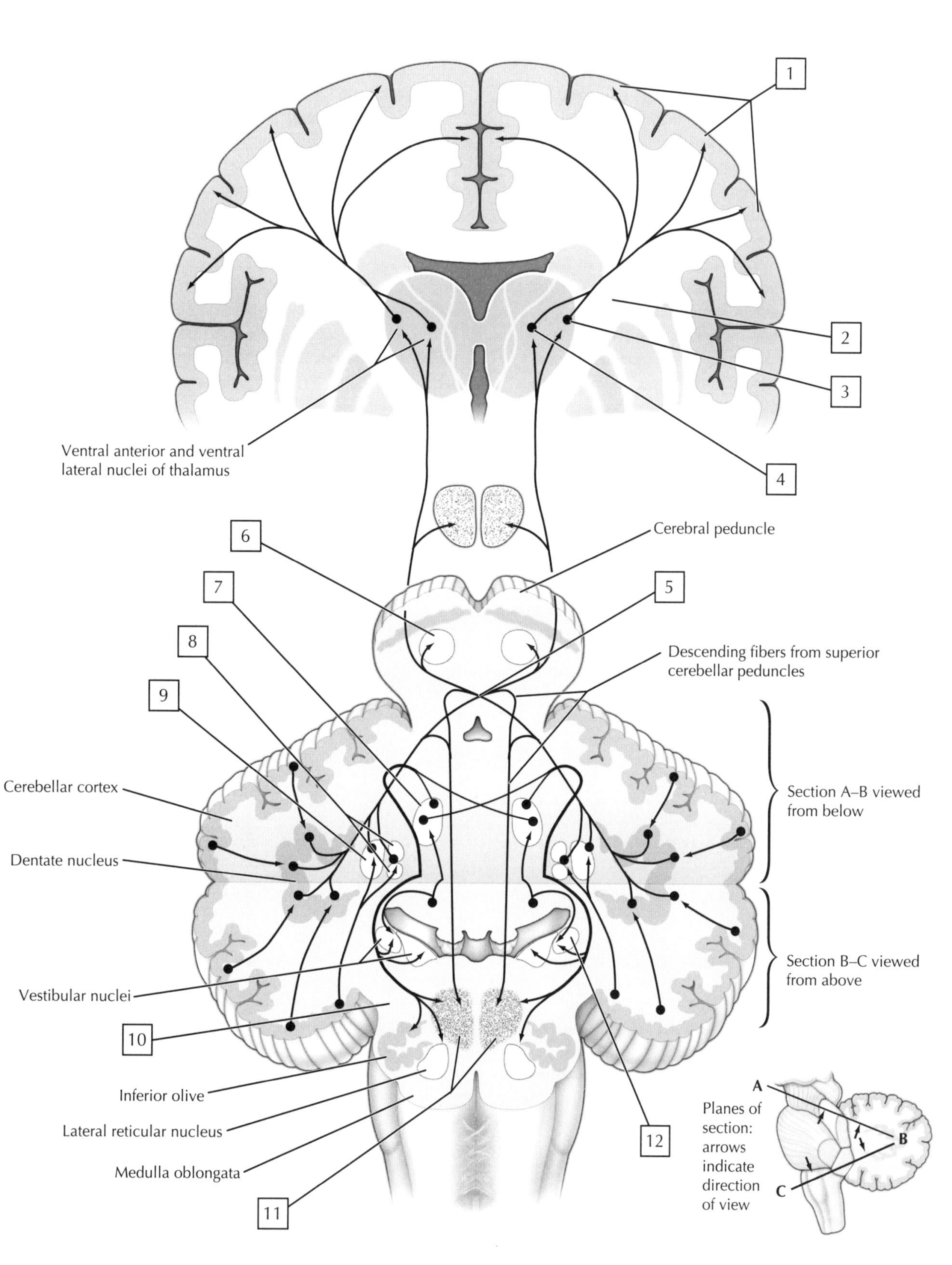
1
2
3
4
Ventral anterior and ventral lateral nuclei of thalamus
6
Cerebral peduncle
7
5
8
Descending fibers from superior cerebellar peduncles
9
Cerebellar cortex
Section A–B viewed from below
Dentate nucleus
Section B–C viewed from above
Vestibular nuclei
10
Inferior olive
Lateral reticular nucleus
Medulla oblongata
12
11
A
Planes of section: arrows indicate direction of view
B
C

10 Schematic Diagram of Cerebellar Efferents to Upper Motor Neurons

This schematic diagram demonstrates the relationship between specific regions of the cerebellar hemispheres, the deep cerebellar nuclei, and the UMN systems. The **vermis**, **flocculus**, and **nodule** project to the **fastigial nucleus**, which in turn regulates the **lateral vestibular nucleus** and **medial pontine and medullary reticular nuclei** that give rise to the lateral vestibular tract and pontine and medullary reticulospinal tracts, respectively. The **paravermis** projects to the **globose and emboliform nuclei**, which in turn regulate the **red nucleus** and its rubrospinal tract. The **lateral cerebellar hemispheres** project to the **dentate nucleus**, which in turn regulates the **ventral anterior (VA) and ventrolateral (VL) nuclei of the thalamus.** These thalamic nuclei project to the **motor premotor**, and **supplemental cortical areas**, which give rise to the **corticospinal tract**. The motor-related cortical areas also give rise to corticopontine projections to the **pontine nuclei** (which provide cortical information to the cerebellum) and the **corticorubral projection** (which contributes to the regulation of the rubrospinal system).

Clinical Note

The cerebellum helps to smooth and coordinate UMN activities. The corticospinal tract regulates fine, skilled movements, especially of the hand and fingers. A large region of the cerebellum and feedback to the cerebellum through the cortico-ponto-cerebellar system is dedicated to this task. The rubrospinal system helps to regulate flexor movements of the extremities, with the paravermis providing cerebellar modulation. The lateral vestibulospinal tract and pontine and medullary reticulospinal tracts help to regulate basic tone and posture, assisted by the vermis and flocculonodular lobes (sometimes called the vestibulocerebellum). Loss of corticospinal and corticorubral regulation leads to decortication (upper extremities flexed, lower extremities extended). Further loss of the rubrospinal tracts leads to decerebration (all four limbs extended). Further loss of vestibulospinal and reticulospinal regulation is usually incompatible with life.

COLOR each of the following structures, using a separate color for each structure.

- ☐ 1. **Motor premotor, and supplemental cortical areas**
- ☐ 2. **Ventral anterior (VA) and ventrolateral (VL) nuclei of the thalamus**
- ☐ 3. **Pontine nuclei**
- ☐ 4. **Red nucleus**
- ☐ 5. **Corticospinal tract**
- ☐ 6. **Corticorubral projections**
- ☐ 7. **Globose and emboliform nuclei**
- ☐ 8. **Dentate nucleus**
- ☐ 9. **Lateral cerebellar hemispheres**
- ☐ 10. **Paravermis**
- ☐ 11. **Flocculus**
- ☐ 12. **Lateral vestibular nucleus**
- ☐ 13. **Medial pontine and medullary reticular nuclei**
- ☐ 14. **Nodule**
- ☐ 15. **Fastigial nucleus**
- ☐ 16. **Vermis**

Schematic Diagram of Cerebellar Efferents to Upper Motor Neurons

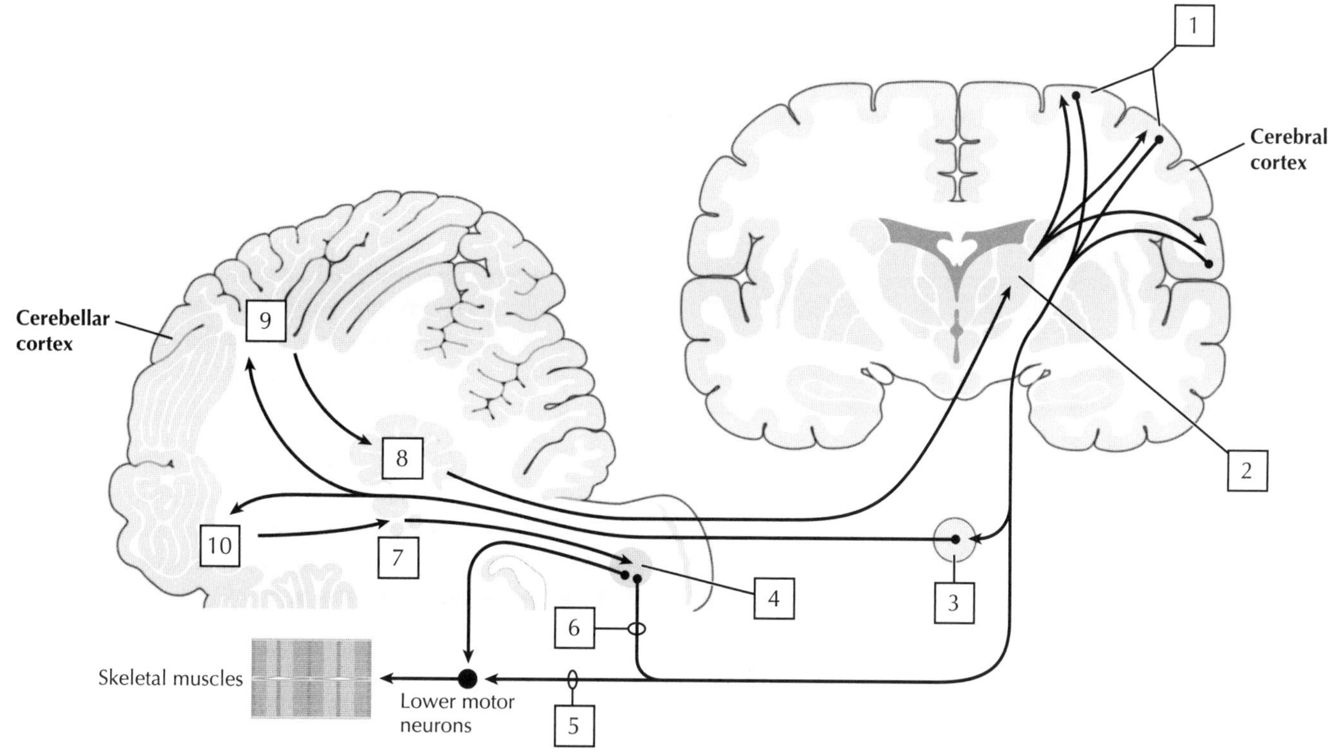

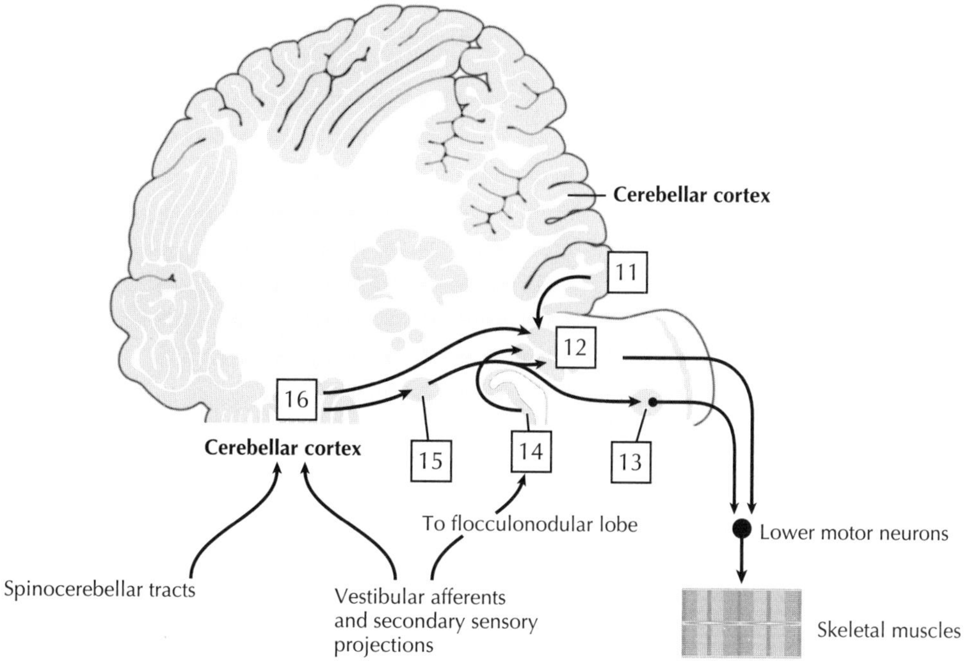

Connections of the Basal Ganglia

The basal ganglia are a group of forebrain nuclei, including the **striatum** (**caudate nucleus**, **putamen**) and the **pallidum (globus pallidus)**; the **subthalamus** (diencephalon) and the **substantia nigra** (midbrain) also are part of the basal ganglia circuitry. This system assists the thalamocortical circuits to select wanted and learned programs of activities and suppress or hold in check unwanted or interfering programs of activity. They are best known clinically for their involvement in movement disorders, but also participate in cognitive, affective, visceral (autonomic), oculomotor, and other activities. The connectivity forms circuits from the cortex to the basal ganglia to the thalamus and back to the cortex.

Widespread areas of the cerebral cortex project to the caudate nucleus and putamen **(corticostriate projections)**. The caudate and putamen send connections to the internal and external segments of the globus pallidus. The **internal segment of the globus pallidus** sends axons to **thalamic nuclei** (VA, VL, centromedian) via the **lenticular fasciculus** and the **ansa lenticularis**. Nuclei VA and VL regulate the cortical areas (4 and 6) that give rise to the corticospinal system and cortical control of other brainstem UMNs. The **external segment of the globus pallidus** is reciprocally interconnected with the subthalamic nucleus. The **substantia nigra pars compacta** gives rise to the **dopaminergic nigrostriatal pathway** (to the caudate nucleus and the putamen)**,** whose damage is involved in Parkinson's disease. The rostral raphe nuclei also send ascending serotonergic axons to basal ganglia structures, including the striatum.

COLOR the following structures, using a separate color for each structure.

- ☐ 1. **Caudate nucleus**
- ☐ 2. **Thalamic nuclei (VA, VL, centromedian)**
- ☐ 3. **Subthalamus (subthalamic nucleus)**
- ☐ 4. **Pars compacta of the substantia nigra**
- ☐ 5. **Internal segment of the globus pallidus**
- ☐ 6. **External segment of the globus pallidus**
- ☐ 7. **Globus pallidus**
- ☐ 8. **Putamen**
- ☐ 9. **Corticostriate projections**
- ☐ 10. **Dopaminergic nigrostriatal pathway**
- ☐ 11. **Substantia nigra**

Clinical Note

Parkinson's disease is a neurodegenerative condition in which dopaminergic neurons of the substantia nigra pars compacta die, and extensive axonal projections of the dopaminergic nigrostriatal pathway are lost. The remaining axons attempt to compensate by releasing more dopamine, which leads to further deterioration of the dopaminergic terminals in the striatum through oxidative damage from toxic metabolites of dopamine. The resultant condition of Parkinson disease causes **bradykinesia** (difficulty initiating or stopping movements), a **resting tremor**, **muscular rigidity** (through all ranges of motion, flexor and extensor, called lead pipe rigidity), and **postural instability**.

Huntington's disease is a progressive inherited (dominant-chromosome 4 with trinucleotide repeats) neurodegenerative disorder involving loss of neurons in the caudate nucleus, some cortical areas, and other structures, with accompanying choreiform movements (brisk dance-like movements), cognitive decline, and affective dysfunction. Other basal ganglia movement disorders include **dystonia**, **athetosis** (slow writhing movements), and **spasmodic torticollis** (writhing movements of neck muscles). **Tourette syndrome** involves tics and involuntary vocalizations, grunts, sometimes bursts of explosive cursing, and hyperactive behavior, often starting in childhood.

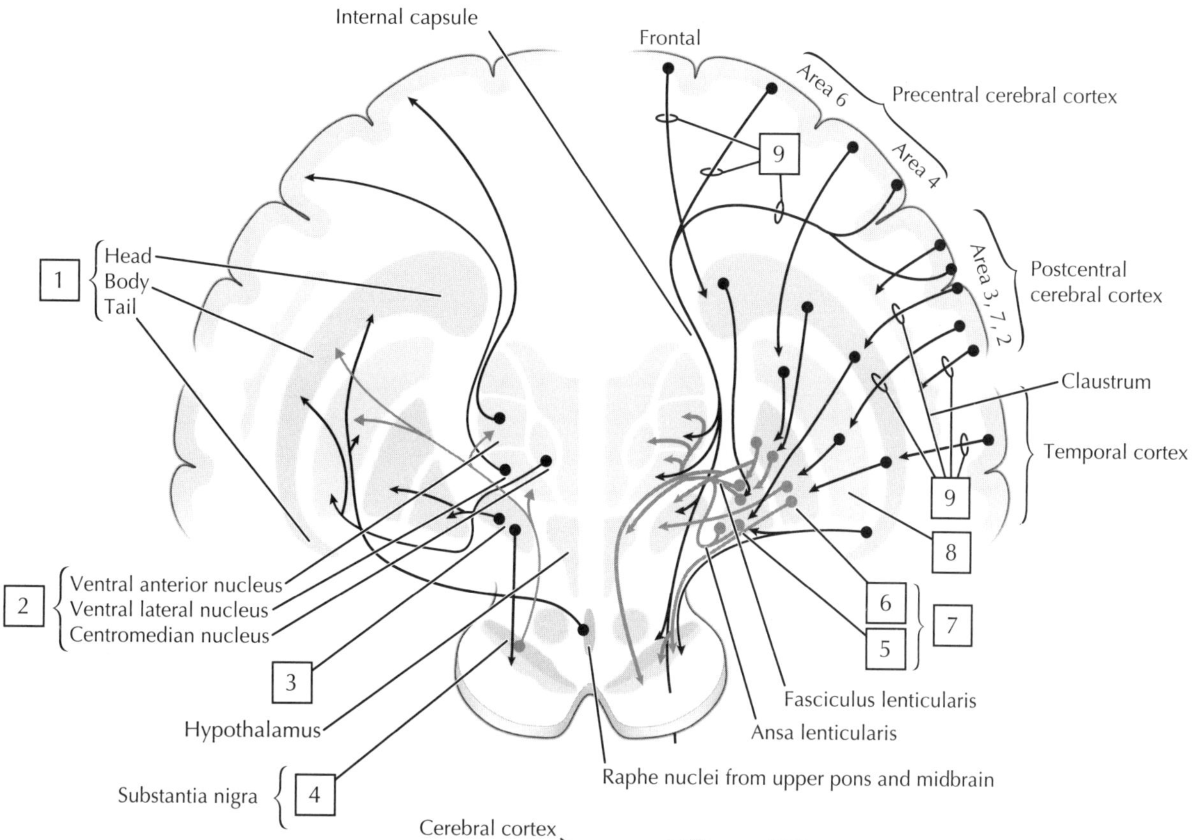

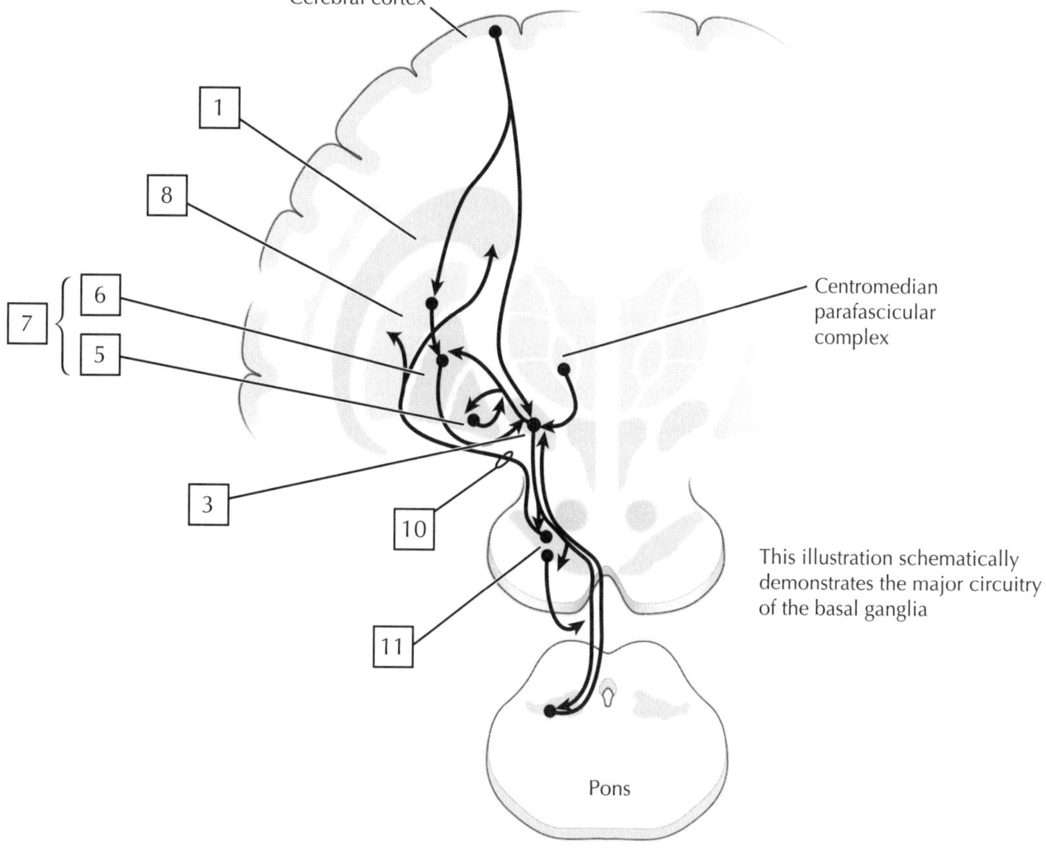

This illustration schematically demonstrates the major circuitry of the basal ganglia

11

Chapter 11 Autonomic–Hypothalamic–Limbic Systems

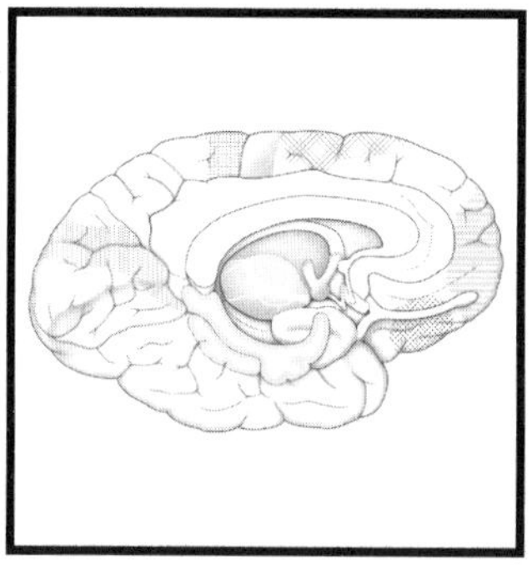
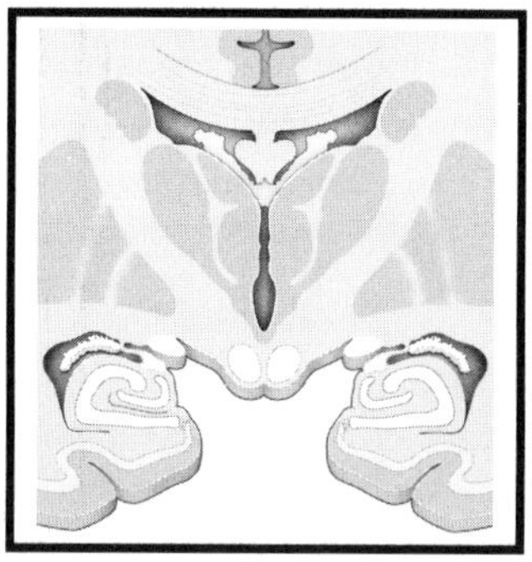
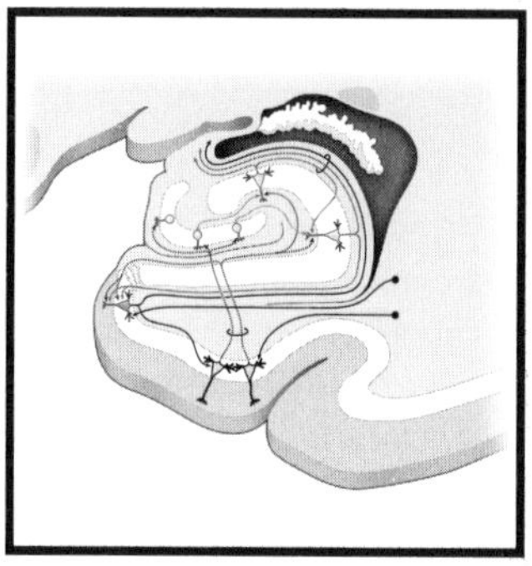
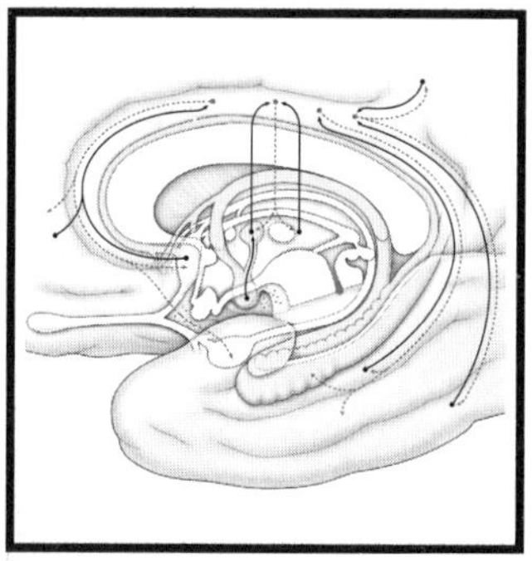

11 General Organization of the Autonomic Nervous System

The autonomic nervous system (ANS) provides regulation of visceral activities, in coordination with neuroendocrine activities, orchestrated by the **hypothalamus**. The ANS consists of a sympathetic division (activational, fight-or-flight system) and a **parasympathetic** division (quiet, homeostatic, reparative system). Some neuroscientists consider the enteric (gut) nervous system as a third component of the ANS; however, the enteric nervous system is a mainly independent peripheral collection of neurons associated with the gut, receiving both sympathetic and parasympathetic inputs, but also functioning autonomously.

The ANS is composed of a two-neuron chain interconnecting preganglionic neurons in the central nervous system (CNS) with ganglion cells in the periphery, which in turn innervate the target tissues, including smooth muscle, cardiac muscle, secretory glands, metabolic tissues (e.g., liver, fat), and immunocytes in primary and secondary lymphoid organs, mucosal-associated (gut, pulmonary) lymphoid tissue, and skin. The sympathetic nervous system is a **thoracolumbar** system, with preganglionic cell bodies found in the **intermediolateral cell column (lateral horn) of the T1–L2 spinal cord**. The myelinated preganglionic axons exit through the ventral roots, traverse the white ramus communicans, and either synapse in the **sympathetic chain ganglia (paravertebral ganglia)** or continue through **splanchnic nerves** to synapse in **sympathetic collateral (prevertebral) ganglia**, closer to the innervated target tissue. Some preganglionic sympathetic axons (T10–L1) travel through splanchnic nerves, synapse directly on **adrenal medullary chromaffin cells**, and regulate the release of epinephrine and norepinephrine as part of the **sympathoadrenal system**. Postganglionic unmyelinated sympathetic axons distribute to the target tissue.

The parasympathetic nervous system is a **craniosacral** system. It arises from preganglionic neurons in the brainstem (**nucleus of Edinger–Westphal [III]**, **superior salivatory nucleus [VII]**, **inferior salivatory nucleus [IX]**, and the **dorsal motor [autonomic] nucleus of the vagus [X]**) and the **intermediomedial cell column** in the **intermediate gray of the S2–S4 spinal cord.** The myelinated axons travel through their respective cranial nerves or sacral nerve roots and pelvic nerves, and synapse in **intramural ganglia,** located close to or within the innervated target tissue. Most of the postganglionic parasympathetic axons also are unmyelinated; ciliary ganglion axonal projections to the ciliary muscle and pupillary constrictor muscle are myelinated

The postganglionic sympathetic axons release norepinephrine as their principal neurotransmitter (with colocalized neuropeptides), which acts on subsets of alpha- and beta-adrenergic receptors on target tissues. The postganglionic parasympathetic axons release acetylcholine as their principal neurotransmitter (with colocalized neuropeptides), which acts on subsets of nicotinic and muscarinic cholinergic receptors. All preganglionic axons release acetylcholine as their principal neurotransmitter to interact with nicotinic receptors on ganglion cells.

COLOR the following structures, using a separate color for each structure.

- ☐ 1. **Nucleus of Edinger–Westphal**
- ☐ 2. **Superior salivatory nucleus**
- ☐ 3. **Inferior salivatory nucleus**
- ☐ 4. **Dorsal motor (autonomic) nucleus of X**
- ☐ 5. **Intermediolateral cell column in the lateral horn**
- ☐ 6. **Intermediate gray of the S2–S4 spinal cord**
- ☐ 7. **Sympathetic chain ganglia**
- ☐ 8. **Splanchnic nerve**
- ☐ 9. **Adrenal medulla (site of chromaffin cells)**
- ☐ 10. **Sympathetic collateral ganglion**
- ☐ 11. **Intramural parasympathetic ganglia**
- ☐ 12. **Hypothalamic regions regulating preganglionic autonomic outflow**

Clinical Note

The balance between sympathetic activation and parasympathetic repair and homeostatic maintenance is critical for the survival of the organism. Sympathetic activation is essential for reacting to danger and aversive internal and external conditions. However, chronic sympathetic activation, as many humans experience from personal, financial, social, and other circumstances (e.g., isolation in an epidemic), may be highly detrimental to the well-being of the individual, contributing to cardiovascular disease, cerebrovascular disease, hypertension, metabolic dysregulation such as type 2 diabetes and metabolic syndrome, and impaired immune responses to viruses and metastatic spread of cancers. Many of the relaxation strategies and "complementary medicine" approaches now in practice for many patients with cancer and other chronic diseases induce a parasympathetic state as a principal component.

General Organization of the Autonomic Nervous System

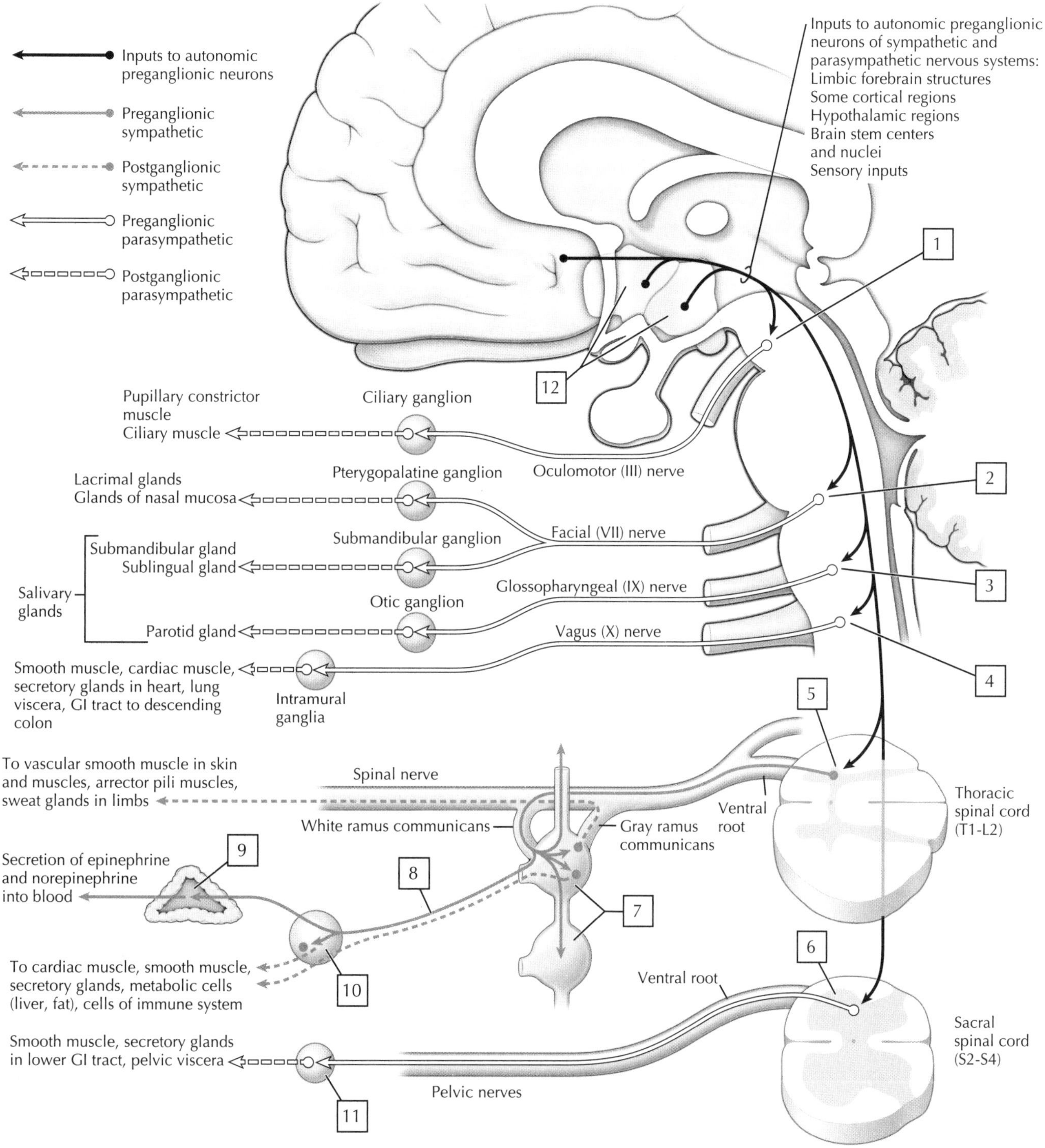

Forebrain Regions Associated With the Hypothalamus

Classical components of the limbic forebrain, including the **amygdaloid nuclei** (emotional responsiveness), the **hippocampal formation** (consolidation of short-term memory), **septal nuclei** (emotional reactivity to environmental stimuli), and others, are notable for utilizing connectivity with the hypothalamus to achieve the visceral/autonomic, neuroendocrine, and motor reactivity needed to accomplish their behavioral goals and intended activities. However, there also are several forebrain areas, both cortical and subcortical, that are important in control of emotional responsiveness, cognition, learning and memory, internal and external responsiveness, decision making, and other activities and behaviors.

Key Regions Associated With Limbic and Cortical Reactivity in the Limbic–Hypothalamic–Autonomic Axis

REGION	FUNCTIONAL ROLES
Prefrontal cortex-dorsolateral (dorsolateral and ventromedial components) See Plate 12.5	Regulates complex cognitive and rational decision making Planning and reasoning, analytical and intellectual ability Anticipatory goal orientation and predicting future outcomes Guiding appropriate social and personal behaviors Determining right from wrong
Orbitofrontal cortex (ventromedial PFC)	Sensory integration (with temporal lobe): smell, taste, touch Rewards, response to winning or losing Cognitive processing and decision making Involved in compulsive behaviors, repetitive behaviors, drives Impulse control and response inhibition, emotional reactivity Modulates body changes associated with emotion (e.g., anxiety) Participates with nucleus accumbens and the amygdala in regulating compulsive behaviors, repetitive behavior, and drives
Anterior cingulate cortex	Helps to regulate affect and emotionally uncomfortable circumstances Helps to detect errors and failure to reach goals Aids in decision making, and anticipation and preparation for activities Helps to regulate physiological processes (heart rate, blood pressure) Interconnects emotional limbic system with cognitive prefrontal cortex
Posterior cingulate cortex	Contributes to human awareness, internally driven cognition Active role in thinking and planning for the future Focusing of attention Participates in episodic memory retrieval Participates in pain awareness
Parahippocampal gyrus	Memory encoding and retrieval Helps navigation in the environment Encodes collective, not individual, environmental scenes Right side: helps to identify social context, such as sarcasm
Entorhinal cortex	Helps with memory and navigation, role in declarative memories (episodic, personal, semantic) and spatial memory Processes familiarity of signals involved in conditioning
Dorsal subiculum	Helps to regulate the hypothalamo–pituitary–adrenal axis
Insular cortex	Role in consciousness, body homeostasis, and perception Role in emotion, empathy, and compassion Perception (body warmth and coldness, abdominal distention, bladder fullness, dyspnea sensation, unpleasant smells) Perception of vestibular sensation, balance, and vertigo Role in laughter, crying, emotional response to music
Uncus, periamygdaloid cortex	Olfaction

For an insightful and fascinating discussion of these cortical areas, see Sapolsky RM. Behave: The Biology of Humans at Our Best and Worst. New York, Penguin Press, 2017.

COLOR the following structures, using a separate color for each structure.

- ☐ 1. **Posterior cingulate gyrus**
- ☐ 2. **Anterior cingulate gyrus**
- ☐ 3. **Prefrontal cortex (especially dorsolateral)**
- ☐ 4. **Hypothalamus**
- ☐ 5. **Orbitofrontal cortex (especially ventromedial prefrontal cortex)**
- ☐ 6. **Uncus**
- ☐ 7. **Amygdala (subcortical nuclei, deep to the cortex)**
- ☐ 8. **Hippocampal formation**
- ☐ 9. **Parahippocampal gyrus**

Clinical Note

Many of these cortical regions are complex, highly interactive with each other, and interconnect emotional, cognitive, and behavioral reactivity, and learning and memory, related to both internal and external conditions. Dysfunction in some of these areas may be involved in psychopathic behavior (e.g., prefrontal), compulsive behavior, depression, autistic spectrum disorder, and many other neuropsychiatric conditions. Some of the regulatory inputs (e.g., noradrenergic, dopaminergic, serotonergic, cholinergic) may drive both normal and abnormal functioning (e.g., depression) of many of these regions.

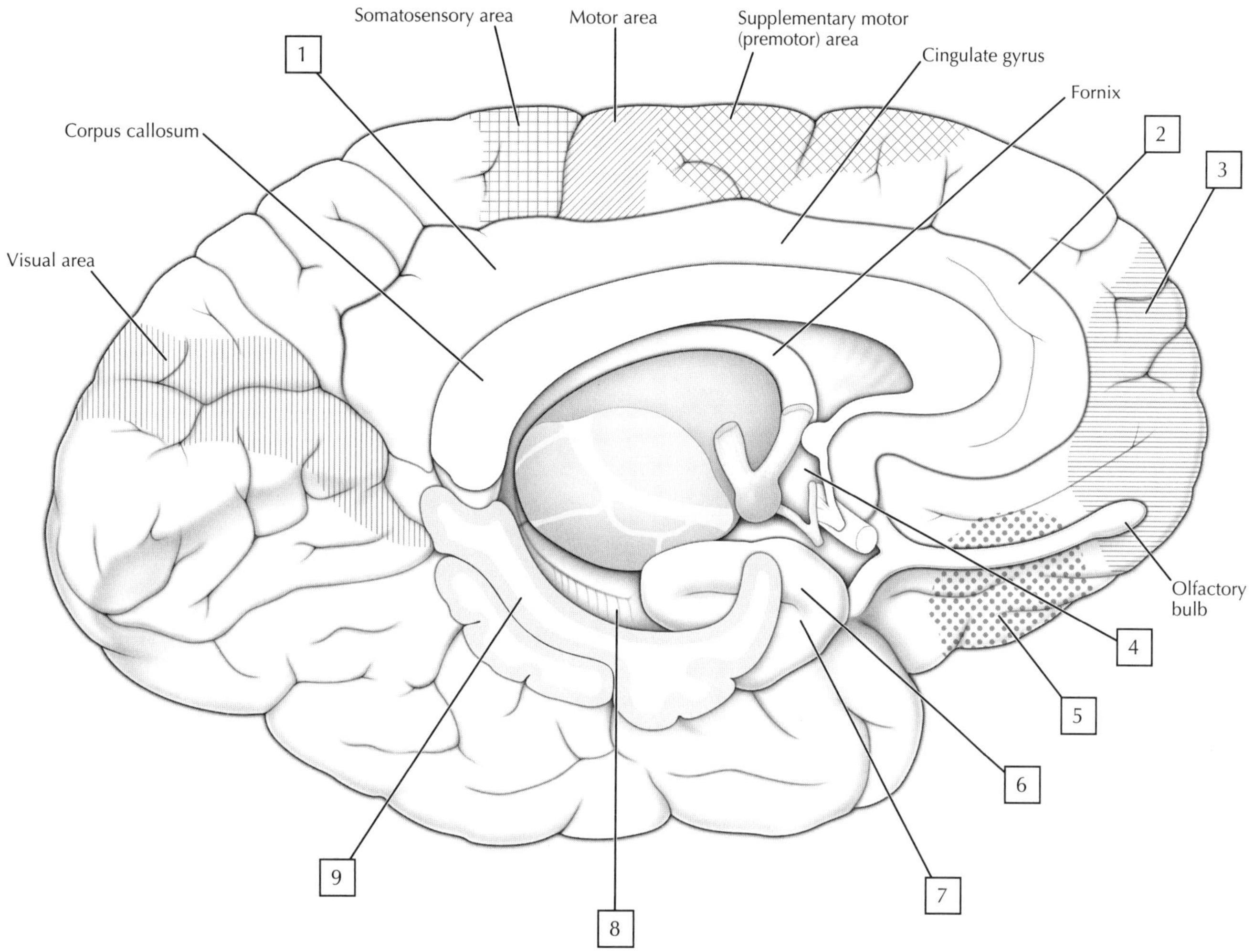
Somatosensory area
Motor area
Supplementary motor (premotor) area
Cingulate gyrus
Fornix
Corpus callosum
Visual area
Olfactory bulb
1
2
3
4
5
6
7
8
9

11 Afferent and Efferent Pathways Associated With the Hypothalamus

The cortical and subcortical forebrain structures, especially those involved in interpreting the external world and the internal milieu, provide emotional context and reactivity, cognitive responsiveness, reactivity based on past associations and memories, and individualized responses to provide optimal behavior in the interest of survival and attention to needs for well-being. Many of these responses require the activation of specific circuits of the hypothalamus (e.g., feeding, drinking, defensive responses, thermoregulation, other visceral functions), as well as achieving a balance between sympathetic activation (fight-or-flight, active engagement) and parasympathetic activation (quiet, homeostatic, reparative state).

Major inputs to the **hypothalamus** arise from the hippocampal formation and subiculum **(fornix)**; amygdaloid nuclei **(stria terminalis, ventral amygdalofugal pathway)**; **prefrontal cortex (both dorsolateral and ventromedial [part of orbitofrontal cortex]); cingulate cortex** (indirectly); **thalamus** (anterior nuclei); the **retina** (to the suprachiasmatic nucleus); and many other forebrain areas. The hypothalamus responds through connections that provide integrated action of visceral autonomic and motor circuits, and neuroendocrine circuits, resulting in appropriate behaviors and physiological activation to achieve the desired end-point effects. These hypothalamic efferent channels include the **descending median forebrain bundle** (mainly sympathetic components), **dorsal longitudinal fasciculus** (mainly parasympathetic components), **mammillotegmental tract** (from mammillary nuclei), and direct descending connections from the paraventricular nucleus (PVN) of the hypothalamus to sympathetic and parasympathetic preganglionic neurons and caudal nucleus solitarius. Connections from the hypothalamus to the neuroendocrine axis are channeled through the neurohypophyseal (supraopticohypophyseal) tract (axons from supraoptic and paraventricular nuclei) for secretion of oxytocin and vasopressin (VP) into the general circulation in the posterior lobe of the pituitary **(hypophysis)**, and through axons that secrete releasing factors and inhibitory factors into the hypophyseal portal system at the contact zone of the median eminence for regulation of release of anterior pituitary hormones.

COLOR the following structures, using a separate color for each structure.

- ☐ 1. **Fornix**
- ☐ 2. **Cingulate cortex**
- ☐ 3. **Thalamus**
- ☐ 4. **Prefrontal cortex**
- ☐ 5. **Hypothalamus (nuclei)**
- ☐ 6. **Orbitofrontal cortex**
- ☐ 7. **Hypophysis (pituitary)**
- ☐ 8. **Ventral amygdalofugal pathway**
- ☐ 9. **Mammillotegmental tract**
- ☐ 10. **Dorsal longitudinal fasciculus**
- ☐ 11. **Descending median forebrain bundle**
- ☐ 12. **Stria terminalis**

Clinical Note

The hypothalamus regulates the release of anterior pituitary hormones (affecting virtually every organ and system of the body), secretes vasopressin (regulating water balance and fluid osmolality) and oxytocin into the systemic circulation in the posterior pituitary gland, and provides neural circuitry for thermoregulation, control of cardiac function and blood pressure regulation (both short and long term), control of appetite and hunger, food intake, body weight and metabolism, aggressive versus passive responses to environmental or internal factors, and modulation of immune responses, to name a few. Damage to hypothalamic mechanisms or neuroendocrine mechanisms (e.g., pituitary adenoma) can result in direct disruption of these key hypothalamic circuits and neurons, producing pathological visceral functions and neuroendocrine responses (e.g., hypothyroidism, amenorrhea, diabetes insipidus). In addition, disruption or abnormal functioning of limbic forebrain input also can drive hypothalamic mechanisms with resultant pathological responses (e.g., anxiety and fear immobilizing the individual's appropriate or adaptive responses to external or internal stimuli).

Afferent and Efferent Pathways Associated With the Hypothalamus

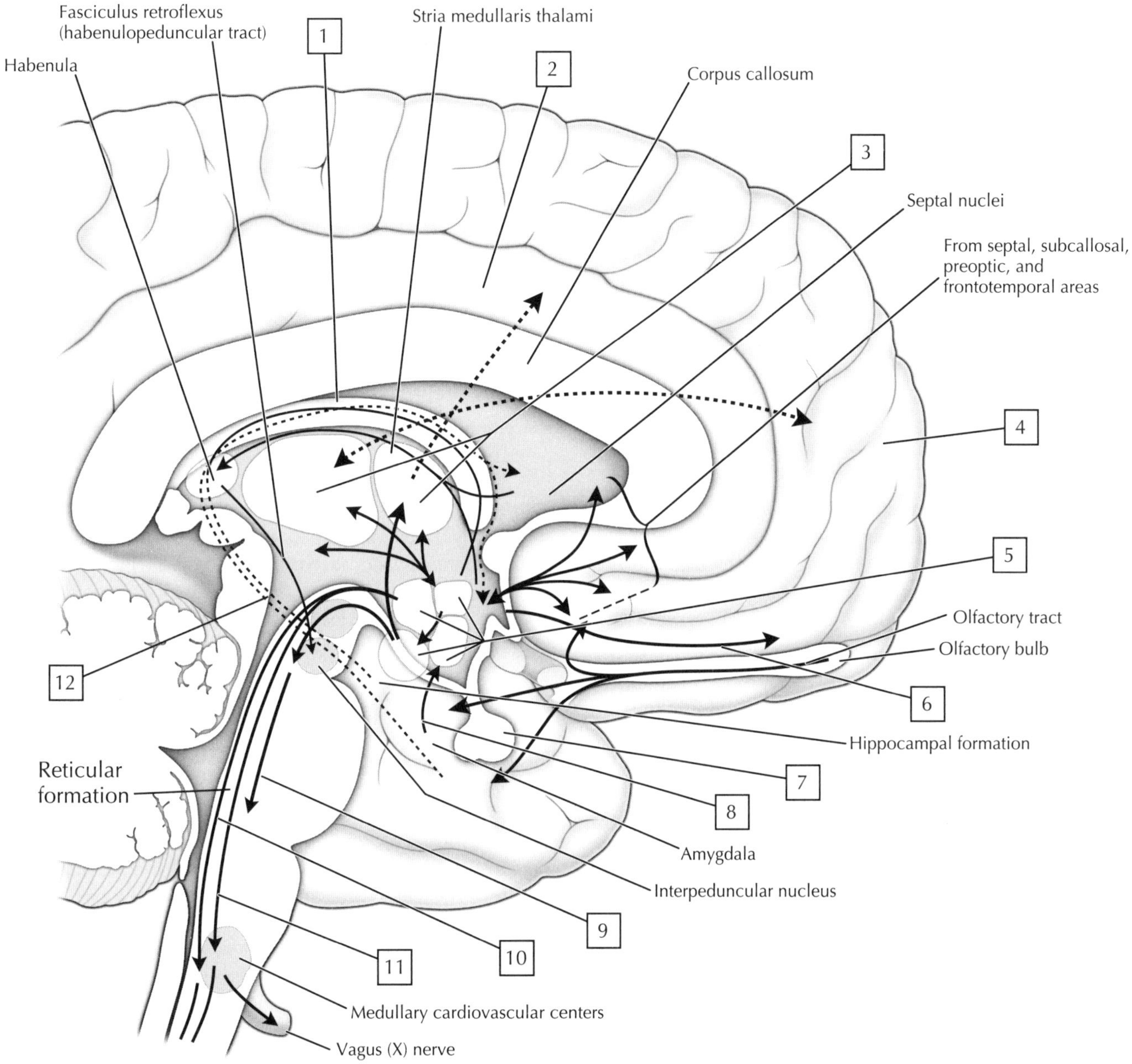

Arrows represent afferent and efferent pathways

11 Paraventricular Nucleus of the Hypothalamus

The **PVN** is a small nucleus in the upper medial region of the **hypothalamus,** sitting along either side of the upper third ventricle. It contains a remarkable collection of chemically specific neurons, many with subsets of connectivity both within the hypothalamus and with far-reaching regions of the CNS. This small nucleus helps to regulate and integrate neuroendocrine, visceral, autonomic, and limbic/emotional functions.

The **magnocellular neurons of the PVN** synthesize both oxytocin and arginine VP (mainly oxytocin) and send axons through the supraopticohypophyseal tract to end on blood vessels in the **posterior pituitary** (neurohypophysis). These hormones are transported by ultrafast axoplasmic transport to this vasculature and are released into the systemic circulation through fenestrated capillaries.

Some **parvocellular neurons in the PVN** synthesize corticotropin-releasing factor (CRF), and some parvocellular neurons synthesize VP. These axons travel in the tuberoinfundibular tract and end on the capillary system of the **hypophyseal-portal vascular system** in the contact zone of the median eminence. The CRF and VP are released into this private circulation system in high concentrations and influence the release of adrenocorticotropic hormone (ACTH) from pituicytes in the **anterior pituitary** (adenohypophysis).

Other **parvocellular neurons** send descending axons to terminate on preganglionic parasympathetic neurons in the **dorsal motor (autonomic) nucleus of the vagus (X)** (control of parasympathetic outflow to thoracic and abdominal viscera), on preganglionic sympathetic neurons in the **intermediolateral cell column in the lateral horn of the T1–L2 spinal cord** (control of sympathetic outflow), and to neurons in the **caudal nucleus solitarius,** a nucleus in the medulla that coordinates the balance of sympathetic–parasympathetic activation. Additional projections from the parvocellular neurons of the paraventricular nucleus are distributed to **amygdaloid nuclei,** the **locus coeruleus** (the source of ascending noradrenergic axons, especially to the hypothalamus, limbic forebrain, and cerebral cortex), and the **parabrachial nuclei.**

COLOR the following structures, using a separate color for each structure.

- ☐ 1. **Paraventricular nucleus (PVN) of the hypothalamus**
- ☐ 2. **Hypophyseal-portal vascular system**
- ☐ 3. **Anterior pituitary (adenohypophysis)**
- ☐ 4. **Posterior pituitary (neurohypophysis)**
- ☐ 5. **Parvocellular neurons in the PVN sending CRF-containing axons to the median eminence**
- ☐ 6. **Nucleus solitarius (nucleus tractus solitarius)**
- ☐ 7. **Intermediolateral cell column in the lateral horn of the T1–L2 spinal cord**
- ☐ 8. **Dorsal motor (autonomic) nucleus of the vagus (X)**
- ☐ 9. **Locus coeruleus in the upper pons**
- ☐ 10. **Parvocellular neuronal projections to the amygdala**
- ☐ 11. **Parvocellular neurons in the PVN sending descending axons to autonomic nucleus**
- ☐ 12. **Magnocellular neurons of PVN projecting to the posterior pituitary**

Clinical Note

In the early days of tracing connections from the hypothalamus to the autonomic and visceral structures in the brainstem and spinal cord, it was presumed that these descending projections were polysynaptic and lacked the precision of motor or sensory connectivity. The focus of attention was directed toward pathways such as the descending median forebrain bundle and dorsal longitudinal fasciculus, with myriad axonal systems entering, leaving, and traversing these bundles. More detailed techniques for anterograde and retrograde transport and for identifying chemically specific neurons (fluorescence histochemistry, immunohistochemistry, in situ hybridization) permitted more accurate tracing of hypothalamic connections. Surprisingly, small neurons in the PVN appeared to coordinate the activational state of sympathetic and parasympathetic systems through direct hypothalamo–medullary and hypothalamo–spinal projections, with additional collaterals communicating with key brainstem autonomic and regulatory systems (locus coeruleus, parabrachial nuclei) and limbic forebrain structures involved in providing emotional connotation of stimuli and perceptions (amygdala). Thus it appears that precise control and connectivity apply as much to the hypothalamo–autonomic axis as it does to the motor and sensory systems.

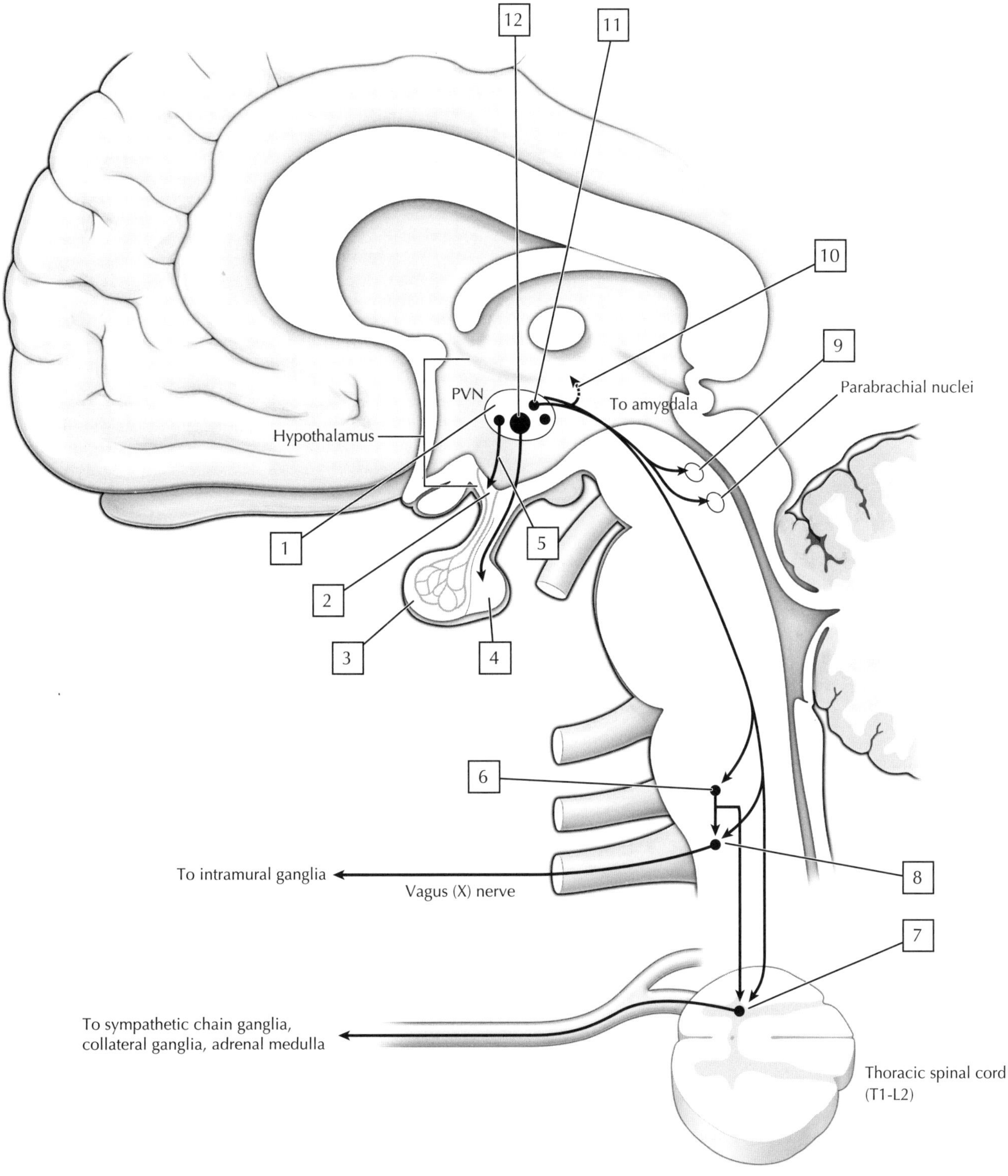
12
11
10
9
Parabrachial nuclei
PVN
To amygdala
Hypothalamus
1
2
3
4
5
6
8
7
To intramural ganglia
Vagus (X) nerve
To sympathetic chain ganglia, collateral ganglia, adrenal medulla
Thoracic spinal cord (T1-L2)

Cytokine Influences on Brain and Behavior

Illness behavior, especially as a consequence of infectious diseases, may include fever, decreased appetite, induction of slow-wave sleep, lethargy, and loss of attention or interest in surroundings. Studies of bidirectional neural–immune signaling have demonstrated that illness behavior is induced by cytokine actions on the brain, especially interleukin (IL)-1β, and can be blocked by an IL-1β receptor antagonist. Cytokines (especially inflammatory cytokines IL-1β, IL-6, tumor necrosis factor-α) and prostaglandin E_2 (PGE_2) have widespread influence on neural functioning; they act especially through the hypothalamus.

Inflammatory cytokines can activate both the hypothalamo–pituitary–adrenal (HPA) axis and the sympathetic nervous system, resulting in peripheral secretion of the two major classes of stress hormones, cortisol and catecholamines (norepinephrine and epinephrine). Chronic activation of the stress axes through this mechanism may increase the likelihood of chronic diseases, such as cardiovascular disease and stroke, metabolic syndrome, type 2 diabetes, and some cancers or their metastases.

Cytokines have many mechanisms by which they may influence brain function: (1) cytokines may directly cross the blood-brain barrier, especially through **cortical cerebral vasculature**; (2) cytokines and PGE_2 may cross into the cerebrospinal fluid (CSF) through circumventricular organs such as the **organum vasculosum of the lamina terminalis (OVLT)**, and activate cells with hypothalamic and visceral connectivity; (3) cytokines may provoke the release of small molecules such as nitric oxide, which can directly cross into the brain, through the **vasculature to the hypothalamus**, and activate neurons; (4) cytokines and PGE_2 may directly activate **vagal afferents** through interactions with **paraganglion cells**, leading to stimulation of neurons in the **caudal nucleus solitarius**, thereby influencing autonomic functions and connections of the PVN; (5) cytokines and PGE_2 may activate **other primary sensory afferents**, may provoke **release of norepinephrine from sympathetic postganglionic axon terminals**, and may modulate the **actions of neurotransmitters with their receptors in target cells**; and (6) cytokines may modulate the **release of pituitary hormones**.

COLOR the following structures, using a separate color for each structure.

- ☐ 1. **Cortical cerebral vasculature**
- ☐ 2. **Organum vasculosum of the lamina terminalis**
- ☐ 3. **Vasculature to the hypothalamus associated with release and actions of nitric oxide and PGE_2**
- ☐ 4. **Site of cytokine modulation of release of anterior pituitary hormones**
- ☐ 5. **Vagal efferents in the viscera**
- ☐ 6. **Paraganglion cells associated with vagal afferents**
- ☐ 7. **Somatic primary sensory afferents activated by cytokines and PGE_2**
- ☐ 8. **Site of cytokine stimulation of release of norepinephrine from postganglionic sympathetic nerves**
- ☐ 9. **Site of cytokine modulation of neurotransmitter signaling in target cells**
- ☐ 10. **Nucleus solitarius (nucleus tractus solitarius)**

Clinical Note

Studies in neural–immune signaling indicate that cytokines, through many of the mechanisms noted above, are capable of gaining access to both the CNS and peripheral regions such as vagal and somatic afferents, target cells, and the anterior pituitary. In the CNS, cytokines such as IL-1β provoke classic characteristics of illness behavior, which enhance a healing milieu. The inflammatory cytokines also provoke extensive changes in CNS neurotransmitter release and signaling, especially with the catecholamines and serotonin. In addition, the inflammatory cytokine in the CNS activates the major stress axes, the HPA system, and the sympathoadrenal system. It is therefore clear that cytokine–brain signaling is a powerful, ongoing form of immune–neural communication. Cytokines other than the inflammatory molecules also have effects on the brain. IL-2 was infused into cancer patients as a component of immunotherapy; in some individuals, IL-2 provoked depression and suicidal ideation. Neural–immune signaling networks are extensive, physiologically important, and bidirectional.

Behaviors Influenced by Cytokines:
Illness behavior
Affective behavior
Cognitive behavior
Autonomic and neuroendocrine regulation

(C) = **Interleukin-1α (IL-1α)**
Other cytokines acting on brain:
IL-6 (interleukin-6)
TNF-α (tumor necrosis factor-α)
IL-2 (interleukin-2)

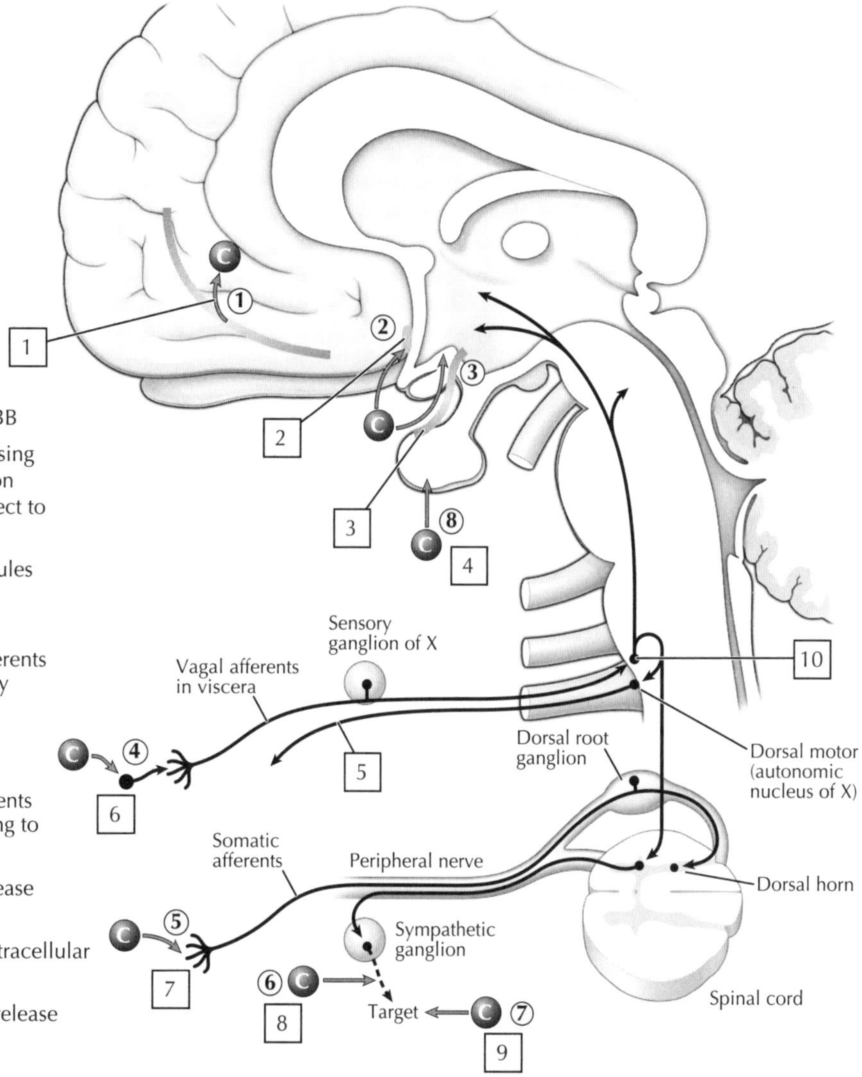

1. Cytokines transported directly across the BBB
2. Cytokines and prostaglandin E_2 (PGE_2) crossing into cerebrospinal fluid at OVLT or acting on cells that release PGE_2 or neurons that project to visceral-autonomic structures
3. Cytokine-stimulated release of small molecules (such as nitric oxide and PGE_2) that directly cross into the brain and act as mediators
4. Cytokine and PGE_2 stimulation of vagal afferents (through paraneurons) that modulate activity in nucleus tractus solitarius, influencing the multiple activities of the paraventricular nucleus and many other sites
5. Cytokine and PGE_2 activation of other afferents that modulate dorsal horn sensory processing to many sites
6. Cytokine modulation of norepinephrine release from sympathetic nerve terminals
7. Cytokine modulation of neurotransmitter intracellular signaling in target cells
8. Cytokine modulation of pituitary hormone release

11 Circumventricular Organs

The circumventricular organs are "the seven windows on the brain," where the structure is either devoid of a blood-brain barrier with the usual tight junctional endothelial appositions or has a modified blood-brain barrier. Some of the circumventricular organs have neurons that respond to incoming humoral or neural signals, and communicate with other CNS structures (e.g., OVLT); others have cells that secrete bioactive molecules into the circulation (e.g., neurohypophysis) and/or the CSF (e.g., area postrema). The circumventricular organs are noted in the following table.

Circumventricular Organs

STRUCTURE	LOCATION AND FUNCTIONAL ROLES
Organum vasculosum of the lamina terminalis (OVLT)	Location: anteroventral region of the third ventricle Contains osmoreceptors, responds to osmotic factors; helps to regulate vasopressin secretion from magnocellular paraventricular nucleus (PVN) and supraoptic nucleus (SON) neurons. Projects to medial preoptic nucleus to help control thirst Angiotensin II stimulates OVLT (and subfornical organ), elevating blood pressure (BP) Produces IL-1β during fever; helps provoke illness behavior Responds to Na^+ and increases lumbar sympathetic and adrenal catecholamine reactivity, elevating BP
Subfornical organ	Location: just below the fornix at rostral end of the third ventricle Senses Na^+ concentration and dehydration; controls water intake Excited by angiotensin II and cholecystokinin; influences water intake and BP, triggers drinking behavior Angiotensin II may help to drive chronic hypertension Responds to glucose during hyperglycemia Responds to ghrelin to increase food intake, responds to satiety signal molecules amylin and leptin, providing a dual feeding response
Subcommissural organ (SCO)	Location: dorsal caudal region of third ventricle, near the aqueduct Ependymal cells produce transthyretin, which helps to move cerebrospinal fluid (CSF), transport thyroid hormone in the blood Secretes transthyretin and other glycoproteins, and basic fibroblast growth factor into adult and fetal CSF; may regulate neuronal stem cell production, neuronal differentiation, and axonal growth and extension Secretes basic fibroblast growth factor: a mitogenic factor and brain repair molecule Secretes SCO-spondin: helps commissural axonal connectivity May be involved in water balance Receives extensive inputs from dopamine, norepinephrine, neuropeptides, CSF factors
Area postrema	Location: at the inferior and posterior limit of fourth ventricle, near obex Detects toxins in the blood, triggers nausea and vomiting; integrates humoral and neural signaling. A lesion prevents detection of poisons and vomiting response, impairs taste aversion Integrates visceral information from vagal and sympathetic afferent inputs; area postrema connects with nucleus solitarius, triggers nausea and vomiting Integrates cardiovascular, feeding, and metabolic responses, osmoregulation and electrolyte balance, and BP control Responds to opiates to trigger nausea and vomiting Transports many substances into and out of the CSF (as do tanycytes)
Pineal	Location: in epithalamus, near the center of the brain Pinealocytes synthesize melatonin (stimulated in dark, inhibited in light) Melatonin synthesized from serotonin, through a rate-limiting enzyme (serotonin *N*-acetyl transferase), regulated by sympathetic norepinephrine input from superior cervical ganglion; pathway for control is retina to suprachiasmatic nucleus to PVN of the hypothalamus to preganglionic neurons in T1–T2 lateral horn or directly to pineal Modulates sleep patterns in circadian rhythms and seasonal rhythms Modulates follicle-stimulating hormone and luteinizing hormone as an "antigonadotropin" response Exogenous melatonin may help to entrain new sleep patterns in jet lag Brainstem parasympathetics, and PVN and other hypothalamic nuclei may directly innervate the pineal, in addition to sympathetics
Median eminence	Location: upper part of the infundibular stem (stalk); lacks neurons Provides a contact zone of capillary loops onto which nerve terminals of the tuberoinfundibular tract secrete hypophysiotropic hormones (releasing and inhibitory factors for anterior pituitary hormones) into the hypophyseal-portal closed vascular system Hypophysiotropic hormones: CRF, gonadotropin-releasing hormone, thyrotropin-releasing hormone, growth hormone-releasing hormone, DA (prolactin inhibitory factor), VP, and many other neuromodulators
Neurohypophysis (posterior pituitary)	Location: posterior region of the pituitary gland, beneath hypothalamus A site where oxytocin and VP are secreted by axon terminals from neurons of PVN and SON into the systemic circulation

COLOR the following structures, using a separate color for each structure.

☐ 1. **Organum vasculosum of the lamina terminalis (OVLT)**
☐ 2. **Median eminence**
☐ 3. **Neurohypophysis (posterior pituitary)**
☐ 4. **Subfornical organ**
☐ 5. **Area postrema**
☐ 6. **Pineal gland**
☐ 7. **Subcommissural organ**

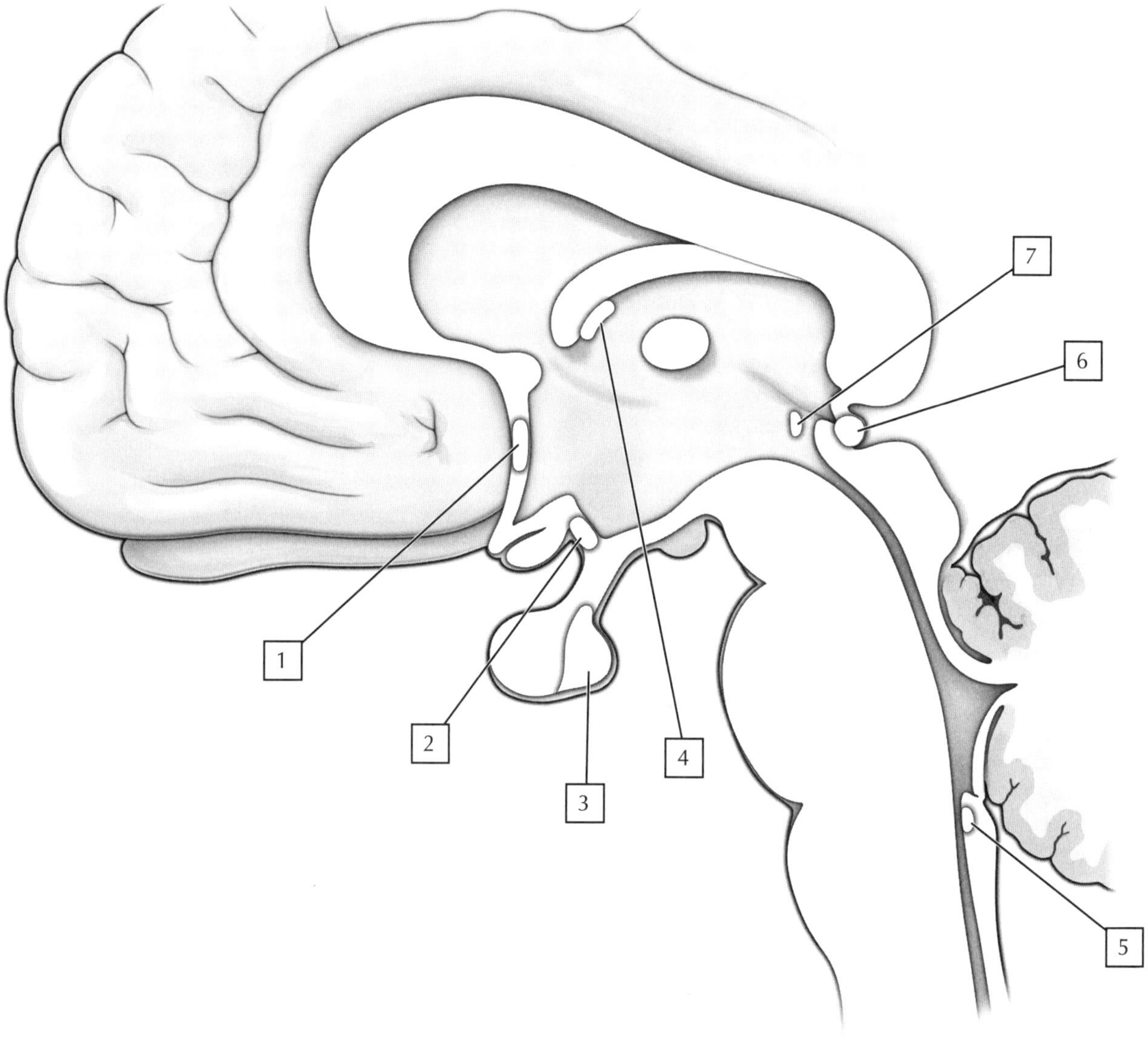
7
6
1
2
4
3
5

Regulation of Anterior Pituitary Hormone Secretion

The **anterior pituitary gland (adenohypophysis)** contains **pituicytes** that synthesize several hormones that either act directly on target organs in the periphery (e.g., growth hormone) or stimulate the release of other hormones from target organs (e.g., **adrenal corticotropic hormone [ACTH]** stimulating the release of **cortisol from the adrenal cortex**). The anterior pituitary hormones include thyroid-stimulating hormone (TSH), ACTH, follicle-stimulating hormone (FSH), luteinizing hormone (LH), prolactin (luteotropic hormone), growth hormone (GH), and melanocyte-stimulating hormone (MSH).

The regulation of the production and release of these anterior pituitary hormones is a complex process involving both CNS circuits and peripheral blood-borne feedback loops. Neurons in the hypothalamus and adjacent regions synthesize releasing factors and inhibitory factors (called hypophysiotropic factors) for the anterior pituitary hormones (e.g., corticotropin-releasing factor [CRF] stimulates the release of ACTH). The **neurons producing the hypophysiotropic factors** are under the influence of **central limbic circuits and neural inputs to the hypothalamus**. These hypophysiotropic factors are transported through axons that travel in the tuberoinfundibular tract (system) and terminate on **fenestrated primary capillaries of the hypophyseal-portal vascular system**. This system forms capillary loops, derived from the superior hypophyseal artery, that are present at the **contact zone of the median eminence** (upper portion of the infundibular stalk). The primary capillary loop coalesces and gives rise to a set of **secondary capillary loops** that delivers very high concentrations of the hypophysiotropic factors to the pituicytes. These secondary capillaries then give rise to the **systemic efferent vasculature from the anterior pituitary** that delivers the anterior pituitary hormones throughout the body.

Both the anterior pituitary hormones and the target organ-produced **hormones circulate back through the systemic vasculature** and signal the parvocellular neurons producing the hypophysiotropic hormones, and the pituicytes, which provides feedback inhibition to regulate the production and release of these hormones.

COLOR the following structures, using a separate color for each structure.

- ☐ 1. **Central limbic circuits and afferents to the hypothalamus that can regulate production of hypophysiotropic factors**
- ☐ 2. **Neurons producing hypophysiotropic hormones (factors)**
- ☐ 3. **Fenestrated primary capillaries of the hypophyseal-portal vascular system**
- ☐ 4. **Secondary capillary loops of the hypophyseal-portal vascular system**
- ☐ 5. **Pituicytes producing specific anterior pituitary hormones**
- ☐ 6. **Anterior pituitary gland (adenohypophysis)**
- ☐ 7. **Systemic efferent vasculature from the anterior pituitary**
- ☐ 8. **Hormones circulating back through the systemic vasculature to the hypothalamus and the anterior pituitary**
- ☐ 9. **Contact zone of the median eminence**

Clinical Note

The balance of the hypophysiotropic factors, their target anterior pituitary hormones, and the peripheral hormones or structures stimulated by them are critical to the well-being and survival of the individual. An imbalance in the thyrotropin-releasing hormone (TRF)–TSH–thyroid hormone system may result in severe metabolic disruption from hypothyroidism or hyperthyroidism. An excess of GH may result in acromegaly (often from a pituitary adenoma), while too little GH may stunt growth and development.

Each of these hormonal circuits has carefully regulated feedback loops to prevent either too much or too little production of hypophysiotropic factors or anterior pituitary hormones. Superimposed on these highly regulated circuits are many central circuits. Limbic and cortical inputs can provoke activation of the HPA axis (and sympathetic axis) and result in an outpouring of stress hormones into the general circulation. A host of chemically specific axonal inputs influences the activity of the hypophysiotropic factor–producing neurons, or influences release and regulation of these factors at the contact zone of the median eminence and also regulates visceral functions.

CRH, Corticotropin-releasing hormone; *FSH*, follicle-stimulating hormone; *GH*, growth hormone; *IGF-1*, insulin-like growth factor 1; *LH*, luteinizing hormone; *MSH*, melanocyte-stimulating hormone; *OXY*, oxytocin; *TSH*, thyroid-stimulating hormone; *VP*, vasopressin.

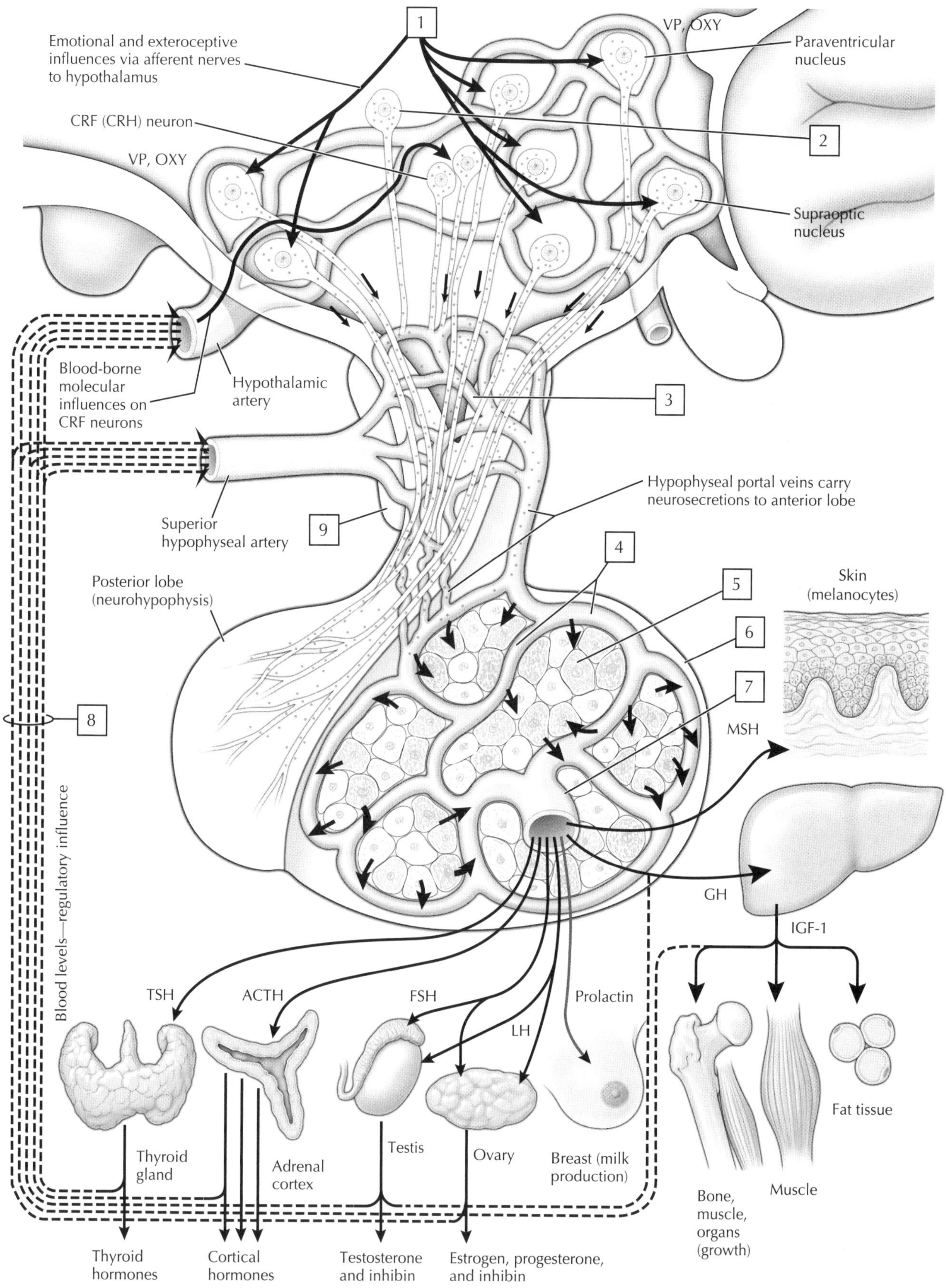
1
VP, OXY
Emotional and exteroceptive influences via afferent nerves to hypothalamus
Paraventricular nucleus
CRF (CRH) neuron
2
VP, OXY
Supraoptic nucleus
Blood-borne molecular influences on CRF neurons
Hypothalamic artery
3
Superior hypophyseal artery
9
Hypophyseal portal veins carry neurosecretions to anterior lobe
4
5
Skin (melanocytes)
Posterior lobe (neurohypophysis)
6
7
MSH
8
Blood levels—regulatory influence
GH
IGF-1
TSH
ACTH
FSH
Prolactin
LH
Fat tissue
Thyroid gland
Adrenal cortex
Testis
Ovary
Breast (milk production)
Bone, muscle, organs (growth)
Muscle
Thyroid hormones
Cortical hormones
Testosterone and inhibin
Estrogen, progesterone, and inhibin

Posterior Pituitary (Neurohypophyseal) Hormones: Oxytocin and Vasopressin

Magnocellular neurons of the **paraventricular nucleus (PVN)** and **supraoptic nucleus (SON)** of the hypothalamus secrete both oxytocin (mainly PVN) and VP (mainly SON). These hormones are synthesized in the cell bodies, are associated with neurophysin carrier proteins, are **rapidly transported down the axons of the supraopticohypophyseal tract** that traverse the **infundibulum (pituitary stalk)**, and are released from nerve terminals that end adjacent to **fenestrated capillaries** of the **inferior hypophyseal arterial system** in the **posterior pituitary gland (neurohypophysis)**. The hormones are secreted through **venous drainage** into the general circulation. These magnocellular neurons of PVN and SON are considered to be neuroendocrine transducer cells. They receive extensive **input from brainstem and forebrain pathways**, from **blood-borne signals through the hypothalamic artery**, and from some circumventricular organs such as the OVLT and the subfornical organ, and release VP and oxytocin into the systemic circulation.

Oxytocin neurons respond to estrogen, ascending neural inputs stimulated by suckling, and signal molecules in the CSF in the third ventricle. Oxytocin stimulates uterine contraction in pregnancy, helps to control uterine bleeding after birth, and stimulates milk let-down into the subareolar sinuses near the nipple during breast feeding. Oxytocin has been reported to promote bonding (especially maternal–infant bonding), trust, and attachment, but also promotes aggressive protective responses in mothers to perceived threats to their infants. Oxytocin also appears to decrease anxiety and protect against stress in a social context.

VP neurons respond to changes in blood osmolarity, secreting VP (also called antidiuretic hormone) in response to high osmolarity, causing the collecting tubules of the kidney to increase water resorption, preventing diuresis. VP is regulated by angiotensin II, especially prominent through delivery from the circumventricular organs such as the OVLT and the subfornical organ. Atrial natriuretic peptide can inhibit VP secretion by blocking the enhancing effect of angiotensin II. Neural afferent pathways to SON, and CSF-borne signals also may influence VP synthesis. VP from parvocellular neurons also is released at the contact zone of the median eminence and works in conjunction with CRF to regulate the release of ACTH from pituicytes in the anterior pituitary gland, with a downstream effect of modulating the release of corticosteroids from the adrenal gland, especially in response to stress.

COLOR the following structures, using a separate color for each structure.

- ☐ 1. **Inputs to PVN and SON from the forebrain**
- ☐ 2. **Blood-borne signals to the PVN and SON through the hypothalamic artery**
- ☐ 3. **Rapid axonal transport of oxytocin and VP down the axons of magnocellular neurons**
- ☐ 4. **Fenestrated capillaries in the posterior lobe of the pituitary**
- ☐ 5. **Inferior hypophyseal artery**
- ☐ 6. **Venous drainage from the posterior pituitary into the general circulation**
- ☐ 7. **Posterior pituitary gland (neurohypophysis)**
- ☐ 8. **Supraopticohypophyseal tract (neurophyophyseal tract)**
- ☐ 9. **Infundibulum (pituitary stalk)**
- ☐ 10. **Supraoptic nucleus (SON) of the hypothalamus**
- ☐ 11. **Paraventricular nucleus (PVN) of the hypothalamus**
- ☐ 12. **Inputs to PVN and SON from the brainstem**

Clinical Note

Disruption of VP transport to the posterior pituitary leads to diabetes insipidus, with high blood sodium (hypernatremia), excess urine production (polyuria), and excess fluid consumption (polydipsia). The patient consumes large volumes of fluid and urinates large volumes of dilute urine. This condition can occur with damage to the pituitary stalk and the supraopticohypophyseal tract, sometimes provoked by a tumor. High alcohol consumption also may mimic this situation.

Excess VP production may occur in a condition called "syndrome of inappropriate antidiuretic hormone secretion (SIADH)." This condition results in excess VP leading to impaired water excretion and increased plasma volume, producing hyponatremia (low sodium) and hypoosmolality in the serum. With chronic SIADH, symptoms may start gradually. Rapid-onset SIADH may result in confusion and disorientation, seizures, muscle weakness, and disrupted motor responses. SIADH can be precipitated by tumors (e.g., small cell carcinoma of the lung), pulmonary infections or bleeding, and medications (antidepressants, some seizure medication, some antibiotics [ciprofloxacin], and some chemotherapeutic agents).

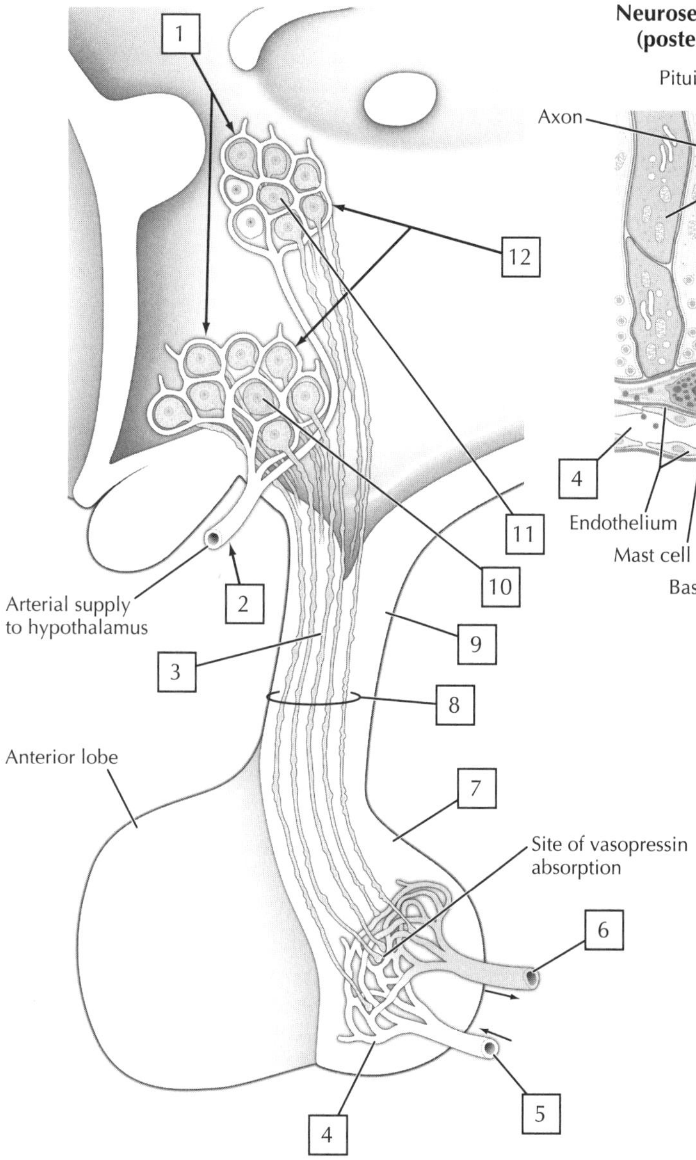

Neurosecretory endings (posterior pituitary)

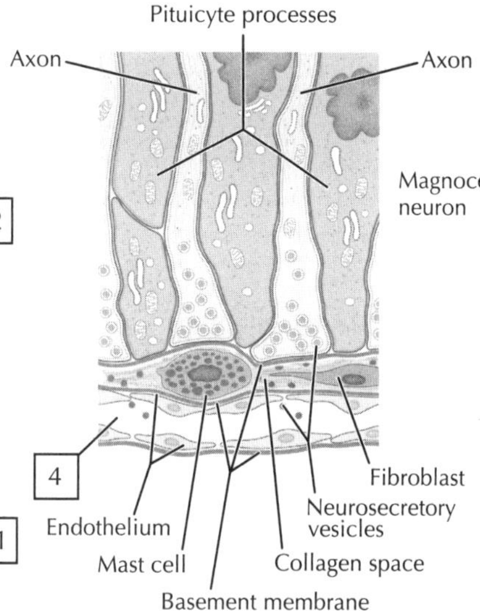

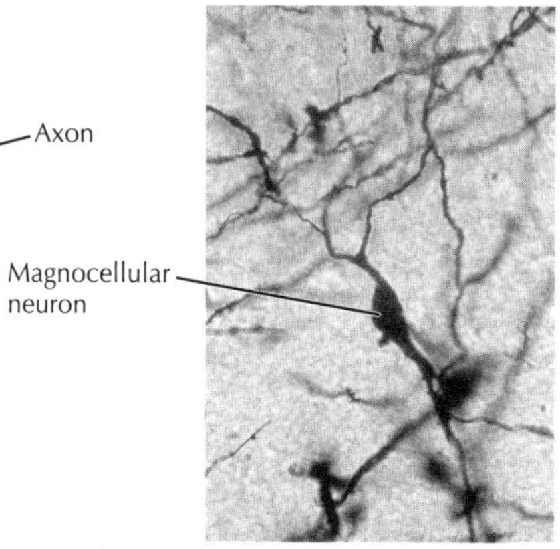

Magnocellular neuron of the supraoptic nucleus demonstrating extensive horizontal and vertical dendritic arborizations. Golgi-Cox stain.

Origin of vasopressin

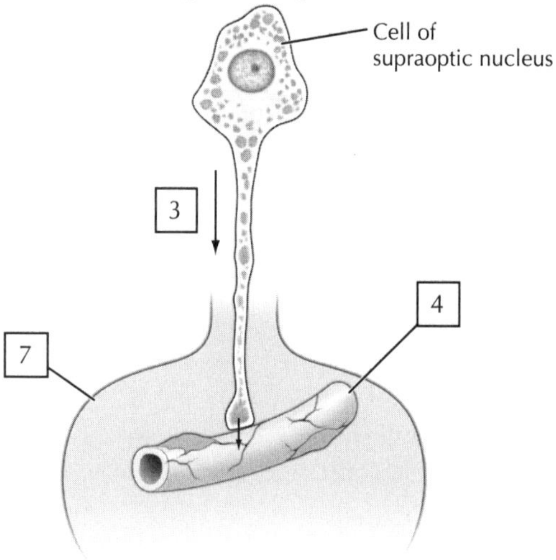

Neuroimmunomodulation

Cells of the immune system in primary lymphoid organs, secondary lymphoid organs, mucosal-associated lymphoid tissue, other sites (e.g., skin), and the circulation are subject to modulatory influences from neurohormones and from peripherally derived autonomic and sensory innervation. Hormones from the **anterior pituitary**, posterior pituitary, and target endocrine organs (e.g., **adrenal cortex and medulla**) act on specific receptors on specific subsets of immunocytes. **Postganglionic sympathetic nerve fibers** (noradrenergic, some independent or colocalized neuropeptides) extensively innervate primary lymphoid organs **(bone marrow, thymus)**, secondary lymphoid organs **(spleen, lymph nodes)**, **mucosal-associated lymphoid tissue**, and many other sites. Many of the nerve terminals end in close apposition to immunocytes (as close as 6 nm), many of which possess cognate receptors for released neurotransmitters from these nerve terminals. Some primary sensory axons (e.g., substance P, calcitonin gene-related peptide, vasoactive intestinal polypeptide, and many others) also innervate lymphoid tissue and can release neurotransmitter from the distal primary sensory process. There is also some **postganglionic parasympathetic innervation** (cholinergic) of some lymphoid tissue.

Many regions of the CNS influence the outflow of innervation to lymphoid organs and immunocytes, including **limbic forebrain sites**, **hypothalamic sites**, **brainstem and spinal cord inputs,** and **blood-borne inputs** (including cytokines that interact with central neural structures).

These autonomic and sensory neurally derived signals and their receptors modulate (1) **individual immunocyte functions** (cell proliferation, migration, gene expression, antigen recognition, presentation, and processing; lymphocyte trafficking and homing); (2) **immune responses** (innate immune responses, especially natural killer cell activity; primary and secondary cell-mediated immune responses and humoral immune responses, Th1 and Th2 cytokine production by T lymphocytes, and immunoglobulin secretion by B lymphocytes); and (3) **responses to immune-mediated diseases** (response to, and clearance of, viral infections; inflammatory responses, autoimmune diseases [e.g., rheumatoid arthritis, lupus, multiple sclerosis exacerbation], metastatic tumor responses, and many other conditions).

Many limbic-related and cortically derived emotional and cognitive perceptions and activities may markedly influence immune responsiveness. Stress from many personal circumstances may inhibit cell-mediated immunity, including antiviral responses and protection from metastases. Examination stress in medical students is associated with diminished cell-mediated immune reactivity, which rapidly recovers in most students, except those who report loneliness and lack of social support. Viewing of humor videos is associated with elevated NK responses, Th1 T cell responses, and GH secretion, which persist for many hours following the viewing of the videos; anticipation of viewing humorous videos is just as enhancing of these responses as the direct viewing itself. It is clear that daily activities and perceptions have an influence of immune-related responses, just as immune responsiveness influence neural responses and neurotransmitter reactivity.

COLOR the following structures, using a separate color for each structure.

- ☐ 1. **Hypothalamic sites influencing neural and hormonal outflow to immune tissue**
- ☐ 2. **Limbic forebrain sites influencing neural and hormonal outflow to immune tissue**
- ☐ 3. **Brainstem sites influencing neural and hormonal outflow to immune tissue**
- ☐ 4. **Anterior pituitary gland (site of production of anterior pituitary hormones)**
- ☐ 5. **Postganglionic sympathetic noradrenergic innervation of primary and secondary lymphoid organs**
- ☐ 6. **Thymus**
- ☐ 7. **Bone marrow**
- ☐ 8. **Postganglionic parasympathetic cholinergic innervation of lung and gut immune tissue**
- ☐ 9. **Spleen**
- ☐ 10. **Lymph nodes**
- ☐ 11. **Mucosal-associated lymphoid tissue (lung and gut)**

Clinical Note

Neural–immune signaling is bidirectional, extensive, regulatory in both directions, and has a profound influence on health and disease. Cytokines can cause illness behavior and change a wide range of neural responses, up to and including depression and suicidal ideation. Hormonal signaling can modulate every aspect of immunocyte function, immune responses, and reactivity to immune-related disease.

Activation of the sympathetic axes may profoundly suppress cell-mediated immune responses, including response to viral infections, susceptibility to infections, response to vaccines, and ability to defend against metastases in many cancers. Chronic stress and its production of high catecholamines in the circulation can suppress natural killer cell activity and Th1 cytokine production that enhances natural killer cell killing. Recent studies of nonspecific β blockers in patients with cancers that may produce metastases (e.g., non–small cell lung cancer, breast cancer, ovarian cancer, colon cancer) have demonstrated fewer metastases with use of nonspecific β blockers, and extended survival (5 years) in women with ovarian cancer.

FSH, Follicle-stimulating hormone; *GA*, glyoxylic acid; *GH*, growth hormone; *LH*, luteinizing hormone; *MALT*, mucosa-associated lymphoid tissue; *MSH*, melanocyte-stimulating hormone; *NA*, noradrenaline; *TSH*, thyroid-stimulating hormone.

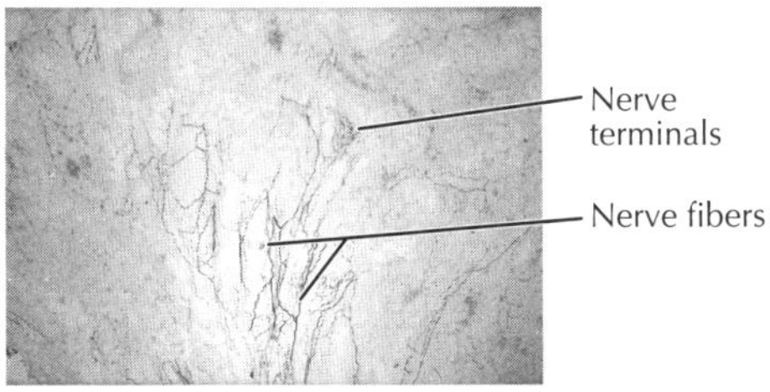

Extensive tyrosine hydroxylase (TH)-positive noradrenergic nerve fibers and terminals in parenchymal regions of the medullary cords and paracortex of a mesenteric lymph node. Immunohistochemical stain for TH.

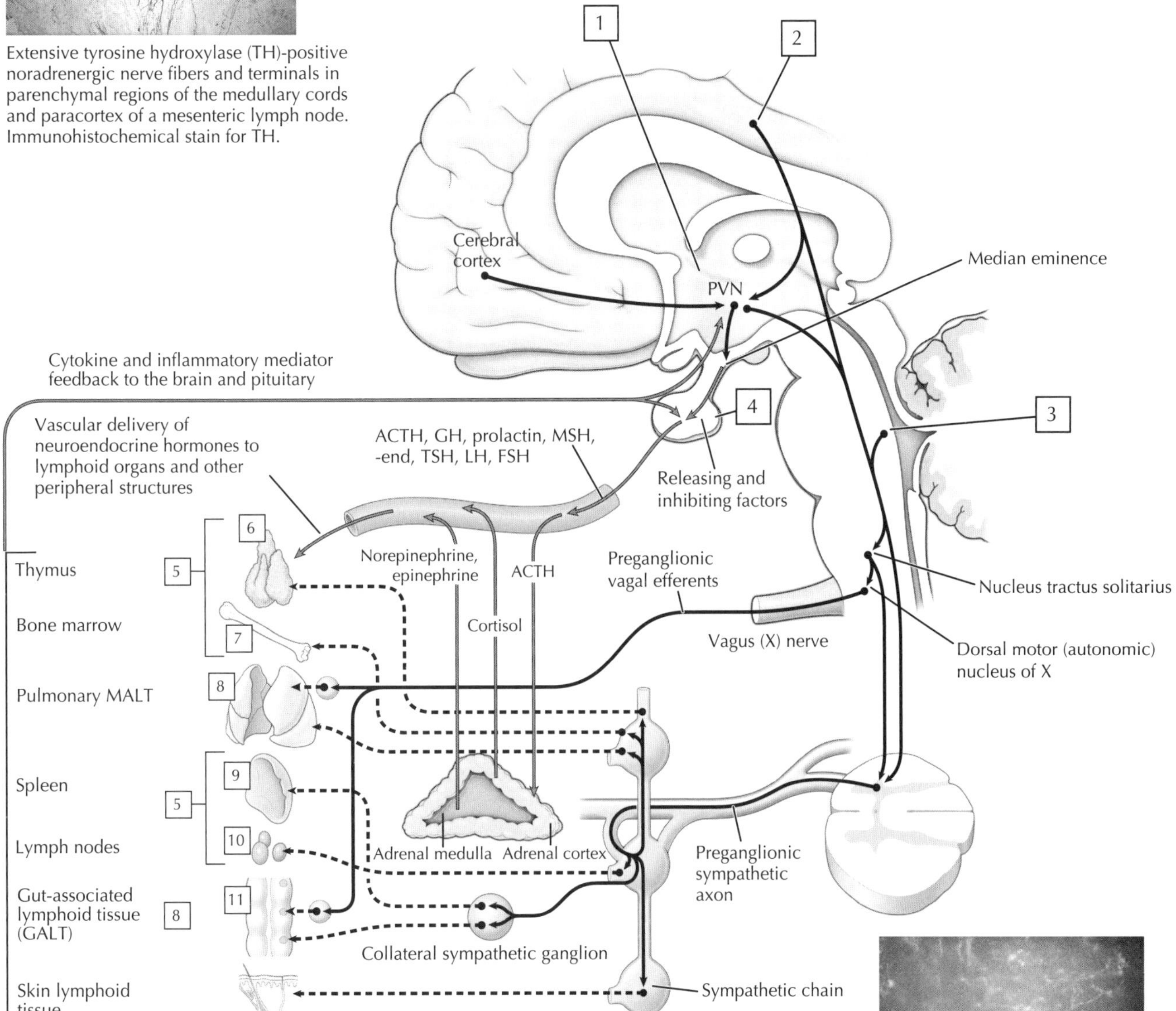

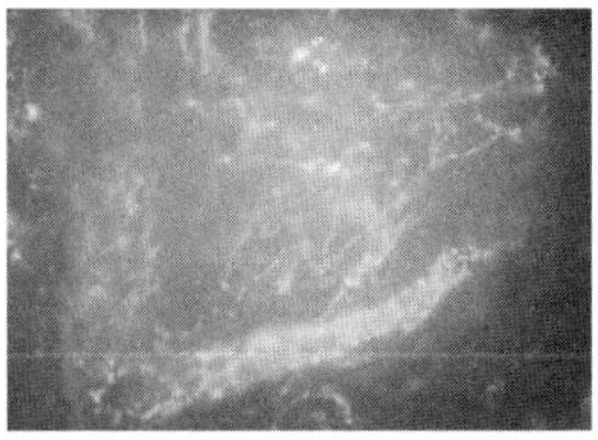

NA postganglionic sympathetic innervation of parenchymal regions of the thymus. GA fluorescence histochemistry.

11 Anatomy of the Limbic Forebrain

The limbic system originally was named as a collection of forebrain structures that surrounded the diencephalon in ring-like fashion. Some of the structures originally viewed as part of the limbic forebrain include the **hippocampal formation** (three-layer cortex) and its associated **fornix,** and the **amygdaloid complex** with its two pathways, the **stria terminalis** and the **ventral amygdalofugal pathway**, both of which have connections with the hypothalamus, as well as other limbic and cortical structures. The hippocampal formation and the amygdala form a C-shape from the temporal lobe around the thalamus into the more anterior forebrain.

The fornix sends projections to the **mammillary nuclei,** which, through the mammillothalamic tract, connect with the **anterior thalamic nucleus.** The anterior thalamic nucleus innervates the **anterior cingulate cortex,** which in turn completes the "**Papez circuit**" back to the hippocampal formation. This Papez circuit was assumed, early on, to be the substrate for memory, but is likely only a small part of the learning and memory systems. The amygdaloid complex of nuclei give rise to the stria terminalis, which sweeps rostrally and then anteriorly, to innervate subcortical structures, including the septal nuclei; the amygdaloid complex also gives rise to the ventral amygdalofugal pathway, which innervates many cortical regions and some subcortical limbic structures. The **septal nuclei** project via the **stria medullaris thalami** to the **habenula,** which has connections with visceral and autonomic structures more caudally.

More recent studies have considered many regions of the cerebral cortex, including the **cingulate**, **prefrontal**, **orbitofrontal**, **entorhinal**, and **periamygdaloid cortex/uncus** olfactory complex as parts of the limbic forebrain, with extensive connections to other parts of the limbic system. The limbic system is collectively the neuronal substrate for regulation of emotional responsiveness and the emotional connotation of stimuli and environmental situations, for individualized responses to both internal and external stimuli, and for integrated memory tasks.

The limbic forebrain expresses its responses through utilization of the hypothalamus and its neuroendocrine and visceral/autonomic connectivity, involving extensive circuitry through the brainstem and its control of preganglionic sympathetic and parasympathetic outflow. Also connected with hypothalamic and limbic forebrain responses are the circumventricular organs with their secretory products, their reaction to molecular messages from the periphery, and their extensive hypothalamic and limbic connectivity.

COLOR the following structures, using a separate color for each structure.

☐ 1. **Septal nuclei**
☐ 2. **Anterior cingulate cortex**
☐ 3. **Anterior thalamic nucleus**
☐ 4. **Fornix**
☐ 5. **Stria terminalis**
☐ 6. **Stria medullaris thalami**
☐ 7. **Habenula**
☐ 8. **Hippocampus**
☐ 9. **Uncus**
☐ 10. **Amygdaloid body (complex, nuclei)**
☐ 11. **Mammillary body (nuclei)**
☐ 12. **Mammillothalamic tract**

Clinical Note

The limbic structures in the temporal lobe may be damaged by trauma in the course of **coup/contrecoup head injury**, a stroke, ischemia, herpes simplex encephalitis, Alzheimer disease, and other conditions. Forebrain trauma may produce bilateral damage to the hippocampal formation, the amygdala, and surrounding structures, named **Klüver–Bucy syndrome** after the psychologist and neuropathologist who discovered the condition in monkeys. The resultant deficits include visual agnosias (inability to recognize objects or faces), hyperorality (tendency to explore objects by mouth), placidity and blunting of emotional responsiveness, indifference to stimuli, undirected hypersexual reactivity, hypermetamorphosis (widespread exploration of everything), compulsive food consumption, and significant short-term memory loss.

Many of these neurobehavioral changes can be attributed to bilateral damage to the anterior temporal lobes, especially the medial portion, including the amygdala and its cortical connections, and the hippocampal formation for memory-related symptoms.

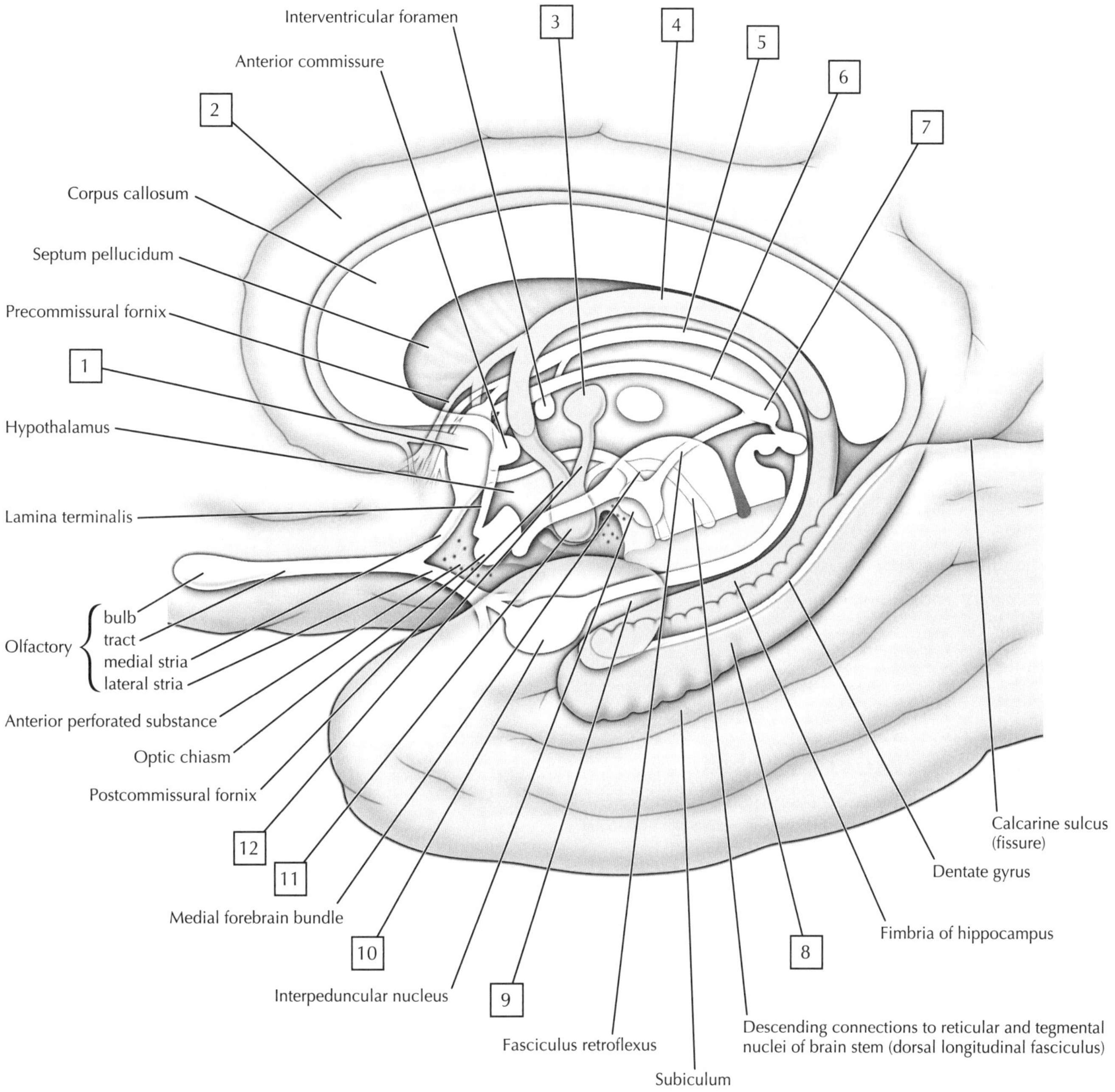
Interventricular foramen
3
4
5
6
7
Anterior commissure
2
Corpus callosum
Septum pellucidum
Precommissural fornix
1
Hypothalamus
Lamina terminalis
Olfactory
bulb
tract
medial stria
lateral stria
Anterior perforated substance
Optic chiasm
Postcommissural fornix
12
11
Medial forebrain bundle
10
Interpeduncular nucleus
9
Fasciculus retroflexus
Subiculum
Descending connections to reticular and tegmental nuclei of brain stem (dorsal longitudinal fasciculus)
8
Fimbria of hippocampus
Dentate gyrus
Calcarine sulcus (fissure)

11 Hippocampal Formation: General Anatomy

The hippocampal formation consists of three structures: (1) the **dentate gyrus,** containing extensive numbers of granule cells; (2) the **hippocampus proper** with its **CA regions** (Cornu Ammonis, or Ammon horn), **CA1–CA4,** containing extensive numbers of pyramidal cells; and (3) the **subiculum.** These structures are intimately interconnected with the adjacent **entorhinal cortex.** The hippocampus was named for its seahorse-shaped structure. It is located in the medial part of the temporal lobe, protruding laterally into the **temporal horn of the lateral ventricle.** The dentate gyrus and hippocampus are three-layered cortical structures, termed "archicortex," distinguishing them from the six-layered "neocortex." The subiculum is a cortical structure whose pyramidal cells receive input from CA1 pyramidal cells, and project to pyramidal cells of the entorhinal cortex.

The hippocampus and subiculum send axonal projections into the **fimbria,** which gives rise to the **fornix** (a C-shaped structure); these axons travel to the hypothalamus (especially the **mammillary bodies or nuclei**), septal nuclei, and other structures. The hippocampal formation has extensive connections with cortical association areas and forebrain structures such as the cingulate cortex.

COLOR each of the following structures, using a separate color for each structure.

- ☐ 1. **Fornix**
- ☐ 2. **Hippocampus proper**
- ☐ 3. **Mammillary bodies (nuclei)**
- ☐ 4. **Fimbria**
- ☐ 5. **Dentate gyrus**
- ☐ 6. **Subiculum**
- ☐ 7. **Entorhinal cortex**
- ☐ 8. **CA regions (color CA1, CA2, and CA3)**
- ☐ 9. **Temporal horn of the lateral ventricle**

Clinical Note

Pyramidal cells in the hippocampus are susceptible to apoptosis (cell death) from glutamate neurotoxicity. Neurons in CA1 (called Sommer's sector) are particularly vulnerable to ischemia (from poor cerebral blood flow or cessation of perfusion from a heart attack) and are among the first neurons to cease functioning without rapid resuscitation (generally within 5 minutes or less after ischemia). Neurons in CA3 are particularly vulnerable to high concentrations of glucocorticoids, both endogenous (cortisol) and exogenous (therapeutic corticosteroids). The combination of ischemia and high glucocorticoids is even more damaging to the hippocampus than either condition separately. This combination may occur without a stroke or heart attack in an elderly individual with marginal cerebral flow (borderline ischemia) who comes into a new setting, such as a hospital or nursing home, and experiences high stress hormone secretion of cortisol, or is receiving corticosteroid therapy. If there is an additional ongoing pathology that produces inflammatory cytokines, those cytokines can further provoke the HPA axis to secrete even more cortisol. The combination of ischemia and corticosteroids may take a borderline tolerable situation to the level of visible symptoms and apoptosis of CA neurons.

The result of this situation is loss of consolidation of short-term memory, confusion, and disorientation, the hallmark of hippocampal damage.

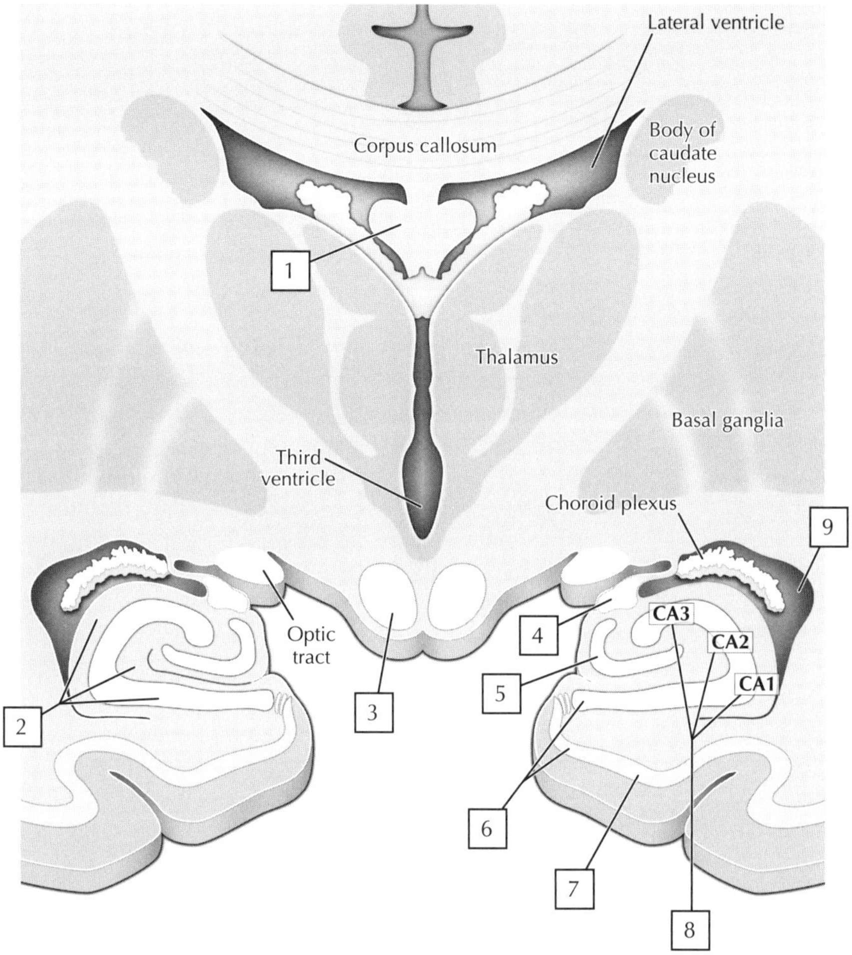

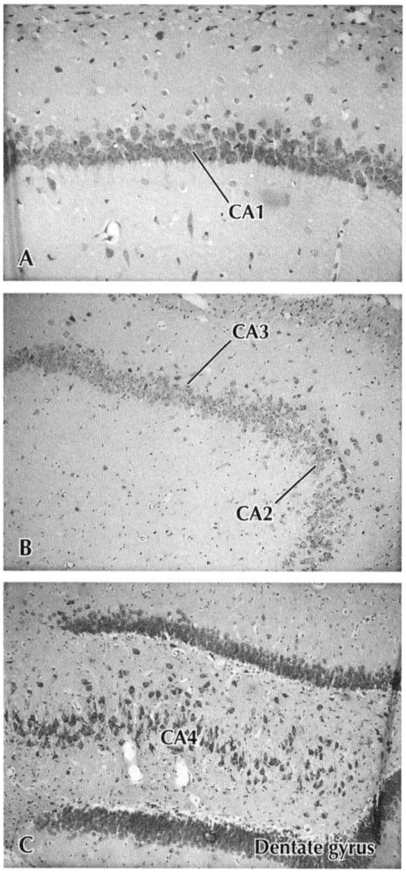

Hippocampal pyramidal neurons in CA1 (**A**), CA2 and CA3 (**B**) and CA4 (**C**) sectors of the hippocampus, and granule cells in the dentate gyrus (**C**). Cell stain.

11 Neuronal Connections of the Hippocampal Formation

The internal circuitry of the hippocampus interconnects with the **entorhinal cortex.** Pyramidal neurons of the entorhinal cortex connect with the granule cell dendrites in the **dentate gyrus. Granule cell axons (mossy fibers)** synapse on pyramidal cell dendrites in **CA3 of the hippocampus.** Pyramidal cell axons in CA3 project to pyramidal cell dendrites in **CA1 (Schaffer collaterals)** and CA2. CA1 pyramidal cell axons project to pyramidal neurons in the **subiculum.** Pyramidal cell in the subiculum sends axons back to pyramidal neurons in the entorhinal cortex. This completes the internal circuitry through the hippocampal formation. The subiculum also sends axons to some nuclei in the amygdala (with reciprocal connections), and to cortical association areas of the temporal lobe. The entorhinal cortex also connects with the CA regions of the hippocampus and with the subiculum via the **perforant pathway.**

Axons from pyramidal neurons in the subiculum and the CA1 and CA3 regions of the hippocampus funnel into the **fimbria** and **alveus,** and give rise to the major efferent pathway from the hippocampal formation, the **fornix.** The axons from the subiculum project to the hypothalamus (mammillary nuclei) and thalamic nuclei through the **postcommissural fornix**. The axons of CA1 and CA3 project to the septal nuclei, the preoptic and anterior regions of the hypothalamus, the anterior cingulate cortex, nucleus accumbens, and association areas of the frontal cortex through the **precommissural fornix**.

Afferent cholinergic axons from neurons in the septal area (medial septal nucleus) traverse the fornix back to the dentate gyrus and CA regions. Extensive **inputs project to the hippocampal formation** from multiple regions of sensory association cortices, prefrontal cortex, insular cortex, some amygdaloid nuclei, and from the uncus (olfaction) via the entorhinal cortex. Thus the hippocampal formation is extensively interconnected with many regions of limbic forebrain, as well as with the hypothalamus. Brainstem projections from noradrenergic neurons in locus coeruleus, and from serotonergic neurons in the rostral raphe nuclei, connect with both the internal components of the hippocampal formation and the target structures connected with the hippocampal formation.

The **entorhinal cortex,** with which the hippocampal formation is connected, also **receives extensive cortical inputs,** including from the association cortex from all sensory modalities, and subcortical inputs from the cholinergic medial septal nucleus, basal forebrain, and amygdala.

COLOR the following structures, using a separate color for each structure.

- ☐ 1. **Alveus**
- ☐ 2. **Schaffer collaterals**
- ☐ 3. **CA1 region of the hippocampus**
- ☐ 4. **Inputs to hippocampal formation (subiculum)**
- ☐ 5. **Cortical (and subcortical) inputs to the entorhinal cortex**
- ☐ 6. **Entorhinal cortex**
- ☐ 7. **Perforant pathway**
- ☐ 8. **Subiculum**
- ☐ 9. **Dentate gyrus**
- ☐ 10. **Mossy fibers**
- ☐ 11. **CA3 region of the hippocampus**
- ☐ 12. **Fimbria**

Clinical Note

Many of the cortical regions of the hippocampal formation, and cortical connections with the hippocampal formation, are highly susceptible to neuronal degeneration in **Alzheimer disease**. Alzheimer disease is a neurodegenerative disease characterized by the accumulation of abnormal **hyperphosphorylated tau proteins** inside of neurons (**neurofibrillary tangles**) and abnormal proteins (**amyloid beta**) outside of neurons, in the parenchyma (**senile plaques**). Disruption of the hippocampal formation circuitry results in the inability to consolidate short-term and intermediate-term memory into long-term memory. Damage to cortical regions in the temporal lobe, and regions of the frontal cortex, cingulate cortex, basal forebrain, and other sites, leads to progressive, severe cognitive decline, accompanying the deficits in consolidation of short-term memory.

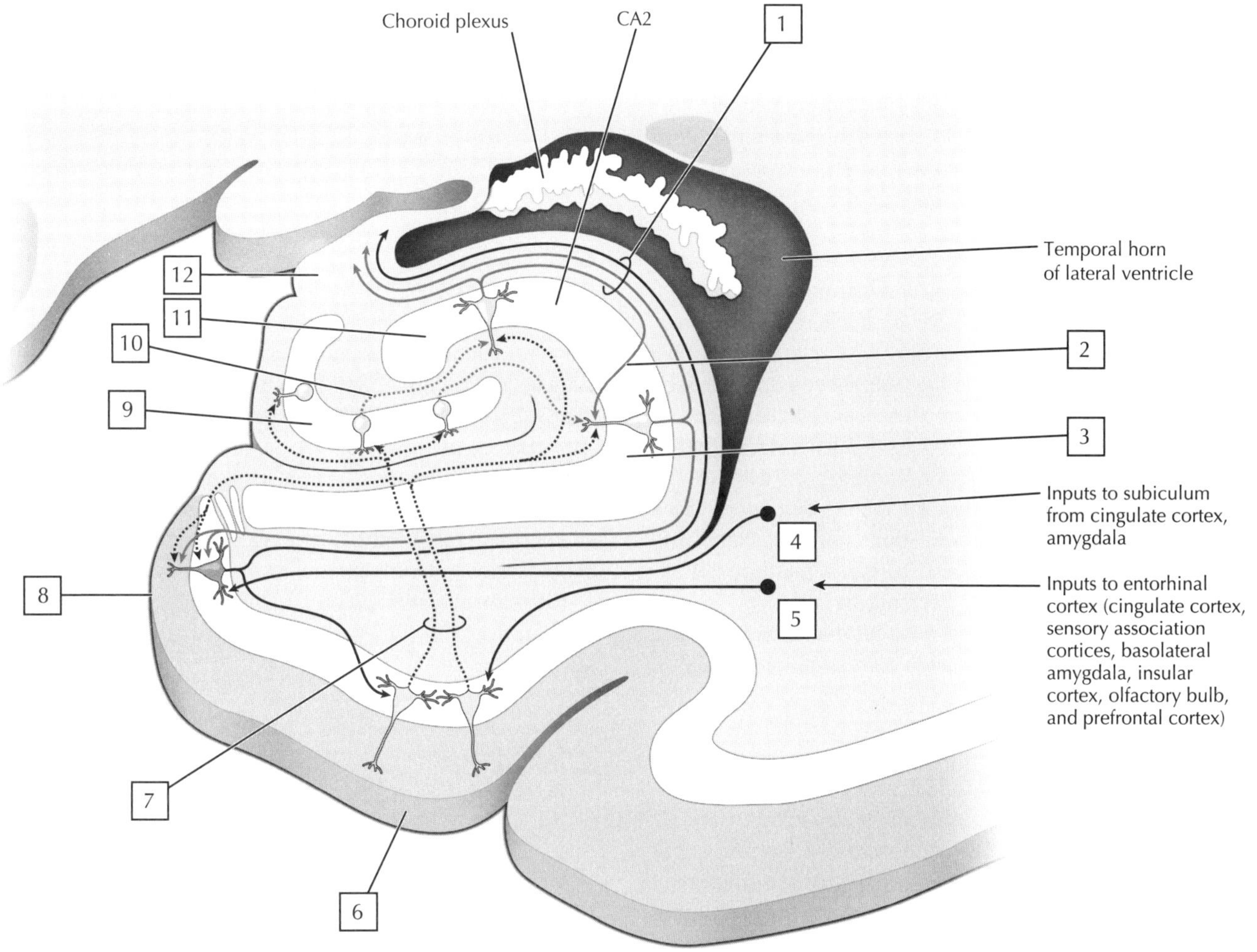
Choroid plexus
CA2
1
Temporal horn
of lateral ventricle
12
11
10
9
2
3
Inputs to subiculum
from cingulate cortex,
amygdala
4
8
Inputs to entorhinal
cortex (cingulate cortex,
sensory association
cortices, basolateral
amygdala, insular
cortex, olfactory bulb,
and prefrontal cortex)
5
7
6

11 Major Afferent Connections of the Amygdala

The **amygdala** is an almond-shaped region in the anterior and medial regions of the temporal lobe. It contains many subcortical nuclei, including the **basolateral** and **corticomedial** groups of nuclei (which receive inputs and give rise to efferent connections with many cortical and subcortical limbic structures), and the **central nucleus** of the amygdala (which mainly sends efferent connections to brainstem regions). Afferent connections with the corticomedial nuclei mainly come from subcortical limbic structures such as: (1) **septal nuclei**; (2) **hypothalamic nuclei** (ventromedial nucleus, lateral hypothalamic area); (3) **thalamic nuclei** (intralaminar nuclei, and medial dorsal nucleus) of the thalamus; (4) the **bed nucleus of the stria terminalis**; (5) the **olfactory bulb**; and (6) many **autonomic nuclei, noradrenergic nuclei, and serotonergic nuclei in the brainstem**. Afferent connections with the basolateral nuclei mainly come from cortical areas, including the **sensory association cortical areas**, **prefrontal cortex**, **cingulate cortex**, and the **subiculum**. The central amygdaloid nucleus receives its input mainly from other amygdaloid nuclei of the corticomedial and basolateral groups.

The amygdaloid complex is associated with the emotional interpretation of both external stimuli and internal states. It provides individual interpretation and emotional responsiveness to stimuli and circumstances, especially those related to fear and aversive situations. Depending on past experience, the sudden presence of a large dog may evoke either fear or a pleasant sense of familiarity. The perception of movement in an elevator assumed to be empty may provoke a fear response with full sympathetic arousal. The amygdala is a major component of fear conditioning, where a neutral stimulus becomes associated with fear or anxiety. Fear conditioning also is seen in posttraumatic stress responses following highly traumatic stimuli.

There may be distinct functional roles for the amygdala on each side. In some studies, stimulation of the right amygdala provoked negative emotions (e.g., fear, sadness), while stimulation of the left amygdala sometimes provoked pleasant emotions. The right amygdala may be associated with episodic memory, with recall of emotional and sensory experiences from a past event; this memory is not necessarily conscious, but may provoke an activational state unconsciously. The emotional arousal provoked by an experience may enhance the strength of memory recall for the event, mediated through the basolateral nuclei, as shown by the work of James McGaugh.

COLOR the following structures, using a separate color for each structure.

- ☐ 1. **Bed nucleus of the stria terminalis**
- ☐ 2. **Cingulate cortex**
- ☐ 3. **Thalamic nuclei (intralaminar, medial dorsal)**
- ☐ 4. **Brainstem inputs**
- ☐ 5. **Subiculum**
- ☐ 6. **Sensory association cortical areas**
- ☐ 7. **Basolateral nuclei of the amygdala**
- ☐ 8. **Corticomedial nuclei of the amygdala**
- ☐ 9. **Olfactory bulb**
- ☐ 10. **Prefrontal cortex**
- ☐ 11. **Septal nuclei**

Clinical Note

Data from observing the effects of **amygdaloid lesions**, such as the **Klüver–Bucy syndrome**, demonstrate the loss of fear, blunting of emotional reactivity to stimuli (even threatening stimuli), inability to recognize familiar objects, and hyperorality. Imaging studies in humans suggest that the amygdala on the left side may be involved in social anxiety, posttraumatic stress, obsessive-compulsive disorder, and the inability to detect fear in the facial expression of others. Some researchers have reported an important role for the amygdala in emotional intelligence and in perceptions of infringement of their "personal space."

Experimental stimulation studies in animal models also suggest a role for the amygdala in aggressive interactions and sexual behavior.

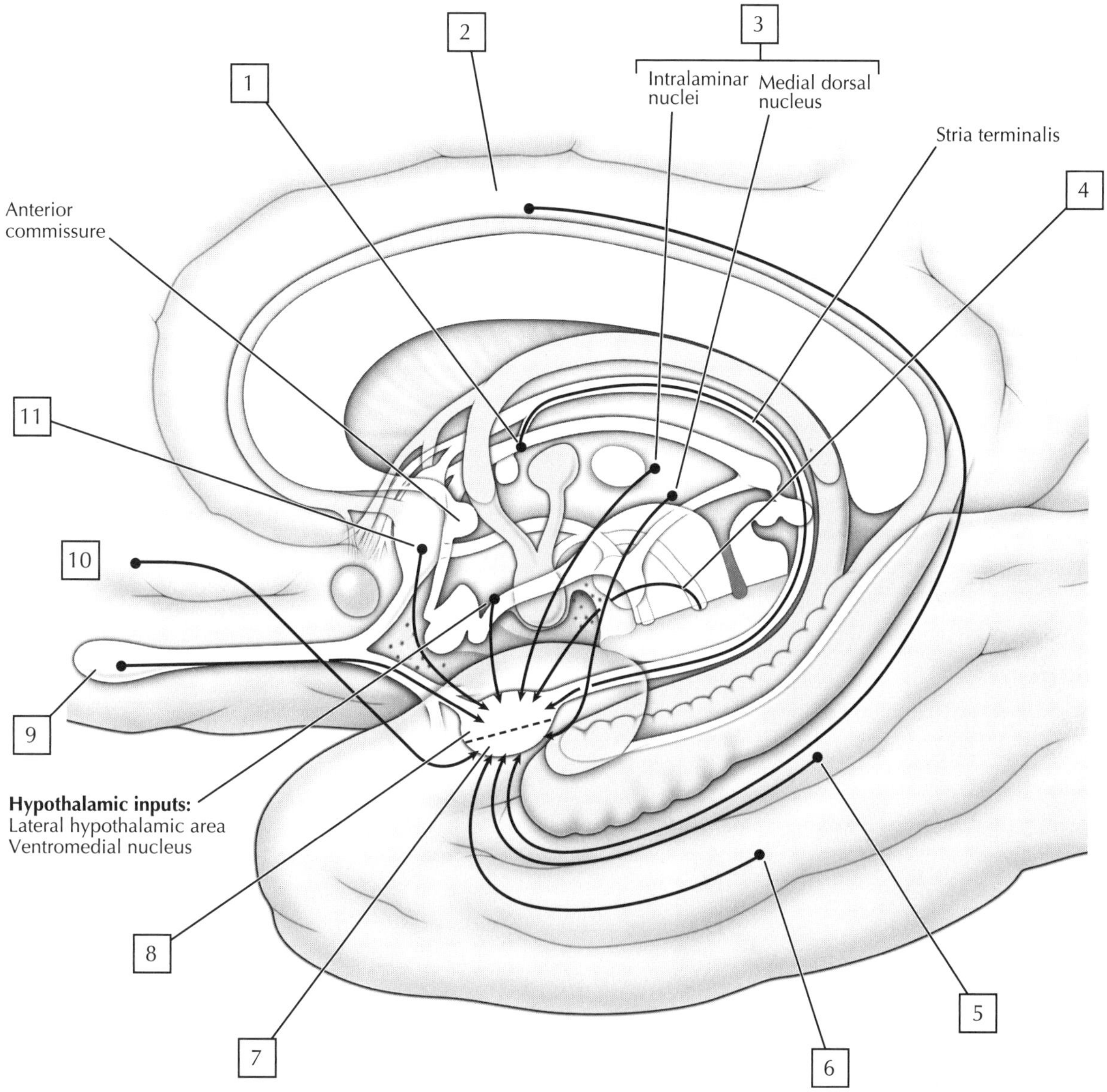
1
2
3
Intralaminar nuclei
Medial dorsal nucleus
Stria terminalis
4
Anterior commissure
11
10
9
Hypothalamic inputs:
Lateral hypothalamic area
Ventromedial nucleus
8
7
6
5

11 Major Efferent Connections of the Amygdala

Efferent connections of the **corticomedial nuclei of the amygdala** project through the **stria terminalis** mainly toward subcortical limbic structures, including: (1) the **septal nuclei**; (2) **the medial dorsal (MD) nucleus of the thalamus**; (3) **hypothalamic nuclei**; (4) the **bed nucleus of the stria terminalis**; (5) **nucleus accumbens**; and (6) the **rostral striatum**, (many of which provide input to the amygdala).

Efferent connections of the **basolateral nuclei of the amygdala** project through the **ventral amygdalofugal pathway** to cortical regions, including the: (1) **frontal cortex**; (2) the **cingulate cortex**; (3) the **inferior temporal cortex**; (4) the **subiculum**; and (5) the **entorhinal cortex**; and to subcortical limbic structures, including: (1) the **septal nuclei**; (2) **hypothalamic nuclei**; and (3) cholinergic **nucleus basalis in the substantia innominata.**

The **central amygdaloid nucleus** receives its input from other amygdaloid nuclei, and projects axons through the **ventral amygdalofugal pathway** to (1) **autonomic and monoaminergic (noradrenergic and serotonergic) nuclei of the brainstem**, (2) **midline thalamic nuclei**, (3) the **bed nucleus of the stria terminalis**, and (4) the cholinergic **nucleus basalis.** This central amygdaloid connectivity provides control over the brainstem and spinal cord machinery needed to carry out the emotionally directed responses and reactivity provoked by amygdaloid activation.

COLOR the following structures, using a separate color for each structure.

- ☐ 1. **Rostral striatum**
- ☐ 2. **Cingulate cortex**
- ☐ 3. **Medial dorsal (MD) nucleus of the thalamus**
- ☐ 4. **Bed nucleus of the stria terminalis**
- ☐ 5. **Stria terminalis**
- ☐ 6. **Pathway to autonomic and monoaminergic nuclei of the brainstem**
- ☐ 7. **Inferior temporal cortex**
- ☐ 8. **Subiculum**
- ☐ 9. **Entorhinal cortex**
- ☐ 10. **Central amygdaloid nucleus**
- ☐ 11. **Basolateral nuclei of the amygdala**
- ☐ 12. **Corticomedial nuclei of the amygdala**
- ☐ 13. **Ventral amygdalofugal pathway**
- ☐ 14. **Nucleus accumbens**
- ☐ 15. **Septal nuclei**
- ☐ 16. **Hypothalamic nuclei**

Clinical Note

Stimulation of the amygdala has occurred during surgery for seizures. Stimulation of the **corticomedial amygdala** results in a freezing response with cessation of all voluntary movement (as may be seen in prey that suddenly detects a predator), automated gestures such as lip smacking, and parasympathetic activation (leading to urination and defecation). Stimulation of the **basolateral amygdala** results in an alerting response, with vigilance and scanning of the environment. This response may be in preparation for fight-or-flight. These reactions reflect the amygdala's direction of brainstem and spinal cord circuitry to achieve the desired behavioral response provoked by the emotional interpretation of environmental stimuli and scenarios. Conditioned fear responses and reactivity to stressful or potentially dangerous situations require the integrated reactivity of the ANS, the neuroendocrine system, and the motor apparatus for behavioral responses.

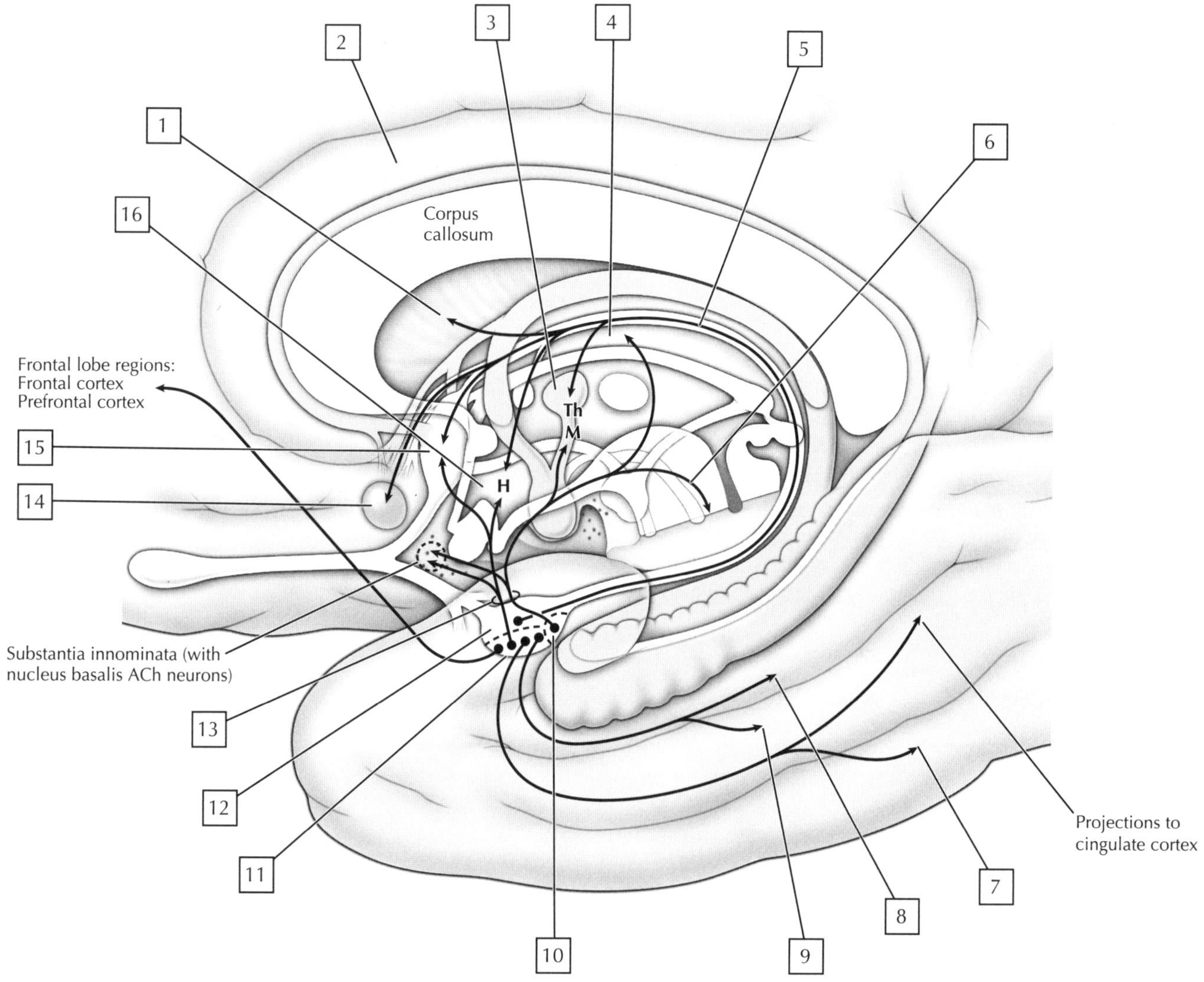

H = Hypothalamus:
Preoptic area
Anterior hypothalamic area
Ventromedial nucleus
Lateral hypothalamic area
Paraventricular nucleus

Th = Thalamus:
Medial dorsal nucleus

M = Midline thalamic nuclei

11 Cingulate Cortex

The **cingulate cortex,** located above the **medial portion of the corpus callosum,** consists of an anterior region, a middle region, and a posterior region. The **anterior cingulate cortex** helps to (1) regulate autonomic and visceral functions (digestion, cardiovascular, respiratory, pupillary responses); (2) regulate affect, and deal with uncomfortable or emotional situations; (3) detect errors and incomplete responses; and (4) aid in decision making and anticipation. The **posterior cingulate cortex**: (1) contributes to awareness, internally driven cognition, and focus of attention; (2) plays a role in thinking and planning for the future; (3) participates in episodic memory retrieval; (4) interconnects emotionally based limbic circuitry with cognitively based prefrontal cortex; and (5) participates in awareness of the severity of pain. Some authors describe a **middle cingulate cortical area** that acts as a premotor and preautonomic control region. Lateralization has been proposed from stimulation studies, with the left side stimulating parasympathetic responses and the right side stimulating sympathetic responses.

Afferents to the cingulate cortex derive from: (1) **association areas of the frontal cortex, parietal cortex, and temporal cortex**; (2) the **subiculum**; (3) **septal nuclei**; and (4) the **medial dorsal and anterior nuclei of the thalamus**. Efferents from the cingulate cortex project to: (1) **association areas** of the frontal cortex, parietal cortex, and temporal cortex; and (2) **limbic forebrain structures** such as the **hippocampus**, the **subiculum**, the **entorhinal cortex**, **basolateral nuclei of the amygdala**, and **septal nuclei**. These limbic forebrain areas, as well as the middle cingulate cortical region, can utilize their hypothalamic and autonomic connectivity to achieve behavioral effects.

COLOR the following structures, using a separate color for each structure.

- ☐ 1. **Anterior cingulate cortex**
- ☐ 2. **Association areas of the parietal cortex**
- ☐ 3. **Posterior cingulate cortex**
- ☐ 4. **Association areas of the temporal cortex**
- ☐ 5. **Subiculum**
- ☐ 6. **Entorhinal cortex**
- ☐ 7. **Hippocampus**
- ☐ 8. **Basolateral nuclei of the amygdala**
- ☐ 9. **Septal nuclei**
- ☐ 10. **Association areas of the frontal cortex**
- ☐ 11. **Medial portion of the corpus callosum**
- ☐ 12. **Medial dorsal and anterior nuclei of the thalamus**

Clinical Note

Lesions in the cingulate cortex may be seen in pathological states, and also have been carried out surgically in an attempt to alleviate responses to severe pain, or to alleviate significant psychiatric disorders such as incapacitating anxiety, obsessive-compulsive disorder, or intractable depression. Lesions of the cingulate cortex lead to indifference to pain, and to other sensations that have a strong emotional connection. Such lesions also produce social indifference and apathy, lack of concern for the future, lack of concern for decision making, and elimination of emotional intonation in speech. Individuals with cingulate cortex lesions undergo significant personality changes.

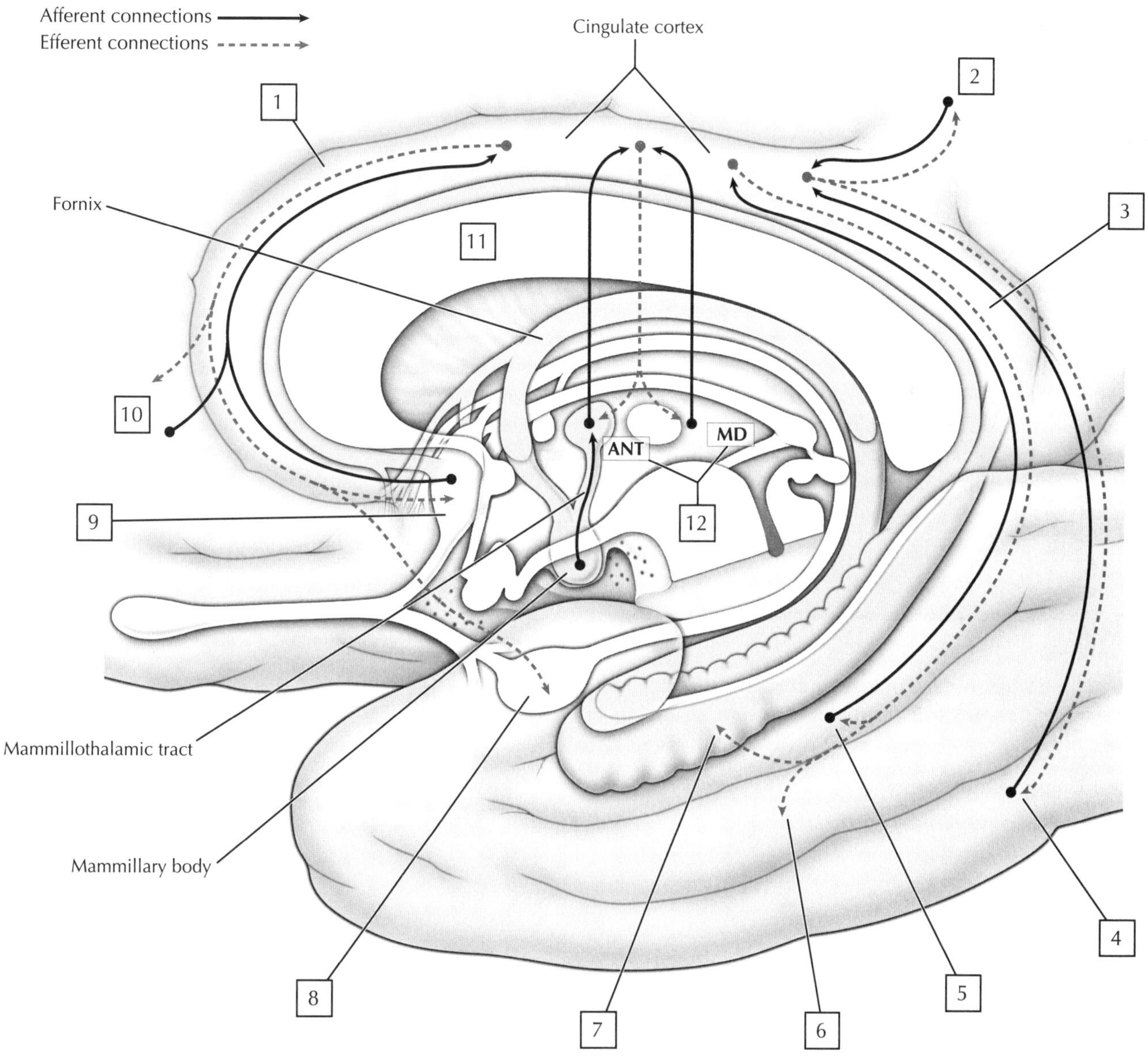

ANT = Anterior nuclei of the thalamus
MD = Medial dorsal nucleus of the thalamus

11 Insular Cortex

The insular cortex is often described as the "fifth lobe" of the brain, located in the lateral fissure, not visible from a lateral view of the brain. It is found lateral to a deeper group of structures, from medial to lateral, consisting of the putamen, external capsule, claustrum, and extreme capsule. The anterior portion of the insular cortex is continuous with the ventromedial prefrontal cortex (vmPFC), part of the orbitofrontal cortex.

Major afferent connections to the insular cortex include: (1) **viscerosensory inputs**, including chemoreceptors (carotid body) and baroreceptors (carotid sinus); (2) **multisensory inputs from cortical circuits** for somatosensory, trigeminal, taste, vision, and interoception, and direct limbic inputs from olfaction; (3) **association cortical inputs** from regions involved in multisensory integration; (4) **cholinergic inputs** from nucleus basalis; and (5) **brainstem inputs** from the periaqueductal gray, parabrachial nuclei, dopaminergic ventral tegmental area, noradrenergic locus coeruleus, and serotonergic rostral raphe nuclei.

Major efferent connections from the insular cortex are mainly reciprocal interconnections with: (1) **limbic forebrain subcortical structures** (basolateral amygdala, lateral bed nucleus of the stria terminalis); (2) **lateral entorhinal cortex**, part of the parahippocampal circuitry; (3) **limbic cortical regions** (medial PFC, anterior cingulate cortex); (4) **nucleus accumbens**, in the basal forebrain; (5) **medial dorsal (MD) nucleus of the thalamus**; (6) the **lateral hypothalamic area**; and (7) the **habenula**.

COLOR the following structures:

- ☐ 1. **Insular cortex (outline of insular cortex in upper figure is ghosted, as it formed laterally)**
- ☐ 2. **Anterior cingulate cortex**
- ☐ 3. **Medial prefrontal cortex**
- ☐ 4. **Ventromedial prefrontal cortex**
- ☐ 5. **Nucleus accumbens**
- ☐ 6. **Lateral hypothalamic area**
- ☐ 7. **Amygdala**
- ☐ 8. **Parahippocampal region (entorhinal cortex)**
- ☐ 9. **Multisensory cortical input**
- ☐ 10. **Bed nucleus of the stria terminalis**
- ☐ 11. **Medial dorsal (MD) nucleus of the thalamus**
- ☐ 12. **Brainstem nuclei**

Clinical Note

The insular cortex plays a role in: (1) consciousness, body homeostasis, and perception (e.g., vestibular sensations, balance, and vertigo); (2) body warmth and coldness; (3) abdominal distension and bladder fullness; (4) sensation of dyspnea; and (5) detection of unpleasant and disgusting smells. The insular cortex links sensory processing with emotional recognition and feelings, and assists with appropriate autonomic and motor reactivity and responses. The insular cortex also aids in risk prediction and decision making related to addictive behaviors and uncertain situations. The insular cortex also plays a role, along with other limbic and cortical structures, in modulating fear and anxiety responses, carrying out socially related behaviors, and in processing complex emotional responses such as empathy, emotional reactions to music, laughter, and crying. Stimulation of the insular cortex can provoke the emotion of disgust, and fMRI studies reveal that the insular cortex is responsive to disgust from noxious sensations as well as disgust for cognitively understood and emotional morally reprehensible situations.

If the insular cortex is damaged or its connections are disrupted, the patient still can perceive sensory information, such as pain, but is unable to respond emotionally to it, showing altered or even absent emotional reactivity.

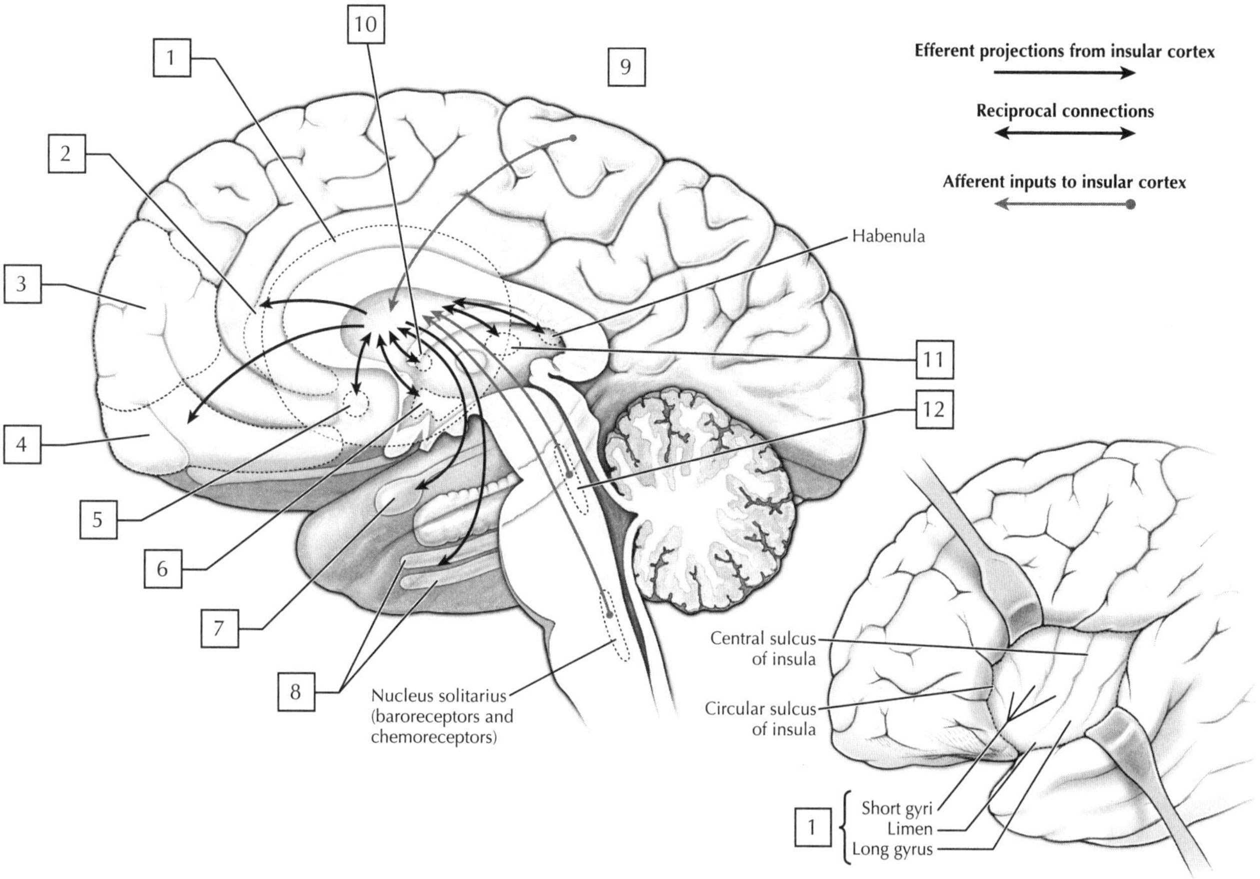
10
1
9
Efferent projections from insular cortex
Reciprocal connections
Afferent inputs to insular cortex
2
3
Habenula
11
12
4
5
6
7
8
Nucleus solitarius
(baroreceptors and
chemoreceptors)
Central sulcus
of insula
Circular sulcus
of insula
1
Short gyri
Limen
Long gyrus

11 The Prefrontal Cortex

The prefrontal cortex (PFC) is an important cortical region that regulates complex cognitive, emotional, and behavioral functions. It is necessary for planning and reasoning involving working memory, carrying out executive functions, regulating anticipatory goal orientation, and predicting future outcomes. Prefrontal cortex also helps to guide appropriate social behaviors. The prefrontal cortex consists of two major functional components, the **dorsolateral prefrontal cortex (dlPFC)** and the **ventromedial prefrontal cortex (vmPFC)**, a major component of the orbitofrontal cortex.

The dlPFC is the rational decision maker, carrying out logical cognitive assessments in an unemotional manner. It carries out complex planning and can inhibit amygdaloid-driven emotionally based activities and behaviors. It is a major site for working memory and deductive reasoning, activities often considered important features of "intelligence," particularly activity of the left lateral prefrontal cortex and its connectivity. A further component of the dlPFC is the capacity to plan strategies such as lying and deception. The dlPFC helps to determine right from wrong, but can override that with behavioral planning.

The dlPFC is connected with many cortical areas, including: (1) **vmPFC**; (2) **primary and secondary sensory cortical association areas** (visual, auditory, somatosensory and trigeminal, taste, olfaction); (3) anterior and posterior **cingulate cortex** and retrosplenial cortex; (4) **premotor cortex**; and (5) **hippocampus**. The dlPFC also is connected with **subcortical areas**, including the striatum, nucleus MD of the thalamus, and lateral cerebellum.

The vmPFC aids in complex sensory integration, particularly from the temporal lobe (smell, taste, touch, vision from the temporal pathway, audition). It participates in reward responses (winning and losing), as well as compulsive behaviors, repetitive behaviors, and drives, working in concert with nucleus accumbens, amygdaloid nuclei, and their dopaminergic inputs. The vmPFC also helps regulate cognitive processing and decision making, especially regarding emotional connotation, expectations, impulse control, and response inhibition. It aids in the perception of pleasure, aggressive behaviors, and other emotional expression. The vmPFC can initiate body changes associated with emotions (e.g., anxiety, anger, aggression).

The vmPFC is reciprocally connected with: (1) **medial dorsal (MD) nucleus of the thalamus**; (2) **many cortical areas** (dlPFC, entorhinal, perirhinal, parahippocampal, other temporal cortical areas); (3) **amygdaloid nuclei** (basolateral and central nucleus); and (4) some areas of the **hypothalamus**. The vmPFC also has extensive inputs from **sensory integration cortex** (pyriform cortex) and many **sensory cortical areas** (somatosensory SI and SII, visual, auditory, taste areas, olfactory cortex – uncus).

COLOR the following structures:

- ☐ **1. Dorsolateral prefrontal cortex (dlPFC)**
- ☐ **2. Ventromedial prefrontal cortex (vmPFC)**
- ☐ **3. Amygdala**
- ☐ **4. Hippocampus**
- ☐ **5. Parahippocampal gyrus, entorhinal cortex, other temporal lobe cortex**
- ☐ **6. Medial dorsal (MD) nucleus of the thalamus**
- ☐ **7. Visual cortex**
- ☐ **8. Somatosensory cortex**
- ☐ **9. Cingulate cortex**
- ☐ **10. Hypothalamus**

Clinical Note

Damage to the dlPFC result in the loss of ambition, motivation, and drive. The patient shows disinterest and loss of attention, with loss of spontaneous activities and conversation. Such damage is accompanied by an increase in depression, addictive behaviors, and indications of major life stressors.

Damage to the vmPFC results in behavioral disinhibition, with aggressive and abusive behaviors. The patient shows poor judgment, decision making, and social interactions. There is an increase in compulsive and addictive behaviors. The patient shows lack of empathy. The classic example of behavioral changes with vmPFC damage (and adjacent frontal areas) is Phineas Gage. In 1848, he was an engineer on a railroad construction project in Vermont. While he was tamping down an explosive, a spark detonated it, driving the long, narrow tamping bar through his left orbit and the top of his skull, destroying the orbitofrontal cortex and other adjacent regions. He survived and recovered, but showed a striking personality change in the remaining 12 years of his life. Friends described him as "no longer Gage." He had been a hard-working, well-liked man before the accident. After, he was described as retaining his intelligence and memory but unable to deal with others emotionally. He became volatile, impatient, disrespectful, profane, and vulgar. In later life he was more functional and better adapted in social situations.

The vmPFC is a component of circuitry involved in neuropsychiatric disorders, including schizophrenia, mood disorders, obsessive-compulsive disorder (OCD), addictive behaviors, and borderline personality disorder.

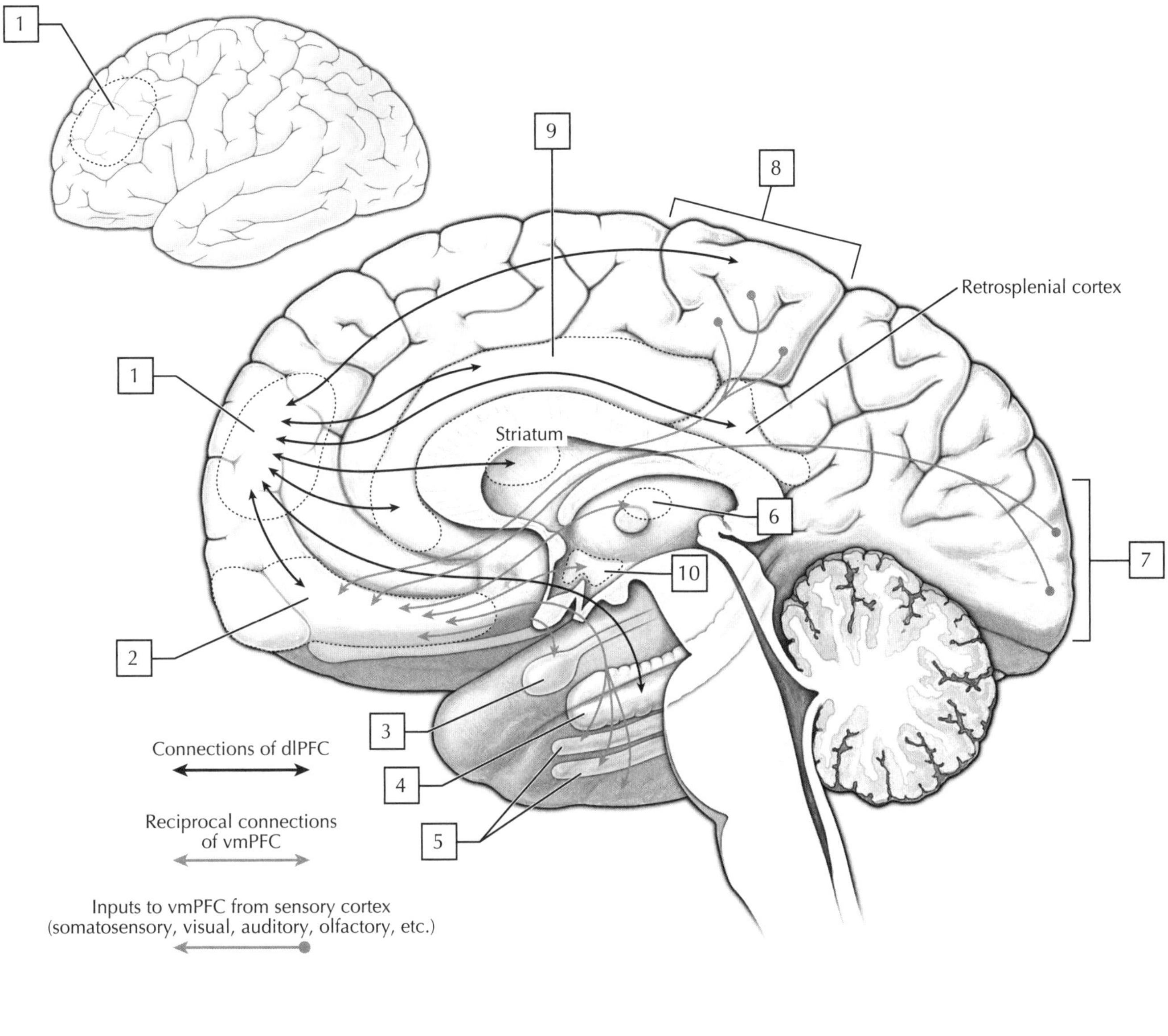
1
9
8
Retrosplenial cortex
1
Striatum
6
10
7
2
3
4
5
Connections of dlPFC
Reciprocal connections of vmPFC
Inputs to vmPFC from sensory cortex (somatosensory, visual, auditory, olfactory, etc.)

11 Olfactory Organization and Pathways

Olfaction is a chemoreceptive sense detected by olfactory receptors located on the distal processes (10–30 **cilia** extending from a large dendrite) of **primary sensory olfactory neurons** located in the **nasal mucosa**. These receptors and their associated neuronal processes are found in the medial and lateral walls of the roof of the nasal cavity. Odorant molecules, sometimes transported by carrier molecules, act on G-coupled protein receptors on these cilia and bring about a slow, depolarizing generator potential.

There is a wide range of odorant receptors, with an estimated 347 functional genes coding for them, up to 3% of the human genome. Each receptor does not code for a single odor; most odorant molecules activate many receptors, permitting coding for the identification of almost limitless numbers of odors.

Primary sensory olfactory **bipolar neurons of the olfactory epithelium** can detect odorant molecules and translate the molecular signaling into neural signaling. The central portion of the axons **(olfactory nerve fibers)** cluster into groups enwrapped by a single Schwann sheath, and pass through the **cribriform plate** and synapse in the **olfactory glomeruli** (complex synaptic configurations) in the glomerular layer of the **olfactory bulb**. The olfactory nerve fibers synapse on the dendrites of **tufted and mitral cells,** the secondary sensory neurons of the olfactory system that give rise to the **olfactory tract** projections. **Periglomerular** cells act as interneurons in the olfactory bulb. **Granule cells** connect with the tufted and mitral neurons and influence their excitability. **Noradrenergic projections** from the locus coeruleus, and **serotonergic projections** from the rostral raphe nuclei, also can modulate the excitability of the tufted and mitral neurons, as well as the periglomerular cells.

The olfactory tract bypasses the thalamus, unlike what occurs in the other sensory systems. The olfactory tract projects axons to the **anterior olfactory nucleus**, **nucleus accumbens**, the **uncus** (primary olfactory cortex) and **periamygdaloid cortex**, corticomedial nuclei of the **amygdala**, and the **lateral entorhinal cortex**. The olfactory cortex is interconnected with the orbitofrontal cortex, insular cortex, hippocampus, and lateral hypothalamus, integrating olfactory processing with important visceral, emotional, and behavioral responsiveness.

COLOR the following structures, using a separate color for each structure.

- ☐ 1. **Olfactory nerve fibers**
- ☐ 2. **Olfactory bulb**
- ☐ 3. **Cribriform plate (of the ethmoid bone)**
- ☐ 4. **Anterior olfactory nucleus**
- ☐ 5. **Olfactory tract**
- ☐ 6. **Bipolar neurons of the olfactory epithelium**
- ☐ 7. **Periamygdaloid cortex**
- ☐ 8. **Lateral entorhinal cortex**
- ☐ 9. **Amygdala**
- ☐ 10. **Uncus**
- ☐ 11. **Granule cells**
- ☐ 12. **Tufted and mitral cells**
- ☐ 13. **Periglomerular cells**
- ☐ 14. **Olfactory glomeruli**

Clinical Note

The primary olfactory neurons can detect thousands of specific molecular configurations for stimulation of unique olfactory signals to the brain. Olfactory information is not sent through detailed analytical circuitry of the thalamus and fine-grained cortical analysis; it goes directly into limbic regions associated with emotional interpretation, behavioral responsiveness, hypothalamic visceral activity for which odors are important, and appropriate autonomic responses. Detection of specific odorant molecules can be channeled to specific limbic regions through components of the olfactory circuitry. The importance of this system for survival is emphasized by the behaviors and activities influenced by olfaction, which includes food acquisition, appetite, territorial defense, relaxation or alertness responses, nausea, reproductive behaviors and many other responses. The reactivity to potentially threatening or dangerous odors must be rapid, appropriate, and able to integrate motor, autonomic, and neuroendocrine components.

The olfactory system can be activated for achieving many beneficial health-related effects. Delivery of odorant molecules by **nasal inhalation** therapeutic delivery devices can alter appetite, bring about relaxation, curb nausea (from cancer chemotherapy, pregnancy), bring about decongestion, support alertness and attention, and many other effects. The olfactory responses are rapid, specific (through specific connectivity from limbic–hypothalamo–autonomic circuits), and long lasting (sometimes 2 hours or longer).

The olfactory and taste system interact extensively, and both are required for a full, satisfying gustatory experience. Anosmia can occur with an olfactory bulb or tract injury, and can be partially precipitated by a cold or allergic rhinitis. The recent epidemic of COVID-19 resulted in many patients losing both senses of smell and taste, sometimes for prolonged periods of time.

The olfactory tract and bulb can be damaged by olfactory groove or sphenoid ridge meningiomas, producing Foster–Kennedy syndrome (ipsilateral anosmia, ipsilateral optic atrophy from pressure injury, and papilledema from increased intracranial pressure). The olfactory bulb and tract also can be damaged by other tumors (gliomas), aneurysms at the circle of Willis, and meningitis.

A unique capability of primary sensory neurons is their ability to undergo continuous replacement and turnover from basal stem cells in the olfactory epithelium.

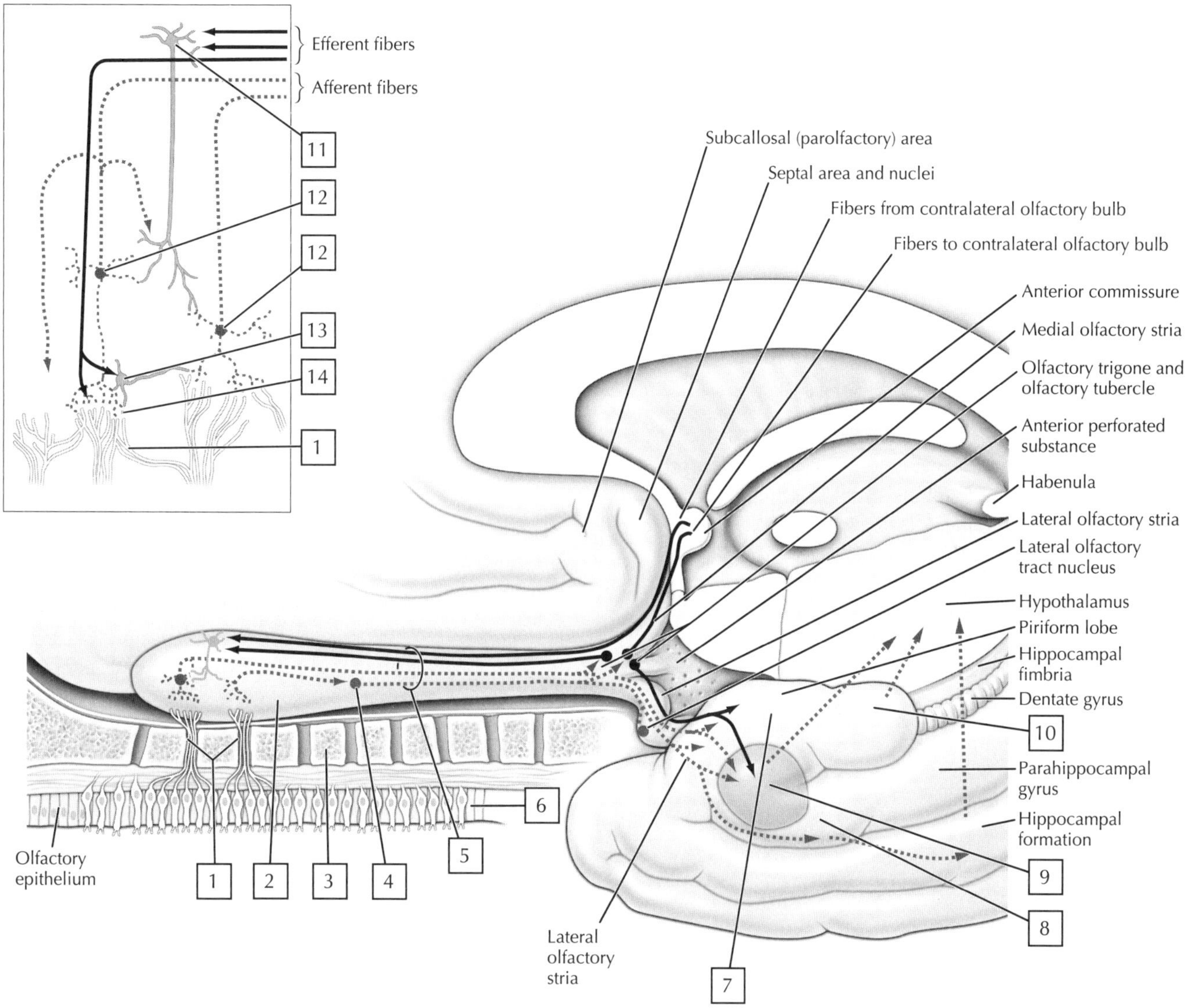
Efferent fibers
Afferent fibers
11
12
12
13
14
1
Subcallosal (parolfactory) area
Septal area and nuclei
Fibers from contralateral olfactory bulb
Fibers to contralateral olfactory bulb
Anterior commissure
Medial olfactory stria
Olfactory trigone and olfactory tubercle
Anterior perforated substance
Habenula
Lateral olfactory stria
Lateral olfactory tract nucleus
Hypothalamus
Piriform lobe
Hippocampal fimbria
Dentate gyrus
10
Parahippocampal gyrus
Hippocampal formation
9
8
7
Lateral olfactory stria
6
5
Olfactory epithelium
1
2
3
4

SECTION III REVIEW QUESTIONS

1. In which of the following situations would you expect to find a loss of both pain sensation and fine, discriminative touch in the same distribution?
   A. A demyelinating lesion in the peripheral nervous system (Guillain–Barré syndrome)
   B. Spinal cord hemisection (Brown–Séquard lesion)
   C. An ischemic stroke in a paramedian branch of the vertebral artery in the lower medulla
   D. A lateral medullary brainstem stroke (posterior inferior cerebellar artery)
   E. An ischemic stroke affecting the posterior limb of the internal capsule

2. Which brainstem lower motor neuron cell group receives only contralateral input from the corticobulbar tract?
   A. CNN III
   B. CNN V
   C. CNN VII for the upper face
   D. CNN VII for the lower face
   E. CNN XII

3. Following a hematoma or edema in the anterior fossa, the brain may herniate, removing the influence of first the forebrain and then the midbrain. The patient demonstrates decerebrate posturing because of uninhibited action of what system?
   A. Corticospinal tracts
   B. Rubrospinal tracts
   C. Lateral vestibulospinal tracts
   D. Medullary reticulospinal tracts
   E. Dentate nucleus projections to the red nucleus

4. What region of the cortex helps to regulate planning and reasoning, anticipatory goal-oriented behavior, and appropriate social behaviors?
   A. Prefrontal cortex
   B. Anterior cingulate cortex
   C. Posterior cingulate cortex
   D. Entorhinal cortex
   E. Insular cortex

5. What region of the cortex plays a role in consciousness, body homeostasis, and body perceptions (e.g., body warmth and coldness, bladder fullness, abdominal distension), and emotional responsiveness such as crying and laughing?
   A. Prefrontal cortex
   B. Orbitofrontal cortex
   C. Posterior cingulate cortex
   D. Parahippocampal cortex
   E. Insular cortex

6. Which circumventricular organ is an important regulator of water balance and thirst?
   A. Organum vasculosum of the lamina terminalis
   B. Subcommissural organ
   C. Area postrema
   D. Pineal gland
   E. Median eminence

7. Which limbic forebrain area is particularly involved in the emotional interpretation of both external and internal stimuli?
   A. Prefrontal cortex
   B. Nucleus accumbens
   C. Hippocampal formation
   D. Amygdala
   E. Entorhinal cortex

8. Which primary sensory tract carries information from a severe toothache? ______________________________

9. Which auditory structure plays a major role for localizing sound laterally in a horizontal plane? ____________________ ________________

10. What tract serves as the major interconnection between the vestibular nuclei and the motor cranial nerve nuclei for eye movements?______________________________

11. What nucleus in the hypothalamus provides regulation of diurnal rhythms? ______________________________ ______________________________

12. Damage to what portion of the visual system will result in a contralateral upper quadrant deficit (quadrantanopia)? ______________________________

13. What region of the brain serves as a control center for vertical and oblique eye movements? __________________ __________________

14. In a patient with a posterior fossa tumor, the examiner finds limb ataxia, dysmetria, dysdiadochokinesia, altered tandem walking, and dysarthria. What structure is damaged? ______ ______________________________

15. What portion of the basal ganglia directly regulates thalamocortical activity? ______________________________ ____________________

16. What substances are secreted into the hypophyseal-portal blood at the contact zone of the median eminence? ______ ______________________________

17. Which circumventricular organ is an important regulator of nausea and vomiting? ______________________________ ____________

18. What region of the hippocampal formation is particularly vulnerable to ischemia? ________________________ ________________________ To high glucocorticoid levels? ________________________

19. Information from which sensory system is processed mainly by limbic structures, and avoids fine-grained analysis by thalamocortical circuitry? ________________________ ________________________

20. An ischemic episode involving the brainstem has damaged the inferior cerebellar peduncle on one side. What would you expect to find on the neurological examination?
    A. Ipsilateral spastic hemiplegia
    B. Contralateral spastic hemiplegia
    C. Ipsilateral ataxia and loss of coordination
    D. Contralateral ataxia and loss of coordination

21. Dorsal column stimulation for severe, intractable pain (or in a less severe setting, rubbing the surface of the body at the site of injury to dampen pain) acts to suppress pain processing in what region?
    A. The dorsal horn of the spinal cord
    B. Nuclei gracilis and cuneatus in the medulla
    C. Brainstem sites where opiate neurons are located (e.g., periaqueductal gray)
    D. Nonspecific thalamic nuclei
    E. Primary sensory cortex

22. Which of the following is a primary sensory tract carrying ipsilateral information from a severe toothache?
    A. Spinothalamic tract
    B. Spinoreticular tract (system)
    C. Descending (spinal) tract of V
    D. Ventral trigeminothalamic tract (trigeminal lemniscus)
    E. Posterior limb of the internal capsule carrying information from the ventral posteromedial nucleus of the thalamus

23. Which sensory modality is least likely to be processed or modulated by the parabrachial nuclei in the brainstem?
    A. Taste
    B. Olfaction
    C. Severe, excruciating pain
    D. Chemical input through circumventricular organs
    E. Auditory

24. What membrane leverages sound waves into mechanical movement through the ossicles?
    A. Tympanic membrane
    B. Round window
    C. Oval window
    D. Basilar membrane in the cochlear duct
    E. Tectorial membrane

25. What auditory structure plays the major role for localizing sound laterally in a horizontal plane?
    A. Lateral lemniscus
    B. Inferior colliculus
    C. Superior olivary nuclei
    D. Medial geniculate body (nucleus)
    E. Auditory radiations

26. What pathway serves as the major interconnection between the vestibular nuclei and the coordination of eye movements?
    A. Medial vestibulospinal tract
    B. Lateral vestibulospinal tract
    C. Tectospinal tract
    D. Medial longitudinal fasciculus
    E. Dorsal longitudinal fasciculus

27. The greatest refraction of incoming light for focusing images on the retina is accomplished by the:
    A. Cornea
    B. Sclera
    C. Lens
    D. Ciliary process
    E. Iris

28. Damage to the parasympathetic portion of the third nerve will result in:
    A. Optic neuritis
    B. Fixed, dilated pupil
    C. Glaucoma
    D. Loss of pain sensation on the cornea
    E. Ipsilateral Horner syndrome

29. Control of diurnal and seasonal rhythms is accomplished by retinal projections from ganglion cells to what structure?
    A. Lateral geniculate nucleus
    B. Superior colliculus
    C. Pretectum
    D. Suprachiasmatic nucleus of the hypothalamus
    E. Pulvinar

30. Damage to what portion of the visual pathway is most likely to result in a contralateral upper quadrantanopia?
    A. Optic chiasm
    B. Optic tract
    C. Lateral geniculate nucleus
    D. Meyer loop in the temporal lobe
    E. Optic radiations near the primary visual cortex

31. A pituitary adenoma that encroaches on the optic chiasm would most likely produce what visual system deficit?
    A. Optic neuritis
    B. Contralateral hemianopia
    C. Upper contralateral quadrantanopia
    D. Bitemporal hemianopia
    E. Visual agnosias

32. Visual agnosias are most closely associated with damage to what region of the cortex?
    A. Occipital cortex
    B. Parietal cortex
    C. Temporal cortex
    D. Frontal cortex
    E. Insular cortex

33. Activation of which of the following fibers would cause the muscle spindle to contract relative to the skeletal muscle fibers?
    A. Ia afferent fibers
    B. Group II afferent fibers
    C. Ib afferent fibers
    D. Gamma motor fibers
    E. Alpha motor fibers

34. Where do fibers of the anterior corticospinal tract cross?
    A. Pyramidal decussation
    B. Ventral tegmental decussation
    C. Anterior white commissure
    D. Anterior commissure
    E. Internal capsule

35. What region of the brain serves as a control center for vertical and oblique eye movements?
    A. Parapontine reticular formation
    B. Superior colliculus
    C. Interstitial nucleus of Cajal
    D. Frontal eye fields
    E. Visual association cortex

36. As a patient decompensates following a head injury, he or she may show a diminished state of consciousness and a pattern of crescendo–decrescendo breathing. This pattern is called:
    A. Cheyne–Stokes breathing
    B. Central hyperventilation
    C. Apneustic breathing
    D. Ataxic breathing

37. During a neurological examination of a patient with a posterior fossa tumor, the examiner finds limb ataxia, dysmetria, dysdiadochokinesia, altered tandem walking, aberrant finger-to-nose testing, and dysarthria. The most likely source of these problems is damage to:
    A. The dorsal and ventral spinocerebellar pathways
    B. The flocculonodular lobes
    C. The cerebellar vermis
    D. The lateral hemispheres of the cerebellum
    E. The corticopontocerebellar system

38. What portion of the basal ganglia directly regulates thalamocortical activity?
    A. Caudate nucleus and putamen
    B. Globus pallidus
    C. Substantia nigra, pars compacta
    D. Subthalamic nucleus
    E. Rostral raphe nuclei

39. What lymphoid organ has direct noradrenergic innervation into the parenchyma and also receives hormonal influences from the anterior pituitary and peripheral target organs?
    A. Bone marrow
    B. Thymus
    C. Spleen
    D. Lymph nodes
    E. Mucosal-associated lymphoid organs
    F. All of the above

40. What region of the cortex helps to regulate navigation through the environment, declarative memories, and spatial memories?
    A. Orbitofrontal cortex
    B. Anterior cingulate cortex
    C. The dorsal subiculum
    D. Entorhinal cortex
    E. Insular cortex

41. What portion of the hypothalamus helps to regulate autonomic activities of the body?
    A. Paraventricular nucleus
    B. Anterior hypothalamic area
    C. Posterior hypothalamic area
    D. Lateral hypothalamic area
    E. All of these areas

42. What substances are secreted into the hypophyseal-portal blood at the contact zone of the median eminence?
    A. Osmotic factors to regulate water balance
    B. Angiotensin II to regulate blood pressure
    C. Oxytocin to regulate uterine contraction and milk let-down
    D. Opiate peptides to regulate pain perception
    E. Releasing factors to regulate release of anterior pituitary hormones

43. Cytokines can regulate some central nervous system functions through which route?
    A. Direct access through cortical vasculature
    B. Through circumventricular organs
    C. Through stimulation of vagal afferents
    D. Through activation of somatic afferents
    E. Through all of these routes

44. Which circumventricular organ acts as a regulatory region for nausea and vomiting?
    A. Organum vasculosum of the lamina terminalis
    B. Subfornical organ
    C. Subcommissural organ
    D. Area postrema
    E. Median eminence

45. What important hormone is secreted by the pineal to help regulate diurnal rhythms and sleep–wake cycles?
    A. Serotonin
    B. Melatonin
    C. Oxytocin
    D. Corticotropins
    E. Melanocyte-stimulating hormone

46. Which of the following regions of the hippocampal formation is particularly vulnerable to ischemia?
    A. Dentate gyrus
    B. CA1 sector of the hippocampus
    C. Subiculum
    D. Entorhinal cortex
    E. Alveus and fimbria

47. The stimulation of which limbic structure results in a response of vigilance and scanning of the environment?
    A. Septal nuclei
    B. Nucleus basalis (of Meynert)
    C. Basolateral amygdala
    D. CA regions of the hippocampus
    E. Subiculum

48. Information from what sensory system is processed mainly by limbic structures and avoids fine-grained analysis by thalamocortical circuitry?
    A. Taste
    B. Vestibular
    C. Trigeminal sensory
    D. Olfactory
    E. Auditory

ANSWER KEY

1. E
2. D
3. C
4. A
5. E
6. A
7. D
8. Descending (spinal) tract of CN V
9. Superior olivary complex
10. Medial longitudinal fasciculus
11. Suprachiasmatic nucleus
12. Meyer loop in the temporal lobe
13. Interstitial nucleus of Cajal
14. Cerebellum, Lateral hemispheres
15. Globus pallidus
16. Releasing factors and inhibitory factors for anterior pituitary hormones
17. Area postrema
18. CA1 region, CA3 region
19. Olfactory
20. C
21. A
22. C
23. E
24. A
25. C
26. D
27. A
28. B
29. D
30. D
31. D
32. C
33. D
34. C
35. C
36. A
37. D
38. B
39. F
40. D
41. E
42. E
43. E
44. D
45. B
46. B
47. C
48. D

Chapter 12 Global Brain Functions and Disorders

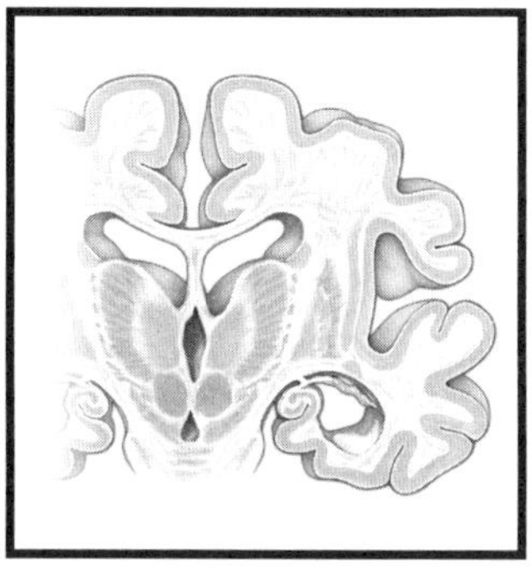
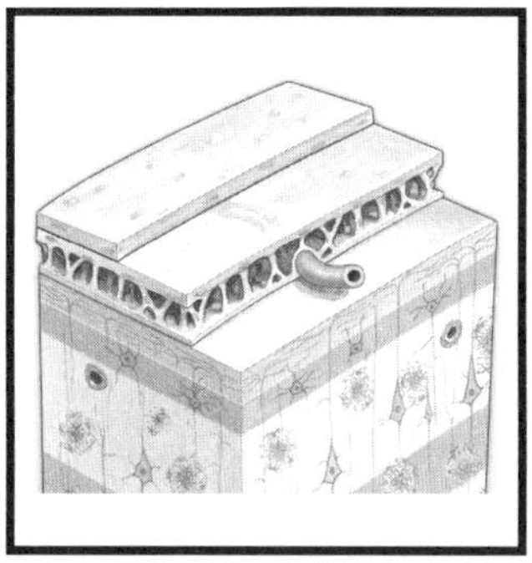
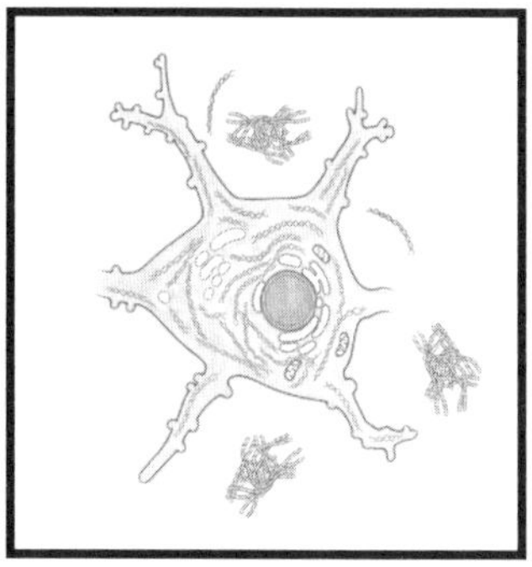
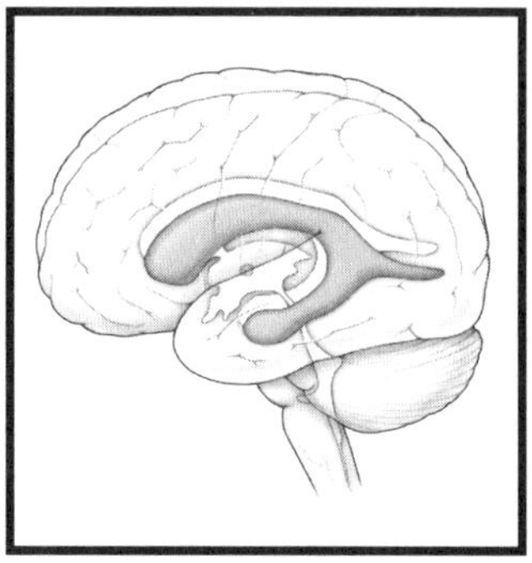

12 Dementia

Dementia is a group of symptoms affecting memory, thought processes, neurophysiological capabilities, and social interactions to a sufficient degree to interfere with daily life. Cognitive dysfunction is a prominent part of dementia and includes memory loss (particularly consolidation of short-term memory) and confabulation (making up components of stories and scenarios), confusion, getting lost, diminished problem-solving and executive functions, impaired reasoning, loss of organizational skills, and inattention. These deficits occur to varying degrees, from mild to severe, with some capabilities more severely affected than others. Psychological changes are also seen, including depression, anxiety, agitation, anger, inappropriate behaviors, and personality changes. Gait alterations and loss of coordination may occur. Psychotic behavior is not a usual component of dementia. Changes in consciousness are not usually seen until very late in the disease. The onset of dementia is usually subacute or chronic. This plate presents five causes of dementia.

1. Alzheimer Disease (AD) is the most common cause of dementia and the focus of intense research efforts. The cortex, particularly association areas, demonstrate atrophy, cortical thinning, and loss of neurons; primary sensory, motor, and visual cortical areas are usually spared. The hippocampus also is atrophied. The affected cortical areas demonstrate aberrant extracellular amyloid-beta protein deposits, called **neuritic plaques**, and intracellular clusters of hyperphosphorylated tau protein, called **neurofibrillary tangles**. It is not definitively determined if these plaques and tangles are causative of Alzheimer symptoms, especially dementia, or if they are a downstream effect of the neuronal damage.

2. Frontotemporal Dementia is characterized by atrophy of the frontal and temporal lobes with loss of neurons and neuronal connections, widened sulci, and atrophied gyri. Patients with frontotemporal dementia show impaired cognitive capabilities, decision-making, and judgment; disinhibition; problems with impulse control; language disorders (expressive aphasia, receptive aphasia, or both); and behavioral and personality changes.

3. Dementia With Lewy Bodies constitute 10% to 15% of dementias. This disorder is accompanied by cognitive alterations, cortical dysfunction such as hallucinations, and many characteristics of a Parkinson-like movement disorder. The Lewy bodies represent clusters of abnormal alpha-synuclein, a synaptic protein, found in regions of the brainstem (especially the substantia nigra, pars compacta dopamine neurons) and many areas of the cerebral cortex. Some patients also demonstrate characteristic neuritic plaques and neurofibrillary tangles as seen in AD. Some patients experience vivid visual hallucinations and striking images of animate objects. The Parkinson-like symptoms may include resting tremor, muscle rigidity, bradykinesia, and postural instability, often accompanied by depression, anxiety, and autonomic dysfunction (orthostatic hypotension, dizziness, syncope).

4. Vascular Dementia is the second most common form of dementia. It may be associated with small or medium-sized vessel disease or large vessel disease. Dementia may follow a single major stroke, or may progress with multiple small infarcts. The gradual occurrence of small vessel disease may damage subcortical white matter (lacunar infarcts) and result in progressive cognitive impairment, loss of attention, inability to focus, slowed thinking, impaired organizational ability, and diminished problem-solving ability. This condition is sometimes described as "multiinfarct dementia."

5. Treatable Dementias may present with cognitive impairment, intellectual decline, and other neurological dysfunction. Causative conditions include traumatic brain injury (TBI), subdural hematomas, brain tumors, normal-pressure hydrocephalus, metabolic encephalopathy, or major depressive disorder. Such dementias may be accompanied by headaches, seizures, gait disturbances, past history of TBI, changes in consciousness or sleepiness (indicative of increased intracranial pressure) or incontinence (often accompanying normal-pressure hydrocephalus). It is necessary to rule out treatable causes of dementia before labeling a patient with a diagnosis such as AD.

COLOR the following structures, using a separate color for each structure:

- ☐ 1. **Frontal lobe gyri showing atrophy**
- ☐ 2. **Temporal and parietal lobe gyri showing atrophy**
- ☐ 3. **Hippocampal atrophy**
- ☐ 4. **Widening of cortical sulci**
- ☐ 5. **Thinning of the cortical mantle**
- ☐ 6. **Atrophy of the olfactory bulbs and tracts**
- ☐ 7. **Atrophy of frontal and temporal lobe cortical areas**
- ☐ 8. **Lewy body in a neuron in substantia nigra, pars compacta**
- ☐ 9. **Intracranial medium-size arterial disease**
- ☐ 10. **Extracranial large-vessel disease**
- ☐ 11. **Subcortical infarcts**
- ☐ 12. **Brain tumor**
- ☐ 13. **Subdural hematoma**

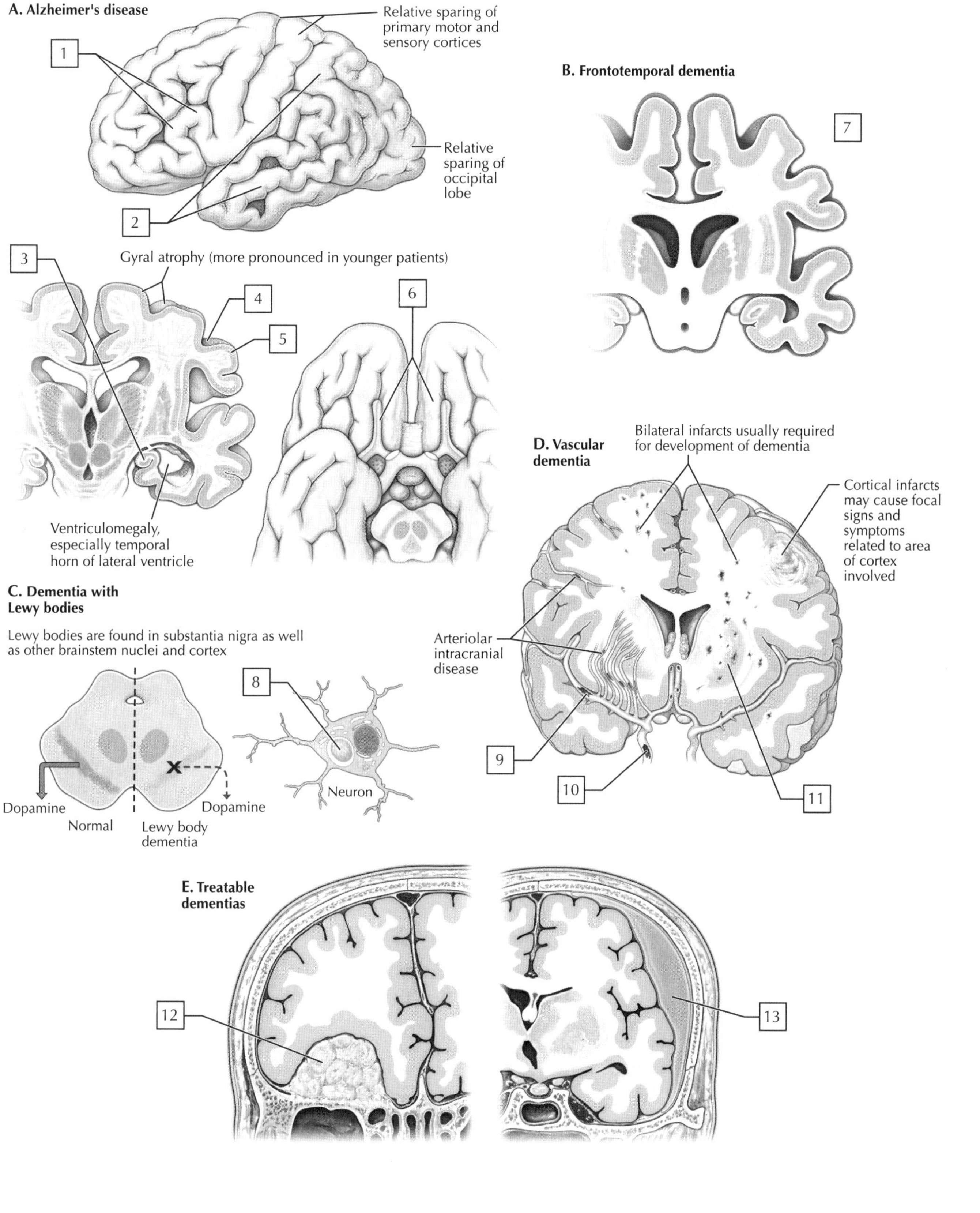
A. Alzheimer's disease
1
Relative sparing of primary motor and sensory cortices
Relative sparing of occipital lobe
2
3
Gyral atrophy (more pronounced in younger patients)
4
5
6
Ventriculomegaly, especially temporal horn of lateral ventricle
B. Frontotemporal dementia
7
C. Dementia with Lewy bodies
Lewy bodies are found in substantia nigra as well as other brainstem nuclei and cortex
8
Neuron
Dopamine
Normal
Lewy body dementia
Dopamine
D. Vascular dementia
Bilateral infarcts usually required for development of dementia
Cortical infarcts may cause focal signs and symptoms related to area of cortex involved
Arteriolar intracranial disease
9
10
11
E. Treatable dementias
12
13

12 Alzheimer Disease

Alzheimer Disease (AD) is the most common form of dementia. Cortical regions (frontal, temporal, parietal) and the hippocampus usually demonstrate the presence of extracellular plaques (aberrant amyloid-beta protein) and intracellular neurofibrillary tangles (hyperphosphorylated tau protein). Although these plaques and tangles are usually described as the characteristic pathological features of affected brain regions in Alzheimer disease, in the classic long-term Nun's study, some subjects with severe cognitive impairment had little or no evidence of plaques and tangles, and some subject with fully intact cognitive abilities had extensive evidence of plaques and tangles. Thus the issue of causation vs. correlation has not been satisfactorily answered.

Neuritic plaques are most abundant in frontal and parietal cortical regions, particularly in upper cortical layers. Amyloid-beta plaques are abundant in the cerebral cortex in many patients, starting in the medial temporal lobe (amygdaloid region, entorhinal cortex), then expanding into the hippocampus and cingulate cortex, and, in later stages, in widespread cortical regions. Hippocampal formation regions most significantly affected include CA1, subiculum, and entorhinal cortex. Neuritic plaques are particularly abundant in layer V of affected cortical regions.

General pathological findings in Alzheimer disease include enlarged ventricles, widened lateral fissure (loss of neurons) and cortical sulci, significant cortical and hippocampal atrophy, loss of cortico-cortical connections, and significant loss of chemically specific neuronal cell groups (noradrenergic locus coeruleus, serotoergic raphe nuclei, cholinergic nucleus basalis) and their widespread connections with both cortical and subcortical areas.

Clinical characteristics of AD include the following: (1) cognitive impairment (e.g., forgetfulness, confusion, impaired concentration, difficulty consolidating new memories, confabulation, impaired math ability, language impairment, and getting lost, even in their own home), (2) behavioral changes (e.g., agitation, irritability, aggressive behavior, lack of restraint verbally and personally, verbal repetition and confused expression, personality changes), (3) mood alterations (e.g., apathy, loneliness, mood swings, anger), (4) neuropsychiatric involvement (e.g., depression), and (5) physiological issues (e.g., impaired gait, movement loss such as arm swinging, altered appetite).

COLOR the following structures, using a separate color for each structure:

- ☐ 1. **Hippocampus**
- ☐ 2. **Nucleus basalis**
- ☐ 3. **Olfactory bulb**
- ☐ 4. **Amygdala**
- ☐ 5. **Locus coeruleus**
- ☐ 6. **Raphe nuclei**
- ☐ 7. **CA1 region of the hippocampus**
- ☐ 8. **Subiculum**
- ☐ 9. **Entorhinal cortex**
- ☐ 10. **Amyloid-beta plaques**
- ☐ 11. **Neurofibrillary tangles**

Clinical Note

AD is a devastating deterioration of the patient significantly affecting the family and caregivers. Intensive research efforts have sought to identify medications that might ameliorate the symptoms of this disease, with the ultimate goal of prevention. However, this disease progresses insidiously, and by the time significant indications of even mild cognitive impairment are present, the disease may have progressed for a decade or more.

Past efforts focused on enhancing cholinergic function; the loss of cholinergic neurons in nucleus basalis and diminished central acetylcholine (ACh) in AD led to therapeutic efforts to enhance ACh function. Enhanced precursor availability was promoted with lecithin treatment. Cholinesterase inhibitors were used to prolong ACh function. Unfortunately, these agents were not successful in restoring memory function or slowing cognitive decline.

Present efforts have focused on using monoclonal antibodies against amyloid-beta protein aggregations (neuritic plaques). The monoclonal antibody aducanumab (injection) leads to binding of amyloid-beta aggregations in the brain. It was approved by the FDA on surrogate evidence related to diminished amyloid-beta presence, with considerable internal dissent over lack of clinical evidence of its effectiveness. A recent review found no clinically significant differences in the antibody (Ab) vs. placebo with the MiniMental State Examination or the Clinical Dementia Rating: Sum of Boxes dementia scales. Unfortunately, this monoclonal Ab had some troubling side effects, such as cerebral edema (35%), cerebral hemorrhages (21%), headaches, confusion, dizziness, and nausea. It was not approved for Medicare reimbursement, and its cost per year was tens of thousands of dollars, plus the need for multiple scans.

The most recent monoclonal antibody targeting amyloid-beta (A-beta) is lecanemab. A placebo-controlled initial 18-month study showed a reduction in A-beta protein in the brain, and a 27% improvement on the cognitive component of the Clinical Dementia Rating Scale Sum of Boxes assessment. This was statistically significant but initially was thought to be of marginal clinical significance. Further evaluation showed positive effects on the cognitive scale, leading to full approval by the FDA in July 2023. Some side effects may occur, such as cerebral edema, brain bleeding (especially patients on anticoagulants), headaches, confusion, and seizures. The listed initial cost is $26,500 per year.

These recent studies of monoclonal Abs show the challenges of the damaging effects of AD. Patients are desperate for treatments, lobbying groups are powerful and politically influential, and the FDA has responded with decisions that are fraught with dissent and lack of clinical efficacy, which many news outlets are promoting as a "breakthrough" for AD treatment. No one has yet addressed the staggering cost of covering these drugs and the myriad scans and medical interactions required, for the millions of patients who would want access to any drug that might benefit AD patients. Coverage may overwhelm CMS in costs to the Medicare-eligible patients. These studies certainly will continue, but we are far from treatments that can stop the progression of or ameliorate AD.

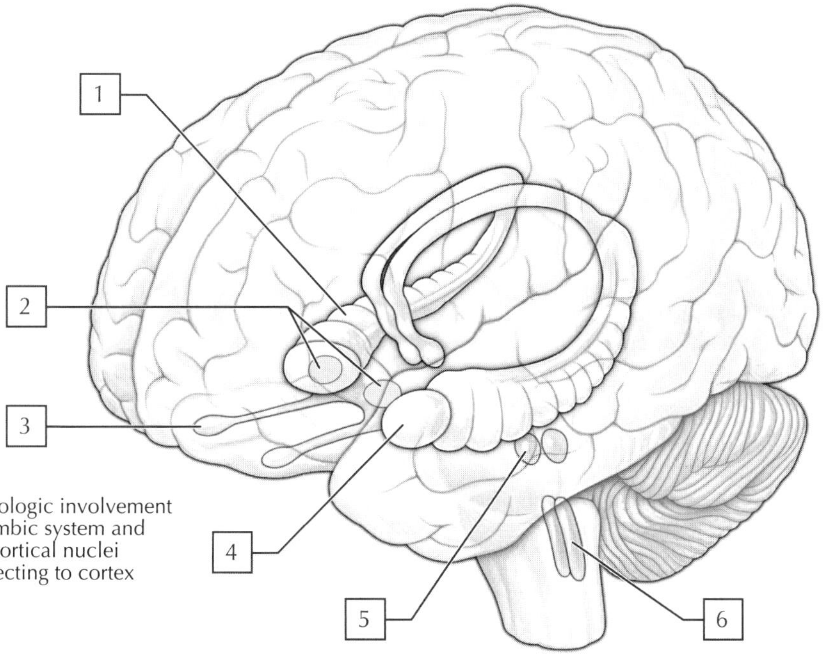

Pathologic involvement of limbic system and subcortical nuclei projecting to cortex

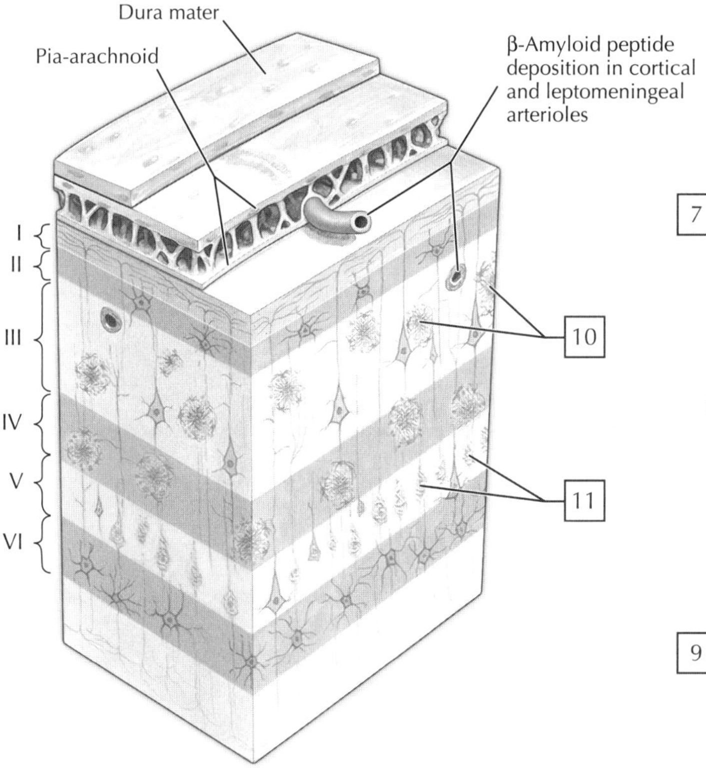

Association cortex

In association cortex, neurofibrillary tangles (NFTs) and synaptic and neuronal loss predominate in layer V. Senile plaques (SPs) occur in more superficial layers

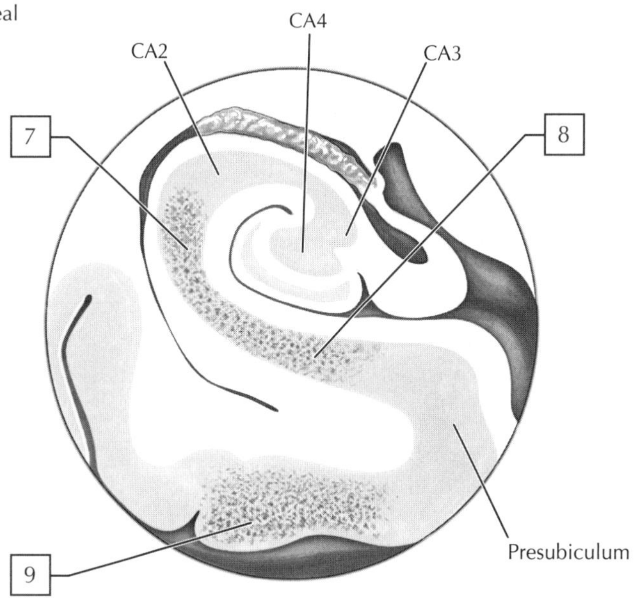

In hippocampus, neurofibrillary tangles, neuronal loss, and senile plaques primarily located in layer CA1, subiculum, and entorhinal cortex

Traumatic Brain Injury

A **concussion** is a traumatic brain injury (TBI) caused by forces impinging on the head that alter brain function but usually do not cause loss of consciousness. More than 1.5 million concussions occur per year in the U.S. associated with athletic activities. When force is applied to the head, the brain experiences a direct effect of the impact (**coup injury**) and an effect opposite the site of the force (**contrecoup**), due to the soft composition of the brain in comparison with the skull, with the brain initially compressing and then snapping back against the opposite portion of the skull. Repeated concussions can cause chronic traumatic encephalopathy (CTE), resulting in serious physical, cognitive, and emotional consequences.

The symptoms of a concussion include memory impairment, physical problems (nausea, headaches, visual impairment), altered thinking, and emotional changes. If a second concussion or trauma occurs before the complete resolution of the first concussion, the damage can be multiplied and magnified, leading to cerebral edema, serious neurological damage, coma, and even death. This long-term consequence is seen following repeated head injuries in football players and other athletes. At first, the seriousness of this condition in contact sports was denied or ignored, but repeated focus on it led to protocols that require an injured player to leave the game for assessment. A continuing challenge is finding the best and most predictive assessments to demonstrate that the effects of the concussion have dissipated, and also predictive tools for indicating which individuals are most vulnerable to repeated neurological injury from concussion.

Mild traumatic brain injury is a head injury with a brief loss of consciousness, retrograde amnesia, but no evidence of identifiable direct brain damage. Studies used for assessment include brain radiographs, magnetic resonance imaging (MRI), computed tomography (CT), and electroencephalograph (EEG), looking for brain injury, bleeds, skull fractures, and abnormal electrical activity. The patient may complain of headaches, difficulty concentrating, memory impairment, difficulty sleeping, irritability and mood swings, and sometimes dizziness and vertigo.

Severe traumatic brain injury may initially result in coma, with structural damage seen on imaging studies (e.g., bleeding, bruising, subdural or epidural hematomas). Subsequent motor and cognitive deficits are often seen, requiring extensive rehabilitative therapy. These deficits include inattention, memory impairment, impulsiveness and agitated behavior from frontal lobe damage, and aphasias.

Chronic traumatic encephalopathy may occur in athletes or other individuals who have experienced repeated head trauma with TBI. There is progressive neuronal deterioration and degenerative brain changes, with the increasing presence of hyperphosphorylated tau protein, similar to that seen in patients with AD, with the presence of neurofibrillary tangles. White matter damage often is seen.

TBI has been a focus in military theaters, with injury from high-velocity rifles, shrapnel, blast injuries, and damage from IEDs (improvised explosive devices). A patient will experience damaging cerebral edema, increased intracranial pressure, and may require mechanical ventilation to survive the injury. With the advent of more sophisticated life-saving medical care in the field, many troops have survived injuries that were not survivable several years ago, with the consequence of serious sequellae, and the need for intensive, long-term therapy.

COLOR the following structures, using a different color for each structure:

- ☐ 1. **Healthy neuron**
- ☐ 2. **Microtubules with associated tau proteins**
- ☐ 3. **Microtubule with tau protein bound to it**
- ☐ 4. **Disintegrating microtubule**
- ☐ 5. **Dissociated tau subunits**
- ☐ 6. **Tau subunits assembling to form neurofibrils**
- ☐ 7. **Aggregated tau proteins within a neurofibrillary tangle**
- ☐ 8. **Damaged/diseased neuron**

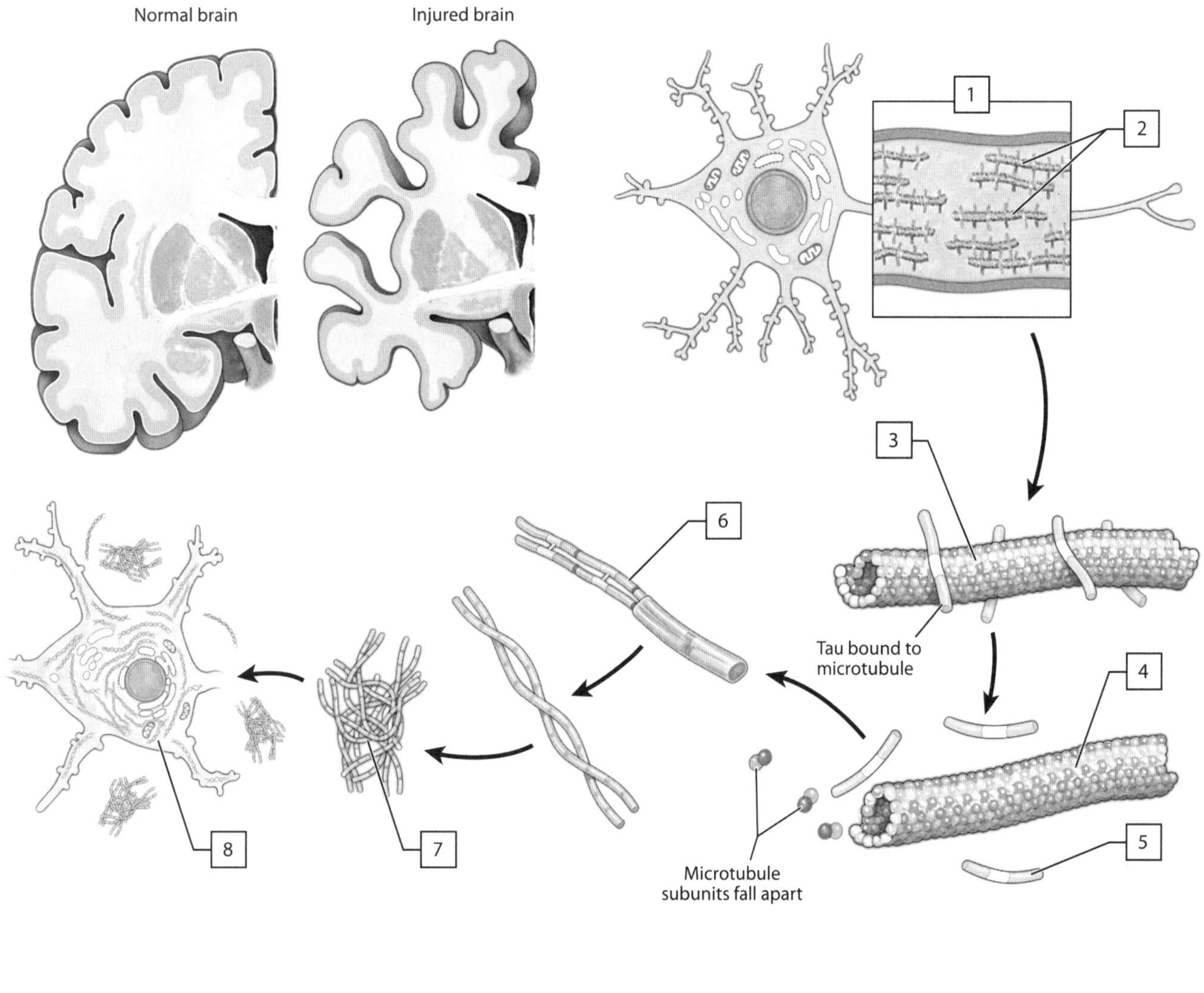
Normal brain
Injured brain
1
2
3
Tau bound to microtubule
4
5
6
7
8
Microtubule subunits fall apart

12 Posttraumatic Stress

Posttraumatic stress (PTS), often termed "posttraumatic stress disorder," is a debilitating and often long-term condition that follows a traumatic or ongoing event. It was initially used to describe traumatic events on a military battlefield (called "**shell shock**" in WWI). It is seen in civilian men and women as well as combat troops. PTS may occur after rape, other violent assaults, life-threatening experiences, and severe trauma.

PTS is characterized by repeated, intrusive recall of the trauma or precipitating event(s), often accompanied by flashbacks, hallucinations, striking perceived images, or nightmares. This is accompanied by hypervigilance, hyperactivity, hyperarousal, a robust startle response, or outbursts of anger displayed toward individuals or circumstances in the environment. Individuals with PTS also may show blunted emotional responses and a sense of detachment in everyday interactions, with hopelessness and a negative attitude. They may exhibit impaired learning and memory, and inattention. These responses often lead to impaired emotional reactivity and cognitive function, with detrimental effects on personal and professional relationships. As sequellae, individuals with PTS may demonstrate problems with depression, substance abuse, and suicidal ideation or attempted suicide. These severe responses may diminish if treatment is successful.

Many therapeutic approaches have been utilized to help individuals with PTS. The main modalities are pharmaceutical (specific serotonin reuptake inhibitors [SSRIs]), behavioral therapy, psychotherapy, or specialized therapy programs, such as equine therapy. The authors have been involved with an equine program pairing a PTS individual and a horse conditioned to work with patients experiencing a variety of challenges (e.g., autism, cancer recovery, sensory impairment); the bonding that occurs with the PTS individual and the horse with which they interact often has a transformative effect, engaging them in support and interactions with the program's counselors, horse trainers, other patients, and caregivers. We have seen this lead to remarkable amelioration of PTS-related responses and problems, bringing the individual to a better mental, emotional, and physical state. We believe such interactions are as powerful an influence on the brain as pharmaceutical or behavioral approaches.

Several chemical changes have been observed in individuals with PTS. There is increased **corticotropin-releasing factor (CRF)**, also called **corticotropin-releasing hormone (CRH)**, in the brain and cerebrospinal fluid (CSF), accompanied by decreased adrenocorticotropic hormone (ACTH) in the anterior pituitary and cortisol in the serum. There is enhanced sensitivity to negative feedback by cortisol. The increased CRH acts on the basolateral amygdala and promotes memory consolidation for traumatic events and is accompanied by elevated norepinephrine in the CSF and brain, which further promotes memory consolidation for fear- and trauma-associated events.

Both the hippocampus and amygdala are involved in the characteristic responses seen in PTS. There is decreased hippocampal volume: elevated CRH and increased sensitivity of CRH receptors in the hippocampus lead to hippocampal cell death (**apoptosis**), a process mediated through NMDA (N-methyl-D-aspartate) glutamate receptors (**excitotoxic cell death**). The damage to the hippocampus leads to blunting of physiological stress responses. The amygdala receives a convergence of damaging hyperstimulation from cranial nerves I (olfactory), II (optic), and VIII (auditory), as continued activation of the nerves from sensory messages involved in the initial trauma drives fear responses to the stimuli and memory of the trauma. A suggested lateralization has been proposed for the amygdala; the left amygdala may be particularly hyperresponsive in PTS. Damage to the amygdala on the right side may lead to loss of fear responses.

Additional CNS regions are involved in the response to PTS. The ventromedial prefrontal cortex (vmPFC) is under-responsive and unable to blunt the overactivity of the amygdala. Autonomic reactivity is driven by the hypothalamus and the bed nucleus of the stria terminalis (BNST). The BNST interconnects with the amygdala and hypothalamus, and drives reactivity to uncertain or unidentified fear, aggressive behaviors, and altered social interactions. The interconnected loops with cortex-basal ganglia-thalamus-cortex promote repeated patterns of movements and responses associated with PTS.

COLOR the following structures, using a separate color for each structure:

☐ 1. **Basal ganglia (caudate nucleus and putamen, globus pallidus)**
☐ 2. **Bed nucleus of the stria terminalis (BNST)**
☐ 3. **Ventromedial prefrontal cortex (vmPFC)**
☐ 4. **Olfactory bulb**
☐ 5. **Optic nerve**
☐ 6. **Amygdala**
☐ 7. **Hippocampus**
☐ 8. **Vestibulocochlear nerve**
☐ 9. **Thalamus**
☐ 10. **Hypothalamus**

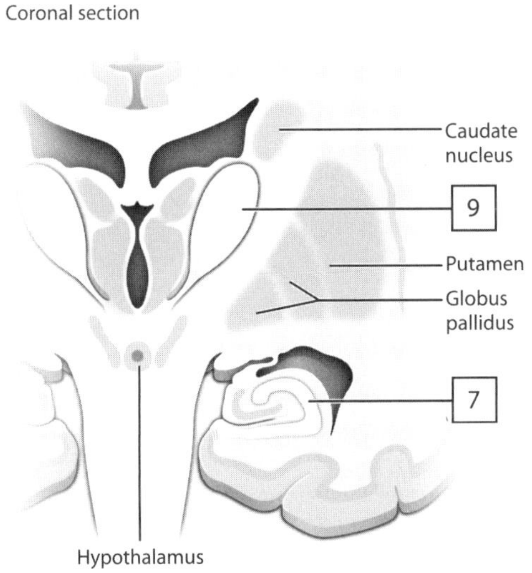
Coronal section
Caudate nucleus
9
Putamen
Globus pallidus
7
Hypothalamus

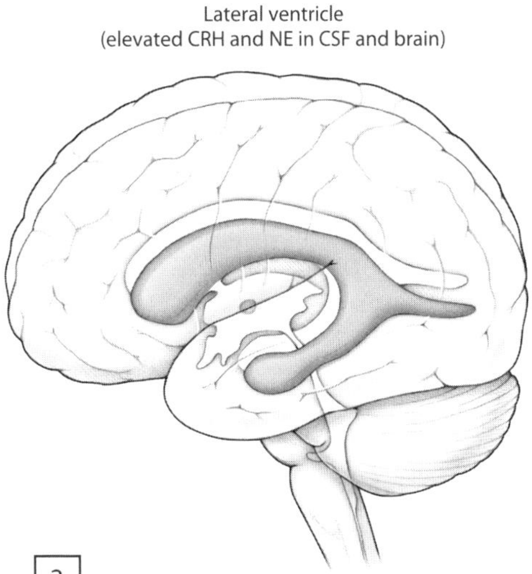
Lateral ventricle
(elevated CRH and NE in CSF and brain)

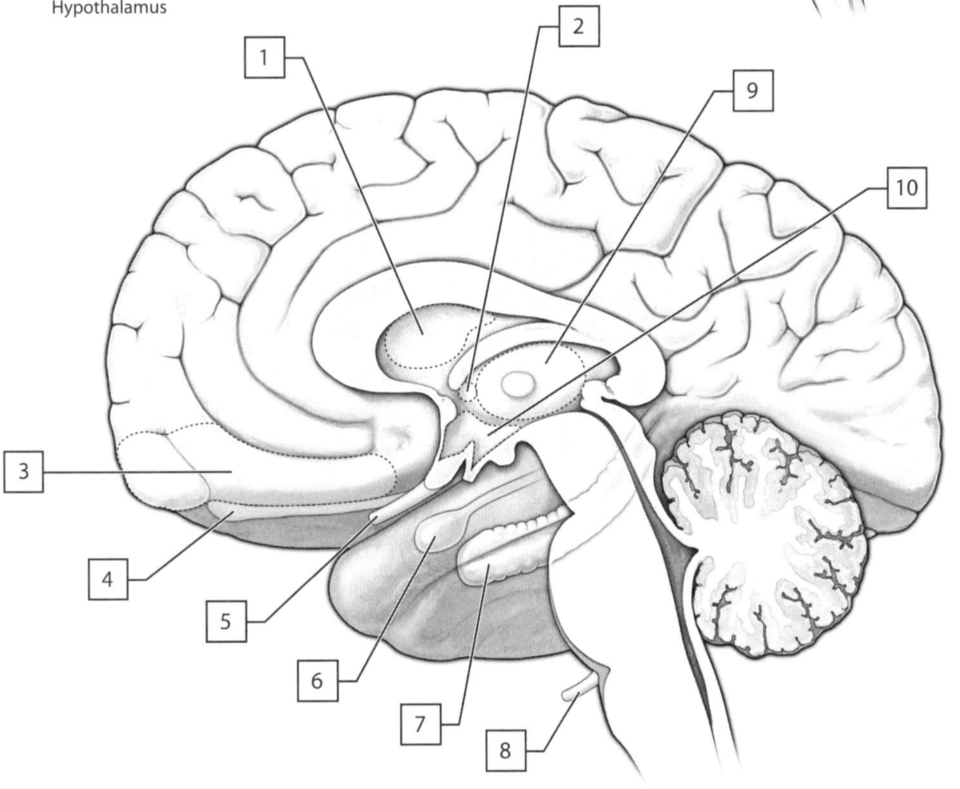
1
2
9
10
3
4
5
6
7
8

Brain Substrates of Addictive Behaviors

Addiction is a compulsion for habit-forming substances (e.g., cocaine, opiates, alcohol, benzodiazepines, nicotine, alcohol) or activities (e.g., smoking, gambling). The *Diagnostic and Statistical Manual of Mental Disorders (DSM-5)*, published by the American Psychiatric Association, recommend use of the term "**substance use disorder**" (SUD) rather than "addiction." **Drug dependence** is physical dependence on a substance, with development of tolerance and withdrawal responses. Addiction refers to both mental and physical reliance on a substance, which becomes the priority of an individual's life. SUD can cause disturbing or irrational behavior in the absence of the substance, leading to intense desire, nervousness, anxiety, and uncontrollable behaviors.

SUD includes physiological and neurological reactivity, especially involving the **mesolimbic and mesocortical dopamine (DA) reward system**. It is driven by internal compulsions, reinforced by environmental influences, and influenced by genetic components through the expression of DA receptor subsets. SUD involves repeated activation of the DA reward system with the substance or activity, driving a three-step cycle: (1) the **rush** or **binge**, producing a **high**, or intoxicating feeling of euphoria; (2) **withdrawal and accompanying adverse effects**; and (3) **anticipation and preoccupation with the next high**. All three phases use the same reward circuitry but with major differences in the activation or inactivation of the mesolimbic and mesocortical DA system. These cyclic changes in the DA system may persist after cessation of the addicting substance or activity. Exposure to the addictive substance often provides stronger motivation, reward, and drive than other positive stimuli.

Brain circuitry involved include nucleus accumbens (reward response); ventromedial prefrontal cortex (vmPFC), subcallosal gyrus (motivation and drive); dorsolateral prefrontal cortex (dlPFC), anterior cingulate cortex (cognitive responses); basolateral amygdala, hippocampus (learning and memory reactions); basal ganglia, nigrostriatal DA circuitry (repetitive and habit-forming responses); and ventral tegmental area (VTA) mesolimbic (to nucleus accumbens, amygdala, hippocampus) and mesocortical (to prefrontal cortex) DA system.

Following substance exposure, initial high amounts of DA are released by the mesocortical and mesolimbic components, affecting mood (nucleus accumbens), motivation (vmPFC), and emotion, learning, and memory (amygdala and hippocampus). The **cognitive control circuitry** (dlPFC and anterior cingulate cortex) cannot block or counter the DA surge, which reinforces the substance use or behavior. The withdrawal response follows prolonged substance use: the amount and release of DA is diminished, removing pleasurable and euphoric responses and initiating negative responses (feelings of tenseness, nervousness, hostility, aggression; altered autonomic responsiveness; change in appetite; dry mouth; insomnia). The adverse response and withdrawal can be reversed only with time, with DA replenished and anticipation of the next high. Anticipation of the next high may be a more powerful stimulus than exposure to the substance itself. This cyclic response may also have environmental influences superimposed on it (e.g., the site of substance exposure), altering the strength of the response.

Susceptibility to addiction may be partially driven by variations in the D1 and D2 receptor subsets, numbers, and expression at specific innervated sites.

Clinical Note

Many drugs of abuse influence neurotransmitter systems and receptors, particularly DA and norepinephrine (NE).

COLOR the following structures, using a separate color for each structure:

- ☐ 1. **Dorsolateral prefrontal cortex (dlPFC)**
- ☐ 2. **Anterior cingulate cortex**
- ☐ 3. **Basal ganglia (caudate nucleus and putamen, globus pallidus)**
- ☐ 4. **Subcallosal gyrus**
- ☐ 5. **Ventromedial prefrontal cortex (vmPFC)**
- ☐ 6. **Nucleus accumbens**
- ☐ 7. **Amygdala**
- ☐ 8. **Hippocampus**
- ☐ 9. **Substantia nigra (nigrostriatal system)**
- ☐ 10. **Ventral tegmental area (mesolimbic and mesocortical dopamine system)**

Stimulants. Amphetamine (alpha-methylphenethylamine) increases the activity of NE and DA systems (and to a lesser extent, serotonin systems). It is taken up by high-affinity carriers into NE and DA terminals, increasing release of the drug, and competes with NE and DA at the high-affinity uptake carrier, prolonging the presence of these neurotransmitters in the synaptic cleft and stimulating postsynaptic receptors. **Methamphetamine** greatly enhances the release of NE and DA. Crystal meth is the most powerful form and may induce cravings after a single encounter. Prolonged use may lead to permanent DA system dysfunction and severe, permanent side effects. **Cocaine** releases DA and NE, flooding the brain through the mesolimbic and mesocortical DA projections. The flood of DA down-regulates the DA receptors, which then upregulate when the exposure is reduced. This may lead to overstimulation, overdose, and death. Crack cocaine is the most addictive form.

Opiates. Oxycodone, hydrocodone, morphine, and **heroin** bind to endogenous opioid receptors. Both endogenous opiates (beta-endorphin, dynorphin, enkephalins) and exogenous opiates may initiate the analgesic and other effects. The most dangerous opiate is **fentanyl**, a synthetic opioid 80 to 100 times stronger than morphine, originally developed for patients with extreme acute or terminal pain from cancer. Unfortunately, manufactured and unregulated fentanyl frequently is added to heroin or other drugs, even cannabis, resulting in powerful addiction, and often overdose and death (~100,000 individuals/year in the United States). Fentanyl exposure can cause rapid shut down of respiration with little warning; only the availability of **naloxone (Narcan)** administration can stop respiratory failure and death. These fentanyl tablets are sometimes manufactured to look like candy, thereby attracting young and naïve users.

Hallucinogens. Lysergic acid diethylamide (LSD) acts by binding serotonergic 5HT 2A receptors with prolonged presence and very slow dissociation, enhancing glutamate release. LSD may provoke psychotic episodes; effects may last for around 12 hours. **Phencyclidine (PCP, angel dust)** provokes feelings of detachment, hallucinations, confusion, disorientation, or other physiological effects. It is similar to **ketamine** and is used as a stimulant, anesthetic, and pain reliever. PCP is a competitive NMDA glutamate receptor antagonist, blocking some glutamate excitatory effects. It is addictive and interacts with DA, opioid, and nicotinic cholinergic receptors.

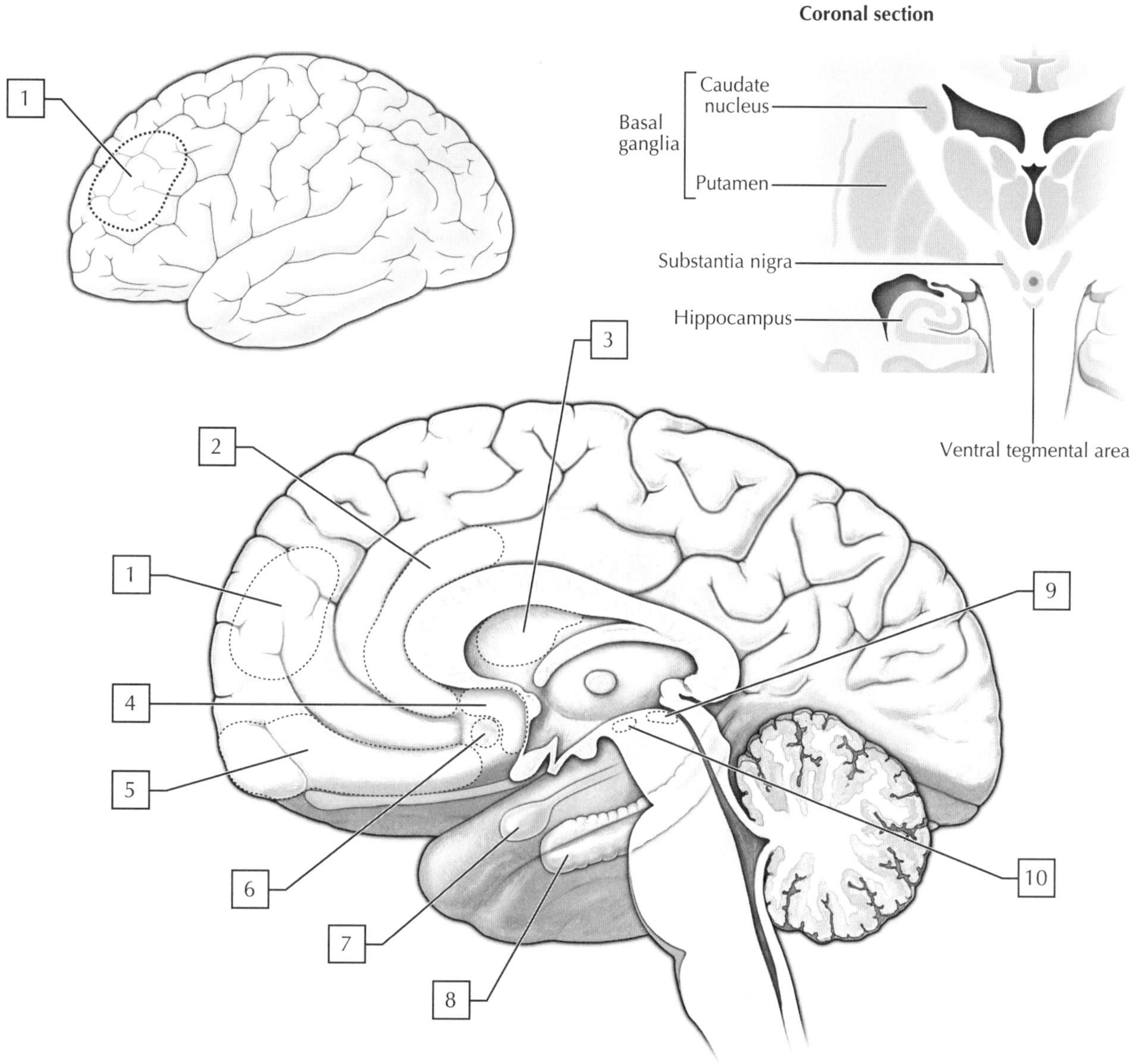
Coronal section
Caudate nucleus
Basal ganglia
Putamen
Substantia nigra
Hippocampus
Ventral tegmental area
1
2
3
1
4
5
6
7
8
9
10

Index

Note: Locators cited are plate numbers. Numbers in regular type indicate the discussion; **boldface** numbers indicate the art in the plate.

B

H

I

J

K

L

M

R

S

Z